Telerehabilitation

PRINCIPLES AND PRACTICE

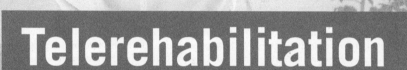

Telerehabilitation

PRINCIPLES AND PRACTICE

EDITOR

Marcalee Alexander, MD

Sustain Our Abilities, Birmingham, AL, USA
Editor-in-Chief, The Journal of Climate Change and Health
University of Alabama at Birmingham School of Medicine,
   Birmingham, AL, USA
Department of Physical Medicine and Rehabilitation,
   Harvard Medical School, Boston, MA, USA

ELSEVIER

Elsevier
1600 John F. Kennedy Blvd.
Ste 1800
Philadelphia, PA 19103-2899

TELEREHABILITATION: PRINCIPLES AND PRACTICE   ISBN: 978-0-323-82486-6

Senior Content Strategist: Humayra Khan
Senior Content Development Specialist: Rishi Arora
Content Development Manager: Somodatta Roy Choudhury
Publishing Services Manager: Shereen Jameel
Senior Project Manager: Umarani Natarajan
Design Direction: Renee Duenow

Printed in the United States of America

Last digit is the print number: 9   8   7   6   5   4   3   2   1

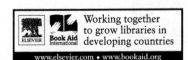

Working together
to grow libraries in
developing countries

www.elsevier.com • www.bookaid.org

Joshua Alexander, MD
Department Chair and Director of Pediatric
  Rehabilitation, Department of Physical
  Medicine and Rehabilitation, University
  of North Carolina School of Medicine,
  Chapel Hill, NC, USA

Marcalee Alexander, MD
Sustain Our Abilities, Birmingham, AL,
  USA
Editor-in-Chief, The Journal of Climate,
  Change and Health
University of Alabama at Birmingham
  School of Medicine, Birmingham, AL,
  USA
Department of Physical Medicine and,
  Rehabilitation, Harvard Medical School,
  Boston, MA, USA

Melodie Anderson, RN
Spinal Cord Injury and Disorders, Hunter
  Holmes McGuire VA Medical Center,
  Richmond, VA, USA

Mohit Arora, PhD, BPT, Diploma (Clinical Research)
Postdoctoral Fellow, John Walsh Centre
  for Rehabilitation Research, The Kolling
  Institute, Faculty of Medicine and Health,
  Sydney Medical School—Northern,
  The University of Sydney, Sydney, NSW,
  Australia

Deborah Backus, PT, PhD, FACRM
Vice President, Research & Innovation
Director of Multiple Sclerosis Research
Crawford Research Institute, Shepherd
  Center, Atlanta, GA, USA

Ines Bersch, PT, PhD
Nottwil Tetrahand®, Swiss Paraplegic Centre,
  Nottwil, Switzerland

Savitha Bonthala, DO
Sam Houston State University, College
  of Osteopathic Medicine, Conroe, TX,
  USA

Teodoro Castillo, MD
Spinal Cord Injury and Disorders, Hunter
  Holmes McGuire VA Medical Center,
  Richmond, VA, USA
Physical Medicine and Rehabilitation,
  Virginia Commonwealth University,
  Richmond, VA, USA

David Crandell, MD
Assistant Professor, Department of Physical
  Medicine and Rehabilitation, Harvard
  Medical School, Boston, MA, USA
Medical Director, Limb Restoration Program,
  Spaulding Rehabilitation Hospital, Boston,
  MA, USA
Director, Amputee Rehabilitation Fellowship,
  Boston, MA, USA

Chanel Davidoff, DO
Donald and Barbara Zucker School
  of Medicine at Hofstra/Northwell,
  Hempstead, NY, USA

Kerry J. Davis, EdD, CCC-SLP
Speech Language Pathologist, Spaulding
  Outpatient Center for Children,
  Foxborough, MA, USA

Giulio Del Popolo, MD
Unit of Neuro-Urology, Azienda Ospedaliero-
  Universitaria Careggi, Florence, Italy

Yannis E. Dionysiotis, MD, MSc, PhD
Senior Consultant, 1st Physical Medicine
  and Rehabilitation Department, National
  Rehabilitation Center EKA, Athens, Greece

Dawn Ehde, PhD
Professor of Rehabilitation Medicine,
  University of Washington—UW
  Medicine, Seattle, WA, USA

Kyle Y. Faget, Esq
Foley & Lardner, LLP, Boston, MA, USA

Fabrizio Fiumedinisi, MD
Nottwil Tetrahand®, Swiss Paraplegic Centre,
  Nottwil, Switzerland

Jan Fridén, MD, PhD
Nottwil Tetrahand®, Swiss Paraplegic Centre, Nottwil, Switzerland

Jacob A. Goldsmith, PhD
Spinal Cord Injury and Disorders, Hunter Holmes McGuire VA Medical Center, Richmond, VA, USA

Ashraf S. Gorgey, MPT, PhD, FACSM, FACRM
Spinal Cord Injury and Disorders, Hunter Holmes McGuire VA Medical Center, Richmond, VA, USA
Physical Medicine and Rehabilitation, Virginia Commonwealth University, Richmond, VA, USA

Daniel Hussey, MD
Department of Physical Medicine and Rehabilitation, Harvard Medical School, Boston, MA, USA
Spaulding Rehabilitation Hospital, Charlestown, MA, USA

Mary Alexis Iaccarino, MD
Department of Physical Medicine and Rehabilitation, Harvard Medical School, Massachusetts General Hospital, Boston, MA, USA
Spaulding Rehabilitation Hospital, Boston, MA, USA

Ingebjørg Irgens, MD
Specialist in Physical Medicine and Rehabilitation, Sunnaas Rehabilitation Hospital Norway, University of Oslo, Oslo, Norway

Nicole B. Katz, MD
Lewis Katz School of Medicine at Temple University, Philadelphia, PA, USA

Sabrina Koch-Borner, PT, MSc
Nottwil Tetrahand®, Swiss Paraplegic Centre, Nottwil, Switzerland

Antonis Kontaxakis, MD
Physical and Rehabilitation Medicine Department, 414 Military Hospital of Special Diseases, Athens, Greece

Radha Korupolu, MD, MS
Department of Physical Medicine and Rehabilitation, The University of Texas Health Science Center at Houston, Houston, TX, USA

Lisa Kozden, MOT, OTR/L, CHT, COMT
Faculty Specialist, Department of Occupational Therapy, Panuska College of Professional Studies, The University of Scranton, Scranton, PA, USA
Owner, Hands For Life Therapy, LLC, Plains, PA, USA

Jennifer Kurz, MD
Department of Physical Medicine and Rehabilitation, Harvard Medical School, Boston, MA, USA
Spaulding Rehabilitation Hospital, Charlestown, MA, USA

Myriam Lacerte, MD

Kate Laver, BAppSc(OT), MClinRehab, CertImpSc, PhD
Flinders Health and Medical Research Institute, Flinders University, Adelaide, Australia

Carl Froilan D. Leochico, PTRP, MD
Clinical Associate Professor, Department of Rehabilitation Medicine, College of Medicine and Philippine General Hospital, University of the Philippines Manila, Manila, Philippines
Consultant, Department of Physical Medicine and Rehabilitation, St. Luke's Medical Center, Global City and Quezon City, Philippines

Susan Maltser, DO
Donald and Barbara Zucker School of Medicine at Hofstra/Northwell, Hempstead, NY, USA

Andria Martinez, MS, OTR/L, CHT
Occupational Therapist, Arizona Burn Center at Valleywise Health, Phoenix, AZ, USA

Ramiro Mitre, MSc
Department of Psychology and Human Relations, Universidad Abierta, Interamericana, Rosario, Argentina
Director, Fundación Neurodiversidad, Rosario, Argentina

Colleen O'Connell, MD, FRCPC
Physical Medicine and Rehabilitation, Stan Cassidy Centre for Rehabilitation, Dalhousie University Faculty of Medicine, New Brunswick, Canada

Kate Osborne, CHIA, BAppSc (Physiotherapy)
Rural Support Service, SA Health, South Australia, Australia

Dana Pagliuco, MS, CCC-SLP
Speech Language Pathologist, Spaulding Outpatient Center for Children, Foxborough, MA, USA

Tiffany Pritchett, MSOT, OTR/L
Clinical Specialist, Department of Occupational Therapy, Spaulding Rehabilitation Hospital, Boston, MA, USA

Camila Quel De Oliviera, Ph.D., BPhys(Honors)
Lecturer, Graduate School of Health, Discipline of Physiotherapy, University of Technology Sydney, Sydney, NSW, Australia

Christina-Anastasia Rapidi, MD, PhD, LFEBPRM
Head of PRM Department, General Hospital "G.Gennimatas", Athens, Greece

Chelsea G. Ratcliff, PhD
Department of Psychology, Sam Houston State University, Huntsville, TX, USA

Bridget Rizik, MD
Physiatrist, Mary Free Bed Rehabilitation Hospital, Grand Rapids, MI, USA

Suzanne Salsman, MD, MSc, FRCPC
Division of Physical Medicine and Rehabilitation, Department of Medicine, Dalhousie University, Halifax, Nova Scotia, Canada

Gianluca Sampogna, MD
Unit of Neuro-Urology, ASST Grande Ospedale Metropolitano Niguarda, Milan, Italy

Silvia Schibli, MD
Nottwil Tetrahand®, Swiss Paraplegic Centre, Nottwil, Switzerland

Jeffrey C. Schneider, MD
Spaulding Rehabilitation Hospital, Spaulding Research Institute, Department of Physical Medicine and Rehabilitation, Charlestown, MA, USA
Medical Director, Burn and Trauma Rehabilitation Program, Harvard Medical School, Boston, MA, USA

Kazuko Shem, MD
Department of Physical Medicine and Rehabilitation, Santa Clara Valley Medical Center, San Jose, CA, USA

Katherine Grace Siwy, MS, OTR/L
Occupational Therapist, Massachusetts General Hospital, Department of Occupational Therapy, Boston, MA, USA

Felicia Skelton, MD, MS
Investigator, Center for Innovations in Quality, Effectiveness and Safety, Michael E. DeBakey VA Medical Center, Houston, TX, USA
Assistant Professor, H. Ben Taub Department of Physical Medicine and Rehabilitation, Baylor College of Medicine, Houston, TX, USA

Michele Spinelli, MD
Unit of Neuro-Urology, ASST Grande Ospedale Metropolitano Niguarda, Milan, Italy

Adam S. Tenforde, MD
Spaulding Rehabilitation Hospital, Spaulding National Running Center, Department of Physical Medicine and Rehabilitation, Harvard Medical School, Charlestown, MA, USA

Debbie Torres, MA
Department of Psychology, Sam Houston State University, Huntsville, TX, USA

Nishu Tyagi, MOT
Research Associate and Occupational Therapist, Department of Telerehabilitation Services, Indian Spinal Injuries Centre, New Delhi, India

Renatos Vasilakis, MD
PRM Department, General Hospital "G. Gennimatas", Athens, Greece

Mitchell Wallin, MD, MPH, FAAN
Associate Professor of Neurology, George Washington University & University of Maryland, Washington, DC, USA
Director, VA Multiple Sclerosis Center of Excellence-East, Baltimore, MD, USA

ACKNOWLEDGMENTS

Telerehabilitation had an unexpected boost because of the Covid-19 pandemic. Although I have been passionate about telerehabilitation for many years as a green, consumer friendly form of health care, the thought of editing a book on the topic never crossed my mind. Coincidentally, in January 2020, a conversation with my friend, Dr. David Cifu, led to a connection with Humayra Khan at Elsevier and this text was conceived. I am very grateful to David and Humayra for this excellent alliance and this book.

The creation of an international volume on a relatively new topic such as telerehabilitation is a difficult task requiring a team of dedicated individuals. As such, I would like to express my appreciation for Umarani Natarajan, Ellen Wurm-Cutter, and Rishi Arora from Elsevier who have provided invaluable patience and support throughout the editorial process.

This book would not have been possible without the incredible team of Sustain Our Abilities, a nonprofit that I lead, which focuses on bringing attention to the concerns of persons with disabilities in relation to climate change and which promotes sustainable health care such as telerehabilitation. Christina Anastasia-Rapidi, Raju Dhakal, Yannis Dionyssiotis, Ingebjorg Irgens, Antonis Kontaxakis, Lisa Kozden, Carl Leochico, Melina Longoni, Ramiro Mitre, Maya Newman, Colleen O'Connell, Adesola Odole, Tiffany Pritchett, Gianluca Sampogna and Nishu Tyagi have been present from the start of this process and have been invaluable throughout this book's development. I feel blessed with their friendship and support. Moreover, any proceeds from this book will go to support the work of Sustain Our Abilities.

As stated, telerehabilitation is a green, patient-friendly form of health care. I am confident it will grow in use due to both patients' and providers' positive experiences and the need for health care organizations to decrease carbon emissions. Fortuitously, as I worked with Humayra on this book, she was also concerned about climate change and referred me to Pascal Leger at Elsevier to discuss my idea for a journal. I am eternally grateful for this connection and to Pascal because, in November 2020, along with Brad Stucky and the rest of the team at Elsevier, we were able to launch The Journal of Climate Change and Health, of which I serve as Editor-in-Chief.

Life is a matter of priorities and while we must all strive for balance, it is inevitable professional activities take time from our family lives. Thus, I must express my love and appreciation for my best friend and husband, Craig Alexander, whose constant support allows me to undertake new challenges and makes my days fulfilled. Finally, I must thank my three wonderful children—Jagger, Sterling, and Graham—whose passions in life and frank discussions of ways I can do things better have taught me more than I could ever have imagined. Moreover, my love for them has galvanized my realization of our need to protect human and planetary health so we can all sustain our abilities. This, in a nutshell, is the true benefit of telerehabilitation.

CONTENTS

Telerehabilitation

PRINCIPLES AND PRACTICE

CHAPTER 1

Introduction

Marcalee Alexander

Imagine a world where you wake up in the morning, eat your breakfast, go out for a run or walk, and then sit down in your home office to see your patients. You don't do this every day of the week, just on the days you choose. After seeing your patients, you might have your own appointments, see your accountant, do the laundry, or see your own physician, which you would also do electronically.

Now imagine you also have a 3-year-old daughter with incomplete tetraplegia. You love her dearly and want her to be as independent as possible, receiving the best medical care and optimal therapies. However, you live 50 miles from the nearest comprehensive rehabilitation center at which she can receive these therapies face-to-face. The prospect of not working so she can attend face-to-face therapy is undesirable, to say the least. Fortunately, that facility has a well-developed telerehabilitation system in place whereby your daughter can receive high-quality one-on-one and group therapies at home, and you have arranged your household so that she can do this. Additionally, her physiatrist and therapists have arranged a system whereby they consult with an academic rehabilitation hospital in another state when they have questions. This allows you and your partner to both work full time and yet participate in activities related to your daughter's rehabilitation needs.

Telerehabilitation is a field in its infancy and the utility of telerehabilitation is evolving. In this book, telerehabilitation is defined as the delivery of medical or rehabilitative care to persons with rehabilitation needs via telecommunication or the internet. The use of telerehabilitation is paramount in terms of ensuring a sustainable and just future for people around the world; however, it has taken significant time for telerehabilitation programs to be established. Although I have personally been fortunate to practice telerehabilitation part-time since 2012, as late as 2019 I visited major cities in the United States and beyond and queried department chairs about whether they were doing telerehabilitation. The answer in most places was a resounding no. Sadly, it took the COVID-19 pandemic, a worldwide disaster, to awaken practitioners and health care systems to the utility of telerehabilitation and for payors to provide reimbursement for services provided. Then, these systems popped up virtually overnight. Moreover, due to necessity, safety, and temporary changes in funding around the world, within months most rehabilitation providers had incorporated telerehabilitation into their practices.

By now millions of people around the world have participated in a telerehabilitation visit as a patient or have observed family members do so; however, it is apparent that thousands of reactive practitioners will not continue to perform telemedicine or telerehabilitation after the COVID-19 crisis is over. In consequence, many people will be disappointed to no longer have the option for telerehabilitation and may be put in a situation where they are anxious to obtain new providers who will provide these services for them. This is unfortunate, because not only is there ease in attending and performing telerehabilitation visits, telerehabilitation is an excellent way to ensure access to health care in both economically privileged large city environments and remote, economically challenged environments, as is seen in the following testimonial:

My first experience with telerehabilitation came in the midst of the major earthquake that struck Nepal in 2015. Our staff at Spinal Injury Rehabilitation Centre were flooded with nearly 150 individuals with new traumatic spinal cord injuries. The quick implementation of telerehabilitation enhanced our services by providing expert support to our interdisciplinary team from international specialists in neurosurgery, orthopedic spine surgery, physical medicine and rehabilitation, pediatric rehabilitation, and spinal cord injury therapy and nursing.

More recently during the COVID-19 pandemic, we again benefited from telerehabilitation services. As we experienced a large outbreak within our centre, telerehabilitation allowed us to continue evaluating, treating, and communicating with inpatient individuals and their families from remote rooms and locations, minimizing infection risks while continuing to provide comprehensive, interdisciplinary care. Simultaneously, we were able to provide outpatient telerehabilitation consultations for our patients in the community, without requiring them to visit the centre during the pandemic. This was especially helpful during times of high viral activity in communities and nationwide lockdowns. During these encounters we were able to provide ongoing rehabilitation care and consultation for individuals with spinal cord injury, including counseling, treatment of acute conditions, and ongoing home therapy sessions.

Given our context in Nepal, where transportation across rugged terrain is both difficult and costly, telerehabilitation has dramatically improved access to care for our patients throughout the country. We have now incorporated telerehabilitation into our routine services. We are actively seeing telerehabilitation reduce costs, improve access to care, and enhance outcomes for individuals with spinal cord injury.

Given our experience, we fully affirm Nepal's national e-health strategy that seeks to integrate smart information and communication technology solutions—like telerehabilitation—within the national health system. We have personally experienced the benefits of digital technologies, which the World Health Assembly acknowledges as major resources to improve public health by promoting universal health coverage and advancing the Sustainable Development Goals.

If telerehabilitation can be effectively implemented in our resource-limited setting, I'm confident it can be beneficially utilized worldwide. This textbook, Telerehabilitation: Principles and Practice, is a critical step forward in making this important resource more accessible to rehabilitation practitioners and patients everywhere.

DR. RAJU DHAKAL, MBBS, MD
CONSULTANT, PHYSICAL MEDICINE AND REHABILITATION
MEDICAL DIRECTOR, SPINAL INJURY REHABILITATION CENTRE, NEPAL

Telerehabilitation is an ideal means to provide care for people with disabilities. Of all populations, those with mobility impairments, impairments in activities of daily living (ADL), sensory, motor, and cognitive dysfunctions have the most difficulty traveling to appointments. Moreover, depending on the impairment, the socioeconomic status, and the individual's physical location, they can have substantial difficulties reaching a specialized center. This is not to say that telerehabilitation can solve all ills. Rather, used prudently, it can be an adjunct to a rehabilitation system of care from prevention, to the emergency room through acute and to outpatient care, and on a lifelong basis. It can also be an effective tool to assist in the provision of research and education, as seen in the vast migration to online professional meetings and consumer education that occurred in 2021. Additionally, it has allowed the possibility for organizations such as Sustain Our Abilities to quickly provide educational resources through venues like Zoom and YouTube to thousands of professionals and persons with disabilities around the world seeking continuing education. Still, if we genuinely want to provide holistic care for persons requiring rehabilitation, we should ensure telerehabilitation includes appropriate education, integrative health care, counseling, and opportunities for therapeutic recreation.

In addition to the benefits of telerehabilitation in increasing access to care and knowledge, there are two other important issues to consider. Currently, the world is moving in the wrong direction with regards to the climate crisis. The UN reports, "Pledges made by so far by countries around the globe to cut greenhouse gas emissions fall strikingly short of the profound changes necessary to avoid the most catastrophic impacts of climate change."[1] A significant advantage of telerehabilitation is that it reduces the need for travel, and systematic replacement of even a portion of rehabilitation care with telerehabilitation would be environmentally beneficial. In my own experience in a small rehabilitation program, adding telerehabilitation services resulted in saving 500,000 miles of driving in 2 years with an associated decrease in greenhouse gases. Finally, time spent in travel is also time that could be used for other purposes, thus saving money, and likely improving quality of life.

Negotiating Telerehabilitation: Principles and Practice

The purpose of this book is to provide a guide for the optimal uses of telerehabilitation and I have sought the most experienced providers in telerehabilitation around the world to participate as chapter authors. They will share a brief overview of the field they practice in or the specific diagnostic area of their expertise. Current and previous research related to the topics will be reviewed, and points about the nuances of telerehabilitation in various areas will be addressed. Research and practice recommendations will be made, because just as telestroke has increased the capacity to save brain function in people with strokes, telerehabilitation, judiciously started prior to planned surgeries or as a way of staying mobile in the community, may be a way to improve health and function. Finally, when appropriate, case reports will be provided to demonstrate various potential experiences in the performance of telerehabilitation.

The book commences with an overview chapter and then moves through groups of diagnosis-based, discipline-specific, and special topic chapters. If you read straight through the whole book you will find repetition as there is in any textbook; however, I believe you will benefit from this repetition and use it to see various opinions on management of different concerns. Moreover, through comparison of these various techniques, we anticipate that you can use creativity in planning how you will perform telerehabilitation.

Telerehabilitation is also designed as an international book. Therefore the authors and coverage of topics are from around the world, allowing the reader to obtain information both from countries where telerehabilitation has been practiced for 10 to 20 years and from countries where it is relatively new. Moreover, while a number of the chapters may be country-centric, as telerehabilitation is just developing, this diversity will add to the richness of the reader's learning experience. I hope you enjoy the text as much as I have enjoyed working with the authors to bring this information to you. *Telerehabilitation* is dedicated to the professionals who work with me at https://SustainOurAbilities.org. Without their support and assistance, this book would not exist. All editor's proceeds from the sale of this book will also go directly to Sustain Our Abilities. To learn more you can reach me at malexander@sustainourabilities.org.

Reference

1. Brady D. United Nations: Countries' pledges to cut emissions are far too meager to halt climate change. *The Washington Post.* 2021. https://www.washingtonpost.com/climate-environment/2021/02/26/un-climate-emissions/

CHAPTER 2

Getting Started: Mechanisms of Telerehabilitation

Kazuko Shem ■ Ingebjørg Irgens ■ Marcalee Alexander

Telerehabilitation (TR) refers to the delivery of rehabilitation via a variety of technologies and encompasses a range of services that include "evaluation, assessment, monitoring, prevention, intervention, supervision, education, consultation, and coaching."[1] The terminology may differ (e.g., teletherapy, teleSCI, telestroke) based on practice settings and business models. The aim of digital technology services that can be offered with TR should be to provide more accessible services and to coordinate and securely transfer knowledge between professionals, care providers, and consumers.

Telecommunication technologies and services are available to provide care for persons with disabilities or in need of rehabilitative services as a part of acute care, subacute care, or long-term follow-up, and TR has been shown to be effective for people with motor and neurological impairments and musculoskeletal conditions.[2] Information and communication technologies that may be used to deliver rehabilitation services include synchronous communication, for example, video and audio conferencing, chat messaging, as well as asynchronous communication, for example, "store and forward" images for consultation, reviewing of data obtained from sensor and wearable technologies at a later time, and nonurgent messaging on patient portals.[3] TR is delivered by a broad range of health care professionals that may include physicians, nurses, occupational therapists, physical therapists, psychologists, respiratory therapists, pharmacists, dieticians, social worker/care managers, and speech-language pathologists.[4] Frequently, family members and caregivers are also involved in TR encounters.

TR services can be performed virtually anywhere rehabilitation services are provided. This can be in the emergency room or at a sporting event, if the local policy includes rehabilitation providers at this stage in a patient's care. TR can also start prior to patient's admission to an acute inpatient rehabilitation program. Using telecommunication technologies, such as videoconference meetings to an acute care hospital, a patient at home, or to a local municipality, can make it possible to personalize and customize an upcoming inpatient stay. Virtual care can also make it easier for inpatients to participate in rehabilitation even if they require isolation for infections or if they are immunocompromised. Evaluating a person's home environment and collaborating with local care providers and thus planning discharge to the patient's community is also an important part of the rehabilitation process that can be facilitated with TR. This is particularly important for persons with lifelong rehabilitation needs that occur in the individual's home or local environment and not in a rehabilitation clinic.

The delivery of TR services can occur in many settings such as clinics, hospitals, homes, schools, therapy offices, long-term care facilities, and other community settings such as worksites. Multiple studies have shown that TR can improve adherence to treatment, improve physical and mental function and quality of life, and reduce health care costs, while maintaining patient satisfaction.[2] Home-based TR may also reduce rehospitalizations and visits to the emergency department. For example, TR can decrease the frequency of exacerbation of conditions like chronic obstructive pulmonary disease (COPD).[5] Therefore any patients with disability who are eligible for in-person rehabilitation should ideally be considered for TR.[6]

Implementation of digital monitoring and TR services can improve the safety and quality of care, and simultaneously increase health care providers' workflow efficiency. Still, the integration of ever-advancing technologies presents challenges to the health care system, and the successful implementation of digital technologies in TR is a complex and time-consuming process. Moreover, as newer digital technologies are deployed, the digital divide may widen and special considerations should be made for vulnerable populations including people with disabilities, migrants, or those that live in rural areas.[7] Participation in TR should especially be encouraged for persons at high risk of complications, those who may have limited access to technology, the elderly, those with low socioeconomic status, and minorities.[6,8]

Key Principles

Rehabilitation professionals and other stakeholders should be aware of the following key principles when developing and implementing a TR program (Table 2.1).

Administrative Principles

Health care organizations and professionals should be aware of guidelines and standards set forth by their nationally recognized associations and other regulatory, credentialing, privileging,

TABLE 2.1 ■ **Four Principles and Three Phases of Implementation for Telerehabilitation Services**

Key Principles	Telerehabilitation Program Phases
Administrative Principles	Development Phase
Regulatory guidelines National and regional standards Policies and procedures Scope of practice Quality of service Risks Viability	Organizational support Funding of service Review of other programs Needs assessment Establish vision, mission, policies Establish procedures and strategies Explore and implement technologies
Clinical Principles	Implementation Phase

Training
   Health care providers
   Patients/families/caregivers
Patient safety
Privacy
	Identify and schedule patients
	Conduct telerehabilitation visits
	Information management and documentation
	Billing and reimbursement

Technical Principles	Evaluation Phase
Appropriate equipment Informational privacy and security Technology maintenance and adaptation	Patient satisfaction Provider feedback Cost analysis
Ethical Principles	
Compliance Codes of ethics Organizational values Autonomy Resource allocation and equitability	

and accrediting requirements for licensing, professional liability, and professional development. Operational and/or contractual requirements should be followed during the implementation of the TR program. Any national and regional laws, professional regulations, and/or organizational policies must be followed with regard to informed consent. The scope of TR services should be established, including types of service being provided, type of technologies, capturing of video, audio, and/or photographic images, record keeping, privacy and security, billing arrangements, and support personnel. Organizations and professionals need to consider policies and/or procedures to determine the client's location at the time of the encounter and establish a secondary mode of communication in the event of communication disruption. This is crucial for safety planning should a medical or domestic emergency arise. Any research activities that may occur with TR programs need to have the research protocol reviewed and approved by the local research/ethical review committee. On a periodic basis, the organization should review the TR program for risks, quality of service, and viability of the program.[1] More detailed legal considerations are covered in Chapter 28.

Clinical Principles

Health care professionals who will be using TR technologies should be trained in the operation and troubleshooting of the equipment they are using and in supporting the patient through troubleshooting their end device. Professionals performing TR services may need to modify educational materials or techniques that can be provided virtually. Having an appropriate facilitator (e.g., caregiver, family member, care manager) and/or interpreter may be necessary to meet the client's needs and to facilitate TR encounters, and any additional persons accompanying and participating in the TR encounter need to be announced, recognized, and approved by both the client and the provider. Clients' safety during TR encounters is paramount. If the professional notices that their client may be experiencing any distress, the virtual encounter may need to be terminated and the client directed to seek an appropriate local health care provider or emergency services.[1]

Technical Principles

Health care organizations and professionals should ensure that the equipment to be used is safe, sufficient, and functioning properly. This may include having ancillary or peripheral devices (e.g., sensor technologies, a blood pressure monitor, digital stethoscopes, etc.) that may be necessary for the encounter. Privacy and security measures should be in place and compliant with organizational, national, and/or local regulatory requirements. Policies and strategies should also be in place to address any need to update or modify the hardware, software, and/or peripheral devices.[1]

Ethical Principles

Organizational values and ethics should be incorporated into the policies and procedures utilized for TR programs, and organizations and/or professionals should comply with any applicable laws, regulations, and codes of ethics. Clients should be informed of their rights and responsibilities and informed consent should be documented. Health care providers and their organizations should also reduce and eliminate any potential conflicts of interest associated with providing TR services.[1]

Precautions to ensure privacy should be considered as they relate to the provider's location (e.g., ensuring headsets are used if the provider is not working from a private office) and using platforms with end-to-end encryption. Furthermore, ensuring the patient is in a therapeutic environment is another nuanced issue, where providers may need to direct the caregiver to leave the room to allow the patient time and space to speak openly about their needs and concerns.

Other ethical considerations include patient autonomy and just and equitable distribution of resources. When using TR methods to a private home, the provider must remain cognizant of potential discomfort a patient may have about being seen in their home environment. Additionally, providers should be prepared to address concerns or refer the patient to resources if the home appears to be unsafe or unfit for a patient. Another prominent issue in the field of TR is the concept of the digital divide and how living in remote locations, poor infrastructure, disability, and lower socioeconomic status can impact the availability of patient-owned TR-enabled devices and access to reliable high-speed Internet. As organizations implement TR, they should consider how they might ensure equitable distribution of services for individuals with these particular barriers.[7]

Types of Telerehabilitation

TR services can be categorized as follows:[2]
- **Synchronous live videoconferencing**—real-time virtual delivery of TR using audio-video technologies.
- **Asynchronous store and forward**—consists of sharing of stored data, such as photographs and radiological images, and recorded visits.
- **eConsult**—electronic messages initiated by a referring provider to a specialist with clinical questions.
- **Remote patient monitoring (RPM)**—personal health and medical information collected on a client at a location is transmitted to a provider at another location for use in care and periodic monitoring of chronic conditions.
- **Mobile health (mHealth)**—the practice of medicine, public health, and education supported by mobile devices such as cell phones and tablet computers.

TR support can also be grouped based on technologies that are used:
- Voice only (telephone or mechanical voice),
- Video plus voice (screen/videoconferencing),
- Computer only (laptop/personal computer [PC]/tablets), and
- Robotic voice or video (mechanical voice and/or animation).

The receivers and the modes of the TR services can be grouped into
- Provider-to-provider (health care workers to health care workers or to other caregivers),
- Direct-to-consumer (health care workers to patients),
- Store and forward (transmission of information to health care receivers or users, not active live communication),
- Web-based treatments (online treatment), and
- Interactive home monitoring (patient educational program).[2]

"Provider-to-provider" TR usually occurs between different departments or hospitals and is frequently used when specialty care is not available where the patient is.[3] One of the most cited "provider-to-provider" TR services is telestroke. Despite stroke being the fifth most common cause of death and the leading cause of long-term disability in the world, and despite and significant advancement in stroke treatment, a limited number of specialists, especially in the rural areas, remains a barrier to evidence-based management.[9] Telestroke programs provide services and management recommendations for patients with acute stroke at a remote site where a stroke physician is not onsite. In spinal cord injury (SCI), the "Hub and Spoke" model is sometimes used between local providers caring for persons with SCI directly and SCI specialists at a distant site, and similar models make sense for other populations of persons with uncommon disabilities.[3,10]

"Direct-to-consumer" TR programs provide health care directly to clients with rehabilitation needs and can be done via synchronous live videoconferencing, telephone, or mHealth if there is the direct management of the clients by health care providers. With the COVID-19 pandemic, "direct-to-consumer" TR programs were implemented urgently in many locations in early

2020, and the number of TR encounters increased exponentially.[7,11] Many examples of "direct-to-consumer" TR exist, for instance follow-up management of musculoskeletal disorders, SCI, or stroke where consumers are evaluated and treated via live videoconferencing, and the health care provider recommends changes to the individual's care. Another example is telemental health, in which a psychologist or a counselor provides counseling via videoconferencing technologies. Speech therapy provided by a speech-language pathologist to the consumer via videoconferencing is also a well-researched service.

Asynchronous "store and forward" TR is frequently used for dermatological conditions like pressure injury (PI) or a rash where photographic images are transmitted to the provider either from the clients themselves or from another provider.[3] Radiological images such as computed tomography images of persons with an acute stroke can be transmitted to a provider at a distant location in a "store and forward" manner. With the advancement of telecommunication technologies, clients can also send video recordings to providers for their review.[12,13] In TR, and in areas where individuals live far from providers, this may be ideal when assessing clients' mobility and equipment needs at their own residences.[13]

Interactive home monitoring or RPM is a TR service in which a client transmits medical information such as blood pressure recordings, weight, glucose levels, catheterization volumes, or nutrition intake to a provider at another location for periodic monitoring to receive timely guidance. Often, this information is submitted to a third-party service that uses nurses or other health care professionals to preliminarily review the data and the physician is only notified in the case of an outlier. A specific example of RPM is the SAPHIRE system for cardiac rehabilitation in which patients exercise using a bicycle with a touch screen and wireless wearable sensors that monitor the patients' blood pressure, oxygen saturation, and electrocardiogram in real-time.[14] RPM is ideal for issues such as blood pressure management for poststroke patients, and for persons with SCI who have orthostatic hypotension and/or autonomic dysreflexia.

Web-based treatments can provide online monitoring and treatment based on the program used. Many online self-help type programs, smartphone apps, and web-based physical therapy exercise interventions have been developed.[3,15] Particularly in cardiac and pulmonary rehabilitation, wearable sensors along with a web app enable patients to monitor pulse oximetry and other vital signs and facilitate self-management.[8,16] In fact, some patients may prefer web or phone-based applications over information provided via computer, and even SMS text messaging has been found to be helpful.[17,18]

Phases in Implementing a TR Program

There are three phases that should occur with developing and implementing a TR program: development phase, implementation phase, and evaluation phase (see Table 2.1).[19]

PROGRAM DEVELOPMENT PHASE

Organizational Support and Funding of the Service

Rehabilitation services should be available for all individuals with disabilities. The organization of health care services should aim to have rehabilitation services available, no matter the geographical location of the consumers or caregivers. Leadership at health care systems including health information management, information technology, credentialing, therapy services, compliance, and billing should be involved early during the integration of telecommunication technologies into all clinical settings in the hospital. Moreover, all members of the multidisciplinary team should ideally be involved in the process of implementation of a TR program. Strong support from the health care organization's leadership, especially financial support, is needed to establish a new TR program. This support ensures sufficient and adequate capacity, reasonable structure, and appropriate expertise in a way that will ensure that quality and patient safety are protected in the health care service. Thus far, around the world, funding to facilitate increased use of TR seems to have been insufficient, but there will undoubtedly continue to be a substantial increase in the use of TR in the future. The need for more TR visits in 2020 has led to an increase in the funding; however, there may still be a problem with the technological solutions between specialized health care services and regional services, including those provided by general health care providers.

Lack of framework and reimbursement had been a significant barrier to widespread adoption of all telemedicine services (including TR services) prior to the COVID-19 pandemic in many countries. Nevertheless, telemedicine expanded quickly in many countries around the world as many changes were made in privacy rulings and reimbursement structures.[20] In the United States, pursuant to authority granted in the Coronavirus Aid, Relief and Economic Security (CARES) Act, the Centers for Medicare and Medicaid Services (CMS) waived the geographic and site of service originating site restrictions for Medicare telehealth services.[21] These flexibilities allowed patients with Medicare to receive treatments from their homes. Additional flexibilities allowing teaching physicians to use synchronous telehealth (audio and video) technology to supervise residents during the pandemic further boosted adoption in academic medical centers and assisted in jump-starting the process of ensuring graduate medical education on this important topic. Similarly, changes in the reimbursement and regulations in countries such as the United Kingdom, Canada, France, and Italy have helped expand telemedicine to reduce patient hospital and clinic visits, allowing health care to be provided expediently via interactive telecommunications around the world (see Chapter 16 for information regarding Italy).

Telerehabilitation Needs Assessment

Worldwide, TR programs have been successfully implemented in many countries but some countries have challenges they may still need to overcome.[22] As noted earlier, there are many different types of TR that can be implemented, which should be reviewed and considered.[2,14,19] The needs of patients and the interest of providers for TR programs should be assessed including possible barriers such as regulatory framework, physical capability, regional broadband infrastructure, and level of technologic proficiency/acceptance of the patient population. In addition, providers should have an awareness of the prevalence of their patients who have telecommunication means and equipment. Performing a needs assessment is appropriate, and some of the more common barriers to implementation of TR are security and privacy issues, concern for the quality of services delivered, lack of evidence to support the effectiveness of TR, reimbursement and billing processes, and technological infrastructure challenges.[22–25]

Establish Vision, Mission, Policies, Procedures, Implementation Strategies

A TR program that involves both originating and distant clinical sites should have a clear and shared vision of the TR program being implemented, and the scope of practice determined.[7,9] The use of TR program leaders (frequently referred to as "champions") has been recommended and these individuals should be identified, developed, and supported. Dedicated rehabilitation clinicians who are passionate about using remote technology and eager to improve health care services by virtual means should be frontliners. Detailed policies and procedures should be written and approved by the health care organization.[19] Moreover, there is an abundance of resources that can be used to establish policies and procedures, such as guidelines from the American Telemedicine Association and the National Consortium of Telehealth Resource Centers in the United States and the World Health Organization.[1,7,26]

Technology, for example videoconferencing, is a useful adjunct in coordination of the rehabilitation process. It can be used to optimize cooperation with local providers, consumer organizations, and other relevant stakeholders. Technology used should provide safe, effective, and predictable interactions that allow specialized health clinicians to share their expertise with providers at a local level. The implementation process should include consumers and other service recipients as active participants and allow the health care system to coordinate follow-up at local and regional levels.[7]

Implementation, however, is not without challenges. Remedying the lack of organizational or facility infrastructure and required videoconferencing software, as well as installation and maintenance of new equipment, take both time and financial support. The coordination of TR can be time-consuming, not only in the initial implementation phase, but also during the maintenance of service delivery. There should be no doubt regarding legal responsibility for service and support, both in hospitals and in the local communities where consumers reside. Privacy, confidentiality, and ethical aspects must also be thoroughly safeguarded before a TR service is initiated. Health care organizations may require providers to obtain additional training and/or be approved for privileges specific to TR. In countries like the United States and Canada,[27] providers must be licensed both in the state/jurisdiction they are practicing and in the state in which the care is being delivered (e.g., when care is provided across state lines) unless within the US Veterans Affairs system that is nationally based and has a legislative exception to this rule. In other countries, providers must also be licensed and the issue of performing health care services across international borders must be evaluated in each possible country-to-country communication. A risk assessment of medicolegal concerns before the initiation of any services is warranted. A prerequisite at the originating sites where the consumers are is a clear understanding of the responsibility of the local providers and for the technologies being used. TR guidelines should be developed and be updated and be continuously available on the organization's web page.[28]

Exploration and Implementation of Technology

Depending on the types of TR to be offered, equipment needs may vary.[2,27] For example, common telecommunication equipment used includes PCs, tablet devices, smartphones, or laptops, and both PCs and laptops may require purchasing of webcams and/or a headset. Multiple platforms, such as Zoom, FaceTime, Microsoft Teams, Doximity, and systems that have patient privacy protection, are available for synchronous visits and there are telehealth systems that are embedded with common electronic medical record systems and their patient portals.[29] If at all feasible, videoconferencing equipment should be provided to all rehabilitation providers including physicians, therapists, nurses, and care coordinators, and training for all participants who will provide services must be completed prior to their participation in a TR program.

A wired connection is preferred over WiFi, and the following minimum bandwidth speeds are recommended for different practice settings by the US Office of Health Information Communication and Technology. Factors to consider are number of users, user locations, real-time transactions, hardware, and storage technology.[30]

- Single physician practice: 4 megabits per second (Mbps)
- Small physician practice (two to three physicians): 10 Mbps
- Nursing home and rural health clinic (approximately five physicians): 10 Mbps
- Clinic/large physician practice (5–25 physicians): 25 Mbps
- Hospital: 100 Mbps
- Academic/large medical center: 1000 Mbps

The American Telemedicine Association guidelines also recommend a minimum of 640×360 resolution and 30 frames per second for videoconferencing.[31]

Instructions and checklists with a focus on ethical issues, professional quality, and safety for the participants should be prepared.[32] Devices being used should have up-to-date security software, and the providers should have a back-up plan in place for an alternate method of communication in case video communication fails. A telemedicine team (TMT) should be available, and staff members on the TR team should be familiar with the TMT services. The TMT members should have specialized technological expertise, be readily available, and be included in all new clinical projects and feasibility studies. Potential errors and complexities regarding new solutions should be addressed promptly. Participating TR members should be included in all parts of the development of the service, and they should continue in maintaining the services after the technology has been implemented.

One challenge is finding ways to organize a seamless workflow and handoffs between disciplines, especially during the first visit for a provider new to TR. That is, a clerk/receptionist may arrive and register the patient first, then a nurse or medical assistant will usually interact with the patient. In an academic setting, a resident physician may see the patient next followed by the attending physician. In a multidisciplinary clinic, physical or occupational therapists may also engage with the patient in real-time, as needed. At the end, the patient usually needs to interact again with the nursing staff to close out the clinic visit and to schedule future appointments. Streamlined coordination between the members of the care team is preferred. When there are challenges with a seamless handoff, it is prudent to provide very direct communication to the consumers so they will know what to expect during these handoffs.[32]

PROGRAM IMPLEMENTATION PHASE

The following section will describe the implementation phase of general routine "direct-to-consumer" TR encounters (Box 2.1). For those interested in establishing a telestroke program with its unique needs for stroke management, the reader is referred to ATA's Practice Guidelines for Telestroke and to Chapter 4.[9]

BOX 2.1 ■ Workflow Prior to and During the Visit.

Prior to the Visit

1. Identify and schedule patient appropriate for TR visit.
2. Confirm the patient has appropriate technologies and ability to connect virtually.
3. Patient should establish a patient portal account if a patient portal is to be used.
4. Confirm contact information including emergency/back-up information.

During Telerehabilitation Visit

Clinic Staff

1. Check the equipment including charging of battery if using a portable device.
2. Patient to log-in to the patient portal, if needed.
3. Check-in patient, check medication list and allergies.
4. Confirm pharmacy information patient uses.
5. Obtain and document vital signs, if available from the patient.

Clinician

1. Clinician joins the visit.
2. Confirm consent to conduct a virtual visit.
3. Inform the patient that the visit is private and confidential.
4. Provide telerehabilitation assessment and care plan.
5. Document assessment and plan and enter orders.

Clinic Staff

1. Electronically provide visit summary.
2. Schedule follow-up appointment.

TR, Telerehabilitation.

Identify and Schedule Patients

Within the electronic medical record and scheduling systems being used, TR providers need to identify and appropriately set up a scheduling system specific to TR. Initially, a provider may need to identify a group of persons with disabilities who have easy access to and who are familiar with using digital technologies to initiate TR programs. Providers should also consider appropriateness of TR encounters versus in-person visits prior to scheduling visits because certain disorders, like musculoskeletal conditions or spasticity, may be better assessed in person. It may also be helpful to have a factsheet available for patients to read regarding how their TR visit will be conducted.[32]

While most return TR visits may be completed within 30 minutes,[33] considering potential technical difficulties and additional time needed to complete documentation etc., additional time may need to be set aside. Many hospital centers will have a practice call for the patient's first visit or have staff assist with patient technical difficulties before the first scheduled appointment to streamline physician visits. Unlike in-person visits, TR visits should be initiated exactly on time, and multiple patients cannot be scheduled during the same time period unless you are having a group visit.

Conducting Telerehabilitation Visits

In some rehabilitation systems, instead of rooming patients as would be done with an in-person appointment, clinic staff/assistants are available and can confirm the virtual clinic visit with the patient, reconfirm the client's full name, date of birth, contact information (telephone numbers, mailing address, email address, emergency contact information), and obtain basic information such as vital signs, medication lists, allergies, and chief complaints.[31,32] Pharmacy information should also be confirmed. In order to have vital signs available for review, patients can be asked to have a blood pressure monitor and a thermometer at home and clinic staff should ask the patients to obtain vital signs prior to the TR visit. For those with respiratory disorders, small portable pulse oximetry monitors are now readily available for purchase. Digital stethoscopes and electrocardiograms can also be used to record lung and cardiac sounds and these data can be transmitted via an application.[16,34,35]

As the provider starts a TR visit, the patient's identity (with two identifiers) along with any other persons (i.e., providers at the originating site, caregivers) should be verified, and informed consent to conduct a TR visit must be obtained and documented (see Chapter 28 for more information).[32] If the patient and the provider do not speak the same language, a certified translation service may need to be connected to the visit. Other health care professionals such as therapists or care managers may join from a third remote site. In such an encounter, the patient should be clearly informed, and their consent must be obtained for the additional professionals to participate in the visit.[1] If multiple people/sites are participating, those who are not speaking should put themselves on mute.[31]

For both patients and the providers, considerations need to be made for the room and physical environment where the TR visits are to be conducted as this will influence the quality of the encounters. Privacy must be ensured as a priority. Both the provider and the patient need to be visible and heard, and any distraction and background noise should be avoided. To improve video quality and ensure the space is well lit, the source of lighting should be behind the screen and webcam and the background should have muted décor to prevent visual disturbances over the camera. Headsets with microphones are preferred to open air microphones as they reduce the likelihood of missed pickups during conversation. The equipment and camera being used should be placed on a stable platform to avoid shaking and wobbling.[31,32]

Eye contact is one of the most important aspects of provider-client interaction. It helps to establish rapport and trust and allows for the use of nonverbal communication. When using a computer monitor with a camera, the camera should be positioned appropriately (about 7 degrees above the eye level) so that one can see the client on the monitor and the camera simultaneously (Fig. 2.1).

Camera Position

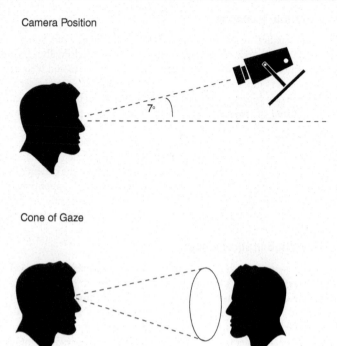

Cone of Gaze

Fig. 2.1 Camera positioning. (Source: Ben-Arieh, D, Charness, N, Duckett K, et al. *A Concise Guide for Telemedicine Practitioners: Human Factors Quick Guide. Eye Contact.* American Telemedicine Association. 2016. Image courtesy of the ATA.)

The provider should replicate eye-contact patterns by looking into the camera frequently. While maintaining focus, the provider should keep oneself centered in the field of view and avoid staring.[36]

Physical examination can be performed virtually as indicated by the patient's symptoms, medical history, and other relevant information. Initial viewing should start with a "passport" shot (include head and top of shoulders),[36] and history and review of symptoms can be obtained with this view. Additionally, the patient's alertness, mental status, facial expressions and symmetry, speech, skin condition, and head position can be observed with this view. Some cranial nerve (CN) functions (e.g., extra ocular movements [CNIII, IV, VI], raising eyebrows [CNVII], opening and closing eyes [CNIII, CNVII], shrugging of shoulders [CNXI], tongue movements [CNXII]) can also be examined relatively easily. Providers may need to guide the patients either verbally or visually for neurological and functional examination.

After the history and physical examination that can be done in the "passport" view is completed, the provider can ask the patient or caregiver to change the camera angle or zoom out so that upper extremities and upper trunk are visible. Muscle strength cannot be tested as objectively during a virtual examination, but providers can still visualize the patients' upper extremity movement and function. For example, providers can ask the patient to "bend your arm at the elbow," "raise your arms above your shoulders," "touch your index finger to your nose," and "touch each of your fingers on both hands to their thumb."

Next, providers should ask the patient and/or caregiver to show a full-length shot of the patient in a sitting position. In this view, like the upper extremity examination, patients can be asked to "bend at the hip," "straighten your knee," "move your foot up and down," and "wiggle your toes." For those patients who can ambulate, the camera can be repositioned so that standing balance (including one leg standing) and gait can be observed. Spasticity and tone may be difficult to assess virtually as providers cannot test reflexes and feel the degree of tone that patients may have. However, involuntary spasms, clonus, and restricted range of motion may be observed and may help guide spasticity management. In addition, more probing interviewing techniques to elicit more information from the patient/family as an indirect assessment, when full physical examination is not available, can also be helpful. For patients who have durable equipment (e.g., wheelchair, commode, shower bench, standing frame, orthoses), the condition of the equipment can be visualized and documented.

Providers are responsible for ensuring the patient's safety and well-being during a TR encounter. If the provider observes their patient to be experiencing significant discomfort or other symptoms that might warrant a rapid in-person assessment, then the virtual encounter should be terminated, and the patient should be instructed to seek a local health care provider for an urgent assessment and management.[1]

Providers should have cultural competency and consider factors that may influence TR encounters such as the client's language, ethnicity, race, age, gender, geographical location, and socioeconomic and cultural backgrounds.[16] The provider should also be updated on any recent significant events (i.e., wildfire, earthquakes, hurricanes) in the client's local community. If the patient is at a remote location, the provider may need to investigate where the patient can obtain laboratory tests, radiological examinations, and/or therapy services. At the end of the visit, the provider should provide a summary of the visit, and an appropriate disposition with plans for future follow-ups should be confirmed with the patient.[32]

Telerehabilitation in Postacute Settings

For rehabilitation during the subacute recovery phase after an event like a stroke or a heart attack, a progressive and protocolized TR program can be planned in addition to the above "direct-to-consumer" care provided virtually by physicians.[4,6] Building upon an existing in-person rehabilitation protocol, patients can receive a progressive TR protocol with multidisciplinary support from their rehabilitation physician, physical and occupational therapists, speech-language pathologist, social worker, and pharmacists.[4] Using an established rehabilitation protocol will minimize any delay in care.[6]

Health Information Management and Documentation

Foremost, that the visit occurred virtually and in what format (video vs. telephone) needs to be documented. The presence of any family members and/or caregivers and any involvement of interpreters should be recorded. Clinical documentation such as chief complaint, subjective reports, history, current medications, allergies, patient education, and assessment and plan should be documented similar to an in-person visit.[32]

However, documentation of the physical examination must be based on what is visible in the video and may need to be more descriptive. For example, rather than having a specific degree measurement of shoulder range of motion with a goniometer as if a visit is done in-person, one may need to document how a patient can raise their arm above shoulder level or not (see Chapter 8 on the use of a goniometer to measure range of motion virtually). Other physical observations including general appearance, speech, facial expression, mood, alertness, and some dermatological findings can be easily observed and documented. In rehabilitation, observation of mobility and assessment of durable equipment is critical and can be also done virtually using synchronous video. Additionally, one must clearly document the time spent on the visit in addition to assessment, planned treatments, recommended actions, and follow-up plans.[32]

Common dermatological conditions including pressure injuries can be assessed and managed using either synchronous or asynchronous visits. If images such as photographs of the skin condition are sent asynchronously by the patient, those images need to be uploaded and associated interactions documented in the patient's medical record.

In most countries, health information, including that obtained during TR encounters, is highly regulated.[12] Documentation and legal record-keeping requirements are discussed in detail in Chapter 28.

Billing and Reimbursement

Prior to providing any services to the patient, they should be made aware of the potential cost. Arrangement for payment and/or insurance authorization should also be made prior to starting the TR visits. These issues are different depending on the country of service and the particular provider. For instance, in the United States, charging for telehealth visits requires adding telehealth specific codes and modifiers (e.g., GT for synchronous live video encounters and GQ for asynchronous "store and forward" services), and the codes differ depending on what services are provided (e.g., physician's consultation/evaluation and management, psychotherapy, nutrition therapy, psychiatry services). Billing requirements, codes, and reimbursement rules change frequently around the world and are beyond the scope of this book; thus providers are recommended to consult their local regulations and organizational guidelines to ensure appropriate practices and coding guidelines are being followed.

The Impacts of COVID-19 on Telerehabilitation and Considerations for the Future

Many countries temporarily or permanently expanded the scope of service and changed policies and reimbursement rules during the COVID-19 pandemic so that telemedicine services could be available more widely to persons needing health care.[7] Some of the changes and waivers that were implemented either temporarily or permanently included initiation of client-to-provider telemedicine where only provider-to-provider telemedicine was allowed previously in countries such as Japan, Republic of Korea, and Vietnam and allowing first-time visits to be done virtually in China and Japan. Remote care was able to be provided outside of local regions in places such as the United States and Canada as in some cases providers not licensed in a particular state/province could practice beyond their licensed area. Moreover, free online telehealth was offered in countries such as China and the Philippines and e-prescription use was expanded in Australia, Malaysia, and the Philippines.[7]

In the United States, previously, there were also no TR codes therapy service providers could use to bill for their TR encounters. Reimbursement for rehabilitation therapy service providers (physical therapists, occupational therapists, and speech-language pathologists) who were not allowed to see and/or needed to avoid seeing their patients in-person during the COVID-19 pandemic was critical, including specific billing codes for therapeutic exercises and activities, neuromuscular reeducation, gait training, group therapeutic procedures, cardiac rehabilitation, wheelchair management training, self-care management training, and so on.[37] In addition to these changes, in the United States and Australia, videoconferencing and audio-only services were reimbursed.

Prior to COVID-19, technologies used for virtual care needed to be fully compliant with the requirements of privacy rules. There was flexibility initiated within the technical framework subsequent to COVID-19 to allow providers to use many different available platforms in countries such as Australia and the United States; however, it is anticipated this will change back in the future so as to ensure care quality and privacy.[7] Medicolegal risk must also be strongly monitored and compliance and risk assessment must be an ongoing concern. Still, flexibility will be needed in the future, especially during times of natural and/or man-made disasters like wildfires, hurricanes, floods, extreme heat and cold spells, and pandemics that may occur.

A different use of TR for "direct-to-consumer" became apparent with COVID-19 and should be considered in future planning. When a considerable risk of infection transmission is present between the provider and consumer, such as occurs with an immunocompromised patient being treated with chemotherapy or posttransplant, TR can be especially beneficial. Moreover, if there is a shortage of health care personnel or resources like personal protective equipment, TR can be preferable to face-to-face care to maintain the capacity for isolation while working on increasing strength, endurance, flexibility, improving speech, assessing changes in medical status, or providing counseling.[38] Additionally, for countries and regions that license practitioners (e.g., physicians, therapists) based on the state or province where they practice (e.g., the United States, Canada), there will be a substantial benefit to have uniformity with professional state licensure requirements so that practitioners can continue to provide care to patients in other states/provinces and improve access to health care services during times of future disasters.[39]

Patients treated remotely may have a low tolerance for therapeutic exercise; thus the following criteria (based on the Japanese Association of Rehabilitation Medicine) or similar guidelines can be used to temporarily pause the performance of remote therapies:

- Resting pulse rate <40 or >120 beats/minute
- Systolic blood pressure at rest <70 or >200 mmHg
- Diastolic pressure at rest >120 mmHg
- Chest pain at rest or with exertion
- Dizziness, cold sweats, nausea, headache, severe fatigue in a sitting position
- Tachypnea >30 beats/minute or shortness of breath
- Oxygen saturation at rest <90%.[38]

PROGRAM EVALUATION PHASE

The program evaluation phase may include quantitative and qualitative data collection, data analysis including cost-saving analysis, assessment of benefits/strengths, challenges/weaknesses/barriers, and recommendations for improvement.[10] With continuously advancing telecommunication technologies, an equipment replacement plan to acquire up-to-date technological tools and software should be established. A network to share experiences and ideas with organizations outside the hospital should be initiated. The American Telemedicine Association and the National Consortium of Telehealth Resource Centers in the United States and the International Society for Telemedicine and eHealth (ISFTeH) provide great resources. Novel and innovative TR projects should quickly result in satisfactory patient outcomes and lead to routine TR services. Active involvement and feedback based on experience and evaluations from consumers, their family members, and regional health care services are beneficial in the development of a sustainable and safe model of long-term care for persons with disabilities.[14] Prior studies have highlighted many positive aspects of TR services such as convenience and promotion of self-awareness and motivation.[40]

Shortly after establishing a TR program, quantitative and qualitative assessment measures should be collected and analyzed. For example, the number of virtual visits conducted should be examined. A successful program should see an incremental increase in the number of virtual visits over time. Satisfaction surveys of consumers should be conducted and potential barriers from the patient's perspective should be examined.[33] Obtaining feedback from the providers is needed to identify any challenges and inefficiencies in the TR program. Benefits and strengths of the TR programs should be highlighted and marketed to consumers and providers.[7]

Common barriers to the use of TR include users' technological challenges and internet connectivity.[22,24,27] For example, consumers may be living in remote areas with poor internet coverage or at locations where there are inadequate secure WiFi connections. Platforms that will directly connect providers and consumers are easier to use and may be similar to making telephone calls, but consumers may struggle to access services if they need to connect using their hospitals' patient portals. The use of commercially already available technologies may be more acceptable to consumers.[40] Older individuals who are not as familiar with using smartphones or internet may be hesitant to use TR services and having providers or caregivers who can assist with setting up the devices may facilitate TR encounters.[24] While the prevalence of smartphones is increasing worldwide,[41] there are still many people, especially in developing countries, who may not have smartphones or internet connections. Finally, the most commonly reported barrier to the use of TR is the lack of national TR policy and laws.[22] Future clinical research can accelerate acquisition of evidence for TR and assist in identifying best practices that are more likely to be adopted and continue to be advanced.[2]

References

1. American Telemedicine Association. *Principles for Delivering Telerehabilitation Services.* American Telemedicine Association; 2017. https://cdn2.hubspot.net/hubfs/5096139/ATA-Telerehabilition-Services.Final_.revised.pdf.

2. Bettger JP, Resnik LJ. Telerehabilitation in the age of COVID-19: an opportunity for learning health system research. *Physical Therapy.* 2020;100(11):1913–1916. https://doi.org/10.1093/ptj/pzaa151.

3. Irgens I, Rekand T, Arora M, et al. Telehealth for people with spinal cord injury: a narrative review. *Spinal Cord.* 2018;56(7):643–655. https://doi.org/10.1038/s41393-017-0033-3. Epub 2018 Mar 7. PMID:29515211. 10.1038/s41393-017-0033-3.

4. Jhaveri MM, Benjamin-Garner R, Rianon N, et al. Telemedicine-guided education on secondary stroke and fall prevention following inpatient rehabilitation for Texas patients with stroke and their caregivers: a feasibility pilot study. *BMJ Open.* 2017;7:e017340. https://doi.org/10.1136/bmjopen-2017-017340.

5. Vasiloupoulou M, Papaiannou AI, Kaisakas G, et al. Home-based maintenance tele-rehabilitation reduces the risk for acute exacerbation of COPD, hospitalizations and emergency department visits. *Eur Respiratory J.* 2017;49:1602129.

6. Moulson M, Vewick D, Selway T, et al. Cardiac rehabilitation during the COVID-19 era: guidance on implementing virtual care. *Canadian J Cardiol.* 2020;30:1317–1321.

7. World Health Organization, Regional Office for the Western Pacific. *Implementing Telemedicine Services During COVID-19: Guiding Principles and Considerations for a Stepwise Approach.* World Heath Organization; 2020. https://iris.wpro.who.int/bitstream/handle/10665.1/14651/WPR-DSE-2020-032-eng.pdf.

8. King D, Khan S, Polo J, et al. Optimizing telehealth experience design through usability testing in Hispanic American and African American patient populations: observational study. *JMIR Rehabil Assist Technology.* 2020;7(2):e16004.

9. American Telemedicine Association. *Practice Guidelines for Telestroke.* American Telemedicine Association; 2017. https://cdn2.hubspot.net/hubfs/5096139/17_NEW_ATA-Telestroke-Guidelines.pdf.

10. Irgens I, Hoff JM, Jelnes R, et al. Telerehabilitation @home: results from a randomized controlled trial in individuals with disability related to spinal cord injury. In press.

11. Irgens I, Bach B, Rekand T, Tornås S. Optimal management of health care for persons with disability related to spinal cord injury: learning from the Sunnaas model of telerehabilitation. *Spinal Cord Ser Cases.* 2020;6:88. https://doi.org/10.1038/s41394-020-00338-6.

12. Peterson C, Watzlaf V. Telerehabilitation store and forward applications: a review of applications and privacy considerations in physical and occupational therapy practice. *Int J Telerehabil.* 2015;6(2): 75–84.

13. Tyagi N, Goel S, Alexander M. Improving quality of life after spinal cord injury in India with telehealth. *Spinal Cord Ser Cases.* 2019;5:70.

14. Peretti A, Amenta F, Tayebati SK, Nittari G, Mahdi SS. Telerehabilitation: review of the state-of-the-art and areas of application. *JMIR Rehabil Assist Technol.* 2017;4(2):e7. https://doi.org/10.2196/rehab.7511. PMID:28733271.

15. Fairman AD, Yih ET, McCoy DF, et al. Iterative design and usability testing of the iMHere system for managing chronic conditions and disability. *Int J Telerehabil.* 2016;8(1):11–20.

16. Rawstorn JC, Ball K, Oldenburg B, et al. Smartphone cardiac rehabilitation, assisted self-management versus usual care: protocol for a multicenter randomized controlled trial to compare effects and costs among people with coronary heart disease. *JMIR Res Protoc.* 2020;9(1):e15022.

17. Frederix I, Hansen D, Coninx K. Medium-term effectiveness of a comprehensive internet-based and patient-specific telerehabilitation program with text messaging support for cardiac patients: randomized controlled trial. *J Med Internet Res*. 2015;17(7):e185.
18. Selzler AM, Wald J, Sedeno M, et al. Telehealth pulmonary rehabilitation: a review of the literature and example of a nationwide initiative to improve the accessibility of pulmonary rehabilitation. *Chronic Respiratory Dis*. 2018;15(1):41–47.
19. Cason J. A pilot telerehabilitation program: delivering early intervention services to rural families. *Int J Telerehabil*. 2009;1(1):29–38.
20. Ohannessian R, Duong TA, Odone A. Global telemedicine implementation and integration within health systems to fight the COVID-19 pandemic: a call to action. *JMIR Public Health Surveill*. 2020;6(2):e18810. https://doi.org/10.2196/18810. Published online 2020 Apr 2. PMCID: PMC7124951. PMID:32238336.
21. Centers for Medicare & Medicaid Services. *General Provider Telehealth and Telemedicine Tool Kit*. https://www.cms.gov/files/document/general-telemedicine-toolkit.pdf. Accessed 08.02.21.
22. Leochico CFD, Espiritu AI, Ignacio SD, Mojica JAP. Challenges to the emergence of telerehabilitation in a developing country: a systematic review. *Front Neurol*. 2020;11:1007. https://doi.org/10.3389/fneur.2020.01007. eCollection 2020. PMID:33013666.
23. Movahedazarhouligh S, Vameghi R, Hatamizadeh N, Bakhshi E, Khatat SMM. Feasibility of telerehabilitation implementation as a novel experience in rehabilitation academic centers and affiliated clinics in Tehran: assessment of rehabilitation professionals' attitudes. *Int J Telemed. Appl*. 2015;2015:468560. https://doi.org/10.1155/2015/468560. Published online 2015 Nov 2.
24. Hale-Gallardo JL, Kreider CM, Jia H, et al. Telerehabilitation for rural veterans: a qualitative assessment of barriers and facilitators to implementation. *J Multidiscip Healthc*. 2020;13:559–570. https://doi.org/10.2147/JMDH.S247267. eCollection 2020.
25. Cason J, Behl D, Ringwalt S. Overview of states' use of telehealth for the delivery of early intervention (IDEA Part C) services. *Int J Telerehabil*. 2012;4(2):39–46.
26. World Health Organization. *Telemedicine: Opportunities and Developments in Member States: Report on the Second Global Survey on eHealth 2009 (Global Observatory for eHealth Series)*. Volume 2. World Health Organization; 2010. https://apps.who.int/iris/bitstream/handle/10665/44497/9789241564144_eng.pdf?sequence=1&isAllowed=y.
27. Øra HP, Kirmess M, Brady MC, et al. Technical features, feasibility, and acceptability of augmented telerehabilitation in post-stroke aphasia-experiences from a randomized controlled trial. *Front Neurol*. 2020;11:671.
28. Federation of Medical Regulatory Authorities of Canada. *Framework on Telemedicine*. Federation of Medical Regulatory Authorities of Canada; 2018. https://fmrac.ca/wp-content/uploads/2019/04/Framework-on-Telemedicine-Final.pdf.
29. American Medical Association. *Telehealth Implementation Playbook*. American Medical Association; 2020. https://www.ama-assn.org/system/files/2020-04/ama-telehealth-implementation-playbook.pdf.
30. HealthIT.gov. What is the recommended bandwidth for different types of health care providers? The Office of the National Coordinator for Health Information Technology; 2019. https://www.healthit.gov/faq/what-recommended-bandwidth-different-types-health-care-providers.
31. Gough F, Budhrani S, Cohn E, et al. Policy: ATA practice guidelines for live, on-demand primary and urgent care. *Telemedicine and e-Health*. 2015;21(3):233–241. http://www.medicalinfo.ch/images/articles/ATA-Practice-Guidelines-for-Live-On-Demand-Primary-and-Urgent-Care.pdf.
32. Rural Health Network Telehealth Working Party. *Guidelines for the Use of Telehealth for Clinical and Non Clinical Settings in NSW*. Agency for Clinical Innovation; 2015. https://www.telemedecine-360.com/wp-content/uploads/2019/02/2015-ACI-telehealth-guidelines.pdf.
33. Sechrist S, Lavoie S, Khong C-M, Dirlikov B, Shem K. Telemedicine using an iPad in the spinal cord injury population: a utility and patient satisfaction study. *Spinal Cord Ser Cases*. 2018;4(1):71. https://doi.org/10.1038/s41394-018-0105-4.
34. Swarup S, Makaryus AN. Digital stethoscope: technology update. *Med Devices (Auckl)*. 2018;11:29–36. https://doi.org/10.2147/MDER.S135882. eCollection 2018.

35. Marshall SG, Shaw DK, Honles GL, Sparks KE. Interdisciplinary approach to the rehabilitation of an 18-year-old patient with bronchopulmonary dysplasia, using telerehabilitation technology. *Respir Care.* 2008;53(3):346–350.
36. Ben-Arieh D, Charness N, Duckett K, et al. *A Concise Guide for Telemedicine Practitioners: Human Factors Quick Guide. Eye Contact.* American Telemedicine Association; 2016. Updated October 3, 2018. https://cdn2.hubspot.net/hubfs/5096139/Eye-Contact-Quick-Guide.final.pdf.
37. Centers for Medicare & Medicaid Services. List of Medicare Telehealth Services effective January 1, 2021-updated August 12, 2021. https://www.cms.gov/Medicare/Medicare-General-Information/Telehealth/Telehealth-Codes. Accessed 8/29/2021.
38. Sakai T, Hoshino C, Yamaguchi R, Hirao M, Nakahara R, Okawa A. Remote rehabilitation for patients with COVID-19. *J Rehabil Med.* 2020;52(9):jrm00095. https://doi.org/10.2340/16501977-2731.
39. Brannon J, Cohn E, Cason J. Making the case for uniformity in professional state licensure requirements. *Int J Telerehab.* 2012;4(1):41–46. https://doi.org/10.5195/IJT2012/6091.
40. Shulver W, Killington M, Morris C, Crotty M. "Well, if the kids can do it, I can do it": older rehabilitation patients' experiences of telerehabilitation. *Health Expect.* 2017;20(1):120–129.
41. Taylor K, Silver L. *Smartphone Ownership Is Growing Rapidly Around the World, but Not Always Equally.* Pew Research Center; 2019. https://www.pewresearch.org/global/2019/02/05/smartphone-ownership-is-growing-rapidly-around-the-world-but-not-always-equally/.

Specific Disorders

CHAPTER 3

Telerehabilitation in Spinal Cord Injury

Kazuko Shem ■ Ingebjørg Irgens ■ Felicia Skelton ■ Marcalee Alexander

Introduction

Spinal cord injury (SCI) causes severe disability and secondary complications with an associated high burden of care.[1] The estimated annual global incidence is 40 to 80 cases per million population. Up to 90% of these cases have traumatic causes, although the proportion of nontraumatic SCI appears to be growing. Most individuals with SCI are males (78%) and the overall average age at injury is 43. Males are the most at risk in young adulthood (20–29 years) and older age (70+ years). Females are the most at risk in adolescence (15–19) and at older age starting in their 60s. Studies report male-to-female ratios of about 2:1 among adults. Many of the consequences associated with SCI do not result from the condition itself, but from inadequate medical care and rehabilitation services, and from barriers in the physical, social, and policy environments.[1]

Common associated conditions experienced in persons with SCI are neurogenic bladder, bowel and sexual dysfunction, neuropathic and musculoskeletal pain, spasticity, pressure injury (PI), orthostatic hypotension, autonomic dysreflexia (AD), respiratory insufficiency, and metabolic and cardiovascular disorders. The top three most frequently reported secondary complications are urinary tract infection (UTI), AD, and PI with incidences of 62%, 43%, and 41%, respectively.[2]

Within the first year after discharge from inpatient acute rehabilitation, persons with SCI develop on average two to three distinct SCI-related complications.[2] As there are an increasing number of aging persons with SCI, cardiometabolic disorders and obesity have become conditions that need to be monitored closely. Preventive measures should be considered after SCI since they may influence cardiovascular health as well as subjective well-being.[3-5] Prevention of secondary conditions is also important since such conditions affect health, "self-management," and quality of life (QoL) as persons with SCI age.[5-10]

Many individuals with SCI live in rural areas without rehabilitation services and must travel hours to see an SCI specialist.[6,7,10,11] There is also a lack of providers in the community who have knowledge and experience treating persons with SCI. These barriers can lead to delays in diagnosis and treatment of secondary complications and may ultimately impede the patient's ability to reintegrate back into the community.[12,13]

Barriers to self-management in persons with SCI include physical limitations, secondary complications, lack of accessibility, caregiver burnout, and lack of funding.[9] Persons with SCI also frequently have extensive needs for disposable supplies and durable medical equipment (DME) and additional needs to document their disabilities for varying purposes (e.g. obtaining disability benefits and disabled parking permits, leave from school/work, documentation of service/emotional support animals, need to fly with medical equipment). These issues present significant challenges for individuals with SCI when they are reintegrating into their community.

In 2016 an international panel of leaders in SCI and telehealth coined the term "telespinalcordinjury" or "teleSCI" at the International Spinal Cord Society (ISCoS) Annual Meeting in Austria.[14] Technological solutions and performing rehabilitation visits via telehealth can mitigate barriers by reducing or eliminating burdens such as the time it takes to travel, the need for caregiver support to travel, and the costs of transportation itself.[15] The following sections describe teleSCI applied for persons with SCIs throughout the continuum of care.

TELESPINALCORDINJURY

TeleSCI allows for low-cost and wide-reaching solutions in providing specialized consultation and therapy to persons with SCI living in rural areas and/or who have transportation difficulties.[15–18] Various forms of technology can be used, ranging from smartphones or tablets that allow for basic audio and visual access to the patient, their caregivers, and their environment to more specialized peripheral devices that allow measurements of vital signs, or more sophisticated examination of limb movements, skin condition, speech, facial expressions, mood, and gait. This is of particular importance for people with SCI that reside in rural areas, whose access to medical services may be limited.[19] The successful integration of teleSCI into traditional in-person health care practices can bridge the discrepancy of quality of care between rural and urban areas, and address issues of lengthy travel and costs that have adverse effects on QoL.[20]

Historically, most studies of telerehabilitation used in the population of people with SCI have been conducted via telephone,[16,21–24] videoconferencing,[17,23,25,26] web-based portal platforms,[27] or data messaging devices.[28] In the United States, the Veterans Health Administration (VHA) was an early adopter of videoconferencing, especially for mental health treatment.[29,30] Today, different telerehabilitation devices are in daily use in many countries around the world, and these telerehabilitation models can reduce the distance needed to consult with SCI specialists. Nevertheless, transportation to local health centers with access to the tools remains a barrier in some places where people do not have adequate internet at their homes or access to a cell phone. In the United States, the VHA has also tried to minimize the "digital divide"[31]—the gap in those who have access to digital devices and the internet and those who do not—by providing tablets and internet access to veterans who are not able to afford devices of their own.[32]

One of the first reports of using teleSCI was in 1999, when telerehabilitation was demonstrated to successfully manage PI.[33] In 2001, Philips et al. compared the standard of care between inpatient care and the use of supporting care using telephone and videoconference.[15] The results showed improved health-related outcomes for patients in the telephone and video group. The European "Thrive" teleSCI project showed no difference in the occurrence of clinical complications when telerehabilitation was used, but there was a higher improvement of functional scores in persons who participated in telerehabilitation interventions.[34]

A number of studies have examined the feasibility and efficacy of care delivery via telerehabilitation to the SCI population.[14,20,35–38] Utilizing and integrating telerehabilitation into treatment practices may offer a unique and low-cost alternative to traditional on-site medical care.[23] Telerehabilitation interventions have also achieved high satisfaction scores for care in persons with SCI and may decrease the rates of rehospitalization after hospital discharge.[34,39] However, despite these benefits and the fact that telerehabilitation has been available for decades, telerehabilitation is still not considered standard of care for this group of people.

INCORPORATING TELESCI INTO A REHABILITATION PRACTICE

Successful implementation of teleSCI requires consideration of several environmental and logistical factors. First, the availability of a private area to conduct the teleSCI visit must be confirmed, as well as access to usable teleconferencing platforms that work with commercially available products (i.e., smartphones and tablets). Effective telehealth visits mirror in-person clinical encounters by being well lit, with the provider centered on the screen, and through efforts to make eye contact by looking directly into the camera to facilitate rapport.

Using TeleSCI for Acute Assessment and Management

Acute care of persons with SCI starts at the scene of an accident if a person sustains a traumatic SCI or at least in the emergency department (ED) when patients arrive with symptoms of SCI. First responders and/or providers in the ED in remote areas may not be familiar with managing persons with acute SCI. Furthermore, an SCI specialist will most likely not be available on-site for the majority of the hospitals in the world to assist critical care providers to manage these patients. Acute care management of SCI involves accurate neurological examination to determine the degree of injury, management of hemodynamic instability and respiratory insufficiency, bladder management, and surgical interventions.[40] While telemedicine is used for acute stroke management,[41] as of yet, teleSCI has not been used routinely for acute SCI care. However, like telemedicine for stroke, it should be possible to use teleSCI to assist with diagnosing and managing persons with acute SCI who are in an ED or in an ICU. Video consultation with acute care facilities is also an appropriate way for rehabilitation facilities to ensure patient stability prior to admission, evaluate for PI, and confirm presumed level and degree of injury. Remote collaboration between different specialists can also be performed between departments and wards during an inpatient stay, and teleSCI can be used for planning the rehabilitation stay for patients needing readmission.[42]

Prognosis and Ongoing Research Studies

After acute SCI, patients should have a neurological examination based upon the International Standards for the Neurological Classification of SCI (Fig. 3.1).[43] In order to facilitate assessment with teleSCI, it is beneficial for patients to have a copy of their neurological examination and to know what date it was performed. After injury, many patients are interested to hear about their prognosis and ongoing clinical trials, and this baseline examination can assist physicians in counseling. With proper assistance, lighting, and positioning of the patient for examination, a repeat neurological examination can also be performed to assess recovery of function. Some physicians may use teleSCI on an ongoing basis to discuss prognosis and neurological recovery with individuals with SCI; however, video-based teleSCI is preferred, which will allow for visualization of the patient's facial expression and reaction to what is being discussed.[44]

TeleSCI in Inpatient Rehabilitation

During inpatient rehabilitation, teleSCI can serve many useful purposes. As shown during the COVID-19 pandemic, it can be used to minimize spreading infections during group meetings between patients and allow providers to see patients without gowning and entering their rooms. TeleSCI can also be used for team conferences across facilities, and it can allow specialists from another facility to see a patient. It has been shown to be useful to use an app to perform a home visit prior to discharge for a patient.[45] It has also been successfully utilized for wheelchair clinics and can effectively be used to allow community-based providers to learn about the needs of the individual with SCI when they return home.[42]

TeleSCI Outpatient Management Applications

Providers with limited experience in working with the SCI population may have inaccurate preconceived notions about the capability of their patients to utilize telehealth platforms, especially if they have not previously interacted with the patient. To avoid these pitfalls, providers should ask patients about their current usage of a smartphone or tablet. Patients who can access the internet for news or emails have a 28 sufficient skill level to use teleSCI services.

In longer term planning for patients with upper-limb mobility impairments, consider recommending accessibility features present on most devices such as voice command, or referring to occupational therapy to identify appropriate adaptive equipment to facilitate independence. During times of crisis where these options may not be feasible, assess if a caregiver is available and

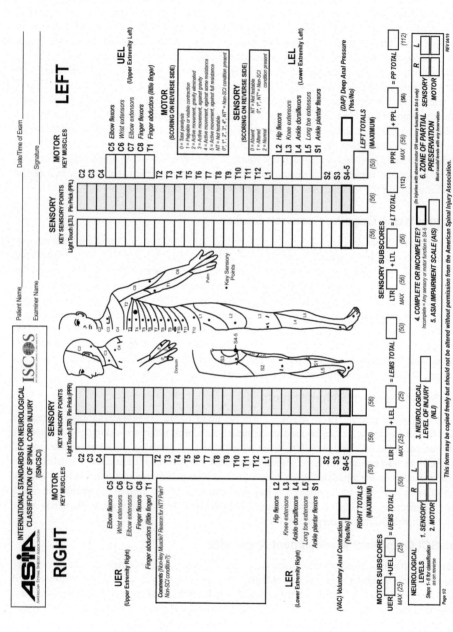

Fig. 3.1 International Standards for Neurological Classification of Spinal Cord Injury 2019 Revision. (Courtesy American Spinal Injury Association: International Standards for Neurological Classification of Spinal Cord Injury, revised 2019; Richmond, VA.)

Muscle Function Grading

0 = Total paralysis

1 = Palpable or visible contraction

2 = Active movement, full range of motion (ROM) with gravity eliminated

3 = Active movement, full ROM against gravity

4 = Active movement, full ROM against gravity and moderate resistance in a muscle specific position

5 = (Normal) active movement, full ROM against gravity and full resistance in a functional muscle position expected from an otherwise unimpaired person

NT = Not testable (i.e. due to immobilization, severe pain such that the patient cannot be graded, amputation of limb, or contracture of > 50% of the normal ROM)

0*, 1*, 2*, 3*, 4*, NT* = Non-SCI condition present *

Sensory Grading

0 = Absent   1 = Altered, either decreased/impaired sensation or hypersensitivity

2 = Normal   NT = Not testable

0*, 1*, NT* = Non-SCI condition present *

Note: Abnormal motor and sensory scores should be tagged with a '' to indicate an impairment due to a non-SCI condition. The non-SCI condition should be explained in the comments box together with information about how the score is rated for classification purposes (at least normal / not normal for classification).

When to Test Non-Key Muscles:

In a patient with an apparent AIS B classification, non-key muscle functions more than 3 levels below the motor level on each side should be tested to most accurately classify the injury (differentiate between AIS B and C).

Movement	Root level
Shoulder: Flexion, extension, abduction, adduction, internal and external rotation Elbow: Supination	C5
Elbow: Pronation Wrist: Flexion	C6
Finger: Flexion at proximal joint, extension Thumb: Flexion, extension and abduction in plane of thumb	C7
Finger: Flexion at MCP joint Thumb: Opposition, adduction and abduction perpendicular to palm	C8
Finger: Abduction of the index finger	T1
Hip: Adduction	L2
Hip: External rotation	L3
Hip: Extension, abduction, internal rotation Knee: Flexion Ankle: Inversion and eversion Toe: MP and IP extension	L4
Hallux and Toe: DIP and PIP flexion and abduction	L5
Hallux: Adduction	S1

ASIA Impairment Scale (AIS)

A = Complete. No sensory or motor function is preserved in the sacral segments S4-5.

B = Sensory Incomplete. Sensory but not motor function is preserved below the neurological level and includes the sacral segments S4-5 (light touch or pin prick at S4-5 or deep anal pressure) AND no motor function is preserved more than three levels below the motor level on either side of the body.

C = Motor Incomplete. Motor function is preserved at the most caudal sacral segments for voluntary anal contraction (VAC) OR the patient meets the criteria for sensory incomplete status (sensory function preserved at the most caudal sacral segments S4-5 by LT, PP or DAP), and has some sparing of motor function more than three levels below the ipsilateral motor level on either side of the body. (This includes key or non-key muscle functions to determine motor incomplete status.) For AIS C – less than half of key muscle functions below the single NLI have a muscle grade ≥ 3.

D = Motor Incomplete. Motor incomplete status as defined above, with at least half (half or more) of key muscle functions below the single NLI having a muscle grade ≥ 3.

E = Normal. If sensation and motor function as tested with the ISNCSCI are graded as normal in all segments, and the patient had prior deficits, then the AIS grade is E. Someone without an initial SCI does not receive an AIS grade.

Using ND: To document the sensory, motor and NLI levels, the ASIA Impairment Scale grade, and/or the zone of partial preservation (ZPP) when they are unable to be determined based on the examination results.

Steps in Classification

The following order is recommended for determining the classification of individuals with SCI.

1. Determine sensory levels for right and left sides.
The sensory level is the most caudal, intact dermatome for both pin prick and light touch sensation.

2. Determine motor levels for right and left sides.
Defined by the lowest key muscle function that has a grade of at least 3 (on supine testing), providing the key muscle functions represented by segments above that level are judged to be intact (graded as a 5).
Note: in regions where there is no myotome to test, the motor level is presumed to be the same as the sensory level, if testable motor function above that level is also normal.

3. Determine the neurological level of injury (NLI).
This refers to the most caudal segment of the cord with intact sensation and antigravity (3 or more) muscle function strength, provided that there is normal (intact) sensory and motor function rostrally respectively.
The NLI is the most cephalad of the sensory and motor levels determined in steps 1 and 2.

4. Determine whether the injury is Complete or Incomplete.
(i.e. absence or presence of sacral sparing)
If voluntary anal contraction = No AND all S4-5 sensory scores = 0 AND deep anal pressure = No, then injury is Complete.
Otherwise, injury is Incomplete.

5. Determine ASIA Impairment Scale (AIS) Grade.

Is injury Complete?   If YES, AIS=A

NO ↓

Is injury Motor Complete? If YES, AIS=B

NO ↓   (No-voluntary anal contraction OR motor function more than three levels below the motor level on a given side, if the patient has sensory incomplete classification)

Are at least half (half or more) of the key muscles below the neurological level of injury graded 3 or better?

NO ↓   YES ↓

AIS=C   AIS=D

If sensation and motor function is normal in all segments, AIS=E
Note: AIS E is used in follow-up testing when an individual with a documented SCI has recovered normal function. If at initial testing no deficits are found, the individual is neurologically intact and the ASIA Impairment Scale does not apply.

6. Determine the zone of partial preservation (ZPP).
The ZPP is used only in injuries with absent motor (no VAC) OR sensory function (no DAP, no LT and no PP sensation) in the lowest sacral segments S4-5, and refers to those dermatomes and myotomes caudal to the sensory and motor levels that remain partially innervated. With sacral sparing of sensory function, the sensory ZPP is not applicable and therefore 'NA' is recorded in the block of the worksheet. Accordingly, if VAC is present, the motor ZPP is not applicable and is noted as 'NA'.

ASIA
AMERICAN SPINAL INJURY ASSOCIATION

ISCOS
INTERNATIONAL SPINAL CORD SOCIETY

INTERNATIONAL STANDARDS FOR NEUROLOGICAL
CLASSIFICATION OF SPINAL CORD INJURY

Page 22

Fig. 3.1 *Continued*

capable of facilitating a teleSCI visit. When setting expectations for the visit, traditional guidance is to recommend parameters (i.e., being dressed and seated upright vs. in bed and ready for a skin examination) to ensure a positive experience. However, for providers who are unfamiliar with the nuances of the SCI population, flexibility is needed. For example, laying prone is typically not allowed in noninjured patients but may be medically required for a patient with a recent muscle flap to the sacrum.

TeleSCI can be used to manage nearly every secondary condition after SCI. In a recent teleSCI program using FaceTime via iPad, different topics were discussed (general/routine SCI follow-up [63%], genitourinary [12%], pain [8%], spasticity [7%], PI [5%], and other uncommon SCI concerns [5%]).[46] Moreover, persons with chronic SCI who present to an ED with acute medical issues could be seen by a specialist in SCI to assist with management of SCI-related problems.

Pressure Injury Management

As already noted, PI management via teleSCI was one of the first areas where video was used to manage secondary conditions seen in persons with SCI.[14,33] With teleSCI being performed with the patient in his or her home, patients do not need to travel and thus avoid the risk of the PI worsening. Furthermore, weight shift techniques can be reviewed via teleSCI. Using video, a provider can observe a patient's methods of weight shift such as tilt-in-space and recline in a power wheelchair, or in a manual wheelchair user, lateral- or forward-lean or full push-up pressure reliefs, and counseling can be provided to correct inadequate weight shifts. More information regarding PI management can be found in Chapter 11.

Neurogenic Bladder, Bowel, and Sexual Dysfunction

Management of neurogenic bladder via teleSCI should be considered, since assessing and recommending interventions for this condition does not necessarily require physical examination.[47] While initial education is often completed during inpatient rehabilitation, ongoing education of patients and caregivers is often needed, and use of teleSCI can spare a patient office visits to complete this. Detailed history taking and counseling are critical for effective bladder management. This knowledge can be conveyed by teleSCI, either by videoconferencing or by telephone. It is recommended that practitioners use the International Standards for the Assessment of Autonomic Function after SCI to ensure the degree of anticipated versus reported voluntary control of sacral autonomic function is adequately documented (Fig. 3.2).[48] Using the autonomic standards as a basis, history on methods of bladder management (including management strategy, frequency of intermittent catheterization if used, and history of incontinence) can be easily obtained using teleSCI. Patients can also be given a urinal to record urination volume in conjunction with residual volumes obtained through catheterizations, and this can be reported to the provider as appropriate. Bladder medication management can also be provided via teleSCI, including monitoring for adverse effects.

UTIs can be managed either with telephone calls or video-based visits as patients do not need to be seen in person for the providers to obtain a history of symptoms of UTI, such as presence of fever and/or chills, increase in spasms, malaise, abdominal discomfort, increases in incontinence, and/or pain on urination.[47] Color, smell, and clarity of urine can be either verbally described by the patients or urine can be visualized using video. Urine sample can be brought to the patient's general physician or local laboratory. However, if urodynamic examination is indicated, the patient will need to see a urologist or a urotherapist in-person.

For bowel management, history is important in guiding providers to manage a patient's bowel function. Using teleSCI, a provider can obtain a detailed history, including frequency and timing of bowel movements, stool consistency, bowel medications being used, diet, fluid intake, and can actually visualize how a bowel program is being done. TeleSCI can also prompt the examiner to

Sacral Autonomic Function

Bladder Emptying	Method Frequency Timing Voluntarily	Yes _____ No _____		
System/Organ	**Scoring**	**Anticipated Function (based on ISNCSCI)**	**Anticipated Functional Score**	**Patient Reported Score**
Awareness bladder fullness	Normal (2)	Any level injury with normal sensation in the T11-L2 and S3-S5 dermatomes		
	Altered (1)	Any level injury with partial preservation of sensation in the T11-L2 and/or S3-S5 dermatomes		
	Absent (0)	NLI at or above T9 and no sensation below		
	Not Tested (NT): indicate reason, other comments			
Ability to prevent bladder leakage	Normal (2)	Normal sensation and motor function in the S3-S5 dermatomes		
	Altered (1)	Partial sensation and motor function in the S3-S5 dermatomes		
	Absent (0)	No sensation and/or motor function at the S3-S5 dermatomes		
	Not Tested (NT): indicate reason, other comments:			
Bowel Emptying	Method Frequency Timing Voluntarily	Yes _____ No _____		
Awareness of bowel fullness	Normal (2)	Normal sensation and motor function in the S3-S5 dermatomes		
	Altered (1)	Partial preservation of sensation and/or motor function in the S3-S5 dermatomes		
	Absent (0)	No motor or sensory function in the S3-5 dermatomes		
	Not Tested (NT): indicate reason, other comments:			

continued

Fig. 3.2 Autonomic Standards Assessment Form. (Courtesy American Spinal Injury Association: International Standards for Neurological Classification of Spinal Cord Injury, revised 2019; Richmond, VA.)

visualize whether the patient is using a commode for their bowel program or whether the bowel program is being done in the bed. Based on the history, medications and bowel program may be adjusted. Hemorrhoids can be diagnosed remotely based on history (e.g., periodic rectal bleeding, blood on stool) and visualization of external hemorrhoids via video or photo. If a patient may need a colostomy, counseling about colostomy and its risks and benefits can be provided via teleSCI, including connecting a peer with colostomy with the patient for peer advice. However, there are

System/Organ	Scoring	Anticipated Function (based on ISNCSCI)	Anticipated Functional Score	Patient Reported Score
Ability to prevent bowel leakage	Normal (2)	Normal sensation and motor function in the S3-S5 dermatomes		
	Altered (1)	Partial sensation and/or motor function in the S3-S5 dermatomes		
	Absent (0)	No motor or sensory function at the S3-5 dermatomes		
	Not Tested (NT): indicate reason, other comments:			
Psychogenic arousal	Normal (2)	Normal sensation at T11-L2 dermatomes		
	Altered (1)	Partial sensation at T11-L2 dermatomes		
	Absent (0)	No sensation at T11-L2 dermatomes		
	Not Tested (NT): indicate reason, other comments:			
Reflex genital arousal	Normal (2)	Normal sensation and reflex function at S3-5 dermatomes		
	Altered (1)	Partial sensation and/or motor function at S3-S5 dermatomes		
	Absent (0)	No sensation or motor function at S3-S5 and absent sacral reflexes		
	Not Tested (NT): indicate reason, other comments:			
Orgasm	Normal (2)	Intact S3-5 sensation and motor function with any degree of preserved sacral reflexes		
	Altered (1)	No S3-5 sensation and/or motor function and preserved sacral reflexes		
	Absent (0)	No motor or sensory function at S3-5 and absent sacral reflexes		
	Not Tested (NT): indicate reason, other comments:			
Ejaculation	Normal (2)	Normal T11-12 sensation and sacral reflexes		
	Altered (1)	Diminished sensation at T11-12 dermatomes and normal sacral reflexes		
	Absent (0)	No sensation at T11-12 dermatomes and absent sacral reflexes		
	Not Tested (NT): indicate reason, other comments:			
Total Score Sacral Autonomic Section				

Fig. 3.2 *Continued*

some occasions when a person with SCI may need an in-person visit, such as rectal examination and radiological imaging. As with bladder management, ongoing education of patient and caregiver is easily facilitated with teleSCI.

Queries about neurogenic sexual function should also be made in conjunction with bladder and bowel function and sexual education can be performed via teleSCI. Chapters 16 and 17 provide complete discussion on neurogenic bladder and bowel, and sexual dysfunction.

Cardiovascular Autonomic Conditions After SCI

AD can be evaluated and managed via teleSCI, as blood pressure measurement and associated symptoms are most critical in managing AD.[49] However, in this case, patients will need to have necessary medications, as well as blood pressure monitors at home, and be able to use them. A diary of blood pressure measurements and pulses over several days with recording of time of the day, associated symptoms, and what activities the patient was doing at the time will be helpful in determining the potential cause of AD and establishing a treatment plan. Similarly, neurogenic orthostatic hypotension can be managed remotely. Depending on the blood pressure measurement and the time of the day when the patient is experiencing hypotension, blood pressure medications like midodrine, fludrocortisone, and/or pseudoephedrine may be prescribed and adjusted remotely.

Pain Management

Pain management, especially for patients with neuropathic pain, usually does not require new physical examination. As pain medications for neuropathic pain are titrated, this can often be done remotely. Moreover, observation of persons with SCI in their home environments can often reveal nuances that can contribute to their pain. In many areas, it is possible for medications to be refilled online so that patients needing regular refills do not need to attend in-person clinic visits just for medication refills.

For those patients who are having musculoskeletal pain, such as shoulder and upper extremity pain—a common secondary condition in persons with SCI—a limited but still worthwhile examination can be done via teleSCI. Using video, a provider can ask the patient to move their upper extremities to see active range of motion (AROM) of shoulders, elbows, and wrists. A modified impingement test and painful arc test can also be done by asking the patient to flex his arm forward and abducting the arm above the shoulder level respectively, and possible rotator cuff tendonitis can be diagnosed. If a caregiver is available at home or if a patient is with a physical therapist, they may also be able to maneuver the patient's limb to see if pain is induced with passive range of motion and at what degree of range of motion. If probable diagnosis of musculoskeletal pain such as rotator cuff tendonitis, elbow bursitis, or de Quervain's tenosynovitis can be determined via teleSCI, conservative treatment such as medications and therapy interventions can be ordered remotely; however, if a patient needs a steroid injection or an imaging study, the patient will need in-person visits.[50]

Utilizing teleSCI for chronic opioid management in patients with severe pain can also be considered. Screening for compliance with treatment, monitoring of pain symptoms, determining risk for opioid use disorder, and opioid medication refill can all be done via audio or audiovisual methods. Urine toxicology screen can also be done locally by the patients or could be taken from a visiting nurse provider. Similarly, opioid weaning can be performed via teleSCI.

Spasticity

Spasticity assessment that can be conducted via telerehabilitation has been described.[51] A caregiver can be coached to perform passive range of motion and to feel for the degree of resistance through the range of motion. Providers can also ask the patients themselves to demonstrate AROM, and the effect of spasticity on the activities of daily living (ADLs) can be also be observed by asking the patients to perform different ADLs. Spasticity management by teleSCI can also be performed to increase or decrease medications. If an individual is on baclofen or another medication, for instance, and lives a distance from a health care provider, tapering the medication by a small dosage and reevaluation in a couple of weeks may be much more beneficial than driving a long distance to an in-person visit. Since most antispasticity medications are oral, teleSCI can be a great adjunct to care.[52] Clearly, if patients need interventions, such as botulinum toxin injection or nerve blocks, or have an intrathecal baclofen pump, then in-person visits will be required.

Venous Thromboembolism

While the risk of deep venous thrombosis (DVT) and pulmonary embolism (PE) is highest in the first few weeks of acute SCI, patients with chronic SCI can remain at a higher risk for DVT and PE throughout their life.[43] Thus a patient may report a new asymmetrical swollen leg via teleSCI. In this case, we recommend the patient is directed to go to the nearest ED for further diagnosis and treatment, in light of the risk of PE. Additionally, it is recommended that the telerehabilitation provider always err on the side of caution, and patients with SCI should always be told to seek emergency care immediately with any chest pain and/or shortness of breath. Still, patients with DVT and/or PE who may need to be on chronic anticoagulation medication can also be managed with teleSCI.

Osteoporosis and Fractures

Osteoporosis is another common complication, and leads to pathological fractures in over half of those with chronic SCI.[53] Persons with SCI may not immediately notice that they may have sustained pathological fractures due to reduced or lack of sensation. While fractures after falling from a wheelchair or from a traumatic event may be obvious, many patients also sustain fractures from low-force impact such as during transfers, range of motion, and ADLs. Patients may notice swelling, redness, and/or bruising of a limb days after the fracture as they may not feel pain from the fracture. With teleSCI, the location of the swelling and associated redness/bruise can be visualized, and the patient can be directed to seek care if appropriate in an ED or told to return to their rehabilitation or general health provider for further follow-up.

Dermatologic Conditions

Common dermatological conditions that are seen in persons with SCI are acne, seborrheic dermatitis, tinea cruris, ingrown toenail, onychomycosis, folliculitis, and drug-induced cutaneous reactions. Except for a severe ingrown toenail that may need surgical intervention, all of these dermatological conditions can be visualized and treated conservatively via teleSCI.

TELETHERAPIES

Telerehabilitation has been utilized to evaluate the maintenance of functional status after rehabilitation, upon discharge to home.[53] Moreover, store and forward telerehabilitation has been utilized after discharge in India to evaluate the patient's status after discharge from acute SCI rehabilitation and to provide and evaluate postdischarge exercise programs.[54] While it is well recognized that home-based exercise programs are effective in improving physical activity and endurance in people with SCI,[55,56] there are few published studies of teletherapy for persons with SCI.[37,57] Some use web-based or virtual games (Nintendo Wii),[57] while in 2014, the first teletherapy videoconferencing program was described by Van Straaten.[37] A 12-week exercise program for rotator cuff and scapular stabilization was designed with physical therapists supervising with personal computers. The exercise program showed reduction in pain and improvement in muscle strength in serratus anterior and scapular retractors and in function based on Shoulder Rating Questionnaire (SRQ) and the Disabilities of the Arm, Shoulder, and Hand (DASH) Index.

Gait can also be assessed via teleSCI. Many persons with SCI also use standing frames at home, which are impossible to bring to an in-person visit. TeleSCI will allow therapists and providers to visualize the patients in their standing frames at home and confirm that the patients are in a good position in their standing frames.

For persons with SCI, tele–occupational therapy can allow visualization of the layout of patients' residences and the condition of DME being used, especially if a person with SCI has more than one piece of DME, such as an electric wheelchair and a manual wheelchair, and may not be able to bring in all their DME to the in-person consultation. The general condition of other

DME, such as hospital beds, commodes, and shower benches, can also be visualized with video and if they are in disrepair, then the need for replacement can be documented.

Ambulant Rehabilitation Team

Some hospitals have ambulatory rehabilitation teams or home care teams that can travel from the rehabilitation hospital to the consumer's home, or to community locations such as assistive aid offices together with the consumer. The Ambulant Rehabilitation Team (ART) can consist of occupational therapists, physical therapists, wound nurses, and/or social workers, amongst other personnel. With this intervention, team members can meet with the local care providers in the consumer's home to discuss and figure out appropriate solutions to increase activity and participation for the consumer. The ART members can also participate in meetings with the municipality care providers and their leaders or in meeting at the assistive aid offices if there are particular concerns that need to be followed up. However, most of these meetings can be performed via teleSCI, giving the ART members more time to spend with the consumers, instead of in their cars.

Telenutrition

Persons with traumatic SCI have a higher prevalence of cardiovascular disease (CVD) and an increased odds of chronic obesity (odds ratio [OR] = 4.05), heart disease (OR = 2.7), hypertension (OR = 2), and diabetes (OR = 1.7), compared with individuals with other traumatic injuries.[58] CVD has become one of the leading causes of death (35%–46%), and the mortality rate due to CVD is 228% higher in persons with SCI than among those without.[59] Hetz et al. found that persons with SCI who considered themselves overweight had more secondary complications, such as fatigue, pain, upper extremity overuse injuries, as well as lower QoL and more depressive symptoms compared with those who did not consider themselves overweight.[5] Barriers to weight management in persons with SCI include lack of established guidelines for weight management specific to SCI, limited wheelchair accessible options to engage in physical activity, difficulties with receiving group counseling, and lack of staffing with expertise in both SCI and nutrition.[60]

Telenutrition (TN) may provide a promising way to address barriers for nutrition management for persons with SCI. In a Veterans Affairs setting, persons with SCI participated in a multidisciplinary CVD risk reduction program. The program consisted of case managers frequently contacting the participants on the telephone and in-person visits by a dietitian, physical therapist, and exercise physiologist. Significant improvements were seen in weight reduction, reduction in plasma insulin levels, and in total cholesterol/high-density lipoprotein (HDL) ratios.[61] In a pilot program using FaceTime, TN was also found to potentially increase healthy eating behaviors in persons with SCI.[62]

Telepsychology

SCI can affect an individual's psychological well-being and compound their physical impairments.[63,64] Mood disorders that affect QoL are common after SCI.[65] Depression has been estimated at 28% in US veterans with SCI as compared with 22% in civilians with SCI.[66,67] Cognitive behavioral therapy (CBT) is a well-established psychological intervention to treat depression and has demonstrated a positive impact on various psychological concerns including depression within the SCI population.[68,69] Telepsychology (TP) for prevention and treatment of psychological disorders with CBT offers many unique physical and psychosocial advantages, such as reduced stress, stigma, inconvenience of travel, and scheduling difficulty, over an in-person appointment with an SCI specialist.[38]

Dorstyn et al. published a systematic review on applications of TP in SCI with a total of 272 participants.[70] The majority of the studies were nonrandomized and uncontrolled, and most of the studies used telephone, with only one using a video format. The telephone counseling studies showed "moderate to large, but non-significant, short-term treatment effects." Psychotherapy has been also offered by telephone and videoconferencing.[15,20,70,71] The major advantage to teleSCI is overcoming the physical barriers, that is, accessibility, transportation, distance and resources, and delivering specialized SCI care directly to the individual in a private and convenient manner. TP can reduce barriers to care as well as facilitate compliance with interventions to reduce depressive symptomology, mitigate secondary associated symptoms (anxiety), and improve QoL in persons with SCI.

Peer Support

In-person and telephone-based peer support for persons with SCI is feasible and effective in increasing life satisfaction, resource awareness and service usage, as well as improving self-management.[24] Although there are no research studies published on the efficacy of peer support conducted via video, peer support is already being conducted via different available platforms.

DEVELOPING A TELEHEALTH SYSTEM OF CARE

An important concept in SCI care is development of a system of care. As such, it is important for teleSCI to be a part of the SCI system of care from prevention through lifelong follow-up.

In the United States, a Hub and Spoke model of telerehabilitation delivery is utilized in the VA. Patients travel to a local health center (spoke) for remote communication with more specialized providers at their assigned SCI center (hub).[26] Although this model dramatically reduces the distance needed to consult with SCI specialists, transportation to "spoke" sites remains a barrier because of the need to travel and reliance on a supporter; thus teleSCI is often used for communications between specialists at the spoke and generalists at the sites. Similar models are present in other countries and rehabilitation systems.

SPECIAL CONSIDERATIONS

Postacute Rehabilitation

After acute inpatient rehabilitation and in the case of shortening of length of stay, home-based postrehabilitation programs by a multidisciplinary team may be beneficial and are frequently provided. The postrehabilitation team can consist of a physiatrist, a visiting nurse, a physical therapist, an occupational therapist, a speech pathologist, a psychologist, a social worker, and/or a case manager. An SCI specialist can coordinate care with the multidisciplinary team via teleSCI by giving guidance on stretching/strengthening, transfer training and ambulation training at home, appropriate DME, supplies, and answering any medical questions that the team members may have. A video visit can be performed when the multidisciplinary team members are visiting the patient at their home. Ongoing education of the patient and their family/caregivers can occur during these video visits.

Aging with SCI

Persons with SCI may experience accelerated aging as compared to their able-bodied peers. The decline in function and/or independence or with potential loss of caregivers that comes with aging makes teleSCI more valuable. With aging, persons with SCI may experience new neurological decline, more musculoskeletal pain, diminished bladder function, worsening constipation, more fragile skin, and diminution of immune function. Depression also has been reported to be more severe for older persons with SCI and for those with longer duration of injury.[72] Persons aging with SCI have increasing needs for assistance as their family members/caregivers age. Therefore attention should be paid not only to the persons with SCI but also to aging family members/caregivers, and teleSCI can be used to address these medical and psychosocial issues on a regular basis.

TeleSCI is a valuable way to minimize the burden on the family/caregivers by decreasing the need to assist the patient to get ready for an in-person appointment, the need to provide transportation, and the time spent at an in-person visit. In addition, both older persons with SCI and their older caregivers may experience challenges with using technology and may require additional support and training with devices to be used for teleSCI.

Adaptive Equipment

Different platforms and technological devices may be used by persons with SCI for teleSCI. For example, the European "THRIVE" project used a dedicated videoconferencing platform comprising a central unit (set-top box), webcam, microphone, remote controller, and multiple cables, and the system was powered by software designed specifically for people with limited manual dexterity.[34] Now that smartphones have become ubiquitous (in 2019, 76% of people in advanced economies and 45% of people in emerging economies owned a smartphone[73]), using more mobile and portable devices like smartphones may be more effective and practical for persons with SCI.[74] However, for some persons with cervical SCI with impaired hand function, smartphones may be too small and challenging, if not impossible, to use. In that case, larger tablet devices can be an option.

For users who have impaired hand function, specialized accessory equipment may be required. Individuals with higher-level cervical injuries (C1–C4) and with very limited or no use of upper extremity function may be unable to access the touchscreen interface of a tablet device. To address this concern, patients can use adaptive equipment such as mouth stick styluses (Fig. 3.3). A mounting bracket with a rotating arm is also useful for providing stability and flexibility in positioning a tablet device (Fig. 3.4). A wheelchair mount is helpful for enabling individuals with high-level injuries that have limited mobility and upper extremity function to access a tablet from the wheelchair. For individuals with injuries at or above C7 level with limited hand function, the use of an adapted stylus such as the ball top or t-shaped stylus (Fig. 3.5) or a u-cuff (Fig. 3.6) can provide access to a tablet's touchscreen. Occupational therapists, special educators, and/or speech therapists can be consulted to assist with training patients on the use of tablet devices and their accessories.[75,76] Most devices have built-in voice control options that are useful for individuals with limited upper extremity function.

Recommendations for Research

QoL in persons with SCI may be diminished more by environmental barriers and inequity of opportunity than by the impairment and secondary consequences of the SCI itself.[9] This suggests that health system factors, such as access and availability of services, need to be improved to create an optimal environment for self-management and wellness among individuals with SCI. Recently published research on teleSCI shows efficacy, improved quality of care, and patient satisfaction using telerehabilitation services and the potential for teleSCI to address accessibility issues.[9,14,39] However, most studies only demonstrate feasibility and improved satisfaction rather than outcomes such as decreased morbidity, prevention of secondary complications, and reduction of health care cost.

Reduced stress, cost, and inconvenience of travel from home to an SCI specialist appointment, which may be difficult to obtain, make teleSCI an extremely favorable alternative to in-person treatment.[38] With the COVID-19 pandemic, teleSCI was given a boost and should undoubtedly be integrated as standard of care. Because teleSCI is a relatively new way to practice medicine in the field of SCI, it does, however, demand further research to evaluate the efficacy and cost savings for both the patients and the health care system.

There are many areas in the system of care for patients with acute SCI that telerehabilitation can be beneficial and more research and resources are necessary. In the emergency and acute phase,

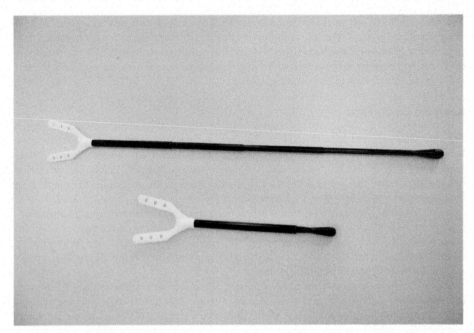

Fig. 3.3 Telescoping mouth stick stylus.

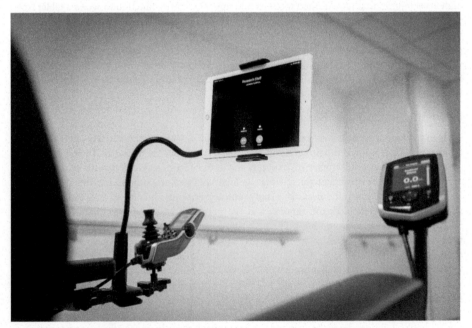

Fig. 3.4 Tyrone gooseneck tablet mounting system.

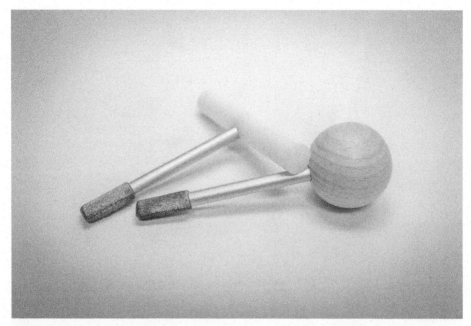

Fig. 3.5 Ball top and t-shaped styluses.

evaluation of the neurological status of the individual with SCI could be performed remotely by the specialist, thereby determining whether transfer to another facility or participation in a research project is appropriate. Telerehabilitation-based SCI physician management could also be performed to the intensive care unit. For patients who are being evacuated at a facility that could cross hundreds or even thousands of miles, a proper transfer of care could be coordinated by the referring and receiving sites and, for individuals with SCI who are already at inpatient facilities, the use of teleSCI could allow non–rehabilitation specialist visits to occur at a remote facility.

After discharge from a rehabilitation facility, teleSCI can be used to document the maintenance of function and the need for readmission; further research could determine the optimal timing and techniques for these interventions. Greater use of telemonitoring of vital signs via telerehabilitation would be optimal for persons with SCIs, and the benefits of telemonitoring on preventing rehospitalization should be studied. As the person with SCI increases their community engagement, teleSCI can be an alternative to face-to-face visits for busy professionals. Finally, as the person with SCI ages, frequent monitoring via teleSCI can allow them to stay at home longer and avoid institutionalization.

Implementation of a telerehabilitation program can be complicated, involving many steps and various stake holders, like consumers, health care providers at the original site and the distant site, compliance, and information services.[26,42] While patients can use their own devices (e.g., smartphones, tablets) these days, hospitals still need to invest in an appropriate Health Insurance Portability and Accountability Act (HIPAA)–compliant telehealth platform for which leadership support will be needed. Greater exploration of the benefits, satisfaction, and potential cost savings of using teleSCI may also provide reasonable justification for medical centers to adopt this technology which will certainly be a large component of the future of SCI management.

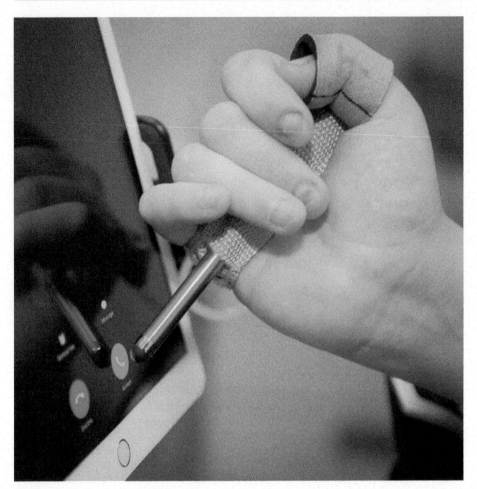

Fig. 3.6 U-cuff with attachable stylus.

CASE STUDY

CJ is a 28-year-old male who sustained a C7 complete SCI in a motor vehicle accident. He underwent an acute rehabilitation program at his rehabilitation facility and was independent with upper body dressing, minimal assistance for lower body dressing, independent bed to wheelchair transfers but contact guard for commode transfers, and minimum assist for car transfers at a wheelchair level after discharge. He lived 100 miles from the rehabilitation center and follow-up after discharge was difficult as he was unable to drive and did not have access to an easy way to return for outpatient care. Additionally, he was taking oxycodone 30 mg daily for pain along with baclofen 10 mg at bedtime for management of his spasticity when discharged home. Following discharge he attended monthly telerehabilitation visits with his physiatrist for management of his medications, and in 3 months was able to be weaned off his oxycodone. He had his baclofen titrated up to 40 mg daily, and with OT and PT his functional status improved over a 6-month period of time to independence at a wheelchair level.

References

1. World Health Organization. *Spinal Cord Injury*. WHO; 2013. https://www.who.int/news-room/fact-sheets/detail/spinal-cord-injury.
2. Stillman MD, Barber J, Burns S, et al. Complications of spinal cord injury over the first year after discharge from inpatient rehabilitation. *Arch Phys Med Rehabil*. 2017;98(9):1800–1805. https://doi.org/10.1016/j.apmr.2016.12.011. Epub 2017 Jan 20. PMID:28115072.
3. Rajan S, McNeely M, Warms C, Goldstein B. Clinical assessment and management of obesity in individuals with spinal cord injury: a review. *J Spinal Cord Med*. 2008;31(4):361–372.
4. Asthagiri H, Wilson J, Frost F. Nutrition in spinal cord injury. In: Kirshblum S, Lin V, eds. *Spinal Cord Medicine*. 3rd ed. New York: Springer Publishing Co; 2019:318–331.
5. Hetz SP, Latimer AE, Arbour-Nicitopoulos KP, Ginis KAM. Secondary complications and subjective well-being in individuals with chronic spinal cord injury: association with self-reported adiposity. SHAPE-SCI Research Group. *Spinal Cord*. 2011;49:266–272.
6. Booth S, Kendall M. Benefits and challenges of providing transitional rehabilitation services to people with spinal cord injury from regional, rural and remote locations. *Aust J Rural Health*. 2007;15:172–178.
7. Cox RJ, Amsters DI, Pershouse KJ. The need for a multidisciplinary outreach service for people with spinal cord injury living in the community. *Clin Rehabil*. 2001;15:600–606.
8. Middleton JW, McCormick M, Engel S, et al. Issues and challenges for development of a sustainable service model for people with spinal cord injury living in rural regions. *Arch Phys Med Rehabil*. 2008;89:1941–1947.
9. Munce S, Straus S, Fehlings M, et al. Impact of psychological characteristics in self-management in individuals with traumatic spinal cord injury. *Spinal Cord*. 2015;54(1):29–33. DOI: 101038sc91. PMID: 26055818.
10. Ronca E, Brunkert T, Koch HG, et al. Residential location of people with chronic spinal cord injury: the importance of local health care infrastructure. *BMC Health Serv Res*. 2018;18:657. https://doi.org/10.1186/s12913-018-3449-3.
11. Hamilton R, Driver S, Noorani S, et al. Utilization and access to healthcare services among community-dwelling people living with spinal cord injury. *J Spinal Cord Med*. 2017;40(3):321–328. https://doi.org/10.1080/10790268.2016.1184828. Epub 2016 May 25. PMID:27221396.
12. Barclay L, McDonald R, Lentin P, Bourke-Taylor H. Facilitators and barriers to social and community participation following spinal cord injury. *Aust Occup Ther J*. 2016;63(1):19–28. 10.1111/1440-1630.12241.
13. Kennedy P, Sherlock O, McClelland M, Short D, Royle J, Wilson C. A multi-center study of the community needs of people with spinal cord injuries: the first 18 months. *Spinal Cord*. 2010;48(1):15–20. https://doi.org/10.1038/sc.2009.65. Epub 2009 Jun 16. PMID:19528997.
14. Irgens I, Rekand T, Arora M, et al. Telehealth for people with spinal cord injury: a narrative review. *Spinal Cord*. 2018;56(7):643–655. https://doi.org/10.1038/s41393-017-0033-3. Epub 2018 Mar 7. PMID:29515211. 10.1038/s41393-017-0033-3.
15. Phillips VL, Vesmarovich S, Hauber R, Wiggers E, Egner A. Telehealth: reaching out to newly injured spinal cord patients. *Public Health Reports*. 2001;116(supp l):94–102.
16. Phillips VL, Temkin A, Vesmarovich S, et al. Using telehealth interventions to prevent pressure ulcers in newly injured spinal cord injury patients post-discharge. Results from a pilot study. *Int J Technol Assess Health Care*. 1999;15(4):749–755.
17. Smith MW, Hill ML, Hopkins KL, et al. A modeled analysis of telehealth methods for treating pressure ulcers after spinal cord injury. *Int J Telemed Appl*. 2012;2012:729492. https://doi.org/10.1155/2012/729492.
18. Yuen HK. Effect of a home telecare program on oral health among adults with tetraplegia: a pilot study. *Spinal Cord*. 2013;51(6):477–481. https://doi.org/10.1038/sc.2012.176. Epub 2013 Jan 15. PMID:23318557.
19. Beatty PW, Hagglund KJ, Neri MT, et al. Access to health care services among people with chronic or disabling conditions: patterns and predictors. *Arch Phys Med Rehabil*. 2003;84(10):1417–1425.
20. Woo C, Guihan M, Frick C, et al. What's happening now! Telehealth management of spinal cord injury/disorders. *J Spinal Cord Med*. 2011;34(3):322–331. https://DOI.org/10.1179/2045772311Y.0000000003.

21. Arora M, Harvey LA, Hayes AJ, et al. Effectiveness and cost-effectiveness of telephone-based support versus usual care for treatment of pressure ulcers in people with spinal cord injury in low-income and middle-income countries: study protocol for a 12-week randomized controlled trial. *BMJ Open.* 2015;5(7):e008369. https://DOI.org/10.1136/bmjopen-2015-008369.

22. Mackelprang JL, Hoffman JM, Garbaccio C, Bombardier CH. Outcomes and lessons learned from a randomized controlled trial to reduce health care utilization during the first year after spinal cord injury rehabilitation: telephone counseling versus usual care. *Arch Phys Med Rehabil.* 2016;97(10):1793–1796. https://doi.org/10.1016/j.apmr.2016.03.002. e1. Epub 2016 Mar 30.

23. Hill ML, Cronkite RC, Ota DT, et al. Validation of home telehealth for pressure ulcer assessment: a study in patients with spinal cord injury. *J Telemed Telecare.* 2009;15(4):196–202. https://DOI.org/10.1258/jtt.2009.081002.

24. Houlihan BV, Brody M, Everhart-Skeels S, et al. Randomized trial of a peer-led, telephone-based empowerment intervention for persons with chronic spinal cord injury improves health self-management. *Arch Phys Med Rehabil.* 2017;98(6):1067–1076. https://doi.org/10.1016/j.apmr.2017.02.005. e1. Epub 2017 Mar 8. PMID:28284835.

25. van de Pol E, Lucas K, Geraghty T, et al. The delivery of specialist spinal cord injury services in Queensland and the potential for telehealth. *BMC Health Services Research.* 2016;16:29. https://doi.org/10.1186/s12913-016-1256-2.

26. Martinez RN, Hogan TP, Balbale S, et al. Sociotechnical perspective on implementing clinical video telehealth for veterans with spinal cord injuries and disorders. *Telemed J E Health.* 2017;23(7):567–576. https://doi.org/10.1089/tmj.2016.0200.

27. Mea DV, Marin D, Rosin C, Zampa A. Web-based specialist support for spinal cord injury person's care: lessons learned. *Int J Telemed Appl.* 2012;2012:861860; https://doi.org/10.1155/2012/861860. Epub 2012 Aug 15.

28. Woo C, Seton JM, Washington M, et al. Increasing specialty care access through the use of an innovative home telehealth-based spinal cord injury disease management protocol (SCI DMP). *J Spinal Cord Med.* 2016;39(1):3–12. https://DOI.org/10.1179/2045772314Y.0000000202.

29. Lindsay JA, Day SC, Amspoker AB, et al. Personalized implementation of video telehealth. *Psychiatr Clin North Am.* 2019;42(4):563–574. https://doi.org/10.1016/j.psc.2019.08.001.

30. Lindsay JA, Hudson S, Martin L, et al. Implementing video to home to increase access to evidence-based psychotherapy for rural veterans. *J Technol Behav Sci.* 2017;2(3-4):140–148. https://doi.org/10.1007/s41347-017-0032-4.

31. Duplaga M. Digital divide among people with disabilities: analysis of data from a nationwide study for determinants of Internet use and activities performed online. *PLoS One.* 2017;12(6):e0179825. https://doi.org/10.1371/journal.pone.0179825. eCollection 2017.

32. Zulman DM, Wong EP, Slightam C, et al. Making connections: nationwide implementation of video telehealth tablets to address access barriers in veterans. *JAMIA Open.* 2019;2(3):323–329. https://doi.org/10.1093/jamiaopen/ooz024. eCollection 2019 Oct.

33. Vesmarovich S, Walker T, Hauber RP, Temkin A, Burns R. Use of telerehabilitation to manage pressure ulcers in persons with spinal cord injuries. *Advances Wound Care.* 1999;12(5):264–269.

34. Dallolio L, Menarini M, China S, et al. Functional and clinical outcomes of telemedicine in patients with spinal cord injury. *Arch Physical Med Rehabil.* 2008;89(12):2332–2341. https://DOI.org/10.1016/j.apmr.2008.06.012.

35. Kroenke K, Krebs EE, Wu J, et al. Telecare collaborative management of chronic pain in primary care: a randomized clinical trial. *JAMA.* 2014;312(3):240–248. https://DOI.org/10.1001/jama.2014.7689.

36. Mercier HW, Ni P, Houlihan BV, Jette AM. Differential impact and use of a telehealth intervention by persons with MS or SCI. *Am J Physical Med Rehabil.* 2015;94(11):987–999. https://DOI.org/10.1097/PHM.0000000000000291.

37. Van Straaten MG, Cloud BA, Morrow MM, et al. Effectiveness of home exercise on pain, function, and strength of manual wheelchair users with spinal cord injury: a high-dose shoulder program with telerehabilitation. *Arch Physical Med Rehabil.* 2014;95(10):1810–1817. e2. https://DOI.org/10.1016/j.apmr.2014.05.004.

38. Shem K, Sechrist SJ, Loomis E, Isaac L. SCiPad: effective implementation of telemedicine using iPads with individuals with spinal cord injuries, a case series. *Front Med.* 2017;4(58). https://DOI.org/10.3389/fmed.2017.00058.

39. Sechrist S, Lavoie S, Khong C-M, et al. Telemedicine using an iPad in the spinal cord injury population: a utility and patient satisfaction study. *Spinal Cord Ser Cases.* 2018;4(1):71. https://DOI.org/10.1038/s41394-018-0105-4.

40. Kirshblum S, Lin V. *Spinal Cord Medicine.* 3rd ed. New York: Springer Publication Co; 2019.

41. Kircher C, Kreitzer N, Adeoye O. Pre and intrahospital workflow for acute stroke treatment. *Curr Opin Neurol.* 2016;29(1):14–19. https://doi.org/10.1097/WCO.0000000000000281.

42. Irgens I, Bach B, Rekand T, Tornås S. Optimal management of health care for persons with disability related to spinal cord injury: learning from the Sunnaas model of telerehabilitation. *Spinal Cord Ser Cases.* 2020;6:88. https://doi.org/10.1038/s41394-020-00338-6.

43. American Spinal Injury Association. International Standards for Neurologic Classification of SCI. 2019.

44. Kirshblum S, Fichtenbaum J. Breaking the news in spinal cord injury. *J Spinal Cord Med.* 2008;31:7–12.

45. Tsai CY, Miller AS, Huang V, et al. The feasibility and usability of a mobile application for performing home evaluations. *Spinal Cord Ser Cases.* 2019;5:76. https://doi.org/10.1038/s41394-019-0219-3.

46. Khong C, Dirlikov B, Lavoie S, et al. SCiPad: patient satisfaction with telemedicine consultations in individuals with a spinal cord injury. *Topics Spinal Cord Inj.* 2019;25(supp 1):34.

47. Linsenmeyer TA. Urological management and renal disease in spinal cord injury. In: Kirshblum S, Lin VW, eds. *Spinal Cord Medicine.* 3rd ed. New York: Springer Publishing Co; 2019:332–356.

48. Wecht JM, Krassioukov AV, Alexander M, et al. International Standards to document Autonomic Function following SCI (ISAFSCI): Second Edition. *Top Spinal Cord Inj Rehabil.* 2021;27(2):23–49. doi:10.46292/sci2702-23

49. Sabharwal S. Cardiovascular dysfunction in spinal cord disorders. In: Kirshblum S, Lin VW, eds. *Spinal Cord Medicine.* 3rd ed. New York: Springer Publishing Co; 2019:212–229.

50. Hogaboom NS, Morse LR, Boninger ML. Overuse injuries and fractures in spinal cord injury. In: Kirshblum S, Lin VW, eds. *Spinal Cord Medicine.* 3rd ed. New York: Springer Publishing Co; 2019:457–471.

51. Verduzco-Gutierrez M, Romanoski NL, Capizzi AN, et al. Spasticity outpatient evaluation via telemedicine: a practical framework. *Am J Phys Med Rehabil.* 2020;90:1086–1091. https://doi.org/10.1097/PHM.0000000000001594.

52. Walker HW, Hon A, Hess MJ. Spasticity management. In: Kirshblum S, Lin VW, eds. *Spinal Cord Medicine.* 3rd ed. New York: Springer Publishing Co; 2019:472–486.

53. Lazo MG, Shirazi P, Sam M, et al. Osteoporosis and risk of fracture in men with spinal cord injury. *Spinal Cord.* 2001;39(4):208–214.

54. Tyagi N, Amar Goel S, Alexander M. Improving quality of life after spinal cord injury in India with telehealth. *Spinal Cord Ser Cases.* 2019;5:70. https://doi.org/10.1038/s41394-019-0212-x.

55. Keyser RE, Rasch EK, Finley M, Rodgers MM. Improved upper-body endurance following a 12-week home exercise program for manual wheelchair users. *J Rehabil Res Dev.* 2003;40(6):501–510. https://doi.org/10.1682/jrrd.2003.11.0501.

56. Latimer AE, Ginis KAM, Arbour KP. The efficacy of an implementation intention intervention for promoting physical activity among individuals with spinal cord injury: a randomized controlled trial. *Rehabil Psychol.* 2006;51(4):273–280. https://DOI.org/10.1037/0090-5550.51.4.273.

57. Coulter EH, McLean AN, Hasler JP, et al. The effectiveness and satisfaction of web-based physiotherapy in people with spinal cord injury: a pilot randomized controlled trial. *Spinal Cord.* 2017;55(4):383–389.

58. Selassie A, Snipe L, Focht KL, et al. Baseline prevalence of heart diseases, hypertension, diabetes, and obesity in persons with acute traumatic spinal cord injury: potential threats in the recovery trajectory. *Top Spinal Cord Inj Rehabil.* 2013;19(3):172–182. https://doi.org/10.1310/sci1903-172. PMID:23960701.

59. Groah SL, Nash MS, Ljungberg IH, et al. Nutrient intake and body habitus after spinal cord injury: an analysis by sex and level of injury. *J Spinal Cord Med.* 2009;32(1):25–33. https://DOI.org/10.1080/10790268.2009.11760749.

60. Locatelli S, Gerber B, Goldstein B, et al. Health care provider practices, barriers, and facilitators for weight management for individuals with spinal cord injuries and disorders. *Top Spinal Cord Inj Rehabil.* 2014;20(4):329–337. https://DOI.org/10.1310/sci2004-329.

61. Myers J, Gopalan R, Shahoumian T, Kiratli J. Effects of customized risk reduction program on cardiovascular risk in males with spinal cord injury. *J Rehabil Research Development.* 2012;49(9):1355. https://DOI.org/10.1682/JRRD.2011.11.0215.

62. Wood S, Khong CM, Dirlikov B, Shem K. Nutrition counseling and monitoring via tele-nutrition for healthy diet for people with spinal cord injury: a case series analyses. [Accepted for publication in *J Spinal Cord Med*].

63. January AM, Zebracki K, Chlan KM, Vogel LC. Mental health and the risk of secondary medical complications in adults with pediatric-onset spinal cord injury. *Top Spinal Cord Inj Rehabil*. 2014; 20(1):1–12. https://doi.org/10.1310/sci2001-1. PMID: 24574817.

64. Arango-Lasprilla JC, Ketchum JM, Starkweather A, et al. Factors predicting depression among persons with spinal cord injury 1 to 5 years post-injury. *NeuroRehabil*. 2010;29(1):9–21. http://DOI.org/10.3233/NRE-2011-0672.

65. Martz E, Livneh H, Priebe M, Wuermser LA, Ottomanelli L. Predictors of psychosocial adaptation among people with spinal cord injury or disorder. *Arch Phys Med Rehabil*. 2005;86(6):1182–1192.

66. Ullrich PM, Smith BM, Blow FC, et al. Depression, healthcare utilization, and comorbid psychiatric disorders after spinal cord injury. *J Spinal Cord Med*. 2014;37(1):40–45.

67. Williams R, Murray A. Prevalence of depression after spinal cord injury: a meta-analysis. *Arch Phys Med Rehabil*. 2015;96(1):133–140.

68. Butler A, Chapman J, Forman E, Beck A. The empirical status of cognitive-behavioral therapy: a review of meta-analyses. *Clinical Psychology Review*. 2006;26(1):17–31. https://DOI.org/10.1016/j.cpr.2005.07.003.

69. Mehta S, Orenczuk S, Hansen KT, et al. An evidence-based review of the effectiveness of cognitive-behavioral therapy for psychosocial issues post-spinal cord injury. *Rehabil Psychol*. 2011;56(1):15–25.

70. Dorstyn D, Mathias J, Denson L. Applications of telecounselling in spinal cord injury rehabilitation: a systematic review with effect sizes. *Clin Rehabil*. 2013;27(12):1072–1083. https://DOI.org/10.1177/0269215513488001.

71. Mozer E, Franklin B, Rose J. Psychotherapeutic intervention by telephone. *Clin Interventions Aging*. 2008;3(2):391–396.

72. Krause JS, Kemp B, Coker J. Depression after spinal cord injury: relation to gender ethnicity, aging and socioeconomic indicators. *Arch Physical Med Rehabil*. 2000;81(8):1099–1109.

73. Taylor K, Silver L. *Smartphone Ownership Is Growing Rapidly Around the World, but Not Always Equally*. Pew Research Center; 2019. https://www.pewresearch.org/global/2019/02/05/smartphone-ownership-is-growing-rapidly-around-the-world-but-not-always-equally/.

74. Kryger MA, Crytzer TM, Fairman A, et al. The effect of the interactive mobile health and rehabilitation system on health and psychosocial outcomes in spinal cord injury: randomized controlled trial. *J Med Internet Res*. 2019;21(8):e14305. https://doi.org/10.2196/14305.

75. Øra HP, Kirmess M, Brady MC, Sørli H, Becker F. Technical features, feasibility, and acceptability of augmented telerehabilitation in poststroke aphasia - experiences from a randomized controlled trial. *Frontiers Neurol*. 2020;11:671. https://doi.org/10.3389/fneur.2020.00671.

76. Øra HP, Kirmess M, Brady MC, Becker F. The effect of augmented speech-language therapy delivered by telerehabilitation on poststroke aphasia - a pilot randomized controlled trial. *Clinical Rehabil*. 2020;34(3):369–381. https://doi.org/10.1177/0269215519896616.

CHAPTER 4

Telerehabilitation in Stroke

Kate Laver ■ Kate Osborne

Introduction

Stroke is defined as an acute episode of focal dysfunction of the brain, retina, or spinal cord which lasts for more than 24 hours or where imaging (computed tomography [CT] or magnetic resonance imaging [MRI]) displays a focal infarction or hemorrhage consistent with the symptoms.[1] This is in contrast to a transient ischemic attack (TIA) where the dysfunction is present for less than 24 hours and there is no evidence of infarction upon imaging.[1] Data show that the incidence rate of stroke is relatively stable over time; this has been attributed to better prevention and management of stroke in higher income countries.[2] However, the prevalence of stroke is increasing and is mostly related to the aging of the world's population.[2] Some studies suggest that the incidence of stroke is higher in rural and remote areas.[3] This must be addressed by policy makers as inequities arise when people in rural and remote areas have poorer access to specialized stroke care and rehabilitation.

Stroke is a leading cause of disability in developed countries.[4] People with stroke may experience a range of symptoms including hemiplegia (weakness on one side of the body), numbness, changes in vision, and changes in speech.[5] These symptoms result in difficulty managing everyday activities and impact the person's abilities to fulfill their life roles. While stroke commonly affects older people (aged 65 or more), approximately 25% of people who experience a stroke are of working age[6] and likely to be involved in paid or volunteer work. Not all of these people will return to work, with research reporting a range of different outcomes varying from 19% to 73% return to work.[7]

Over the last 20 years, there have been improvements in acute therapies and treatments for stroke.[8] However, most people still experience symptoms that may last for weeks, months, or for the rest of their lives.[9] Rehabilitation addresses impairment, activities, and participation with the overarching goal of maximizing quality of life.[10] It should involve goal setting to identify relevant goals of therapy and individualized care to assist the person to achieve their goals with the support of a multidisciplinary team.[11] Rehabilitation programs are resource intensive as they involve a number of different health professionals often providing individualized (1:1) therapy. Where resources are scarce[12] not all people who would benefit from rehabilitation are able to access such programs, with data suggesting that access to inpatient rehabilitation ranges between 13% and 57%.[12] Inequities in access exist internationally and may be influenced by the severity of the stroke, predicted discharge destination, cognitive impairment, and whether the person lives in a regional or remote area.

Rehabilitation therapies aim to both maximize function in areas of the brain (on the basis of neuroplasticity theories) and use compensatory approaches to maximize independence despite deficits.[9] Research suggests that recovery is dose dependent[13] and clinicians are encouraged to offer services that provide ample opportunity for practice. This remains a challenge in clinical practice and studies suggest that people in rehabilitation spend much of the day inactive and alone.[14] Providing self-directed or home-based exercise programs is often recommended; however, a number of barriers to self-directed exercise programs exist.[15]

Organization of stroke care and health services varies by country. In most Western countries, people are initially admitted to an acute stroke unit. Pathways from acute care may include home (with or without follow-up rehabilitation services), inpatient rehabilitation, or a long-term care facility. People with stroke have reported that transitions in care (e.g., hospital to home) can be difficult and that they feel abandoned and unsupported when they are discharged home.[16] People have also reported that there are gaps in the rehabilitation offered after formal services cease. Of those that survive the stroke and are alive 1 year following stroke (62%), most (80%) remain impaired and require help from informal carers (family) or professional carers.[17]

Telerehabilitation Models for Stroke

Telerehabilitation may be used to aid in assessment, rehabilitation, and support following discharge from an acute hospital or inpatient rehabilitation service. It is commonly used around the times of transition to provide support and rehabilitation in the home upon discharge. It may also be used as a way of offering rehabilitation services to who are people in the chronic phase after stroke yet still have stroke-related symptoms and ongoing rehabilitation goals. Important trials are presented in Table 4.1.

TABLE 4.1 ■ **Key Trials Conducted in Telerehabilitation for People After Stroke**

Study, Country	N	Intervention	Comparison	Findings
Cramer et al. (2019)[18] **United States**	124	Telerehabilitation program that was designed to improve upper limb function and utilized on-screen games	Clinic-based therapy (matched dose)	Therapy participation resulted in improved arm function in both those who received home-based telerehabilitation and those who received clinic-based rehabilitation. Telerehabilitation was not inferior to in-person rehabilitation.
Hassett[19] **Australia**	300	The intervention group used technological devices to address mobility and physical activity goals, individually prescribed by a physiotherapist. Devices included virtual reality video games, activity monitors, and handheld computer devices for 6 months in hospital and at home.	Usual care	People who received the intervention had improved mobility at 6 months. Note that this study included people with stroke as well as other conditions requiring rehabilitation.
Boter (2004)[20] **Netherlands**	536	Case management after discharge from hospital: three telephone calls and a home visit over a duration of up to 24 weeks	Usual care	No significant difference between groups except for one item on the SF36 measure of quality of life

Continued

TABLE 4.1 ▪ **Key Trials Conducted in Telerehabilitation for People After Stroke—Cont'd**

Study, Country	N	Intervention	Comparison	Findings
Mayo et al. (2008)[21] **Canada**	190	Case management: home visits and phone calls for 6 weeks after discharge from hospital	Usual care	No significant differences between groups
Rochette et al. (2013)[22] **Canada**	186	Phone calls to discuss family functioning and risk factors after discharge from hospital (WE CALL)	Phone number provided and patient asked to call if they had any queries (YOU CALL)	Both groups improved over time; however, people in the WE CALL group reported high satisfaction with the intervention, whereas those in the YOU CALL group rarely made contact.
Meltzer et al. (2018)[23] **Canada**	53	Aphasia therapy provided via telerehabilitation	Aphasia therapy provided in person	Both groups showed beneficial effects of training and the difference between telerehabilitation and in person was not significantly different with the exception of one measure, the confidence rating scale for aphasia where the in-person group reported higher scores.
Lloréns et al. (2015)[24] **Spain**	31	Virtual reality system used within the home which aims to improve balance. Includes remote monitoring and phone call checks	Virtual reality system used within the clinic	No significant difference between groups in terms of patient outcomes
Lawson et al. (2020)[25] **Australia**	46	Modified version of the Monash Memory Skills Group delivered via videoconferencing	Same program delivered in the home or clinic	Participants in both groups had improvements in goal attainment and key subjective outcomes of everyday memory and prospective memory.
Van Den Berg et al. (2016)[26] **Australia**	63	Caregiver-mediated training program with support via telehealth, a tablet, and exercise applications	Usual care	Patients who received telerehabilitation had higher scores on a measure of instrumental activities of daily living, fewer readmissions, and caregivers reported higher levels of self-efficacy.

Telerehabilitation services for stroke to date can be categorized around the following key themes.

ASSESSMENT

Researchers and therapists have shown interest in developing new techniques or methods to remotely assess people after stroke. For example, the eHAB program involves a suite of measurement tools including goniometers to measure range of movement.[27] A variety of home monitoring systems also exist and may monitor health status, including blood pressure, heart rate, blood sugar, and mood (through patient-completed surveys). Researchers and clinicians are also interested in whether existing assessment tools or outcome measures can be administered using telerehabilitation communications. For example, the Chedoke-McMaster Stroke Assessment Activity Inventory is one tool that is used in stroke rehabilitation settings which has been adapted for telephone administration.[28]

DELIVERY OF TRADITIONAL MODELS OF REHABILITATION IN THE HOME ENVIRONMENT

Several studies have examined how traditional rehabilitation services could be delivered using information and communication technologies.[29,30] In these studies, therapists undertake the traditional rehabilitation process (goal setting and therapy interventions) but use simple video-conferencing techniques as the medium rather than being in the clinic or the person's home. Telerehabilitation is desirable as an alternative to clinic- or home-based rehabilitation as it may be more cost-effective (reduces travel time) and can be offered to people who live great distances from rehabilitation services (so more accessible). Forducey and colleagues reported that a telerehabilitation program involving 12 treatment sessions with a physiotherapist and occupational therapist was as effective as when delivered in person.[29] This study was conducted several years ago and involved use of a desktop videophone. Results showed that there was no significant difference between groups on key functional outcomes, suggesting that telerehabilitation was as effective as in-person rehabilitation.

TRIALING INNOVATIVE MODELS OF CARE

Coaching

Changing the mode of service delivery provides an opportunity to also change the model of service delivery. It has been suggested that telehealth provides an opportunity to think about what should be done rather than what is currently done in practice. As people who receive telerehabilitation services are typically living in their own home, there is an opportunity to focus on rehabilitation goals and activities that are more relevant and contextually appropriate. It is also an opportunity to use approaches that empower the person after stroke to take control of their recovery and rehabilitation.

A telerehabilitation initiative in Canada introduced and evaluated several different models of telerehabilitation. In one study a Stroke Coach program was evaluated. The Stroke Coach program was designed to meet key principles, including being patient centered, highly accessible, timely, and community based.[31] The telephone was chosen as the preferred mode of intervention delivery based on statistics that showed that telephones were one of the most widely used technologies in that population and that people were interested in receiving health education via the phone. The program commenced with two phone calls in the first month after discharge and then monthly calls for 6 months. The program included lifestyle coaching, stroke self-management, and self-monitoring and was offered over seven phone consultations and five follow-up calls. People who received the intervention reported that it was helpful in overcoming low mood, encouraging them to be more physically active, and making better diet choices.[31]

Use of Avatars to Promote Engagement

Clinical practice does not necessarily adjust to the speed of changes in technology. People are still discharged home after stroke with paper-based educational leaflets or written home exercise programs. Avatar technology is being trialed as a more innovative method of educating people about their condition and healthy behaviors.[32] Some work has been done to develop mHealth applications that utilize avatars to encourage patients to remain engaged in rehabilitation activities after stroke. Aljaroodi and colleagues described a process of co-design in which they set out to design the "Regain" app that was able to communicate in a way that promoted engagement, selected appropriate rehabilitation activities, and contained features that nudged the user to complete the prescribed activities.[33] The research group designed a program that involved self-avatars (avatars that visually resembled the user); however, the program has not yet been evaluated. There is great potential to develop this area of stroke rehabilitation; however, significant evaluation will be necessary and the issue of human versus avatar interaction should be considered.

Transition Support to Improve Mood and Quality of Life

Depression is common after stroke, with approximately 25% of people experiencing depression within 2 years of having a stroke.[34] Clinical guidelines recommend that people who appear to have changes in their mood after stroke should be assessed and that antidepressants, psychological therapies, and exercise should be considered as part of intervention.[35] Services have been trialed to support people after discharge with the aim of improving mood and supporting the transition home. Kirkness et al. showed that a brief psychosocial intervention (the Living Well with Stroke program) could be delivered effectively over the phone and that people who received the intervention reported fewer depressive symptoms over time.[36] It should be noted that while several telerehabilitation interventions have tested transitional support, few have reported positive outcomes. Our metaanalysis containing six randomized trials with 1146 participants showed that telerehabilitation services to support the person upon transition home were not more effective than usual care in altering depressive symptoms.[37] Researchers should also consider whether alternative approaches or more intense support is required to show a beneficial effect.

Promoting Stroke Recovery at Scale

The incidence of stroke in developing countries has increased over time. The consequences of stroke are long term and often significant levels of disability mean that low- and middle-income countries are unable to offer widespread and accessible rehabilitation programs. Research is underway to trial whether information and communication technologies can be used to aid recovery and rehabilitation efforts in low- and middle-income countries as a way of offering services at low cost to a large group of stroke survivors. For example, a smartphone-enabled, carer-supported educational intervention for stroke survivors is currently being tested in India.[38] Even in countries that are considered high income, the concept of improving care outcomes for a large group of stroke survivors using low-cost approaches is appealing. In the iVERVE trial, researchers are testing whether personalized electronic self-management support (sent via personalized text messages or emails) can better support the person to achieve their goals.[39] Outcomes of this study are not yet known.

Incorporating Family and Caregiver Support

Upon discharge from hospital or inpatient rehabilitation, the patient's family will ultimately become more involved in care (and may experience increased carer burden). Family may also be involved in encouraging and supporting the person to complete their rehabilitation therapies. Caregiver-mediated training (in which the patient and carer are educated about which activities are appropriate and the carer supports and supervises the person to perform their rehabilitation with e-health support) has been identified as a promising way of augmenting therapy with beneficial outcomes for the stroke survivor.[26] The CARE4STROKE intervention consists of an 8-week program, executed with a caregiver, and use of an e-health application that presents prescribed and tailored exercise programs. Between sessions, the person and caregiver are encouraged to make contact with the therapist via the phone, videoconferencing, or email. Trials of the CARE4STROKE intervention have had mixed results. A trial involving 63 stroke survivors in Australia found that those who received CARE4STROKE had improved extended activities of daily living (ADL) and fewer readmissions over 12 months,[26] whereas a trial involving 66 people after stroke in the Netherlands did not find that those involved in the intervention had significantly better outcomes on mobility or function compared with those in the usual care group.[40]

Using Combinations of Innovative Technologies Including Gaming and Wearable Sensors

Various telerehabilitation applications have incorporated virtual reality programs to increase the level of innovation for people participating in home-based rehabilitation programs. These telerehabilitation programs assume that the person with stroke will enjoy using the virtual reality program and therefore be more likely to participate in home-based therapy. While there is some research that suggests that virtual reality can be enjoyable, this may not always be the case and may not apply to all individuals. The therapist can monitor the person's performance and how much time they spend in the program from a distance. The AMOUNT trial used a pragmatic approach and tested whether the tailored prescription of affordable digital technologies results in better outcomes for people admitted to aged care and neurological rehabilitation units.[19] They used a suite of devices including commercial exergaming applications, activity monitors, and specialized rehabilitation programs and commenced intervention in the hospital and continued upon discharge home with remote support from trial staff.

Practice

In practice, the key principles of telerehabilitation remain.

USE OF TELEREHABILITATION FOR INITIAL CONSULTATION PURPOSES

Initial consultations in rehabilitation include multidisciplinary assessment and goal setting, all of which can take place using telerehabilitation technologies.

Swallowing, Speech, and Communication Assessment

Clinical swallowing examinations can be conducted remotely using telehealth. A study in Australia used a trained assistant who assisted the client.[41] The speech pathologist was able to remotely screen for dysphagia risk and review client progress; however, having the correct software and hardware was important (including good lighting, free standing speakers, lapel microphones, and web cameras). A separate study involved the Teleswallowing approach that was developed in the United Kingdom and also uses a trained assistant who assists the person being assessed. This person could be a nurse, care worker, or therapy assistant.[42] A number of studies have demonstrated that assessment of aphasia can successfully be conducted remotely.[43] Furthermore, studies that compared remote versus in-person assessment reported that there were no significant differences between the results obtained in each setting.[44]

Physical Assessment

Uptake of mobility and balance assessments conducted via telehealth appears variable, with clinicians possibly reluctant to do this because assessment can be "hands on" and may present risk of falls. Many specialist mobility and gait assessment clinics have used trained assistants to be present with the client to help and ensure safety.[45] However, this may not always be required and studies have shown that in other health conditions it is possible to conduct a remote assessment of lower limb function and mobility where the patient can safely follow instructions.[46] Multiple specific assessment tools have been tested via remote administration including the Tinetti Performance-Oriented Mobility Assessment, Six Meter Walk Test, Timed Up and Go, Sit to Stand, and Forward Reach Test.[47] Venkataraman and colleagues used standard videoconferencing equipment (desktop computers) and showed that teleassessment of mobility (assessed using the Tinetti Assessment) was feasible, valid, and reliable.[47] It is also possible that a carer or family member could assist the person where they are able to do so and the person is at risk of falls or that the environment could be structured for safety (e.g., exercises while standing at the kitchen bench). As previously mentioned, the eHAB system includes features such as a goniometer that may assist with remote assessment of physical function.

Upper Limb and Hand Assessment

Worboys and colleagues compared telehealth hand function assessment (using standard videoconferencing equipment) with traditional clinical model assessment and found that agreement between the two methods of assessment was high and that clinical decisions made using telehealth were comparable to those made in traditional clinic settings.[48]

Home Assessment

Home assessments conducted by occupational therapists can be time-consuming, require a vehicle, and may involve extensive travel. In a review of the use of information and communication technology within occupational therapy home assessments, we found that therapists are both developing new technologies to facilitate assessments and using simple and accessible equipment to conduct home assessments.[49] Studies to date have shown feasibility of assessing the home remotely. However, traditional in-home assessment appears to be more sensitive in identifying hazards. Whether or not this makes a difference to patient outcomes is unknown. Implementation of this approach in practice has been shown to lead to increased capacity of occupational therapists to conduct home assessments for more people.

USE OF TELEREHABILITATION IN DISEASE MANAGEMENT, SECONDARY STROKE PREVENTION, AND SELF-MANAGEMENT PROGRAMS

There are a few examples of applications being used to promote healthy lifestyle, reduce risk of subsequent stroke, and assist with self-management; however, they have reported limited success to date and are therefore not in a position to be widely implemented yet. Adie and James evaluated whether four telephone calls (over 4 months) could help with risk factor management and resulted in changes in blood pressure, statin use, and cholesterol. The intervention was based on social cognitive theory and used a motivational interviewing approach; however, they found no difference in outcomes between groups at 6 months.[50] Gillham and Endacott similarly found that secondary prevention support delivered in part via the telephone did not significantly alter the person's readiness to change behavior after TIA or minor stroke.[51] Chronic disease self-management programs have not been rigorously tested in people with stroke via telerehabilitation although studies to date suggest that this is possible, can feasibly include group activities, and may have positive outcomes on self-efficacy and lifestyle in people after stroke.[52-54]

USE OF TELEREHABILITATION FOR THERAPY PURPOSES

Rehabilitation therapies including physiotherapy, occupational therapy, cognitive and communication therapies, and psychosocial interventions have all been tested through telerehabilitation and in randomized controlled trials. In most cases, the usual therapeutic approach is simply adapted by the therapist for remote delivery. This involves a less hands-on approach and structuring the environment and communication methods to develop rapport. Therapies may involve screen sharing or sending and receiving information to complete some therapy tasks. Only in some cases does the intervention involve more sophisticated technologies such as virtual reality.

When Compared With In-Person Rehabilitation

Metaanalyses of randomized trials show that to date there have been no significant differences in outcomes between groups where one group received telerehabilitation therapy and the other group received in-person therapy.[37] This applies for outcomes of independence in ADL, balance, and upper limb function. However, the grade of evidence is considered low as there are few studies, and the studies that do exist feature some characteristics that place them at risk of bias. Overall, the implication for practice is that telerehabilitation can be used in place of in-person therapy in cases where this seems feasible. This assumes that the person can use the technology (or has someone who can help) and the intervention can be delivered remotely without placing the person at risk of harm (e.g., falls).

When Compared With Usual Care

The evidence for using telerehabilitation as an additional therapy to improve the quality of care is less positive.[37] Metaanalyses have shown that the addition of a telerehabilitation to usual care has not resulted in improved ADL function or upper limb function and has not reduced depressive symptoms or improved quality of life. The grade of evidence for these outcomes is also low to moderate as there are few studies and those studies that do exist are at risk of bias. The implication for practice is that considerable thought should be given before health service managers develop and implement new telerehabilitation programs as an add-on service with the goal of improving care. As there are few studies it is important to conduct more research in the area as it is quite possible that the mode of therapy (e.g., telephone rather than videoconference) and low dose of therapy could play a strong role in the failure of these studies to date.

Special Considerations

Some extra telerehabilitation considerations are required for stroke survivors as they are usually older, may be less technologically literate, may have visual impairment, and may have cognitive or communication impairments.

For clients with communication issues, including people with aphasia, it may be useful to have supported conversation tools on hand (i.e., maps, rating scales, pictures). Consider sending materials in advance so that the person has them with them. Stick with simple technology and ensure rapport through chatting informally at the start. Be aware of what is required to help the person understand and use gesturing, written key words, and diagrams. Monitor the speed of your own speech and allow time for processing. Consider fatigue levels and minimize background noise which will make the person work harder.

For clients with cognitive issues, it is important to minimize distractions. Check in regularly to monitor fatigue and seek support from family members when required. Take advantage of the person being in their own environment and the ability to perform contextually relevant activities. Use notes or a follow-up email to reiterate key information shared.

For clients with visual issues, it is important to determine whether they can see you and you can see all of them, as visual field deficits and neglect can be a barrier to communication. Ensure that the lighting is appropriate for the client and there is no background clutter.

When the client needs "hands-on" help, check whether there is a carer or helper who can be present. Can the person be instructed in using their own hands to test or guide? Can the environment be set up to support the person (e.g., standing at a bench for balance support)?

Control and scheduling. Multidisciplinary rehabilitation programs often involve multiple therapy sessions per day. Patient-centered care models place the person (and possibly their family) centrally in planning therapy and working in collaboration. Therapists and physicians must consider that telerehabilitation sessions should be properly scheduled in advance as if the professional was planning to visit the person in their own home. This ensures that both the professional and the patient are properly prepared and the person with stroke can have control over their day and fit in other important roles such as spending time with friends or leisure activities. Some telerehabilitation programs include features to assist with scheduling although this is not common. For example, the program may contain a calendar that shares the person's availability for treatment sessions, displays when they are seeing other health professionals, enables the clinician to book the appointment, and provides the person with reminders. A review of features of telerehabilitation devices found that only approximately one-third of devices contained this feature.[55] Morris tested a scheduling app (Anna Cares) within a clinical service.[25] An avatar (named Anna) communicates with the person about their schedule and provides reminders about who is providing therapy and for what purpose (e.g., speech therapy). Evaluation found that while therapists could see the benefit of the app for patients, there were challenges in using the app particularly when their work schedule was unpredictable, or they needed to frequently cancel and reschedule. They also felt that benefits were most apparent when the whole team and patient were using the app and in that case, it could be quite effective.

A summary of important considerations when establishing telerehabilitation is presented in Box 4.1.

BOX 4.1 ■ Top Tips for Setting Up

Top Tips for Setting Up a Telerehabilitation Session for Someone With Stroke

1. Book the session (including rooms and technology) ensuring clinician/s and consumer/s all have the required equipment and resources they need to successfully complete the aims for the specific session. Be clear about the best location for the session to ensure safety and quality of outcomes.
2. Prepare the consumer by ensuring they have consented to a telehealth consult and are aware they can stop at any point.
3. Prepare for the clinical session by ensuring you have all documentation and tools easily accessible (having a dual screen at the clinician end allows you to have documents ready to share easily).
4. Ensure you have a back-up plan if technology fails. Is there a helpline or local support person who can help troubleshoot? Will you revert to telephone or reschedule if unable to resolve?
5. At the beginning of the session ensure all present are introduced including anyone off-screen who may be able to see or hear the session.
6. Depending on the rehabilitation goals you may spend considerable time interacting with, teaching, and encouraging carers, so be prepared to take on a coaching role.
7. Telehealth is a modality and offers a way to effectively connect with consumers remotely. Utilize your existing expertise, problem solving, and skill set in partnership with others in the call to meet the goals.
8. Documentation should include that the session was undertaken via telehealth and any extra considerations that were made to accommodate the modality.

IMPLEMENTATION: LESSONS LEARNT FOLLOWING IMPLEMENTATION OF A TELEREHABILITATION SERVICE IN A STATE HEALTH SERVICE

Telerehabilitation commenced in South Australian (SA) Health in 2013 in partnership with Flinders University and Commonwealth research grant funding. Initial research demonstrated the feasibility of using off-the-shelf equipment to provide rehabilitation via telehealth. Following this, a significant financial investment was made across the system to embed telerehabilitation into all public adult rehabilitation services in SA, with 15 new positions created to support effective implementation and ongoing service delivery. Statewide clinical leads in Allied Health and Nursing and a Statewide program manager were established to support the local support teams with information and communication technology, nursing and administration staff who were employed in the Local Health Networks and provide "at-the-elbow" support for clinical teams. A large investment was also made in regard to hardware and software. Over time the SA Health telerehabilitation loan iPad fleet has grown to include 500 devices and consumers and clinicians have access to more than 200 applications that can be tailored (and managed remotely) to target individual consumer goals.

Telerehabilitation has become an expected part of a consumer's rehabilitation journey and many anticipated barriers were overcome. Consumer survey feedback data obtained by SA Health indicates that more than 80% of consumers participating in telerehabilitation agree or strongly agree that they have received the same standard of care from telerehabilitation as from in-person care and would be willing to participate in telerehabilitation in the future.

Embedding sociotechnical changes in complex health systems is an adaptive challenge and team cultures, individual mindsets, and behaviors need to be considered.

- *Provide flexible training and development approaches and assist teams to modify processes and procedures to embed the telehealth modality into existing and new care pathways.*
- *Co-design with individual teams and professions to discuss their "wicked challenges" and problem solve where technology can help address these challenges.*
- *Keep the technology as easy to use as possible and monitor and address technical challenges in real time. The "at-the-elbow" support model means that there are staff trained to assist with problem-solving connection issues and providing support to both clinicians and consumers.*
- *Match the technology to the session requirements. Simple videoconferencing equipment may be all that is required for a "check-up" consultation and review, whereas a speech or cognition therapy session may require two separate devices at the consumer end and peripherals such as a document camera at the clinician end.*
- *Consider consumer empowerment and trust in others to assist in completing what the clinician historically would have done themselves.*

The following strategies can improve clinician confidence when using telehealth:

- *Provide technical training and a chance to practice using the technology with peers before the first patient experience. Supplement training with "how to" guides, troubleshooting resources, and mock videos of telerehabilitation in practice.*
- *Establish clinical simulations with mock patients so that clinicians can practice the "clinical translation" elements of telehealth, as well as use of the technology.*
- *Provide case studies for staff using telehealth to share their successes and challenges. These can then be recorded and uploaded for staff to review at a later date and can be used for orientation and confidence building with new staff.*
- *Aim to make a clinician's first sessions successful as this assists with engagement and sustainability.*
- *Foster belief in telehealth. Confident clinicians who believe in this modality can adapt their experience into the telehealth environment and engage their consumers in shared problem solving to meet session goals.*

- *Reassure staff about patient confidentiality. Some staff may need additional conversations about consumer empowerment and consent to assist confidence building in the modality.*
- *Tailor education to individual learning styles. Clinicians are individuals and will have their own individual learning styles and innate confidence in technology.*
- *Do not be concerned about age being a barrier. Consumers of any age (and technological literacy/ experience) can participate with the right instructions and support framework and many older community members are quite chuffed that they achieve telehealth.*
- *Remember to keep the technology as simple as possible!*

Now that the SA Health telerehabilitation service has successfully integrated stroke telereha-bilitation services into the health service we are looking at how we may continue to improve our service. Our future vision is to:

- *Start looking at integrating home monitoring equipment for earlier supported discharge after stroke. This approach is currently used successfully in chronic disease management but there is limited evidence to date on acute hospital substitution.*
- *Explore the potential of new applications for stroke rehabilitation as they become available. We are interested in applications where avatars provide coaching to help people achieve their goals. We are also interested in programs that further empower the consumer to direct their therapy, for example, the consumer is able to communicate their goals and the app is able to respond with suggested thera-peutic activities that may help achieve these goals.*

Recommendations

RECOMMENDATIONS FOR PRACTICE

Evidence suggests that where appropriate (i.e., the person is able to use the technology and there is no concern about communication or adverse events), telerehabilitation services for stroke may be used instead of in-person rehabilitation. The present evidence does not suggest that telere-habilitation improves the quality of care as compared to face-to-face care. Several studies have shown that some services, particularly those that involve a few phone calls to support the person's mood at the time of transition from hospital to home, do not seem beneficial.

RECOMMENDATIONS FOR RESEARCH

Although one of the key advantages of telerehabilitation for health services is reduced cost and travel time, few studies have tested cost-effectiveness in stroke populations. Randomized con-trolled trials in this area should routinely collect data relating to the costs of care for each group. In some situations the cost may not be less for telerehabilitation where expensive technologies are purchased and therapy assistants are required to be with the person at their home to provide hands-on assistance.

While there is an increasing volume of research, there are still relatively few randomized trials in the field. As such, the grade of evidence is low to moderate in most cases, meaning that further research is likely to have an important impact on our confidence in the estimate of effect and is likely to change the estimate. More research is required to test different approaches (including physical communication and cognitive and psychosocial intervention) and to look at how increased dose can be achieved. Approaches that empower the person and use techniques such as coaching and motivational interviewing to achieve significant behavior change are also likely to be beneficial.

CASE STUDY

Mr. Evan Dragon is a 72-year-old farmer who lives 800 km away from Adelaide (the nearest capital city). While sitting in the garden one morning, his wife Glenda noticed sudden changes to his speech and movement. The SA telestroke service provides 24/7 neurologist consultant support via videoconferencing with all country hospital emergency departments. The Royal Flying Doctor Service was able to transport Evan to his closest rural hospital, where he underwent a CT scan. A clot was located that was able to be treated locally with tenecteplase.

Evan stayed in the rural hospital for 2 weeks as an inpatient, where the rehabilitation team introduced him (and his wife Glenda) to the idea of telerehabilitation for his return home. He was loaned a tablet device (iPad) that was used to track his physical exercise program during his inpatient stay. He was provided with applications that could be used for self-directed therapy, especially on the weekends when the rehabilitation team was minimally staffed. Evan and Glenda were very glad that the tablet device had been set up by the therapists to make it easy to access and understand as they did not have a lot of previous experience with technology.

Prior to discharge from hospital Glenda took the iPad home and was able to video call the occupational therapist and walk around the home to discuss what physical changes were needed for Evan to return home safely. A decision was made by Glenda and the occupational therapist that a ramp at the front door and some rails through the house would assist Evan and luckily Glenda knew a local tradesperson who was able to assist with this quickly.

On discharge from hospital, Evan's goals included walking increased distances, continued improvement in upper limb function, improved clarity of speech, and return to driving. Evan was able to use his loaned iPad to connect via video with members of the multidisciplinary team for therapy 3 days per week for the next 8 weeks with improvements noted in all areas. Physiotherapy and occupational therapy were mainly undertaken in the kitchen where there was plenty of bench space to use for support while Evan went through his exercises. A range of household objects such as tins of food were used as weights and Evan's daily step count was monitored using a wrist-based activity monitoring device (Fitbit) that had also been provided on discharge from hospital. Speech pathology and discussions with the rehabilitation specialist were either undertaken at the dining table or in the lounge.

Evan was hoping to return to driving. In order to access the "fitness-to-drive" assessment, Evan and Glenda returned to the rural hospital that was a 600-km round trip rather than the 1600-km trip that would have been required if they needed to get to Adelaide. The rehabilitation nurse undertook a range of assessments and then linked via video with the rehabilitation specialist based in Adelaide.

Six months after Evan's stroke he and Glenda used their son's iPad to link with the rehabilitation specialist to discuss how Evan was doing and whether there were any further therapy goals that could require another program of telerehabilitation.

References

1. Sacco LR, Kasner ES, Broderick PJ, et al. An updated definition of stroke for the 21st century: a statement for healthcare professionals from the American Heart Association/American Stroke Association. *Stroke*. 2013;44:2064–2089. https://doi.org/10.1161/STR.0b013e318296aeca.

2. Feigin VL, Norrving B, Mensah GA. Global burden of stroke. *Circ Res*. 2017;120:439–448. https://doi.org/10.1161/CIRCRESAHA.116.308413.

3. Joubert J, Prentice LF, Moulin T, et al. Stroke in rural areas and small communities. *Stroke*. 2008;39:1920–1928. https://doi.org/10.1161/STROKEAHA.107.501643.

4. Mozaffarian D, Benjamin EJ, Go AS, et al. Executive summary: heart disease and stroke statistics-2016 update: a report from the American Heart Association. *Circulation*. 2016;133:447–454. https://doi.org/10.1161/CIR.0000000000000366.

5. Hankey GJ, Blacker DJ. Is it a stroke? *BMJ*. 2015;350:h56. https://doi.org/10.1136/bmj.h56.

6. Australian Institute of Health and Welfare. *Cardiovascular Disease in Women—a Snapshot of National Statistics*. 2019. Canberra.

7. Treger I, Shames J, Giaquinto S, et al. Return to work in stroke patients. *Disabil Rehabil*. 2007;29:1397–1403. https://doi.org/10.1080/09638280701314923.

8. Hankey GJ. Stroke. *Lancet*. 2017;389:641–654. https://doi.org/10.1016/S0140-6736(16)30962-X.

9. Cramer SC, Wolf SL, Adams HP, et al. Stroke recovery and rehabilitation research: issues, opportunities, and the National Institutes of Health StrokeNet. *Stroke.* 2017;48:813–819. https://doi.org/10.1161/STROKEAHA.116.015501.

10. World Health Organization. *The Need to Scale Up Rehabilitation.* World Health Organization; 2017. https://apps.who.int/iris/handle/10665/331210.

11. Wade DT. *What is rehabilitation? An empirical investigation leading to an evidence-based description.* London, England: SAGE Publications Sage UK; 2020.

12. Lynch EA, Cadilhac DA, Luker JA, et al. Inequities in access to inpatient rehabilitation after stroke: an international scoping review. *Top Stroke Rehabil.* 2017;24:619–626.

13. Schneider EJ, Lannin NA, Ada L, et al. Increasing the amount of usual rehabilitation improves activity after stroke: a systematic review. *J Physiother.* 2016;62:182–187. https://doi.org/10.1016/j.jphys.2016.08.006.

14. Selenitsch NA, Gill SD. Stroke survivor activity during subacute inpatient rehabilitation: how active are patients? *Int J Rehabil Res.* 2019;42:82–84.

15. Findorff MJ, Wyman JF, Gross CR. Predictors of long-term exercise adherence in a community-based sample of older women. *J Women's Health.* 2009;18:1769–1776.

16. Luker J, Murray C, Lynch E, et al. Carers' experiences, needs, and preferences during inpatient stroke rehabilitation: a systematic review of qualitative studies. *Arch Phys Med Rehabil.* 2017;98:1852–1862. e1813.

17. Anderson CS, Linto J, Stewart-Wynne EG. A population-based assessment of the impact and burden of caregiving for long-term stroke survivors. *Stroke.* 1995;26:843–849.

18. Cramer SC, Dodakian L, Le V, et al. Efficacy of home-based telerehabilitation vs in-clinic therapy for adults after stroke: a randomized clinical trial. *JAMA Neurol.* 2019;76:1079–1087.

19. Hassett L, van den Berg M, Lindley RI, et al. Digitally enabled aged care and neurological rehabilitation to enhance outcomes with Activity and MObility UsiNg Technology (AMOUNT) in Australia: a randomised controlled trial. *PLoS Med.* 2020;17:e1003029.

20. Boter H. Multicenter randomized controlled trial of an outreach nursing support program for recently discharged stroke patients. *Stroke.* 2004;35:2867–2872.

21. Mayo NE, Nadeau L, Ahmed S, et al. Bridging the gap: the effectiveness of teaming a stroke coordinator with patient's personal physician on the outcome of stroke. *Age Ageing.* 2008;37:32–38.

22. Rochette A, Korner-Bitensky N, Bishop D, et al. The YOU CALL–WE CALL randomized clinical trial: impact of a multimodal support intervention after a mild stroke. *Circ Cardiovasc Qual Outcomes.* 2013;6:674–679.

23. Meltzer JA, Baird AJ, Steele RD, et al. Computer-based treatment of poststroke language disorders: a non-inferiority study of telerehabilitation compared to in-person service delivery. *Aphasiology.* 2018;32:290–311.

24. Lloréns R, Noé E, Colomer C, et al. Effectiveness, usability, and cost-benefit of a virtual reality-based telerehabilitation program for balance recovery after stroke: a randomized controlled trial. *Arch Phys Med Rehabil.* 2015;96:418–425. e412.

25. Lawson DW, Stolwyk RJ, Ponsford JL, et al. Telehealth delivery of memory rehabilitation following stroke. *J Int Neuropsychol Soc.* 2020;26:58–71.

26. Van Den Berg M, Crotty M, Liu E, et al. Early supported discharge by caregiver-mediated exercises and e-health support after stroke: a proof-of-concept trial. *Stroke.* 2016;47:1885–1892.

27. NeoRehab. *NeoRehab.* https://www.neorehab.com/. 2020. Accessed 16.09.20.

28. Barclay R, Miller PA, Pooyania S, et al. Development of a telephone interview version of the Chedoke-McMaster stroke assessment activity inventory. *Physiother Can.* 2016;68:216–222.

29. Forducey PG, Glueckauf RL, Bergquist TF, et al. Telehealth for persons with severe functional disabilities and their caregivers: facilitating self-care management in the home setting. *Psychol Serv.* 2012;9:144.

30. Lin K-H, Chen C-H, Chen Y-Y, et al. Bidirectional and multi-user telerehabilitation system: clinical effect on balance, functional activity, and satisfaction in patients with chronic stroke living in long-term care facilities. *Sensors.* 2014;14:12451–12466.

31. Sakakibara BM, Lear SA, Barr SI, et al. *A Telehealth Intervention to Promote Healthy Lifestyles After Stroke: the Stroke Coach Protocol.* London, England: SAGE Publications Sage UK; 2018.

32. Wonggom P, Kourbelis C, Newman P, et al. Effectiveness of avatar-based technology in patient education for improving chronic disease knowledge and self-care behavior: a systematic review. *JBI Database System Rev Implement Rep.* 2019;17:1101–1129.

33. Aljaroodi HM, Adam MT, Chiong R, et al. *Empathic Avatars in Stroke Rehabilitation: a Co-designed mHealth Artifact for Stroke Survivors.* International Conference on Design Science Research in Information System and Technology: Springer; 2017:73–89.

34. Jørgensen TSH, Wium-Andersen IK, Wium-Andersen MK, et al. Incidence of depression after stroke, and associated risk factors and mortality outcomes, in a large cohort of Danish patients. *JAMA Psychiatry.* 2016;73:1032–1040. https://doi.org/10.1001/jamapsychiatry.2016.1932.

35. Stroke Foundation *Clinical Guidelines for Stroke Management.* Melbourne, Australia: Stroke Foundation; 2019. https://strokefoundation.org.au/What-we-do/For%20health%20professionals%20and%20researchers/Clinical-guidelines.

36. Kirkness CJ, Cain KC, Becker KJ, et al. Randomized trial of telephone versus in-person delivery of a brief psychosocial intervention in post-stroke depression. *BMC Res Notes.* 2017;10:500. https://doi.org/10.1186/s13104-017-2819-y.

37. Laver KE, Adey-Wakeling Z, Crotty M, et al. Telerehabilitation services for stroke. *Cochrane Database Syst Rev.* 2020;1:CD010255.

38. Sureshkumar K, Murthy G, Kuper H. Protocol for a randomised controlled trial to evaluate the effectiveness of the "Care for Stroke" intervention in India: a smartphone-enabled, carer-supported, educational intervention for management of disabilities following stroke. *BMJ Open.* 2018;8:e020098.

39. Cadilhac DA, Busingye D, Li JC, et al. Development of an electronic health message system to support recovery after stroke: Inspiring Virtual Enabled Resources following Vascular Events (iVERVE). *Patient Prefer Adherence.* 2018;12:1213.

40. Vloothuis JDM, Mulder M, Nijland RHM, et al. Caregiver-mediated exercises with e-health support for early supported discharge after stroke (CARE4STROKE): a randomized controlled trial. *PLoS One.* 2019;14:e0214241. https://doi.org/10.1371/journal.pone.0214241.

41. Ward EC, Burns CL, Theodoros DG, et al. Evaluation of a clinical service model for dysphagia assessment via telerehabilitation. *Int J Telemed Appl.* 2013;2013:918526.

42. Morrell K, Hyers M, Stuchiner T, et al. Telehealth stroke dysphagia evaluation is safe and effective. *Cerebrovasc Dis.* 2017;44:225. https://doi.org/10.1159/000478107.

43. Hall N, Boisvert M, Steele R. Telepractice in the assessment and treatment of individuals with aphasia: a systematic review. *Int J Telerehabil.* 2013;5:27–38. https://doi.org/10.5195/ijt.2013.6119.

44. Hill AJ, Theodoros DG, Russell TG, et al. The effects of aphasia severity on the ability to assess language disorders via telerehabilitation. *Aphasiology.* 2009;23:627–642.

45. Hoffman NB, Prieto NM. Clinical video telehealth for gait and balance. *Fed Pract.* 2016;33:34–38.

46. Richardson BR, Truter P, Blumke R, et al. Physiotherapy assessment and diagnosis of musculoskeletal disorders of the knee via telerehabilitation. *Journal of Telemedicine and Telecare.* 2016;23:88–95. https://doi.org/10.1177/1357633X15627237.

47. Venkataraman K, Amis K, Landerman LR, et al. Teleassessment of gait and gait aids: validity and inter-rater reliability. *Physical Therapy.* 2020;100:708–717. https://doi.org/10.1093/ptj/pzaa005.

48. Worboys T, Brassington M, Ward EC, et al. Delivering occupational therapy hand assessment and treatment sessions via telehealth. *J Telemed Telecare.* 2017;24:185–192. https://doi.org/10.1177/1357633X17691861.

49. Ninnis K, Van Den Berg M, Lannin NA, et al. Information and communication technology use within occupational therapy home assessments: a scoping review. *Br J Occup Ther.* 2019;82:141–152.

50. Adie K, James MA. Does telephone follow-up improve blood pressure after minor stroke or TIA? *Age Ageing.* 2010;39:598–603. https://doi.org/10.1093/ageing/afq085.

51. Gillham S, Endacott R. Impact of enhanced secondary prevention on health behaviour in patients following minor stroke and transient ischaemic attack: a randomized controlled trial. *Clin Rehabil.* 2010;24:822–830. https://doi.org/10.1177/0269215510367970.

52. Taylor DM, Stone SD, Huijbregts MP. Remote participants' experiences with a group-based stroke self-management program using videoconference technology. *Rural Remote Health.* 1947;2012:12.

53. Jaglal SB, Haroun VA, Salbach NM, et al. Increasing access to chronic disease self-management programs in rural and remote communities using telehealth. *Telemed J E Health.* 2013;19:467–473. https://doi.org/10.1089/tmj.2012.0197.

54. Taylor DM, Cameron JI, Walsh L, et al. Exploring the feasibility of videoconference delivery of a self-management program to rural participants with stroke. *Telemed J E Health.* 2009;15:646–654. https://doi.org/10.1089/tmj.2008.0165.
55. Hosseiniravandi M, Kahlaee AH, Karim H, et al. Home-based telerehabilitation software systems for remote supervising: a systematic review. *Int J Technol Assess Health Care.* 2020;36:113–125. https://doi.org/10.1017/S0266462320000021.

CHAPTER 5

Telerehabilitation in Brain Injury

Mary Alexis Iaccarino ▦ Bridget Rizik ▦ Myriam Lacerte

Introduction

Traumatic brain injuries (TBIs) encompass those injuries that cause a disruption in normal functioning of the brain when it is exposed to some direct or indirect external force (bump, blow, jolt) or a penetrating injury. This is a diverse group of injuries ranging from mild, transient perturbations to devastating structural injuries with severe and long-lasting disability. Across injury severity, the clinical presentation can also vary as TBI can cause a wide variety of symptoms in multiple domains including physical symptoms, cognitive challenges, and psychological disturbances. Those that suffer TBI may engage the health care system in one or more clinical environments and interface with many types of providers including emergency rooms, critical care, acute and subacute inpatient rehabilitation, outpatient rehabilitation, and medical outpatient clinics, among others. In addition, those with long-term sequelae will continue to rely on the health care system over their lifetimes to manage chronic disease-related issues and downstream complications.

Telerehabilitation

Telehealth and telerehabilitation are poised to serve an important role in helping to provide care to TBI patients. Given the breadth of needs of those with TBI, the variety of health care providers and settings in which they may seek care, and the chronic nature of some injuries, there are many uses for telerehabilitation. While some of these uses are well established and their effectiveness studied, others may be underdeveloped. The gap between current roles of telehealth and future uses may be related to a multitude of factors, including limitations in technology resources, lack of infrastructure or institutional support, reimbursement for care, and limits of physical examination maneuvers and accurate diagnostic assessments that may portend liability issues. This chapter will explore current and future uses for telerehabilitation in the TBI population by drawing on what is present in the TBI literature, as well as experience in other areas of neurological and rehabilitative care. We will provide practical guidance for deployment of telerehabilitation for people with TBI, examine special populations, and explore clinical caveats to this mode of health care.

Practice

ACUTE CARE EMERGENCE AND CRITICAL CARE MANAGEMENT

Telehealth can play an important role in providing access to specialist care for trauma patients that may have sustained TBI. One such potential role is in providing triage-based care to rural and underserved health care settings in which the need for surgical intervention or higher level of care can be rapidly determined through virtual consultation. This methodology has been best illustrated in the stroke community, in which teleconsultation between local emergency room staff and specialty stroke providers is used to determine injury severity, early interventions, and need for patient transfer when presenting with stroke symptoms. In addition, teleradiology services are used to read emergent neuroimaging studies that may diagnose TBI and aid decision-making for neurosurgical intervention.[1]

While triage of neurocritical care emergencies in TBI is not well studied, teleneurology or telestroke has already been used extensively for neurocritical care and emergent stroke.[2] A study utilizing telestroke technology reported improved triage, faster intervention times, and better functional outcomes in patients evaluated virtually.[3] Teleneurosurgical practice may also have a role in the management of acute brain injuries. Studies performed in the United States have shown cost-reduction benefits while maintaining good outcomes when using telerehabilitation in the setting of neurocritical emergencies such as intracranial hemorrhage. In addition, remote neurosurgical consultation may facilitate cost savings by limiting unnecessary transfers to tertiary care centers from outlying hospitals.[4,5] In addition, telehealth may have a role in neurosurgical follow-up care as a substitute for an in-person clinic visit.[6] A similar approach has been shown to be clinically valuable and cost-effective in the burn and trauma literature.[7] For neurological intensive critical care units (ICU) with less critical care clinicians available, telemedicine allows the ICU to expand coverage for neurocritical emergencies. A metaanalysis compared outcomes before and after establishing tele-ICU services and found reductions in hospital lengths of stay and mortality with tele-ICU.[8] Thus the care of the acute TBI patient can be enhanced by multiple telerehabilitation adaptations.

ACUTE CARE REHABILITATION CONSULTATION SERVICE

Early access to dedicated and experienced rehabilitation providers is important for those with brain injuries. However, a recent survey of acute care facilities worldwide found there may be limited access to this type of care in the acute hospital environment.[9] Rehabilitation teleconsultations from provider to provider or provider to patient may serve a critical role in expanding opportunities for early rehabilitation specialty care. Options for rehabilitation teleconsultation to the acute care setting can occur in real-time (synchronous), in which the consulting rehabilitation provider can speak to the patient and primary clinician and conduct an assessment. Alternatively, "e-consultation" (asynchronous) allows rehabilitation providers to provide advice to treating providers regarding specific aspects of care, relying on review of the medical records to provide recommendations and guidance.

Many lessons from acute teleneurology can serve as a model for the continued evolution of telerehabilitation in acute settings, especially while performing consults on brain injury patients. Teleneurology has been used to assess patients with stroke, Parkinson's disease, epilepsy, and other neurological diseases as part of acute inpatient care.[10,11] In an assessment of hospitals with teleneurology, lengths of stay were reduced and there was no difference in subsequent mortality or additional costs and utilization following discharge. In addition, telemedicine assessment and diagnosis was found to be similar to in-person evaluation.[12] This model could be mirrored in telerehabilitation consultations of the brain injury patient.[13] In brain injury telerehabilitation, real-time videoconferencing providing two-way audiovisual input between patients and clinicians may allow the consulting rehabilitation provider to be most impactful in their consultation recommendations. Asynchronous or e-consultation may be less valuable to answer diagnostic questions or facilitate an overall plan of care but may have utility in triaging a specific treatment question.

There are a variety of new technologies that might serve to enhance telerehabilitation of TBI patients in acute care. Telerehabilitation consultation may be enhanced through the use of technologies such as a movable cart with a pan-tilt-zoom camera, high-resolution screen, and a computer positioned at the site of patient care. Additional features such as the ability to connect via a web browser–based system to control the camera from a remote site may enable better communication with the patient and may allow the provider to perform elements of the neurological examination with or without a telepresenter at the bedside.[13]

IN THE FIELD REMOTE ASSESSMENT

While brain injuries that result in prolonged loss of consciousness, amnesia, and profound motor and sensory deficits necessitate evaluation in emergency room settings, there is a large subset of individuals with TBI who may present with more mild symptoms for which the need to seek immediate medical care is less obvious. This is a common scenario in sports environments and military settings in which concussions or mild TBI frequently present with subtle findings. Proper triage of these injuries is important to facilitate removal from high-risk activities and avoid repetitive and overlap head traumas in those that are concussed. Teleconcussion could play a role in triaging those patients that may be symptomatic from mild head injuries.

Remote monitoring for TBI during game play is common in professional sports using spotter and video replay. In addition, teleconcussion sideline assessments have been proposed for cases in which a concussion-trained health provider is not present, which applies in many youth and recreational sporting events. A study by Vargas et al. in 2017 investigated the feasibility of teleconcussion for sideline concussion assessments with a cohort of 11 consecutive male collegiate football players with a suspected concussion. The Standardized Assessment of Concussion, King-Devick test, and modified Balance Error Scoring System were used for remote assessment. A remote neurologist assessed each athlete using a telemedicine robot with real-time, two-way audiovisual capabilities, while a sideline provider performed a simultaneous face-to-face assessment. The results showed a high agreement between remote and face-to-face providers on examination findings, suggesting that teleconcussion assessment may be feasible.[14]

When discussing the acute management of brain injury in the field, there is much to gain from military medicine. For example, in the United States, the Defense and Veterans Brain Injury Center has utilized a remote cognitive assessment system that allows clinicians in the field to gather cognitive information more rapidly. TBI specialists at distant sites then can review this information and work with other clinicians to develop treatment strategies and return-to-duty recommendations.[15]

At present the most readily available and realistic use of remote assessment for acute injuries in the field is likely in the triage process. Performing a complete and thorough neurological examination that provides a high level of accuracy in making a diagnosis may not be feasible at this point. In studies of acute neurological examination and diagnosis in non-stroke patients, there is good interrater reliability for remote examination, though accuracy is less established.[13,16] Thus remote assessment and examination may assist in determining the need for immediate transfer to a hospital versus watchful observation in the field, when in-person assessment is not available, but it is unlikely to fully replace in-person care.

PHYSICAL EXAMINATION

While examination of the brain-injury patient will be different based on the rehabilitation specialist and the goals of the evaluation, there are some universal themes that may optimize the remote TBI evaluation. Due to challenges with attention, concentration, and impulse control experienced after TBI, both patient and provider should be in a distraction-free environment with limited background noise or interruptions. When possible, technology should be optimized for sensory symptoms such as light and noise sensitivity, hearing loss, and visual impairments. For those with moderate-to-severe physical and cognitive difficulties, visits should be conducted with a caregiver or assistant with the patient. Prior to beginning the assessment, equipment, supplies, or other resources should be obtained. Examples of these may include pencil and paper for cognitive testing, assistive devices such as bracing and other durable medical equipment that may be evaluated for its use and fit, and medication lists or prescription bottles to conduct a medication reconciliation. At the close of the visit, providing written instructions and summary of the visit recommendations can assist those with organization and memory difficulties.

Performing a complete neurological examination solely via telerehabilitation, particularly when evaluating muscle tone, strength, sensation, and reflexes, is not possible currently. For cases of teleconsultation in which the patient is in a health care facility or clinic, a nurse practitioner, physician assistant, registered nurse, or other allied health professional may be trained to perform a neurological examination (i.e., a "telepresenter") during the teleconference examination or in front of the camera. In the case of telerehabilitation for patients at home a family member may be able to assist with some physical examination maneuvers such as range of motion. Apart from physical examination, telerehabilitation may play an important role in evaluating the cognitive and psychological aspects of TBI and are discussed below.

USE OF TELEREHABILITATION IN DISEASE MANAGEMENT

There are a variety of opportunities to incorporate telerehabilitation into the management of TBI across the spectrum of disease and the course of care. The evidence to support use of telerehabilitation is explored here but is limited. There are likely uses that are reasonable in this population but have yet to be studied or widely published. The advantage of incorporating telerehabilitation into disease management can include increased access to specialty care, convenience for patients and providers, reduction in care barriers such as time for travel and appropriate transportation, cost-effectiveness, and timeliness of care delivery.

Access to specialty care and appropriate guidance about brain injury is critical to patient success. An important aspect of disease management is education of the patient, family, or other providers. Guidance on expectant management and natural history of the injury can assist with planning care needs, behavioral modifications, environmental adaptation, and treatment interventions. Telerehabilitation allows for ready access to professionals who can provide appropriate education at any stage of brain injury recovery. Particularly as the understanding of brain injury evolves from one of a static injury toward brain injury as a chronic condition, education throughout the duration of recovery may play a role in reducing symptoms and enhancing function.

In a review of existing literature on the effects of education in both mild and moderate-severe injuries, Hart et al. noted increased patient self-efficacy and investment in one's own rehabilitation in those who received formal education about their injuries.[17] In a broader systematic review of interventions for mild TBI, there was sufficient agreement amongst studies to suggest that patient-centered interaction and the delivery of symptom-related information support recovery from mild TBI symptoms.[18] And in another systematic review of psychological interventions for mild TBI, the authors concluded that, though difficult to quantify, most studies agree that active educational treatment is favored over no treatment.[19] Though there are fewer studies regarding virtual delivery of education, initial results suggest that a web-based format may be a valuable adjunct to traditional education strategies.[17] Active, patient-centered education either remotely or in person seems to be an important factor in recovery from brain injuries along the entire continuum of care.

Another potential role of telerehabilitation in the brain injury population is in assistance with initiation and monitoring of pharmacotherapy. Individuals with acquired brain injuries often experience physical, cognitive, and emotional sequelae including but not limited to seizures, spasticity, pain, fatigue, sleep disturbances, depression, and agitation.[20-22] One aspect of management is pharmacological—acutely and chronically, with single or multiple pharmacological agents. In one cross-sectional, multicenter evaluation of patients with acquired brain injury admitted to inpatient postacute rehabilitation, 479 of 484 patients were on a medication of some kind, and perhaps even more notably, 80% of patients (387 of 483) were prescribed six or more medications at the examined point in admission.[21] In addition, studies on pharmacotherapy following brain injury demonstrate a high prevalence of prescription medications not only acutely, but also chronically. Yasseen et al. evaluated subjects between 7 and 24 years post-injury, finding that 58.9% (178) continued to take prescription medications, with 44% (70) taking three or more. Most prevalent medication types were anticonvulsants, antidepressants, analgesics, and anxiolytics.[23] Titration of these types of medication requires information from patients and caregivers on current symptoms and side effects. However, much of this can be garnered without in-person assessment and can be completed via telerehabilitation. In other aspects of care, such as spasticity management, in-person physical examination may be needed to determine medication titration. While data are lacking on remote pharmacotherapy intervention and medication titration, one might surmise that ready access to a specialist, as afforded by telehealth, would facilitate timely medication initiation, earlier recognition and reporting of side effects, and reduce unnecessary polypharmacy. Further data are needed to support this use case.

While some aspects of the diagnostic physical examination may not be amenable to telerehabilitation, psychological and cognitive diagnostic assessments may be reasonable to conduct using telerehabilitation. This is of particular significance to the brain injury population, who commonly experience neurobehavioral, cognitive, and emotional changes following injury. Regarding cognitive screening tools, studies have found that the Mini-Mental State Examination performed remotely versus in-person did not differ significantly either in scoring or in interrater reliability.[24,25] Broader neuropsychological testing batteries, too, appear reliable via the virtual domain.[26] In one study, 32 subjects underwent a total of 12 visual, verbal, and performance tests; most measures ultimately demonstrated high correlation between in-person and remote assessment.[27] A larger validation study by Cullum et al. in 2014, the largest of its kind at the time, included 202 subjects and utilized the Mini-Mental Status Examination, Hopkins Verbal Learning Test-Revised, Digit Span forward and backward, short form Boston Naming Test, Letter and Category Fluency, and Clock Drawing. This study demonstrated highly similar results when comparing virtual to in-person assessments. Importantly, this study included 83 individuals with cognitive impairment, with no significant difference in conclusions.[28] This is certainly of significance when extrapolating to the brain injury population, where cognitive impairment may be a perceived barrier to the utilization of telerehabilitation resources. A 2020 systematic review across teleneuropsychology summarized that virtually conducted neuropsychological assessments, although challenging, appear valid and present an opportunity to increase accessibility to cognitive services and support.[29]

USE OF TELEREHABILITATION FOR THERAPY

There is a robust collection of literature demonstrating the effectiveness of virtual physiotherapy in general rehabilitation, but a paucity specific to brain injury. A systematic review by Ownsworth et al. acknowledged the limitations of brain injury–specific telerehabilitation research, identifying only 13 eligible studies, with significant heterogeneity amongst them.[30] Conclusions noted promising feasibility, cost-effectiveness, and improvement in certain functional outcomes—though more studies were needed for definitive efficacy statements.[30] Another systematic review focusing on improving cognitive function and quality of life in individuals with TBI also denoted limitations in the current literature on remote cognitive rehabilitation due to lack of standardized protocol between studies. Despite these limitations, the authors concluded that remote cognitive therapies may be beneficial regardless of the specific interventions utilized between therapists.[31] Similar difficulties exist in tele-based physical therapy, in which individual studies have reported benefits of remote physiotherapy in the brain injury population, but standardized protocol and parameters have yet to be established, limiting generalizability and application on a wider scale.[32]

While data in telerehabilitation therapies are lacking in brain injury, data from non–brain injury studies could be extrapolated and applied to the brain injury population. A systematic review of poststroke telerehabilitation deemed telerehabilitation at least as effective as in-person therapies for motor and higher cortical deficits as well as poststroke depression.[33] In another study including 81 individuals with brain injury, stroke, or multiple sclerosis, subjects were randomized to month-long programs either utilizing a computerized activity desk directed at upper extremity retraining versus a "usual care" group. Improvements in the Action Research Arm Test and Nine Hole Peg Test were similar between treatment arms, indicating that the home-based training might be an equivalent alternative to in-person therapies. Of note, individuals with serious cognitive and behavioral problems were excluded from this trial.[34] Though studies focused specifically on brain injury are needed, research in other areas of neurorehabilitation offers guidance and encouraging results thus far.

Importantly, remote opportunities for ongoing therapy appear to be an area of interest to affected individuals and their caregivers: in a survey of 71 individuals with acquired brain injury in the community, a majority indicated strong interest in a variety of telerehabilitation options including instructing home-based physical therapies, activities of daily living (ADL) training, and cognitive exercises.[35] In addition, patients reported satisfaction with teletherapy interventions. A recent survey issued to 205 patients undergoing virtual therapy indicated an overall positive response from subjects. Across patient demographics and patient-centered metrics, the large majority of responses were "excellent" or "very good" (93.7%–99%), indicating a high degree of patient acceptance, and suggesting value in future telerehabilitation.[36] Patient interest, support, and satisfaction are critical factors of therapeutic relationships and virtual care appears to be an acceptable, even desirable or preferable option, to patients.

Interventions such as physical and occupational therapy and speech-language pathology also play an important role in the assessment and modification of the home environment. From initial transition home to ongoing, unfolding developments, therapists provide evaluation and counseling to optimize the home setting. Such home modifications have been shown to improve the health and safety of subjects with a variety of health conditions.[37] These home evaluations are traditionally done in person, which may be limited by personnel, location, time, and other resources. Several studies have assessed the feasibility of performing these assessments remotely, utilizing both novel and existing technologies. Initial results suggest at-home versus remote assessments are nearly equivalent, and at least worth exploring as potential adjuncts or alternatives when in-person evaluations are not feasible.[37–39] Individuals who have sustained brain injuries may benefit from an assortment of home modifications for ease, efficiency, and safety, from installation of new equipment (e.g., railings, ramps) to modifying an existing setup (e.g., reorganizing shelves, removing tripping hazards). Beginning or continuing this process remotely may be an opportunity for increased therapist presence in the home, and in turn, an improved home environment.

Special Considerations

PEDIATRIC POPULATION

There are unique populations who may necessitate special considerations in discourse of telerehabilitation. For example, the pediatric population poses additional challenges in terms of their functional abilities to utilize technology. Depending on developmental age, caregiver presence may be required to facilitate virtual visits, provide collateral, or assist with examination techniques. Despite these barriers, initial studies suggest both feasibility and efficacy of virtual interventions for youth with brain injuries.[40–42] One randomized controlled trial relying on an online problem-solving intervention even demonstrated long-term benefits in everyday executive function following its use.[42] Some studies have attempted to utilize computerized games as aids to the rehabilitation process, which might be a favorable option to the adolescent population in particular; however, generalizability has not been definitively confirmed.[43] Telehealth may also be an opportunity to foster family or friend engagement, with a chance for parents, siblings, and other caregivers to partake in the rehabilitation process of a pediatric patient. This is an area of remote medicine that would benefit from further investigation.

MILITARY POPULATION

Members of the military are another population meriting special attention in this discussion. Telerehabilitation is already widely utilized in the military for diagnosis, acute treatment, and long-term rehabilitation.[15,44,45] TBIs, particularly mild TBIs, are common in modern warfare due to increased exposure to powerful weaponry and explosives. For example, the United States estimates that 15% to 20% of veterans from the Iraq and Afghanistan wars have sustained at least one TBI.[45] For this reason, there may be greater demand for TBI services in active duty military and veterans that can be alleviated by telehealth.

CAREGIVERS

Caregivers of patients with brain injuries may also benefit from telehealth. Caregivers share in the burden of injuries and illnesses affecting their loved ones, particularly those caring for people with TBI. It is estimated that 28.5% of the US adult population or 65.7 million people provide "informal" caregiving for an adult relative.[46] Caregiver socialization and support could be an area of opportunity for remote interventions. There also may be educational or training benefits for caregivers as they learn to tend to an individual with brain injury. As questions, concerns, and challenges arise in the home environment, caregivers may look for advice from professionals and peers. As such, this too may be a population who would benefit from the accessibility, continuity, and social opportunities made possible by remote medicine. A 2012 systematic review concluded that telehealth programs for families of individuals with brain injuries are both feasible and effective, with the large majority reporting positive outcomes.[47] Though there were limited direct comparisons to face-to-face encounters, those that did include in-person encounters as a control found no significant difference in caregiver outcome.[47]

Limitations

BEHAVIORAL DISTURBANCES, PSYCHOSIS, OR SELF-HARM

In some types of brain injuries, patients may have co-occurring severe behavioral disturbances, mood disorders with psychotic features, self-harm behaviors, or even suicide risk.[48,49] Using telerehabilitation with brain injury patients suffering from these types of psychological sequela presents a unique challenge for patient safety. There are little data on telerehabilitation in this subpopulation of brain injury. Yet, in patients with psychosis without TBI, videoconferencing afforded patients a higher degree of comfort because the perceived distance of the interaction was less anxiety-provoking and may reduce overstimulation triggered by some in-person interactions.[50] In addition, telerehabilitation may allow better insight into the patient's daily life by assessing their homes and living environments, thus better informing diagnosis and treatment. Nevertheless, it is critical for the clinician to weigh the benefits of the telerehabilitation visit with the potential risks of remotely triaging or managing unstable and serious mental health symptoms. If telerehabilitation is used, additional precautions may be considered for a patient at risk of harming himself/herself or others; for example, this may include confirming a patient's location at the beginning of the visit, having a plan for maintaining the telerehabilitation connection to the patient, and knowing how to guide emergency services to a patient in the event of crisis.

COGNITIVE AND SENSORY DEFICITS

Patients with brain injuries can often present with hearing loss, visual impairment, or other sensory difficulties that could impede virtual care. For example, patients with reduced hearing are at a disadvantage if using telephone communication, mainly due to the absence of visual cues and a narrower range of speech frequencies. Sound quality and visual input can vary widely across different telecommunication devices such as landline, cellular phone, and videoconference. Low-quality sensory input may affect a brain-injured person's ability to provide a history, perform physical examination maneuvers, or participate in cognitive testing. Lighting quality and the patient's screen size are also important factors when assessing this subset of patients with visual impairments or symptoms. When testing these patients, providers should not assume intact sensory abilities.[51] At a minimum the examiner should inquire about hearing and vision prior to a telerehabilitation visit. Patients should be prompted to use hearing aids, glasses, and other assistive devices during the examination.

ELDERLY PATIENTS

Older adults with TBI experience higher morbidity and mortality and tend to have a slower recovery.[52] On average, they also have worse functional, cognitive, and psychosocial outcomes months or years post-injury than their younger counterparts.[53,54] It is commonly believed that elderly patients may show reluctance to adopt a novel technology and this could be compounded by the effect of a brain injury. However, a recent study has found that 65% of the geriatric population would be willing to trial current technological advancements such as virtual reality.[55] In addition, telerehabilitation can easily be extended to elder care centers and residential facilities, where staff can assist with the technology required to complete a telerehabilitation visit successfully.[56] It also appears that establishing videoconferencing integrated with a local health care service such as a primary care physician[57] may significantly improve elderly persons' behavior and also reduce the caregivers' burden.[58] Findings suggest that the delivery of videoconferencing is feasible, acceptable, and beneficial to older adults in the chronic phase after TBI and stroke.[59]

UNDERSERVED POPULATIONS WITH TBI

Increasing access to specialty care is an important benefit of telerehabilitation and can improve health care disparities in underserved TBI populations. Recent research has shown that non-Hispanic Black and Hispanic patients are less likely to receive follow-up care and rehabilitation following a TBI compared with non-Hispanic White patients.[60] Compared with insured White patients, insured Black patients had reduced odds of discharge to rehabilitation as did insured Hispanics and insured Asians. Telerehabilitation has also been shown to reduce location-based disparities in care. Not only can telerehabilitation make care more accessible to patients who live in remote or inaccessible areas, but it also can improve access to those who are unable to drive following their injuries and can reduce reliance on family members and caregivers to attend medical and therapy visits. In addition, telehealth may assist patients of lower socioeconomic status who have limited means to afford adaptive transportation, sick leave from work, or childcare. While reducing some barriers to underserved populations, telehealth may also create barriers with socially or economically disadvantaged groups. Those of lower socioeconomic status or who suffer financial hardship may have limited access to technologies (internet access, tablets, smartphones, computers) needed to participate in their visit. Every effort should be made to reduce barriers to telehealth care for these groups, including but not limited to offering telehealth platforms that are verbal only and do not require a camera, using telehealth applications that do not require downloads or an email address, and providing technical support or orientation to technology prior to the visit.

FUTURE DIRECTIONS

Telerehabilitation in the rehabilitation setting is in its infancy. While some diagnoses and domains of care are developing quickly, such as stroke care, TBI telerehabilitation has had comparatively little research to validate its use. Nonetheless, the uses for telerehabilitation in TBI are many, spanning early triage through the acute care, inpatient rehabilitation, and outpatient rehabilitation settings. Future work is needed to determine the most impactful telerehabilitation uses and compare them to in-person care. In addition, there is a need to develop technology interfaces that may assist or improve physical examination assessment and therapeutic interventions such as robotics and virtual reality. Finally, more work is needed to improve access to telehealth services, including wider adoption of telerehabilitation by private and government health care organizations, optimization of regulations to broaden telerehabilitation services, and development of telerehabilitation interfaces that are accessible to all including underserved and marginalized TBI specialty populations.

CASE STUDY

Jon is a 52-year-old married salesman and avid cyclist who suffers a helmeted road biking accident, sustaining depressed skull fracture with epidural hematoma, bifrontal intraparenchymal hemorrhage, and diffuse axonal injury. He is taken by ambulance to a small regional medical center where a computed tomography scan shows the aforementioned injuries. Remote teleradiology and teleneurosurgery services evaluate the imaging, determining that Jon requires transfer for urgent surgical intervention.

Two weeks after injury, Jon remains in the intensive care unit, awake and confused despite medical optimization. A telerehabilitation consultation is conducted due to lack of in-person specialists. With assistance of an in-person speech therapist, the physician remotely conducts a neurological and cognitive examination and provides recommendations for agitation management and arousal. One week later, the telerehabilitation physician conducts a follow-up remote assessment. Jon's agitation improves; he is more awake but still confused. The physician recommends inpatient acute rehabilitation and has an extensive discussion with Jon's wife about his disposition.

Two months later, Jon is ready to leave inpatient rehabilitation. Since he lives 3 hours from the rehabilitation facility, a virtual home assessment is conducted by physical and occupational therapy to help his wife optimize the home environment and obtain necessary equipment. Jon's discharge plan includes twice monthly in-person rehabilitation with physical, occupational, and speech therapy with twice weekly telerehabilitation sessions in his home to reduce the travel burden on his wife. He also has telerehabilitation follow-up by his physiatrist to titrate medications for sleep, attention, and headaches.

One year later, Jon has made a good recovery. He is independent with activities of daily living and needs supervision for complex tasks such as managing his finances. He has returned to driving but only drives short distances due to fatigue. He wants to return to work. Jon's physiatrist arranges for remote sessions with vocational rehabilitation services to discuss return to work. He ultimately returns to part-time work in online advertising sales. He has weekly virtual cognitive rehabilitation sessions to work on strategies and skills needed for his job. He appreciates the virtual sessions so that he limits time away from his new job.

Overall, Jon and his wife are grateful for the role telerehabilitation has played in his care. Telerehabilitation enhanced Jon's care by allowing rapid triage of his injuries, early rehabilitation intervention in the ICU, assistance with inpatient rehabilitation admission, and long-term multidisciplinary follow-up care in his home.

References

1. Olldashi F, Latifi R, Parsikia A, et al. Telemedicine for neurotrauma prevents unnecessary transfers: an update from a nationwide program in Albania and analysis of 590 patients. *World Neurosurg.* 2019;128:e340–e346. https://doi.org/10.1016/j.wneu.2019.04.150.
2. Meyer BC, Lyden PD, Al-Khoury L, et al. Prospective reliability of the STRokE DOC wireless/site independent telemedicine system. *Neurology.* 2005;64(6):1058–1060. https://doi.org/10.1212/01.WNL.0000154601.26653.E7.
3. Kepplinger J, Dzialowski I, Barlinn K, et al. Emergency transfer of acute stroke patients within the East Saxony telemedicine stroke network: a descriptive analysis. *Int J Stroke.* 2014;9(2):160–165. https://doi.org/10.1111/ijs.12032.
4. Kahn EN, La Marca F, Mazzola CA. Neurosurgery and telemedicine in the United States: assessment of the risks and opportunities. *World Neurosurg.* 2016;89:133–138. https://doi.org/10.1016/j.wneu.2016.01.075.
5. Planchard R, Lubelski D, Ehresman J, et al. Telemedicine and remote medical education within neurosurgery. *J Neurosurg Spine.* 2020;33(4):549–552. https://doi.org/10.3171/2020.5.spine20786.
6. Reider-Demer M, Raja P, Martin N, et al. Prospective and retrospective study of videoconference telemedicine follow-up after elective neurosurgery: results of a pilot program. *Neurosurg Rev.* 2018;41:497–501. https://doi.org/10.1007/s10143-017-0878-0.
7. Liu YM, Mathews K, Vardanian A, et al. Urban telemedicine: the applicability of teleburns in the rehabilitative phase. *J Burn Care Res.* 2017;38(1):e235–e239. https://doi.org/10.1097/BCR.0000000000000360.
8. Wilcox ME, Adhikari NKJ. The effect of telemedicine in critically ill patients: systematic review and meta-analysis. *Crit Care.* 2012;16(4):R127. https://doi.org/10.1186/cc11429.
9. Cnossen MC, Lingsma HF, Tenovuo O, et al. Rehabilitation after traumatic brain injury: a survey in 70 European neurotrauma centres participating in the CENTER-TBI study. *J Rehabil Med.* 2017;49(5):395–401. https://doi.org/10.2340/16501977-2216.
10. Kane RL, Bever CT, Ehrmantraut M, et al. Teleneurology in patients with multiple sclerosis: EDSS ratings derived remotely and from hands-on examination. *J Telemed Telecare.* 2008;14(4):190–194. https://doi.org/10.1258/jtt.2008.070904.
11. Ahmed SN, Mann C, Sinclair DB, et al. Feasibility of epilepsy follow-up care through telemedicine: a pilot study on the patient's perspective. *Epilepsia.* 2008;49(4):573–585. https://doi.org/10.1111/j.1528-1167.2007.01464.x.
12. Craig J, Chua R, Russell C, et al. A cohort study of early neurological consultation by telemedicine on the care of neurological inpatients. *J Neurol Neurosurg Psychiatry.* 2004;75(7):1031–1035. https://doi.org/10.1136/jnnp.2002.001651.
13. Wechsler LR. Advantages and limitations of teleneurology. *JAMA Neurol.* 2015;72(3):349–354. https://doi.org/10.1001/jamaneurol.2014.3844.
14. Vargas BB, Shepard M, Hentz JG, et al. Feasibility and accuracy of teleconcussion for acute evaluation of suspected concussion. *Neurology.* 2017;88(16):1580–1583. https://doi.org/10.1212/WNL.0000000000003841.
15. Girard P. Military and VA telemedicine systems for patients with traumatic brain injury. *J Rehabil Res Dev.* 2007;44(7):1017–1026. https://doi.org/10.1682/JRRD.2006.12.0174.
16. Craig JJ, McConville JP, Patterson VH, et al. Neurological examination is possible using telemedicine. *J Telemed Telecare.* 1999;5(3):177–181. https://doi.org/10.1258/1357633991933594.
17. Hart T, Driver S, Sander A, et al. Traumatic brain injury education for adult patients and families: a scoping review. *Brain Inj.* 2018;32(11):1295–1306. https://doi.org/10.1080/02699052.2018.1493226.
18. Comper P, Bisschop SM, Carnide N, et al. A systematic review of treatments for mild traumatic brain injury. *Brain Inj.* 2005;19(11):863–880. https://doi.org/10.1080/02699050400025042.
19. Snell DL, Surgenor LJ, Hay-Smith EJC, et al. A systematic review of psychological treatments for mild traumatic brain injury: an update on the evidence. *J Clin Exp Neuropsychol.* 2009;31(1):20–38. https://doi.org/10.1080/13803390801978849.
20. Gualtieri CT. Pharmacotherapy and the neurobehavioural sequelae of traumatic brain injury. *Brain Inj.* 1988;2(2):101–129. https://doi.org/10.3109/02699058809150936.

21. Cosano G, Giangreco M, Ussai S, et al. Polypharmacy and the use of medications in inpatients with acquired brain injury during post-acute rehabilitation: a cross-sectional study. *Brain Inj*. 2016;30(3):353–362. https://doi.org/10.3109/02699052.2015.1118767.

22. Knottnerus AM, Turner-Stokes T, van de Weg FB, et al. Diagnosis and treatment of depression following acquired brain injury: a comparison of practice in the UK and the Netherlands. *Clin Rehabil*. 2007;21(9):805–811. https://doi.org/10.1177/0269215507079129.

23. Yasseen B, Colantonio A, Ratcliff G. Prescription medication use in persons many years following traumatic brain injury. *Brain Inj*. 2008;22(10):752–757. https://doi.org/10.1080/02699050802320132.

24. Timpano F, Pirrotta F, Bonanno L, et al. Videoconference-based mini mental state examination: a validation study. *Telemedicine J E Health*. 2013;19(12):931–937. https://doi.org/10.1089/tmj.2013.0035.

25. Ciemins EL, Holloway B, Coon PJ, et al. Telemedicine and the mini-mental state examination: assessment from a distance. *Telemedicine J E Health*. 2009;15(5):476–478. https://doi.org/10.1089/tmj.2008.0144.

26. Parsons TD. *Clinical Neuropsychology and Technology: What's New and How We Can Use It*. New York: Springer; 2016:1–190. http://doi.org/10.1007/978-3-319-31075-6.

27. Jacobsen SE, Sprenger T, Andersson S, et al. Neuropsychological assessment and telemedicine: a preliminary study examining the reliability of neuropsychology services performed via telecommunication. *J Int Neuropsychol Soc*. 2003;9(3):472–478. https://doi.org/10.1017/S1355617703930128.

28. Munro Cullum C, Hynan LS, Grosch M, et al. Teleneuropsychology: evidence for video teleconference-based neuropsychological assessment. *J Int Neuropsychol Soc*. 2014;20(10):1028–1033. https://doi.org/10.1017/S1355617714000873.

29. Marra DE, Hamlet KM, Bauer RM, et al. Validity of teleneuropsychology for older adults in response to COVID-19: a systematic and critical review. *Clin Neuropsychol*. 2020;34(7-8):1411–1452. https://doi.org/10.1080/13854046.2020.1769192.

30. Ownsworth T, Arnautovska U, Beadle E, et al. Efficacy of telerehabilitation for adults with traumatic brain injury: a systematic review. *J Head Trauma Rehabil*. 2018;33(4):E33–E46. https://doi.org/10.1097/HTR.0000000000000350.

31. Betts S, Feichter L, Kleinig Z, et al. Telerehabilitation versus standard care for improving cognitive function and quality of life for adults with traumatic brain injury: a systematic review. *Internet J Allied Heal Sci Pract*. 2018;16(3), Article 9.

32. O'Neil J, van Ierssel J, Sveistrup H. Remote supervision of rehabilitation interventions for survivors of moderate or severe traumatic brain injury: a scoping review. *J Telemed Telecare*. 2020;26(9):520–535. https://doi.org/10.1177/1357633X19845466.

33. Sarfo FS, Ulasavets U, Opare-Sem OK, et al. Tele-rehabilitation after stroke: an updated systematic review of the literature. *J Stroke Cerebrovasc Dis*. 2018;27(9):2306–2318. https://doi.org/10.1016/j.jstrokecerebrovasdis.2018.05.013.

34. Huijgen BCH, Vollenbroek-Hutten MMR, Zampolini M, et al. Feasibility of a home-based telerehabilitation system compared to usual care: arm/hand function in patients with stroke, traumatic brain injury and multiple sclerosis. *J Telemed Telecare*. 2008;14(5):249–256. https://doi.org/10.1258/jtt.2008.080104.

35. Ricker JH, Rosenthal M, Garay E, et al. Telerehabilitation needs: a survey of persons with acquired brain injury. *J Head Trauma Rehabil*. 2002;17(3):242–250. https://doi.org/10.1097/00001199-200206000-00005.

36. Tenforde AS, Borgstrom H, Polich G, et al. Outpatient physical, occupational, and speech therapy synchronous telemedicine: a survey study of patient satisfaction with virtual visits during the COVID-19 pandemic. *Am J Phys Med Rehabil*. 2020;99(11):977–981. https://doi.org/10.1097/phm.0000000000001571.

37. Stark S, Keglovits M, Arbesman M, et al. Effect of home modification interventions on the participation of community-dwelling adults with health conditions: a systematic review. *Am J Occup Ther*. 2017;71(2). https://doi.org/10.5014/ajot.2017.018887.

38. Ninnis K, Van Den Berg M, Lannin NA, et al. Information and communication technology use within occupational therapy home assessments: a scoping review. *Br J Occup Ther*. 2019;82(3):141–152. https://doi.org/10.1177/0308022618786928.

39. Cheng S, Lau R, Mak E, et al. Benefit-finding intervention for Alzheimer caregivers: conceptual framework, implementation issues, and preliminary efficacy. *The Gerontologist*. 2014;54(6):1049–1058.

40. Corti C, Urgesi C, Poggi G, et al. Home-based cognitive training in pediatric patients with acquired brain injury: preliminary results on efficacy of a randomized clinical trial. *Sci Rep*. 2020;10(1):1–15. https://doi.org/10.1038/s41598-020-57952-5.

41. Corti C, Poggi G, Romaniello R, et al. Feasibility of a home-based computerized cognitive training for pediatric patients with congenital or acquired brain damage: an explorative study. *PLoS One.* 2018;13(6):e0199001. https://doi.org/10.1371/journal.pone.0199001.

42. Kurowski BG, Wade SL, Kirkwood MW, et al. Long-term benefits of an early online problem-solving intervention for executive dysfunction after traumatic brain injury in children: a randomized clinical trial. *JAMA Pediatr.* 2014;168(6):523–531. https://doi.org/10.1001/jamapediatrics.2013.5070.

43. Zickefoose S, Hux K, Brown J, et al. Let the games begin: a preliminary study using Attention Process Training-3 and Lumosity™ brain games to remediate attention deficits following traumatic brain injury. *Brain Inj.* 2013;27(6):707–716. https://doi.org/10.3109/02699052.2013.775484.

44. Yurkiewicz IR, Lappan CM, Neely ET, et al. Outcomes from a US military neurology and traumatic brain injury telemedicine program. *Neurology.* 2012;79(12):1237–1243. https://doi.org/10.1212/WNL.0b013e31826aac33.

45. Martinez RN, Hogan TP, Lones K, et al. Evaluation and treatment of mild traumatic brain injury through the implementation of clinical video telehealth: provider perspectives from the Veterans Health Administration. *PM R.* 2017;9(3):231–240. https://doi.org/10.1016/j.pmrj.2016.07.002.

46. Olson S. *The Role of Human Factors in Home Health Care: Workshop Summary.* Washington, D.C: The National Academies Press; 2010.

47. Clement PF, Brooks FR, Dean B, et al. Supporting family members of people with traumatic brain injury using telehealth: a systematic review. *Behav Sci (Basel).* 2018;13(1):51–62. https://doi.org/10.1097/00001199-200206000-00005.

48. Teasdale TW, Engberg AW. Suicide after traumatic brain injury: a population study. *J Neurol Neurosurg Psychiatry.* 2001;71(4):436–440. https://doi.org/10.1136/jnnp.71.4.436.

49. Bahraini NH, Simpson GK, Brenner LA, et al. Suicidal ideation and behaviours after traumatic brain injury: a systematic review. *Brain Impair.* 2013;14(1):92–112. https://doi.org/10.1017/BrImp.2013.11.

50. Sharp IR, Kobak KA, Osman DA. The use of videoconferencing with patients with psychosis: a review of the literature. *Ann Gen Psychiatry.* 2011;10(1):14. https://doi.org/10.1186/1744-859X-10-14.

51. Al-Yawer F, Pichora-Fuller MK, Phillips NA. The Montreal cognitive assessment after omission of hearing-dependent subtests: psychometrics and clinical recommendations. *J Am Geriatr Soc.* 2019;67(8):1689–1694. https://doi.org/10.1111/jgs.15940.

52. Whitehouse KJ, Jeyaretna DS, Enki DG, et al. Head injury in the elderly: what are the outcomes of neurosurgical care? *World Neurosurg.* 2016;94:493–500. https://doi.org/10.1016/j.wneu.2016.07.057.

53. Gardner RC, Dams-O'Connor K, Morrissey MR, et al. Geriatric traumatic brain injury: epidemiology, outcomes, knowledge gaps, and future directions. *J Neurotrauma.* 2018;35(7):889–906. https://doi.org/10.1089/neu.2017.5371.

54. Cuthbert JP, Harrison-Felix C, Corrigan JD, et al. Epidemiology of adults receiving acute inpatient rehabilitation for a primary diagnosis of traumatic brain injury in the United States. *J Head Trauma Rehabil.* 2015;30(2):122–135. https://doi.org/10.1097/HTR.0000000000000012.

55. Narasimha S, Madathil KC, Agnisarman S, et al. Designing telemedicine systems for geriatric patients: a review of the usability studies. *Telemed J E Health.* 2017;23(6):459–472. https://doi.org/10.1089/tmj.2016.0178.

56. De Luca R, Bramanti A, De Cola MC, et al. Cognitive training for patients with dementia living in a Sicilian nursing home: a novel web-based approach. *Neurol Sci.* 2016;37(10):1685–1691. https://doi.org/10.1007/s10072-016-2659-x.

57. Velayati F, Ayatollahi H, Hemmat M. A systematic review of the effectiveness of telerehabilitation interventions for therapeutic purposes in the elderly. *Methods Inf Med.* 2020;59(2-03):104–109. https://doi.org/10.1055/s-0040-1713398.

58. Calabrò RS, Bramanti A, Garzon M, et al. Telerehabilitation in individuals with severe acquired brain injury rationale, study design, and methodology. *Medicine (Baltimore).* 2018;97(50):e13292. https://doi.org/10.1097/MD.0000000000013292.

59. Beit Yosef A, Jacobs JM, Shenkar S, et al. Activity performance, participation, and quality of life among adults in the chronic stage after acquired brain injury—the feasibility of an occupation-based telerehabilitation intervention. *Front Neurol.* 2019;10:1247. https://doi.org/10.3389/fneur.2019.01247.

60. Asemota AO, George BP, Cumpsty-Fowler CJ, et al. Race and insurance disparities in discharge to rehabilitation for patients with traumatic brain injury. *J Neurotrauma.* 2013;30(24):2057–2065. https://doi.org/10.1089/neu.2013.3091.

CHAPTER 6

Telerehabilitation in Cancer Care

Chanel Davidoff ▪ Susan Maltser

There are more than 16.9 million cancer survivors in the United States as of 2019 and the number is projected to reach to more than 22 million by year 2030,[1] with the global burden expected to rise to nearly 27 million by year 2040.[2] At the same time, the 5-year relative survival rate for all cancers combined continues to rise in the United States, which reflects the aging population, advances in treatments, and improvements in screening and detection.[3]

Research has demonstrated that cancer survivors experience a complex variety of functional impairments as a consequence of disease burden and treatment toxicity.[4] These impairments can lead to long-term functional decline, precipitate psychological distress, and negatively impact quality of life if left untreated. The growing number of elderly cancer survivors[5] highlights the need for better access to rehabilitative services,[6] as well as developing alternative models of care to overcome critical shortages of rehabilitation providers in order to improve outcomes in cancer patients.

Advances in technology have pushed the boundaries of medicine, shifting the way care is being delivered. Telemedicine uses a variety of technological applications to support clinical practice by enhancing communication and expanding accessibility. It has reached multiple medical disciplines and has recently expanded to the fields of oncology and rehabilitation, referred to as "teleoncology" and "telerehabilitation," respectively. This chapter discusses the practical applications of telerehabilitation in the rehabilitation of cancer patients with emphasis on impairment screening, diagnosis of complications, exercise considerations, symptom monitoring, and multidisciplinary collaboration.

The Current State of Cancer Rehabilitation

The term "cancer survivor" is defined by the National Coalition for Cancer Survivorship as individuals living with, through, and beyond cancer. Whether it is at the time of diagnosis, during active treatment, in remission, or nearing end-of-life, the cancer survivor experience encompasses the entire scope of the care continuum. As the number of cancer survivors continues to rise internationally, there is increased attention to the health and well-being of this population. Further, the prevalence of elderly cancer survivors (65 and older) currently reaches 60% of the cancer patients and is expected to increase respectively with the aging of the US population, significantly contributing to the number of expected survivors.[5]

Cancer survivors experience a variety of treatment or disease-related adverse effects at any point of their journey, which may disrupt essentially any organ system and manifest as profound physical impairments. Elderly survivors may have preexisting comorbidities with unique survivorship needs, further adding to the demand and complexity of care. To meet these demands, survivorship care models have shifted focus to a more holistic, patient-centered approach, providing comprehensive and multidisciplinary services to effectively address the needs of cancer survivors of all ages and stages of care. As a result, cancer rehabilitation has had increased recognition in light of the rising demands for screening, identifying, and mitigating potential side effects in individuals living with cancer. The field is supported by a growing body of research that has demonstrated the positive effects of cancer rehabilitation and physical activity on functional prognosis and cancer-specific mortality[7,8] as well as improvements in quality of life and reported pain scores.[9,10] For this reason, new comprehensive cancer rehabilitation care models are being implemented throughout the course of cancer treatment in efforts to optimize physical function and prevent disability among cancer survivors.[6]

Despite ongoing evidence demonstrating efficacy and safety of cancer rehabilitation, cancer patients continue to have unmet needs due to underutilization of services.[11] A study by Cheville et al. found that outpatient oncologists were less likely to address functional deficits such as gait or balance dysfunction.[12] The study underscores the importance of integrating cancer rehabilitation specialists into oncology care in order to properly screen for impairments and better identify rehabilitation needs before dysfunction escalates to disability. This evolving model of survivorship care has raised interest in improving health care delivery to allow for this integration to occur. One of those efforts involves incorporating telerehabilitation into traditional cancer care.

Teleoncology

Telemedicine was initially implemented in cancer care with the aim of redistributing the workforce of oncology specialists to areas that lack specific services. With immediate access to care, teleoncology can improve patient health outcomes, allowing for early detection of anticipated complications, decreased time and cost of transportation, lessened caregiver burden, and better adherence to therapies.[13]

The growth of teleoncology has resulted in multiple changes to cancer care as summarized in Table 6.1. Despite these benefits, the adaptation of telerehabilitation into clinical practice has remained a challenge as a result of clinical, technical, legal, and administrative consequences.[18]

Impact of COVID-19 on Cancer Care

In December 2019, the outbreak of the novel coronavirus Sars-CoV-2, referred to as COVID-19, resulted in a state of global emergency affecting over 200 countries and classified as pandemic by the World Health Organization (WHO).[19] This highly virulent disease characterized by rapid spread, multiorgan dysfunction, and varying degrees of illness[20] raised concern for those who are immunocompromised or have multiple comorbidities, such as individuals with active cancer.

Emerging evidence has shown that patients with cancer have an increased risk for contracting COVID-19[21] and, if infected, are more likely to develop severe symptoms (acute respiratory distress requiring ventilation)[22] with a higher 30-day mortality rate.[23] Government-mandated physical distancing, diversion of medical resources, lack of preparedness plans, and concern for inadvertently spreading infection made it increasingly difficult for cancer patients to receive care. Physicians were compelled to adapt to telemedicine models in an attempt to mitigate viral transmission and preserve health care resources while minimizing disruption of cancer care.

As a response to the COVID-19 pandemic, the US federal government set forth emergency waivers and stimulus packages to allow for ease of care delivery in the midst of a health crisis. Centers for Medicare & Medicaid Services (CMS) made several changes to improve virtual health care access by allowing more flexibility with regulations and better reimbursement rates.[24] These changes allowed for prompt adaptation of telemedicine in the setting of cancer care.

Similar to acute cancer management, rehabilitation and survivorship care services were significantly impacted as a result of the COVID-19 pandemic. Various cancer rehabilitation

TABLE 6.1 ■ **Telerehabilitation Interventions in Cancer Care.**[a]

Remote office visits	Primary oncologist meets with patients using synchronous (real-time communication) methods via telephone or virtual videoconferencing. Can reduce transportation costs and time. Extends services to rural sites.
Patient communication	The physician is able to communicate with patients asynchronously (in between visits) to transmit data such as lab results, images, and other reports, as well as answer patient inquiries and triage complaints.
Tele-education	Provides remote continuing education opportunities for rural oncology practitioners. Promotes multidisciplinary collaboration. For patients, virtual education sessions may include lifestyle modification, smoking cessation, psychosocial support, presurgical information sessions, wound care, and pre-habilitation.
Chemotherapy supervision	Wearable technologies such as heart monitors and skin sensors provide periodic monitoring of vital signs during active treatment.
Symptom monitoring	Mobile applications and portable interactive tools can provide more frequent engagement and monitoring of symptoms that may otherwise be overlooked and underdiagnosed.
Interprofessional care	Bundling of services such as radiology, pathology, oncology in a visit to enhance the patient experience and access to care in a timely manner with less frequent office visits.
Telegenetics	Provide virtual genetic counseling for patient and families to identify possible carriers. With telemedicine, more family members are able to be engaged in the visit.
Telepathology	Remote viewing of tissue pathology and cytology. Pathologists and cytologists do not have to remain onsite during long procedures, making them more available for remote reviewing of specimens in multiple sites. Can provide real-time feedback on molecular analysis and histochemical testing.
Clinical trial engagement	Extending access to those living in distant areas. Improve interest, eligibility, participation, engagement, adherence, and follow-up for clinical trials.
Multidisciplinary tumor board	Increase interprofessional participation in tumor board meetings by overcoming distance barriers. Facilitate engagement from multiple health professionals to discuss treatment plans for patients.
Telerehabilitation	Applications in acute rehabilitation and ambulatory rehabilitation clinics to provide remote and immediate communication with interdisciplinary teams, acute care specialties, and primary care providers[14] Functional assessment in the context of home environment Monitoring exercise tolerability and progress Web-based home exercise programs[15,16]

[a]Referenced from Sirintrapun and Lopez (2018).[17]

strategies used to screen, diagnose, and manage cancer-related impairments often require physical, in-person visits such as a physical evaluation of functional deficits, manual therapies for lymphedema, electrodiagnostic testing to investigate neurological symptoms, and various interventional procedures to address cancer-related pain. The benefits of these rehabilitation interventions had to be weighed against risk for contracting COVID-19, and although telerehabilitation has its setbacks, it offers an opportunity to meet the rehabilitative needs of patients living with cancer.

Evidence and Implications for Telerehabilitation in Cancer Management

Over the years, telerehabilitation has mostly existed in the context of neurological rehabilitation, providing remote therapies and monitoring progress in stroke patients.[25] In this setting, telerehabilitation was shown to be an effective, alternative way of providing therapy and improving patient outcomes after stroke.[26] Similar to stroke patients, physical activity levels in cancer patients are significantly reduced (33%–60% decline) after diagnosis, necessitating ongoing therapeutic intervention.[27]

The use of telerehabilitation services in cancer care remains limited. This can be attributed to the fact that, in general, exercise-based rehabilitation programs are not yet part of the standard of care for cancer patients, and, therefore, are not regularly recommended by oncologists.[28] Additionally, there may be hesitancy to refer a patient to remote rehabilitation programs versus supervised face-to-face programs due to the perceived fragility and medical complexity of this population. Nevertheless, there is emerging evidence to support the use of telerehabilitation in cancer rehabilitation as an effective, accessible, feasible, and cost-effective alternative to traditional care.

EFFICACY

Improvements in function, patient-reported symptoms, satisfaction surrounding care, and quality of life measures support the efficacy of telerehabilitation in oncology. About one-fifth of the elderly population undergoing chemotherapy can experience a decline in activities of daily living (ADLs).[29] Further, the functional decline trajectory in a patient with advanced disease in the last year of life is much steeper compared to other diseases.[30] Collaborative telerehabilitation, such as remote monitoring and web-based exercises, is useful in minimizing functional regression and improving overall functional capacity in cancer patients. These interventions have been successfully applied in individuals with advanced cancer[31] and those undergoing chemotherapy.[32] Additionally, the functional improvements derived from remote therapies have been shown to be maintained months after completion of a program.[25,27,33] Another advantage of telerehabilitation for the purpose of improving function is the ability to observe the home environment. By doing so, rehabilitation specialists can better assess equipment needs and address barriers to ADLs.

Despite improvements in treatments, cancer patients continue to experience a high symptom burden long after completing treatments.[34] Symptoms are highly variable, with the most common symptoms being pain, fatigue, and depression.[35] Due to the multifactorial nature of these symptoms, frequent assessment and patient engagement is imperative. A collaborative telerehabilitation care model with a principle physician, nursing staff, and therapists can be advantageous for making these assessments. These comprehensive and multidisciplinary assessments have resulted in improvements in pain and depression scores.[36] For patients undergoing chemotherapy, symptom monitoring can screen for toxicity-related side effects. Automated symptom monitoring and remote support in between follow-up visits has resulted in reduced symptom burden and improved symptom outcomes for patients undergoing chemotherapy.[37,38]

Telerehabilitation enhances the quality of care received by cancer patients. One metaanalysis by Chen et al. looked into the effect of telehealth interventions on quality of life and psychological outcomes in breast cancer patients and found that patients who received telehealth interventions had improved quality of life scores, less depression, and less perceived stress compared to usual care.[39] These results have been replicated in patients with head and neck cancer[40] who experience significantly reduced quality of life due to treatments resulting in facial disfigurement, speech complications, and swallowing dysfunction.[41]

Patient health care experience, including satisfaction with care, is a core focus of interest in medicine and is part of the Institute for Health Care Improvement "Triple Aim" initiative for optimizing health system performance.[42] As the use of telerehabilitation emerges in oncology, patient satisfaction outcomes assume the upmost importance in order to support and maintain delivery of care through these platforms. From a patient perspective, telehealth has been found to be well accepted and satisfactory due to its relative ease of use and ability to improve communication between providers.[43]

ACCESSIBILITY

According to the WHO, issues with treatment adherence in cancer care are multifaceted and often occur as a result of patient-related, condition-related, treatment-related, socioeconomic-related, and health system–related factors.[44] Patients with physical disability related to cancer benefit from easier access to care. Telerehabilitation addresses access barriers by providing opportunities to conduct visits and therapies remotely. Ease of follow-up with telerehabilitation also influences treatment and exercise adherence. Telerehabilitation appears to be an ideal solution to meet the accessibility needs of cancer patients by promoting compliance with clinic visits, exercise programs, and treatment regimens. For example, reducing the frequency of travel to treatment or clinic settings will not only improve follow-up compliance but also ease caregiver burden. Inconsistencies with medication administration due to the complexity of treatment or presence of uncontrolled side effects can be addressed through remote education and symptom monitoring.

From an exercise perspective, the ideal exercise program for this population is one that is well tolerated, safe, and sustainable. Telerehabilitation can improve adherence to exercise due to the inherent flexibility of delivering programs to best fit a patient's lifestyle. The added benefit of symptom monitoring can allow for exercise prescription adjustments based on tolerability.

FEASIBILITY AND SAFETY

Although telerehabilitation has been recognized as a valuable and effective method of delivering care, little is known about the feasibility of these interventions in clinical practice. A systematic review investigating the use of videoconferencing (a form of telemedicine) in clinical oncology supports the feasibility for assessing, monitoring, and managing oncology patients through this intervention.[45] In fact, patients with advanced cancer with moderate functional impairments were able to tolerate an individualized walking and resistance training program delivered via telephone for 6 months with good tolerability and no reported adverse events.[31] Other administrative, clinical, technical, and ethical-related factors need to be considered for delivering telerehabilitation services as outlined by the American Telemedicine Association.[46]

HEALTH CARE UTILIZATION AND COST-EFFECTIVENESS

The cost of cancer care in the United States is projected to increase by 34% by 2030 and is estimated to reach nearly $246 billion based on population aging and cancer survivor prevalence.[47] According to Commonwealth 2019 analysis of Organisation for Economic Co-operation and Development data, the United States spends nearly twice as much on health care compared to other high-income countries.[48] In the United States, health care costs are nearly four times greater compared to non-cancer cohorts,[49,50] especially in the elderly population[51] and those with more advanced disease.[52] It is difficult to compare health care utilization and hospital expenditures among individuals with cancer across nations given the heterogeneity of cancer cohorts, inconsistency with international data sources, and differences in health policies and payment models. With that being said, some data suggest that health care expenditures for individuals with cancer and nearing the end of life were highest in the United States, Norway, and Canada.[53]

Patients with advanced cancer may contribute to rising health care costs due to hospitalization readmissions and frequent emergency room visits for uncontrolled adverse symptoms and functional loss related to disease or treatments.[54] Telerehabilitation can be useful for facilitating transition care of cancer patients after hospitalization by providing a more suitable method of postacute care follow-up and ensuring rehabilitative services are in place. The results from the Collaborative Care to Preserve Performance in Cancer (COPE) trial support telerehabilitation and its efforts to reduce the economic burden of cancer by addressing pain and functional loss early on as a means to decrease hospital lengths of stay and restore function in this highly symptomatic population.[31]

Practical Applications of Telerehabilitation in Cancer Rehabilitation

Cancer rehabilitation has become an increasingly relevant field, playing an integral role in survivorship care. This section discusses the practical applications of telerehabilitation into the clinical practice of cancer rehabilitation such as addressing preexisting barriers, conducting virtual visits, and integration of a telerehabilitation model throughout the course of cancer care.

ADDRESSING CANCER REHABILITATION BARRIERS WITH TELEREHABILITATION

Despite all the benefits, expansion of cancer rehabilitation across diverse clinical settings has met considerable challenges. Current advocates of cancer rehabilitation have explored these barriers and suggested they may occur as a result of deficits in knowledge, access, and adherence.[55] The emerging use of telerehabilitation provides unique opportunities to overcome these barriers and enhance the impact of cancer rehabilitation in the field of oncology.

Knowledge barriers result from the lack of awareness of rehabilitative services by oncologists and patients, ambiguity of referral practices, and uncertainty of roles. Telerehabilitation can fill knowledge gaps by extending educational services from already established cancer rehabilitation programs to health systems, clinicians, and community clinics regarding current, evidence-based practices of the field.

Incorporating telerehabilitation services can relieve financial and time constraints associated with traveling and, as a result, relieve the burden of multiple clinic and therapy visits. Moreover, the cancer rehabilitation workforce has an exclusive presence in mostly large academic, tertiary care centers.[56] Telerehabilitation can be used to expand this limited workforce to serve in areas in need of such programs.

Lastly, other barriers to cancer rehabilitation fall under issues with adherence. Examples include patient motivation to participate, activity intolerance, and lack of support and oversight. Remote technology, such as the use of wearable sensors for activity tolerance,[57] mobile applications for symptom monitoring,[58] and web-based exercise programs[32] for support and accountability for home exercises, has been shown to address these issues and promote positive behavior change.

THE VIRTUAL VISIT: FROM CONSULTATION TO DISEASE MANAGEMENT

Virtual visits can be conducted synchronously (physician and patient engage in real-time communication via live video or audio platforms) or asynchronously (transmitting, reviewing, and storing clinical data such as images, results, or reports reviewed at later times).[17] Although in practice both approaches are used interchangeably, recent attention on telerehabilitation has focused on synchronous visits since they maintain the patient-physician relationship reminiscent of an in-person clinic visit. Maintaining good patient rapport is imperative in the cancer population as it facilitates an environment where patients feel comfortable asking questions and are open to reporting adverse symptoms.

The virtual visit, conducted through video interface, is essentially identical to in-person visits in terms of flow and content of the encounter, except the inability to use tactile techniques for a physical examination. Virtual adaptations to the conventional physical examination have been proposed in the setting of telerehabilitation in the outpatient setting that allow physicians to provide a comprehensive evaluation.[59] Physical examination of a patient with cancer may vary significantly depending on tumor type, stage, treatments endured, and presence of comorbidities. Although examination of multiple systems is critical in this population, the cancer rehabilitation evaluation tends to put more focus on neurological, musculoskeletal, and functional aspects of the examination. Table 6.2 provides examples of virtual examination modifications with respect to common cancer rehabilitation conditions. Table 6.3 describes various functional assessment scales and measurement tools that may aide in the virtual examination.

TABLE 6.2 ■ Addressing Common Cancer-Related Rehabilitation Conditions in the Virtual Visit

System	Specific Condition	Virtual Evaluation and Assessment Tools	Virtual Management and Follow-up Plan
Functional	General performance	KPS, ECOG	Communication with oncology regarding treatment plan, referral for nutrition for weight management, referral for pre-habilitation if indicated. Provide durable medical equipment (DME). OT and PT prescriptions
	Mobility	TUG test	
	Self-care and ADLs	Barthel index, home assessment	
Systemic	Cancer-related fatigue	BFI, FACIT-F	Education, exercise program, medications
	Dyspnea/ deconditioning	RPE, CDS	Rule out PE, metastasis. Refer to pulmonary rehabilitation and PFT measurements
Head and neck (H&N)	Trismus	Direct observation, mouth opening measurement (patient can use fingers and document in "finger breadths"). Inquire about food intake and weight loss.	Trismus exercises, referral to SLP, prescription for jaw stretching device
	Dystonia	Direct observation for muscle contraction, instruct patient to perform neck range of motion (ROM), and palpation of tender areas	Stretching exercises, evaluate for trigger point, and Botulinum toxin injections

(Continued)

TABLE 6.2 ■ **Addressing Common Cancer-Related Rehabilitation Conditions in the Virtual Visit—Cont'd**

Musculoskeletal	Bone metastasis	Assessment of new pain, observation of functional pain	Referral for imaging. Communication with primary oncology team. If known metastasis, referral for appropriate exercise interventions and bracing as needed. Orthopedic assessment for long bone metastasis
	Amputation	Wound inspection, ROM of limb, mobility observation	Therapy and prosthetic prescription
	Shoulder tendonitis	ROM, shoulder and arm special tests	PT prescriptions, medications as appropriate, referral for imaging if no improvement
	Adhesive capsulitis	Shoulder ROM, shoulder and arm special tests	PT prescriptions, medications, referral for injection as appropriate
	Myopathy	Direct observation for atrophy, strength testing with squat and wall push up	Review steroid use, PT prescriptions, DME as appropriate
	Post-mastectomy/ thoracotomy pain	Incision evaluation, assessment for scar dysfunction/pain, muscle atrophy observation, evaluate for axillary cording by instructing patient to palpate axilla	PT prescriptions, medications, and injection as appropriate
	Scapular winging	Direct observation of scapula and shoulder girdle during wall push up	PT prescription, referral for NCS/EMG as appropriate
Soft tissue	Lymphedema	Direct observation for edema, skin color, and texture. Measurement by patient comparing to contralateral limb if measuring tape available. Facial lymphedema in H&N cancer	Venous duplex as needed, prescription for manual lymphatic drainage (MLD) as needed, garment prescriptions
	Radiation fibrosis syndrome	Direct observation for atrophy, skin changes, muscle contraction, ROM restrictions. Progressive dysphagia in H&N cancer	PT prescriptions, medications, and injection as appropriate, bracing as appropriate. SLP for swallow dysfunction
	Graft vs. host disease	Assess for maculopapular rash, abdominal cramps with diarrhea	Refer to oncology for management

(Continued)

TABLE 6.2 ■ Addressing Common Cancer-Related Rehabilitation Conditions in the Virtual Visit —Cont'd

Neurological	Chemotherapy-induced peripheral neuropathy	Instruct patient to assess sensation and strength, CIPNAT, FACT/GOG-Ntx	Education on neuropathy, compensatory strategies, PT/OT prescription, bracing as needed, DME
	Compression neuropathy/plexopathy	Instruct patient to assess sensation and strength, special tests.	Education, referral for NCS/EMG, compensatory strategies, PT/OT prescription, bracing as needed, referral to surgery as needed
	Cognitive impairment	FACT-COG, MOCA, assess IADLs, home assessment	Referral to neuropsychology, compensatory strategies, medications when appropriate
	Speech and swallow dysfunction	Language evaluation, screen for dysphagia	Referral to speech and language pathology; consider imaging if symptom is new complaint

ADL, Activities of daily living; *BFI*, brief fatigue inventory; *CDS*, cancer dyspnea scale; *CIPNAT*, chemotherapy-induced peripheral neuropathy assessment tool; *ECOG*, Eastern Cooperative Oncology Group; *FACIT-F*, functional assessment of chronic illness therapy–fatigue scale; *FACT-COG*, functional assessment of cancer therapy–cognitive function; *FACT/GOG-Ntx*, functional assessment of cancer therapy/gynecologic oncology group neurotoxicity; *IADL*, instrumental activities of daily living; *KPS*, Karnofsky performance scale; *MOCA*, Montreal cognitive assessment; *NCS/EMG*, nerve conduction study/electromyography; *OT*, occupational therapy; *PE*, pulmonary embolism; *PFT*, pulmonary function tests; *PT*, physical therapy; *RPE*, rating of perceived exertion scale; *SLP*, speech language pathology; *TUG*, timed up and go.

TABLE 6.3 ■ Functional Assessment Scales and Measurement Tools for the Virtual Visit.[a]

Karnofsky performance scale (KPS)	Two widely used methods to measure the general performance of adult patients with cancer to perform ordinary tasks. Commonly used by oncologists to track performance changes with treatment[60,61]
Eastern Cooperative Oncology Group (ECOG) performance status	
Timed up and go (TUG) test	A timed measurement of balance and mobility to assess risk of falling. Has been shown to correlate with treatment-related functional decline in elderly adults with cancer[62]
Brief fatigue inventory (BFI)	A nine-item questionnaire to assess subjective fatigue. Shown to be a reliable, rapid tool to assess fatigue level in cancer patients[63]
Functional assessment of chronic illness therapy –fatigue scale (FACIT-F)	Self-reported questionnaire used to assess self-reported fatigue and anemia-related concerns for individuals with cancer[64]
Borg rating of perceived exertion scale (RPE)	Self-reported effort during physical activity. Can be used to assess issues related to cardiovascular capacity[65]
Cancer dyspnea scale (CDS)	Self-rated, 12-item scale to evaluate perceived dyspnea in cancer patients[66]

(Continued)

TABLE 6.3 ■ Functional Assessment Scales and Measurement Tools for the Virtual Visit.[a]—Cont'd

Barthel index (BI)	Self-reported or observed score assessing independence for activities of daily living[67]
Chemotherapy-induced peripheral neuropathy assessment tool (CIPNAT)	Self-reported questionnaire evaluating occurrence, frequency, severity, and distress of neurotoxicity symptoms and their impact on functional activities[68]
Functional assessment of cancer therapy/gynecologic oncology group neurotoxicity (FACT/GOG-Ntx)	An 11-item scale that addresses issues with neuropathy in the setting of chemotherapy and assesses level of impact on quality of life[69]
Functional assessment of cancer therapy–cognitive function (FACT-COG)	A 38-item questionnaire addressing cognitive impairment related to treatment[70]
Montreal cognitive assessment (MOCA)	A commonly used cognitive screening tool. Shown to be well tolerated in brain tumor population[71]

[a]Referenced from Gilchrist et al. (2009).[72]

Due to the complexity of an oncological examination, it is wise to first obtain a thorough history in order to guide the virtual examination appropriately. For example, knowing a patient underwent a mastectomy with subsequent treatment with taxane chemotherapy and radiation to the chest would direct the examiner to focus on the chest wall around the surgical site and area in field of radiation, extremities (especially the upper ipsilateral extremity for any range of motion restrictions), as well as a neurological examination (to assess for chemotherapy-related neuropathy).

RED FLAG SIGNS AND SAFETY CONSIDERATIONS

Even with a focused virtual examination, evaluators must be mindful of certain oncological "red flag" signs or symptoms that may suggest disease progression or worsening existing adverse effects. Evidence or endorsement of any red flag signs or symptoms listed in Fig. 6.1 should trigger prompt referral or close follow-up with a clinician in person.

Additionally, it is essential to consider patient ability and safety when performing a virtual examination, especially during ambulation and balance assessments. Given the safety concerns highlighted in Fig. 6.1, it is advised that the patient have supervision or assistance from a caregiver prior to performing the virtual examination. If assistance is unavailable, risky and technical examination maneuvers should be deferred until the patient is seen physically in the clinic.

TELEREHABILITATION MODEL FOR CANCER REHABILITATION

Essential components of cancer rehabilitation include identification of impairments, preservation of function, mitigation of adverse effects, promotion of physical activity, and coordination of care with essential health care providers. Cancer rehabilitation delivery models have evolved from shared-care and nurse-led delivery models[73] to the prospective surveillance model (PSM),[74] and, more recently, the impairment-driven model (IDM).[75]

Shared-care delivery occurs during the transition from active treatment to survivorship care in which there is a transfer of information from specialists to the primary care provider who then

Red Flag Signs

- New neurological changes
  - Bowel/Bladder dysfunction
  - New weakness
- Functional or nocturnal pain
- Swelling or redness
- New dyspnea on exertion or cyanosis
- New or progressive gait dysfunction
- New or persistent headaches
- New communication or swallow dysfunction
- New cognitive changes

Safety Considerations

- Impaired balance, coordination, sensation, or proprioception
- History of falls
- Cognitive impairments
- Weight bearing or ROM restrictions
  - Spinal, sternal, hip precautions from recent surgical procedure
- Orthostasis or autonomic dysfunction
- Lab abnormalities (cytopenias)

Fig. 6.1 Red flag signs and safety considerations in the cancer patient during a virtual visit.

assumes responsibility of the patient's needs moving forward.[73] Clinical nurses play a central role in the delivery of posttreatment care, including symptom management, psychosocial support, and advanced care planning. However, these earlier models are not widely implemented nowadays due to confusion regarding specific roles and responsibilities of providers.

Novel models have focused on the concept of early detection and prevention of impairments to counteract potential long-lasting dysfunction. The PSM has been developed and applied in the setting of breast cancer and is described as a proactive and comprehensive approach to early identification and management of physical impairments and promotion of health behaviors throughout the trajectory of care.[74] The PSM has been influential to the construct of the IDM, which offers similar goals to the PSM, but with the extended focus on screening for physical, cognitive, and psychological impairments that may further affect quality of life.[75]

Telerehabilitation builds on these previous models and functions as a tool to disseminate current rehabilitative services. The telerehabilitation model aims to improve access to rehabilitation specialists and facilitate ongoing rehabilitation support for cancer patients before, during, and after treatment. Fig. 6.2 depicts the telerehabilitation framework throughout the progression of care—at the time of diagnosis, during active treatment, or in a period of survivorship (includes those in remission or with advanced disease). The role of telerehabilitation during each stage is further divided into components for remote intervention, functional assessment, patient education, therapies, and interdisciplinary involvement. The table in Fig. 6.2 can be used as a guide to structure a telerehabilitation visit based on where the patient is on the continuum of care when they are referred for rehabilitation evaluation.

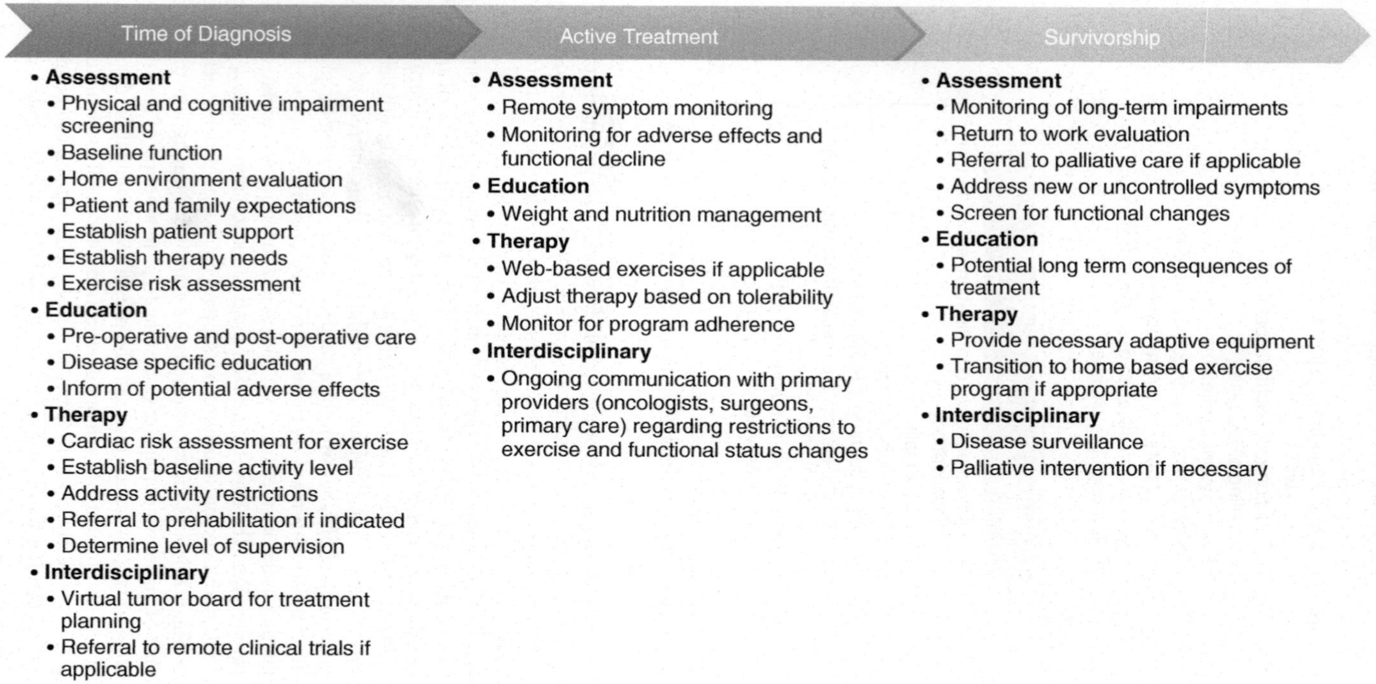

Time of Diagnosis

- **Assessment**
  - Physical and cognitive impairment screening
  - Baseline function
  - Home environment evaluation
  - Patient and family expectations
  - Establish patient support
  - Establish therapy needs
  - Exercise risk assessment
- **Education**
  - Pre-operative and post-operative care
  - Disease specific education
  - Inform of potential adverse effects
- **Therapy**
  - Cardiac risk assessment for exercise
  - Establish baseline activity level
  - Address activity restrictions
  - Referral to prehabilitation if indicated
  - Determine level of supervision
- **Interdisciplinary**
  - Virtual tumor board for treatment planning
  - Referral to remote clinical trials if applicable

Active Treatment

- **Assessment**
  - Remote symptom monitoring
  - Monitoring for adverse effects and functional decline
- **Education**
  - Weight and nutrition management
- **Therapy**
  - Web-based exercises if applicable
  - Adjust therapy based on tolerability
  - Monitor for program adherence
- **Interdisciplinary**
  - Ongoing communication with primary providers (oncologists, surgeons, primary care) regarding restrictions to exercise and functional status changes

Survivorship

- **Assessment**
  - Monitoring of long-term impairments
  - Return to work evaluation
  - Referral to palliative care if applicable
  - Address new or uncontrolled symptoms
  - Screen for functional changes
- **Education**
  - Potential long term consequences of treatment
- **Therapy**
  - Provide necessary adaptive equipment
  - Transition to home based exercise program if appropriate
- **Interdisciplinary**
  - Disease surveillance
  - Palliative intervention if necessary

Fig. 6.2 Applications of a telerehabilitation model through the cancer care continuum.

EXERCISE AND THERAPY RECOMMENDATIONS VIA TELEREHABILITATION

Exercise therapy in cancer is an extensive and emerging field within oncology. It is well established that cancer survivors benefit from physical activity, reflected in improvements seen in aerobic fitness, muscle strength, quality of life, and decreased fatigue.[76] Additionally, physical activity is shown to be effective in mitigating cardiorespiratory decline associated with cancer and its treatments.[77]

General exercise and rehabilitation guidelines for cancer survivors have been published by multiple national and international organizations. Notably, the recommendations established by the American College of Sports Medicine and other international stakeholder organizations recommend moderate intensity aerobic activity for at least 30 minutes a day and 3 days a week to achieve health-related benefits.[78]

The use of telerehabilitation for therapy purposes promotes and engages cancer survivors in physical activity by providing ease of access. Moreover, if safety is a concern, a telerehabilitation consult can be utilized for medical evaluation by rehabilitation health care professionals (physiatrists, physical therapists, exercise physiologists) prior to therapies to help determine the appropriate level of supervision and inform of any necessary precautions, modifications, or contraindications to exercise. Likewise, remote monitoring (via sensors, mobile application, or telephone inquiry) throughout participation in a program can address any issues related to tolerability, which can prompt necessary modifications.

Special Population Considerations

HEALTH CARE DISPARITIES

Differences in cancer prevalence, mortality, and cancer-related complications continue to exist despite advances in oncological management.[1] These health disparities in cancer survivors have been well established in the literature and are based on age, gender, racial/ethnic backgrounds, socioeconomic status, and geographic factors.[3,79,80] Additionally, there are disproportionately fewer cancer rehabilitation services received in low socioeconomic or minority groups, resulting in undertreated impairments.[4]

Telerehabilitation offers a promising opportunity to reduce disparities by overcoming barriers of access and communication with providers.[81] Extending remote access can increase participation of various patient populations in clinical trials, addressing disparities that exist in cancer and rehabilitation research. Although telerehabilitation aims to bridge the gap between health care disparities in cancer, consideration should be made regarding the inherent "digital divide" that telerehabilitation can potentially evoke.[82] In particular, demographics such as age, income, education level, and race have been linked to discrepancies with digital access and literacy.

ADVANCED DISEASE

Advanced cancer is defined as cancer that is unlikely to be cured or controlled with treatments.[83] The characteristics of patients with advanced cancer are considerably diverse, which can be distinguished by the burden of their disease (locally advanced or metastatic), functional performance status, or management plan (palliative vs. curative). As a result, patients with advanced cancer experience profound physical impairments and debilitating functional loss throughout their cancer trajectory. Notably, most advanced cancer patients have impairments that could be amenable to traditional rehabilitation, yet only a third of them receive appropriate care.[4] The goal of rehabilitation in advanced disease and end-of-life care is to attenuate functional decline, mitigate symptoms, reduce caretaker dependency, and preserve psychological well-being.[84] Rehabilitation is often integrated with palliative services in order to preserve physical and cognitive function, ease discomfort of symptoms, and provide emotional support as an individual approaches the end of life.

Telerehabilitation has been a promising intervention for this population, owing to improvements in pain, functional loss, and quality of life. Low-tech interventions such as telephone or web-based applications have been instrumental in addressing patient concerns of pain and function without the inconveniences of additional appointments. In the COPE trial mentioned earlier in this chapter, Cheville et al. concluded that individuals with advanced stage cancer were able to tolerate and even benefited from a telephonically delivered exercise instruction that consisted of a walking program and resistance training.[31] Telerehabilitation can serve as an adjunct to palliative services and provide patients and families additional support at home.

Recommendations

As the evidence for telerehabilitation continues to evolve, further research is warranted to evaluate cost-effective and practical methods of delivering rehabilitative cancer care. Efforts should be made to determine the impact of comprehensive telerehabilitation models on patient and system-based outcomes. Once established, future directions should consider the expansion of telerehabilitation services to all types and stages of cancer.

Conclusion

In summary, the application of telemedicine to cancer rehabilitation has been shown to be a feasible and effective way to deliver services to a population at risk for functional decline. The ability to engage with patients and families remotely has the potential to enhance patient satisfaction, ease caregiver burden, bridge health care disparities, and improve quality of life.

CASE REPORT

HISTORY OF PRESENT ILLNESS

A 71-year-old female presented with progressive left hemiparesis and fatigue. Imaging revealed two contrast enhancing lesions with surrounding edema in the right hemisphere (deep thalamic and basal ganglia into the right temporal lobe). She underwent a biopsy that was consistent with glioblastoma multiforme. She then completed a 6-week course of chemoradiation with temozolomide in early January. Treatment course was complicated by left lower extremity deep vein thrombosis during chemoradiation therapy, now on Xarelto. Two years later, she was noted to have worsening fatigue and left-sided weakness. Subsequent imaging demonstrated increased edema surrounding her tumor. As a result, her treatment regimen switched to Avastin.

She was referred to physiatry for left shoulder weakness and left upper extremity pain extending to her hand. Shoulder pain was exacerbated with movement noted during range of motion exercises with physical therapy.

On review of systems, she states that she is very fatigued from her treatments and has been sleeping more than usual. Family has noticed difficulty with short-term memory since completing radiation. She denies difficulty swallowing.

Functionally, she continues to have difficulty walking and requires minimum assistance for transfers, ambulation, and activities of daily living from her husband. She is able to take a few steps with a walker.

VIRTUAL EXAMINATION

Husband able to provide supervision and hands-on assistance during virtual examination as indicated.
    General appearance: Patient appears alert but fatigued
    Systemic: No distress. Breathing comfortably.

Neuro:
- Cognition: Alert, awake, and oriented to person, place, and time. Slow processing. Follows one-to two-step commands with moderate accuracy. Attention impaired due to fatigue.
- Speech: Hypophonic speech. Word finding difficulty. Naming, repetition, and comprehension intact.
- Cranial nerves: No facial asymmetry. Grossly, extraocular muscles appear intact with horizontal and vertical gaze.
- Strength: Left shoulder flexion and elbow flexion require assistance from husband. Elbow extension performed against gravity. Grip strength reportedly diminished. Spontaneous movement noted in left lower extremity although unable to perform against gravity.
- Sensation: Hyperesthesia throughout left upper extremity.
- Coordination: Performed with husband's assistance. Impaired finger to nose on left side.

Extremities: No swelling in upper or lower extremities.

Musculoskeletal: Decreased active range of motion of left shoulder, restricted <90 degrees with horizontal adduction, internal and external rotation.

Function: Unable to ambulate independently, requires minimum assistance from husband. Foot drop noted on left during attempted ambulation. Standing balance is fair and requires contact guard from husband.

Mood: Flat affect and guarded.

GENERAL PERFORMANCE

ECOG score 3—capable of only limited self-care; confined to bed or chair more than 50% of waking hours.

REHABILITATION ASSESSMENT AND PLAN

1. **Hemiparesis**—continue current home physical therapy. Prescribed left shoulder sling and instructed to wear during therapy. Prescription for ankle foot orthosis for left foot drop. Add occupational therapy to focus on activities of daily living and hand function. Follow-up to assess medical equipment needs.
2. **Shoulder pain likely due to hemiparesis**—prescribed lidocaine patch to left shoulder. Discussed sling use as above. Tylenol as needed for pain.
3. **Neuropathic pain**—begin gabapentin 300 mg at bedtime. Medication side effect profile reviewed, including drowsiness. Medication may also help with sleep.
4. **Fatigue**—provided patient and family education that fatigue is multifactorial resulting from radiation, chemotherapy, inactivity, and poor sleep. Discussed plan to add light activity in chair and to continue physical therapy. Optimizing sleep cycle to improve daytime fatigue. Provided brief fatigue inventory questionnaire and instructed to complete for baseline assessment.
5. **Cognitive dysfunction**—cognitive evaluation ordered. Discussed trialing a stimulant if there is no improvement.
6. **Follow-up**—instructed to follow-up in 4 weeks to assess functional progress and medication tolerance.

References

1. Miller KD, Nogueira L, Mariotto AB, et al. Cancer treatment and survivorship statistics. *CA Cancer J Clin.* 2019;69(5):363–385. https://doi.org/10.3322/caac.21565.
2. Bray F, Ferlay J, Soerjomataram I, et al. Global cancer statistics 2018: GLOBOCAN estimates of incidence and mortality worldwide for 36 cancers in 185 countries. *CA Cancer J Clin.* 2018;68(6):394–424. https://doi.org/10.3322/caac.21492.
3. American Cancer Society. *Cancer Facts & Figures.* American Cancer Society; 2020. https://cancer.org/content/dam/cancer-org/research/cancer-facts-and-statistics/annual-cancer-facts-and-figures/2020/cancer-facts-and-figures-2020.pdf.
4. Cheville AL, Troxel AB, Basford JR, et al. Prevalence and treatment patterns of physical impairments in patients with metastatic breast cancer. *J Clin Oncol.* 2008;26(16):2621–2629. https://doi.org/10.1200/JCO.2007.12.3075.

5. Parry C, Kent EE, Mariotto AB, et al. Cancer survivors: a booming population. *Cancer Epidemiol Biomarkers Prev.* 2011;20(10):1996–2005. https://doi.org/10.1158/1055-9965.EPI-11-0729.

6. Alfano CM, Cheville AL, Mustian K. Developing high-quality cancer rehabilitation programs: a timely need. *Am Soc Clin Oncol Educ B.* 2016(36):241–249. https://doi.org/10.1200/edbk_156164.

7. Marciniak CM, Sliwa JA, Patrick G, et al. Functional outcome following rehabilitation of the cancer patient. *Arch Phys Med Rehabil.* 1996;77(1):54–57.

8. Lemanne D, Cassileth B, Gubili J. The role of physical activity in cancer prevention, treatment, recovery, and survivorship. *Oncol (Williston Park).* 2013;27(6):580–585.

9. De Groef A, Penen F, Dams L, et al. Best-evidence rehabilitation for chronic pain part 2: pain during and after cancer treatment. *J Clin Med.* 2019;8(7):979. https://doi.org/10.3390/jcm8070979.

10. Reis AD, Pereira PTVT, Diniz RR, et al. Effect of exercise on pain and functional capacity in breast cancer patients. *Health Qual Life Outcomes.* 2018;16(1):58. https://doi.org/10.1186/s12955-018-0882-2.

11. Thorsen L, Gjerset GM, Loge JH, et al. Cancer patients' needs for rehabilitation services. *Acta Oncol (Madr).* 2011;50(2):212–222. https://doi.org/10.3109/0284186X.2010.531050.

12. Cheville AL, Beck LA, Petersen TL, et al. The detection and treatment of cancer-related functional problems in an outpatient setting. *Support Care Cancer.* 2009;17(1):61–67. https://doi.org/10.1007/s00520-008-0461-x.

13. Pennell NA, Dicker AP, Tran C, et al. mHealth: mobile technologies to virtually bring the patient into an oncology practice. *Am Soc Clin Oncol Educ B.* 2017;37:144–154. https://doi.org/10.1200/edbk_176093.

14. Song K, Khan F. Cancer rehabilitation during the COVID-19 pandemic: an overview of special considerations. *J Int Soc Phys Rehabil Med.* 2020;3(2):38. https://doi.org/10.4103/jisprm.jisprm_10_20.

15. Timmerman JG, Tönis TM, Wouters MWJM, et al. Towards cancer rehabilitation at home. Design of a telerehabilitation service for lung cancer patients. *J Thorac Oncol.* 2013. https://doi.org/10.1097/01.JTO.0000438438.14562.c8. Published online.

16. Galiano-Castillo N, Ariza-García A, Cantarero-Villanueva I, et al. Agreement between telerehabilitation involving caregivers and face-to-face clinical assessment of lymphedema in breast cancer survivors. *Support Care Cancer.* 2014;22(1):253–258.

17. Sirintrapun SJ, Lopez AM. Telemedicine in cancer care. *Am Soc Clin Oncol Educ Book.* 2018;38:540–545. https://doi.org/10.1200/edbk_200141.

18. Gogia SB, Maeder A, Mars M, et al. Unintended consequences of tele health and their possible solutions. Contribution of the IMIA Working Group on telehealth. *Yearb Med Inform.* 2016(1):41–46. https://doi.org/10.15265/iy-2016-012.

19. World Health Organization. Coronavirus Disease (COVID-19). *World Health Organization.* 2020. https://www.who.int/emergencies/diseases/novel-coronavirus-2019.

20. Guan W, Ni Z, Hu Y, et al. Clinical characteristics of coronavirus disease 2019 in China. *N Engl J Med.* 2020;382:1708–1720. https://doi.org/10.1056/NEJMoa2002032.

21. Yu J, Ouyang W, Chua MLK, et al. SARS-CoV-2 transmission in patients with cancer at a tertiary care hospital in Wuhan, China. *JAMA Oncol.* 2020;6(7):1108–1110. https://doi.org/10.1001/jamaoncol.2020.0980.

22. Liang W, Guan W, Chen R, et al. Cancer patients in SARS-CoV-2 infection: a nationwide analysis in China. *Lancet Oncol.* 2020;21(3):335–337. https://doi.org/10.1016/S1470-2045(20)30096-6.

23. Kuderer NM, Choueiri TK, Shah DP, et al. Clinical impact of COVID-19 on patients with cancer (CCC19): a cohort study. *Lancet.* 2020;395(10241):1907–1918. https://doi.org/10.1016/S0140-6736(20)31187-9.

24. Centers for Medicare & Medicaid Services. *Medicare Telemedicine Health Care Provider Fact Sheet.* Centers for Medicare & Medicaid Services; 2020. https://www.cms.gov/newsroom/fact-sheets/medicare-telemedicine-health-care-provider-fact-sheet.

25. Peretti A, Amenta F, Tayebati SK, et al. Telerehabilitation: review of the state-of-the-art and areas of application. *JMIR Rehabil Assist Technol.* 2017;4(2):e7. https://doi.org/10.2196/rehab.7511.

26. Cramer SC, Dodakian L, Le V, et al. Efficacy of home-based telerehabilitation vs in-clinic therapy for adults after stroke: a randomized clinical trial. *JAMA Neurol.* 2019;76(9):1079–1087. https://doi.org/10.1001/jamaneurol.2019.1604.

27. Irwin ML, Crumley D, McTiernan A, et al. Physical activity levels before and after a diagnosis of breast carcinoma: the health, eating, activity, and lifestyle (HEAL) study. *Cancer.* 2003;97(7):1746–1757. https://doi.org/10.1002/cncr.11227.

28. Silver JK, Stout NL, Fu JB, et al. The state of cancer rehabilitation in the United States. *J Cancer Rehab.* 2018;1:1–8.

29. Kenis C, Decoster L, Bastin J, et al. Functional decline in older patients with cancer receiving chemotherapy: a multicenter prospective study. *J Geriatr Oncol.* 2017;8(3):196–205. https://doi.org/10.1016/j.jgo.2017.02.010.

30. Teno JM, Weitzen S, Fennell ML, et al. Dying trajectory in the last year of life: does cancer trajectory fit other diseases? *J Palliat Med.* 2001;4(4):457–464. https://doi.org/10.1089/109662101753381593.

31. Cheville AL, Moynihan T, Herrin J, et al. Effect of collaborative telerehabilitation on functional impairment and pain among patients with advanced-stage cancer: a randomized clinical trial. *JAMA Oncol.* 2019;5(5):644–652. https://doi.org/10.1001/jamaoncol.2019.0011.

32. Ariza-Garcia A, Arroyo-Morales M, Lozano-Lozano M, et al. A web-based exercise system (e-cuidatechemo) to counter the side effects of chemotherapy in patients with breast cancer: randomized controlled trial. *J Med Internet Res.* 2019;21(7):e14418. https://doi.org/10.2196/14418.

33. Galiano-Castillo N, Arroyo-Morales M, Lozano-Lozano M, et al. Effect of an Internet-based telehealth system on functional capacity and cognition in breast cancer survivors: a secondary analysis of a randomized controlled trial. *Support Care Cancer.* 2017;25(11):3551–3559. https://doi.org/10.1007/s00520-017-3782-9.

34. Deshields TL, Potter P, Olsen S, et al. The persistence of symptom burden: symptom experience and quality of life of cancer patients across one year. *Support Care Cancer.* 2014;22(4):1089–1096. https://doi.org/10.1007/s00520-013-2049-3.

35. Carr D, Goudas L, Lawrence D, et al. Management of cancer symptoms: pain, depression, and fatigue. *Evid Rep Technol Assess (Summ).* 2002(61):1–5. https://doi.org/10.1037/e439612005-001.

36. Kroenke K, Theobald D, Wu J, et al. Effect of telecare management on pain and depression in patients with cancer: a randomized trial. *JAMA.* 2010;304(2):163–171. https://doi.org/10.1001/jama.2010.944.

37. Mooney KH, Beck SL, Wong B, et al. Automated home monitoring and management of patient-reported symptoms during chemotherapy: results of the symptom care at home RCT. *Cancer Med.* 2017;6(3):537–546. https://doi.org/10.1002/cam4.1002.

38. Kearney N, McCann L, Norrie J, et al. Evaluation of a mobile phone-based, advanced symptom management system (ASyMS©) in the management of chemotherapy-related toxicity. *Support Care Cancer.* 2009;17(4):437–444. https://doi.org/10.1007/s00520-008-0515-0.

39. Chen YY, Guan BS, Li ZK, et al. Effect of telehealth intervention on breast cancer patients' quality of life and psychological outcomes: a meta-analysis. *J Telemed Telecare.* 2018;24(3):157–167. https://doi.org/10.1177/1357633X16686777.

40. van den Brink JL, Moorman PW, de Boer MF, et al. Impact on quality of life of a telemedicine system supporting head and neck cancer patients: a controlled trial during the postoperative period at home. *J Am Med Inform Assoc.* 2007;14(2):198–205. https://doi.org/10.1197/jamia.M2199.

41. De Boer MF, McCormick LK, Pruyn JFA, et al. Physical and psychosocial correlates of head and neck cancer: a review of the literature. *Otolaryngol - Head Neck Surg.* 1999;120(3):427–436. https://doi.org/10.1016/S0194-5998(99)70287-1.

42. Institute for Healthcare Improvement. The IHI Triple Aim. http://www.ihi.org/Engage/Initiatives/TripleAim/pages/default.aspx; Accessed 15.09.20.

43. Kruse CS, Krowski N, Rodriguez B, et al. Telehealth and patient satisfaction: a systematic review and narrative analysis. *BMJ Open.* 2017;7(8):e016242 https://doi.org/10.1136/bmjopen-2017-016242. Published online 2017 Aug 3.

44. De Geest S, Sabaté E. Adherence to long-term therapies: evidence for action. *Eur J Cardiovasc Nurs.* 2003;2(4):323. https://doi.org/10.1016/S1474-5151(03)00091-4.

45. Kitamura C, Zurawel-Balaura L, Wong RKS. How effective is video consultation in clinical oncology? A systematic review. *Curr Oncol.* 2010;17(3):17–27. https://doi.org/10.3747/co.v17i3.513.

46. Richmond T, Peterson C, Cason J, et al. American Telemedicine Association's principles for delivering telerehabilitation services. *Int J Telerehabilitation.* 2017;9(2):63–68. https://doi.org/10.5195/ijt.2017.6232.

47. Mariotto AB, Robin Yabroff K, Shao Y, et al. Projections of the cost of cancer care in the United States: 2010-2020. *J Natl Cancer Inst.* 2011;103(2):117–128. https://doi.org/10.1093/jnci/djq495.

48. Tikkanen R, Abrams MK. U.S. Health Care from a Global Perspective, 2019: Higher Spending, Worse Outcomes? *The Commonwealth Fund.* https://www.commonwealthfund.org/publications/issue-briefs/2020/jan/us-health-care-global-perspective-2019; Accessed 02.11.20.

49. Park J, Look KA. Health care expenditure burden of cancer care in the United States. *Inquiry*. 2019;56: 1–9. https://doi.org/10.1177/0046958019880696.

50. Singleterry J. *The Costs of Cancer Care: Addressing Patient Costs*. American Cancer Society Cancer Act Network; 2017. https://www.fightcancer.org/sites/default/files/Costs of Cancer - Final Web.pdf.

51. Stafford RS, Cyr PL. The impact of cancer on the physical function of the elderly and their utilization of health care. *Cancer*. 1997;80(10):1973–1980. https://doi.org/10.1002/(SICI)1097-0142 (19971115)80:10<1973::AID-CNCR15>3.0.CO;2-V.

52. Price RA, Stranges E, Elixhauser A. *Cancer Hospitalizations for Adults, 2009: Statistical Brief #125*. Healthcare Cost and Utilization Project (HCUP) Statistical Briefs [Internet]. Rockville, MD: Agency for Healthcare Research and Quality (US); 2006. https://www.ncbi.nlm.nih.gov/books/NBK92614/.

53. Bekelman JE, Halpern SD, Blankart CR, et al. Comparison of site of death, health care utilization, and hospital expenditures for patients dying with cancer in 7 developed countries. *JAMA*. 2016;315(3): 272–283. https://doi.org/10.1001/jama.2015.18603.

54. Longacre CF, Nyman JA, Visscher SL, et al. Cost-effectiveness of the Collaborative Care to Preserve Performance in Cancer (COPE) trial tele-rehabilitation interventions for patients with advanced cancers. *Cancer Med*. 2020;9(8):2723–2731. https://doi.org/10.1002/cam4.2837.

55. Stubblefield MD. The underutilization of rehabilitation to treat physical impairments in breast cancer survivors. *PM R*. 2017;9(9):S317–S323. https://doi.org/10.1016/j.pmrj.2017.05.010.

56. Cheville AL, Mustian K, Winters-Stone K, et al. Cancer rehabilitation: an overview of current need, delivery models, and levels of care. *Phys Med Rehabil Clin N Am*. 2017;28(1):1–17. https://doi.org/10.1016/j.pmr.2016.08.001.

57. Shen J, Naeim A. Telehealth in older adults with cancer in the United States: the emerging use of wearable sensors. *J Geriatr Oncol*. 2017;8(6):437–442. https://doi.org/10.1016/j.jgo.2017.08.008.

58. Pennell NA, Dicker AP, Tran C, et al. mHealth: mobile technologies to virtually bring the patient into an oncology practice. *Am Soc Clin Oncol Educ B*. 2017;37:144–154. https://doi.org/10.1200/edbk_176093.

59. Verduzco-Gutierrez M, Bean AC, Tenforde AS, et al. How to conduct an outpatient telemedicine rehabilitation or prehabilitation visit. *PM R*. 2020;12(7):714–720. https://doi.org/10.1002/pmrj.12380.

60. Karnofsky D, Burchenal J. The clinical evaluation of chemotherapeutic agents in cancer. In: MacLeod CM, ed. *Evaluation of Chemotherapeutic Agents*. New York: Columbia University Press; 1949:196.

61. Oken MM, Creech RH, Tormey DC, et al. Toxicity and response criteria of the Eastern Cooperative Oncology Group. *Am J Clin Oncol*. 1982;5(6):649–655. PMID: 7165009. https://pubmed.ncbi.nlm.nih.gov/7165009/. Accessed October 24, 2020.

62. Verweij NM, Schiphorst AHW, Pronk A, et al. Physical performance measures for predicting outcome in cancer patients: a systematic review. *Acta Oncol*. 2016;55(12):1386–1391. https://doi.org/10.1080/028 4186X.2016.1219047.

63. Mendoza TR, Wang XS, Cleeland CS, et al. The rapid assessment of fatigue severity in cancer patients: use of the brief fatigue inventory. *Cancer*. 1999;85(5):1186–1196. https://doi.org/10.1002/(SICI)1097-0142(19990301)85:5<1186::AID-CNCR24>3.0.CO;2-N.

64. Butt Z, Shei Lai J, Rao D, et al. Measurement of fatigue in cancer, stroke, and HIV using the Functional Assessment of Chronic Illness Therapy - Fatigue (FACIT-F) scale. *J Psychosom Res*. 2013;74(1):64–68. https://doi.org/10.1016/j.jpsychores.2012.10.011.

65. Borg G. Psychophysical scaling with applications in physical work and the perception of exertion. *Scand J Work Environ Health*. 1990;16 suppl 1:55–58. https://doi.org/10.5271/sjweh.1815.

66. Tanaka K, Akechi T, Okuyama T, et al. Development and validation of the cancer dyspnea scale: a multidimensional, brief, self-rating scale. *Br J Cancer*. 2000;82(4):800–805. https://doi.org/10.1054/bjoc.1999.1002.

67. Mahoney FI, Barthel DW. Functional evaluation: the Barthel index. *Md State Med J*. 1965;14:61–65. PMID: 14258950. https://pubmed.ncbi.nlm.nih.gov/14258950/.

68. Tofthagen CS, McMillan SC, Kip KE. Development and psychometric evaluation of the chemotherapy-induced peripheral neuropathy assessment tool. *Cancer Nurs*. 2011;34(4):E10–E20. https://doi.org/10.1097/NCC.0b013e31820251de.

69. Calhoun EA, Welshman EE, Chang CH, et al. Psychometric evaluation of the Functional Assessment of Cancer Therapy/Gynecologic Oncology Group - Neurotoxicity (Fact/GOG-Ntx) questionnaire for patients receiving systemic chemotherapy. *Int J Gynecol Cancer*. 2003;13(6):741–748. https://doi.org/10.1111/j.1525-1438.2003.13603.x.

70. Jacobs SR, Jacobsen PB, Booth-Jones M, et al. Evaluation of the functional assessment of cancer therapy cognitive scale with hematopoietic stem cell transplant patients. *J Pain Symptom Manage.* 2007;33(1): 13–23. https://doi.org/10.1016/j.jpainsymman.2006.06.011.

71. Olson RA, Chhanabhai T, McKenzie M. Feasibility study of the Montreal Cognitive Assessment (MoCA) in patients with brain metastases. *Support Care Cancer.* 2008;16(11):1273–1278. https://doi.org/10.1007/s00520-008-0431-3.

72. Gilchrist LS, Galantino ML, Wampler M, et al. A framework for assessment in oncology rehabilitation. *Phys Ther.* 2009;89(3):286–306. https://doi.org/10.2522/PTJ.20070309.

73. Hewitt M, Greenfield S, Stovall E. *From Cancer Patient to Cancer Survivor.* Washington, DC: National Academies Press; 2005. https://doi.org/10.17226/11468.

74. Stout NL, Binkley JM, Schmitz KH, et al. A prospective surveillance model for rehabilitation for women with breast cancer. *Cancer.* 2012;118(suppl 8):2191–2200. https://doi.org/10.1002/cncr.27476.

75. Silver JK, Baima J, Mayer RS. Impairment-driven cancer rehabilitation: an essential component of quality care and survivorship. *CA Cancer J Clin.* 2013;63(5):295–317. https://doi.org/10.3322/caac.21186.

76. Fuller JT, Hartland MC, Maloney LT, et al. Therapeutic effects of aerobic and resistance exercises for cancer survivors: a systematic review of meta-analyses of clinical trials. *Br J Sport Med.* 2018;52:1311. https://doi.org/10.1136/bjsports-2017-098285.

77. Scott JM, Zabor EC, Schwitzer E, et al. Efficacy of exercise therapy on cardiorespiratory fitness in patients with cancer: a systematic review and meta-analysis. *J Clin Oncol.* 2018;36(22):2297–2304. https://doi.org/10.1200/JCO.2017.77.5809.

78. Campbell KL, Winters-stone KM, Wiskemann J, et al. Exercise guidelines for cancer survivors: consensus statement from International Multidisciplinary Roundtable. *Med Sci Sport Exerc.* 2019;51(11): 2375–2390. https://doi.org/10.1249/MSS.0000000000002116.

79. Dean LT, Gehlert S, Neuhouser ML, et al. Social factors matter in cancer risk and survivorship. *Cancer Causes Control.* 2018;29(7):611–618. https://doi.org/10.1007/s10552-018-1043-y.

80. Hendren S, Chin N, Fisher S, et al. Patients' barriers to receipt of cancer care, and factors associated with needing more assistance from a patient navigator. *J Natl Med Assoc.* 2011;103(8):701–710. https://doi.org/10.1016/S0027-9684(15)30409-0.

81. Gonzalez BD. Promise of mobile health technology to reduce disparities in patients with cancer and survivors. *JCO Clin Cancer Inform.* 2018;2:1–9. https://doi.org/10.1200/cci.17.00141.

82. van Dijk JAGM. Digital divide: impact of access. In: *The International Encyclopedia of Media Effects*; 2017. https://doi.org/10.1002/9781118783764.wbieme0043.

83. National Cancer Institute. Definition of Advanced Cancer - NCI Dictionary of Cancer Terms. https://www.cancer.gov/publications/dictionaries/cancer-terms/def/advanced-cancer; Accessed 26.10.20.

84. Cheville A. Rehabilitation of patients with advanced cancer. *Cancer.* 2001;92(suppl 4):1039–1048. https://doi.org/10.1002/1097-0142(20010815)92:4+<1039::AID-CNCR1417>3.0.CO;2-L.

CHAPTER 7

Telerehabilitation for Persons With Amputations

David Crandell

Introduction

Using telerehabilitation for the management of patients with limb loss and amputations enhances the care of a challenging patient population. This care may begin after an acute inpatient rehabilitation stay following an amputation or, just as importantly, as a presurgical virtual consultation. In either case, telerehabilitation can be a valuable initial phase of the rehabilitation process. Using available technology, telerehabilitation provides timely and quality clinical care that can improve the functional outcome of patients with limb loss throughout their lifespans. As with other diagnoses and other disciplines, telerehabilitation can also provide an opportunity to connect clinical experts to patients in more remote or underserved areas with a concomitant goal of reducing health care disparities.

Telerehabilitation advantages include (1) timely access to care, (2) improved clinical communication and transitions between locations of care, and (3) reduced or streamlined travel for patients with limb loss and mobility impairments and their families.[1] Telerehabilitation affords practicing clinicians an opportunity to observe how patients ambulate, navigate, and participate in activities of daily living (ADLs) in their homes. This provides essential information and improves recommendations for mobility equipment, assistive devices, and home environment modifications, to improve safety and facilitate greater independence. Prior to the use of telerehabilitation, this knowledge was only gained by performing house calls.

Patients can experience limb loss throughout their lifespan, and caring for the individual, not what is missing, is a core principle of amputee rehabilitation. Patients who experience an amputation present with many unique challenges beyond their respective limb loss. Most patients with lower-limb amputation have an expected impact on mobility. Upper limb loss can dramatically impact an individual's ability to perform ADLs and thus their overall independence and their ability to work and play. Unlike a traumatic amputation, a single or first amputation may be part of an ongoing pathophysiological process, leading to additional amputations and impairment. Medical management of comorbidities, for example, coronary heart disease, renal insufficiency, and neuropathies, is essential for the patients' overall health and for prevention of secondary amputations. Others who develop pain or skin issues may also require revision surgeries, restarting the preprosthetic rehabilitation process. The psychological loss experienced by these patients also needs acute management, counseling, and peer mentor support. Education throughout the rehabilitation process is key to a safe return to their community, work, and avocational pursuits. Due to many factors, including local environments, health care access, and the increase of individuals with diabetes mellitus, vascular disease, trauma, and cancer, the number of patients with amputations is expected to grow.

Although not unique to rehabilitation care, the interdisciplinary team plays an essential role in the management of the patient experiencing an amputation. For limb loss patients, the interdisciplinary team consists of a physiatrist, physical therapist (PT), occupational therapist (OT), and prosthetist. This team, along with the patient and family, should meet in real time to listen, examine, discuss, and plan the course of pre- and prosthetic rehabilitation. The interdisciplinary team can be expanded to include advanced practice providers (physician assistants/nurse practitioners), psychologists, case managers, surgeons, wound care nurses, engineers, and recreational therapists, as needed. Interdisciplinary team membership may change or shift over time to reflect the patient's needs and goals, and telerehabilitation can promote access to the required team as a foundation of the system of care.

Telerehabilitation Experience in a US Military/Veterans System of Care

In the United States, the health care system for the military, the largest national health care system in the country, encompasses all aspects of care for active duty members and veterans. With the possibility of both polytrauma—including traumatic amputations incurred as part of their service—and a lifetime that may include the development of dysvascular disease and complications of limb loss, the Veterans Administration (VA) and Department of Defense (DoD) have developed extensive clinical practice guidelines for the rehabilitation of individuals with lower-limb amputation.[2] This highly advanced and innovative care in amputation rehabilitation has included the use of a telerehabilitation approach in their amputee clinics model system of care for many years. VA-based telerehabilitation often focuses on advanced mobility training with an emphasis on community-based, adaptive sports and recreation involvement.

In 1998, a monthly clinic run by the Milwaukee VA team was developed in a rural medical facility 206 miles away from Milwaukee, Wisconsin (a larger city). The rural clinic was attended by a PT, a community prosthetist, and a patient. Physical examination, directed by the physiatrist in Milwaukee, was performed either by the PT or the prosthetist. Challenges included technical issues, such as broken video equipment resulting in clinic cancelation and relocation to a different building, and clinician difficulty with controlling a remote camera. The small clinic limited gait assessment and the echoing sound quality at times interfered with communication. Perhaps the greatest challenge felt by the clinician was in assessing skin conditions on the residual and intact limbs. Despite the challenges, the patient satisfaction survey indicated a high level of satisfaction.[3] The VA continued with early investigation, investment, and research that demonstrated that telerehabilitation can be effective and practical for many individuals. A 2004 study showed improved outcomes for veterans with lower-limb ulcers for whom trips to the clinic are too difficult.[4]

The VA's telehealth services have evolved with the mission to "provide the right care, at the right place and at the right time" and, through technology, meet the needs of those with limb loss. Since 2008 there has been steady growth in the VA's teleamputation services. The VA currently provides different types of teleamputation services with the interdisciplinary team amputee clinic as the most common. At the interdisciplinary amputee clinic provider site, the team is joined by the patient and a telepresenter who is at the patient site. The telepresenter is typically a PT or nurse, who assists in the telerehabilitation visit, by serving as the team's "hands", and supports the technical and administrative functions needed. Services provided can include the initial patient evaluation and follow-up visits, prosthesis(es) and rehabilitation prescriptions, new prosthesis "checkout" after delivery, and follow-up for comorbidities and complications involving the residual and/or unaffected extremities. Amputee support groups and direct peer support are also conducted under the structure of the VA telerehabilitation system.

Telerehabilitation in a Civilian Amputee Program: A Rapid Changeover Due to COVID-19

The Limb Restoration Program (LRP) based at Spaulding Rehabilitation Hospital (SRH) in Boston is a principal program of the Department of Physical Medicine and Rehabilitation (PMR) at Harvard Medical School. As a free-standing, inpatient rehabilitation facility, SRH admits new patients with limb loss from tertiary acute care hospitals in the city, region, nation, and internationally. Patients receive early postoperative rehabilitation including postoperative wound care, edema control, and residual limb shaping. Patients participate in preprosthetic training with several hours of intensive PT and OT daily. Amputee education, psychological counseling, and dispositional planning are all components of the program. Upon successful completion of the inpatient stay, patients return for follow-up in the Limb Restoration Clinic (LRC) after several weeks. This postdischarge visit allows the clinical team to evaluate residual limb healing and ongoing rehabilitation training needs. In consultation with their surgeons, the readiness to begin the prosthetic phase of their rehabilitation is determined and initial prosthetic prescriptions generated. Patients return to the LRC for prosthetic checkout once they have received their prosthesis to confirm proper fit and function before initiating prosthetic therapy training.

The success of the LRP within the amputee system of care is directly linked to visits to the LRC, held weekly. Here, in a first-floor clinic space with one large examination room outfitted with a set of parallel bars and a wall-length mirror, as well as an adjoining consultation room, a meaningful therapeutic milieu is established to enable outpatients to be seen in follow-up. Additionally, new inpatient amputees can meet prospective prosthetists, and all patients can learn about adaptive sports and ongoing research activities with the LRP. The LRC typically work with 10 or 12 patients in a half-day session, requiring a high level of administrative coordination amongst the patients and their respective prosthetists. This physical setting has historically and practically allowed decision-making with the patient, physicians, therapists, and prosthetists in real time to establish the "gold standard of interdisciplinary care." The timing of the LRC is also linked to a monthly amputee support group for both inpatients and outpatients.

Despite the relative satisfaction of all participants in the LRC, several gaps and challenges in the delivery of "pre-telerehabilitation" amputee care have been identified. For example, not all patients live locally; some live outside the state or country. It is sometimes "too long a drive" to get to the LRC, and the hospital is not fully accessible by public transportation. The LRC is not available every day of the week, so scheduling conflicts arise, especially for patients on hemodialysis. The LRC works with a number of community-based prosthetists who are strongly encouraged to free up time in their busy offices to attend the clinic. If the clinic starts running behind, or if the patient cancels at the last minute, prosthetist team members may be frustrated with the loss of operational efficiency. Some patients simply cannot participate in the LRC. Patients who are acutely hospitalized in referring institutions are not currently able to access the LRC for valuable presurgical consultation, and so they miss out on postsurgical rehabilitation planning and expectation management.

The global health care response to COVID-19 led to accelerated adoption of telerehabilitation worldwide and at SRH. During the early "shutdown," with no weekly typical LRC possible, managing the amputee patients changed "as we knew it." Patients' appointments had to be canceled, prescriptions for prostheses were put on hold, and patients could not be evaluated for therapy needs. The impact on the amputee inpatients was also significant, including the prohibition of family visits and training, no amputee peer visitation, and elimination of the monthly amputee support group. Having an established hospital network telehealth system operational for several years, virtual visits allowed the LRP to quickly pivot to embrace telerehabilitation.

Without the ability to have scheduled outpatients come to the hospital, the LRC quickly became fully virtual. Patients were seen in their homes with the use of their computers, smartphones, and occasionally, the smartphones of their visiting nurses or therapists. Each patient's respective prosthetist was able to join the interdisciplinary telerehabilitation visit according to a published schedule. Initially the number of patients scheduled was reduced out of caution, but this was quickly advanced as the team gained experience, which allowed patient volume to closely match pre–COVID-19 numbers. The conversion of the LRC to a telerehabilitation model did require enhanced coordination with regular preclinic communication among the interdisciplinary team members. This allowed the LRC to run on schedule and ensure timely connections with patients and providers.

Later in the spring of 2020, with overall improvements in the local COVID-19 response, universal mask usage, and a decrease in community viral spread, the hospital was able to reopen clinics to outpatients. The LRC team was able to triage during preclinic meetings to determine which patients should be seen in person and which patients could continue to be seen virtually. In-person visits continued to have all prosthetists participate virtually (which continued in 2021). Other hybrid versions of the telerehabilitation visits included clinic visits with the patient attending outpatient therapy sessions and/or visits to their prosthetist's office. These hybrid models have continued since then (Fig. 7.1).

Early amputee telerehabilitation observations included patient satisfaction with regular follow-up during the pandemic. Patients reported being very comfortable and happy to see the team and their prosthetists virtually "on the computer" and to know that everyone was working together. Seeing patients in clinic, at their therapy sessions, and/or at the prosthetist's offices allowed for the direct observation of the patient's gait. The prosthetists also acknowledged improved satisfaction when they were able to sign in and out of clinic while in their respective offices. Thus

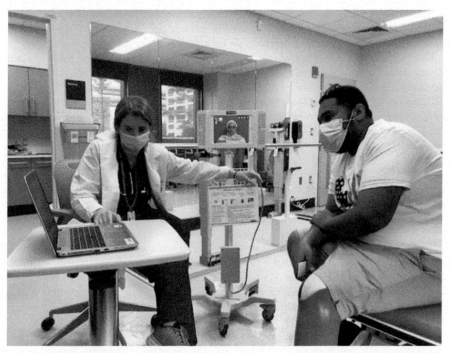

Fig. 7.1 Hybrid telerehabilitation clinic. An international patient present in the limb restoration clinic utilizing telerehabilitation for real-time interactions with their prosthetist (off-site) and an interpreter (off-site).

telerehabilitation created less work disruption for them, with improved efficiency as they avoided unnecessary trips to the hospital when the patient canceled at the last moment.

Delivering on some of the LRP core components affecting the new amputee inpatients also required telerehabilitation solutions during the pandemic. Early challenges to family training were solved by a hospital-wide initiative utilizing iPads and staff to directly connect during dedicated training sessions with therapy and nursing. After an initial delay, amputee peer mentoring visits were reestablished virtually, utilizing this SRH system or the patient's own smart phone. Formerly, inpatient amputees had learned about the different prosthetic companies in the community and had the ability to meet with multiple local prosthetists in person, as a meet-and-greet activity. This LRP component has slowly been converted to online introductions.

PRACTICALITIES OF TELEREHABILITATION WITH AMPUTEE PATIENTS

A targeted physical examination should be considered an essential element of any telerehabilitation visit.[6] Being able to perform a virtual physical examination and gait analysis on a patient with limb loss is helped if a structured evaluation is incorporated. This includes a general survey of the residual limb: level of amputation, residual limb length, shape, surgical incision, skin grafting, wounds, and examination of the contralateral limb (Box 7.1). Assessing both upper and lower limb strength can be done with provider-directed techniques.[7] There should also be enough room to permit gait assessment with a full body view of the patient walking, with or without a device, both toward and away from the camera. A family member at home or the prosthetist in their office controlling the camera placement is typically needed.

The examination of common bony pressure areas, sensory loss, and vascular status, other than skin color or wound status, poses practical telerehabilitation challenges. If the patient has difficulty

---

BOX 7.1 ■ Amputee Telerehabilitation Structured Evaluation

General survey of the residual limb
  Level of amputation
  Residual limb length (affects prosthetic fitting), shape (bulbous/conical)
  Surgical incision healing, retained staples or suture, redness
  Skin grafting, scarring, adherence (patient self-test)
  Wounds (observe removed dressings or socks)
  Vascular status: color, warmth (patient or other to test)
  Prosthetic concerns: bony prominences, limited soft tissue coverage
General survey of the contralateral limb
  Wounds, color
Lower limb strength
  Residual limb: hip extension/abduction, knee flexion/extension
  Contralateral limb: as above, plus ankle dorsiflexion/plantar flexion/inversion/eversion
Upper limb strength
  Shoulder depression, pectoralis, and latissimus
  Elbow flexion/extension
  Hand or partial hand grip strength
  Hand dexterity (observe for any intrinsic muscle atrophy)
Range of motion
  Bilateral hips: flexion, extension, abduction
  Bilateral knees: flexion, extension
  Partial feet: dorsiflexion, plantarflexion, inversion, eversion
Gait assessment in both directions, coming and going, with or without devices and/or assistance

donning or doffing their prosthesis, the prosthesis does not fit, or the patient is immobile (without a set of parallel bars and skilled PT), then the gait and/or functional mobility assessment may not be possible. The inability to solve prosthetic fit issues in person, such as adjusting the patient's prosthesis length or alignment, can also limit the practicality of the telerehabilitation visit. Capturing still photographs during the virtual physical examination and videos during the gait assessment, and uploading this data into the electronic medical record directly can improve the patient's documentation and be a key quality and functional measure of the patient's longitudinal care.

FUTURE CLINICAL AND RESEARCH RECOMMENDATIONS

An important component of rehabilitation is providing specialized training for new amputees to learn to use their prostheses correctly and safely. At Spaulding, the therapy Boost program was established in 2019 to meet these needs, and to give timely and intensive upfront prosthetic training as a group to boost the transition to more customary outpatient physical and occupational therapy, including some small bootcamp-style group exercise sessions. This highly successful program was paused during the COVID-19 pandemic. As the program was able to reopen gradually with a reduced number of participants due to the need for social distancing, the original design was modified to encompass a more one-on-one model, still meeting the needs of the patients while preserving the group-inspired workout motivation. Moving forward, the Boost program is looking to include telerehabilitation Peloton-like sessions where patients can log on from home or potentially in small groups at therapy facilities within the SRH network.

The incidence of patients with upper-limb amputation or loss is significantly lower than lower-limb amputations. There is limited experience among OTs and prosthetists, even in Boston where the level of surgical expertise is high, including partnering institutions performing a number of hand transplantations. After initial fitting and training, many patients require specialized therapy and support before they can fully integrate the new devices into daily routines.[8] Some advanced prosthetic technologies can be challenging to even experienced OTs who may have never worked with a specific novel prosthetic device. Telerehabilitation has been utilized to bridge this gap in our program, allowing timely and regular remote consultations to occur between our therapist and a regional subspecialized OT who is also a prosthetic expert and upper extremity amputee. The subspecialized OT, who has given in-person training to our occupational therapy staff in the past, is now able to offer this training virtually to increase the level of local expertise with our institution.

In light of the benefits of telerehabilitation, physiatrists, OTs, and PTs should have the orientation, education, training, and continuing education to ensure that they have the necessary competencies for the efficient and quality provision of telerehabilitation services.[9] Telerehabilitation training is important for rehabilitation professionals and should be incorporated into educational programs for therapists and PMR residents. Moreover, similar educational training should be available to clinicians already in practice, and the efficacy of this training should be evaluated.

In summary, the use of telerehabilitation can improve the quality of amputee rehabilitation care and patient satisfaction whether in the hospital, home, therapy gym, or prosthetist's office. Telerehabilitation can facilitate the interdisciplinary teamwork required to manage amputee patients effectively, albeit not exclusively.

Telerehabilitation can also help meet the needs of the growing amputee rehabilitation population and is essential to respond to changing needs of the patients and their environment locally, nationally, and internationally.

CASE STUDY

Mr. V has been followed in the LRP for the past 2 years. He is an 80-year-old retired truck driver with a number of comorbidities (diabetes, hypertension, and advanced peripheral arterial disease). Despite multiple revascularization surgeries, he developed acute left lower-limb ischemia, resulting in the need for a left below-knee amputation. Unfortunately, soon after his surgery, his residual limb developed distal ecchymosis and blister formation consistent with a failure to heal requiring a left above-knee amputation (AKA) on February 14, 2019. He was admitted to the inpatient amputee rehabilitation program at SRH several days later.

Four months later, after initial success with his left AKA rehabilitation, Mr. V developed right-sided critical limb ischemia due to a thrombosed right femoral artery bypass. With no revascularization options, he underwent a right AKA. His warfarin was discontinued as his right leg grafts were removed with the amputation. He was readmitted for interdisciplinary amputee rehabilitation, now as a bilateral AKA. At the time of his discharge a few weeks later, he required contact guard assistance to transfer to a wheelchair.

Several weeks later Mr. V was accompanied by his daughter to his postdischarge LRC visit. He had been at home receiving services, including a home health aide two times/week to help primarily with bathing. He had no recorded falls and used a bedside commode for toileting. He was experiencing phantom pain in his right AKA, taking Gabapentin three times per day as well as Tramadol, as needed.

Mr. V was followed closely and he remained interested and motivated in moving forward with prosthetic rehabilitation despite his age and the energy requirements needed to walk with bilateral, high-level amputations. At 1 year from his initial amputation, he was successfully fitted with bilateral AKA prostheses and was able to stand in the parallel bars in the clinic. He was admitted again to the inpatient program for 2 weeks of intensive gait training and was discharged home walking with assistance during the first week of March 2020.

Having successfully completed his intensive inpatient gait training with his bilateral AKA prostheses in March 2020, Mr. V was to continue with outpatient physical therapy two times per week. Unfortunately, due to initial COVID-19 restrictions, this plan for outpatient therapy was unavailable. He was limited to the exercises that PT had given him during his hospitalization.

At his first postdischarge telerehabilitation virtual visit in April 2020, Mr. V reported that without therapy, he had a significant increase in pain in both thighs throughout the day and this was worse when he was sitting in the wheelchair. Due to the pain in his thighs and worsening phantom pain, he had not been wearing his prostheses. This did not happen during his recent inpatient stay. He had been able to wear his prosthetic liners and noted a slight decrease in pain when he put them on. As this was his first telerehabilitation visit, the telerehabilitation setup in his home did not allow the full team to evaluate him with his prostheses on and walk.

Two weeks later, a second telerehabilitation visit was conducted. Mr. V reported that his pain was better with an increase in his Gabapentin (prescribed during his last telerehabilitation visit). He had been able to walk approximately 50 steps during the past week when his PT was able to come to his house. The interdisciplinary team was able to perform a physical examination with the help of family members positioning a phone. This revealed no skin or prostheses issues. The team was also able to observe his gait with both prostheses and using a rolling walker with family providing contact guard assist. He was very happy about walking and hoped to break his record for steps during his next PT session.

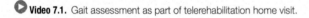 **Video 7.1.** Gait assessment as part of telerehabilitation home visit.

References

1. Scholten J, Poorman C, Culver L, et al. Department of Veterans Affairs Polytrauma Telerehabilitation: twenty-first century care. *Phys Med Rehabil Clin N Am.* 2019;30(1):207–215.
2. Amputation Clinical Practice Guidelines. Dept of Veterans Affairs, D. of D. VA/DoD Clinical Practice Guideline for Rehabilitation of Individuals with Lower Limb Amputation. 2017. https://www.healthquality.va.gov/guidelines/Rehab/amp/.
3. Kosasih JB. Challenges in telemedicine prosthetic clinic. *Am J Phys Med Rehabil.* 2005;84(3):205.
4. Rintala DH, Krouskop TA, Wright JV, et al. Telerehabilitation for veterans with a lower-limb amputation or ulcer: technical acceptability of data. *J Rehabil Res Develop.* 2004;41:481–490.
5. Prvu Bettger J, Thoumi A, Marquevich V, et al. COVID-19: maintaining essential rehabilitation services across the care continuum. *BMJ Global Health.* 2020;5:e002670.

6. Benziger CP, Huffman MD, Sweis RN, et al. The telehealth ten: a guide for patient-assisted virtual physical examination. *Am J Med*. 2021;134(1):48–51.
7. Laskowski ER, et al. The telemedicine musculoskeletal examination. *Mayo Clin Proc*. 2020;95(8): 1715–1731.
8. Whelan LR, Wagner N. Technology that touches lives: teleconsultation to benefit persons with upper limb loss. *Int J Telerehab*. 2011;3(2):19–21.
9. Brennan D, et al. A blueprint for telerehabilitation guidelines. *Int J Telerehab*. 2010;2(2):31–34.

CHAPTER 8

Telerehabilitation in Burns

Katherine Grace Siwy ■ Andria Martinez ■ Jeffrey C. Schneider

Telerehabilitation

Burn rehabilitation focuses on maximizing patient outcomes and ensuring that patients achieve as many functional goals as possible. Rehabilitation of the burn patient encompasses positioning and orthosis management, scar management, exercise prescription, education, and management of symptoms that impair function.[1] These areas of burn care can be further divided in subcategories; positioning and orthoses prescription for specific parts of the body, pressure therapy, scar mobilization, endurance and strength training, and formal education on patient needs. Customarily, burn rehabilitation is performed via in-person sessions with immediate feedback and information exchange between the patient and provider.[1]

The evolution of technology has equipped health care providers with the tools to provide high-quality care via telehealth. The burn care field has widely adopted the many types of telehealth to deliver specialty care to patients for reasons such as distance, pandemics, limited access, and cross communication with the medical system at large.[2,3] Telehealth has demonstrated its value over time and has shown that it can be a critical tool that can positively impact patient outcomes. This is especially true for telerehabilitation. Utilization of tele-burn rehabilitation significantly decreased outpatient visits, improved quality of treatment for smaller burn injuries, improved care for major burn injuries, and allowed for allocation of burn resources across the entire continuum of care.[4,5] Telerehabilitation has demonstrated its ability to parallel in-person therapy sessions due to its versatility and availability.[2,3] Comparable supporting data regarding quality and success of tele-burn rehabilitation has been shown within the literature.[4,5]

The use of telehealth as a means of impactful service delivery has been well documented in the literature since as early as the 1990s across many domains of health care, including neurology, cardiology, trauma, critical care, and diabetes.[5,6] A literature review demonstrates the utilization of tele-burn rehabilitation since 1999, however with limited subjects.[5] Tele-burn rehabilitation was initially utilized to drive specialized service delivery to rural areas in the form of follow-up visits with synchronous videoconferencing when possible.[7-10] However, subsequently tele-burn rehabilitation has expanded from follow-up visits to include evaluations and therapy interventions from many specialized burn disciplines.

Moreover the literature has demonstrated positive outcomes for patient satisfaction, travel reduction, decreased cost, and increased specialized services for patients who live in rural areas or at longer distances from a burn center.[6,11] Studies have shown cost savings in travel for patients living greater than 2 miles from the medical center. Studies also suggest improved access for those patients with limited mobility or access to transportation. Time efficiencies were also shown allowing maximizing effectiveness of time spent with visits as well as early discharge, allowing more open beds for greater inpatient volume.[11] It should be noted that at this time, literature has not been published that demonstrates the longitudinal efficacy and impact of tele-burn rehabilitation to this special patient population. Additionally the overall impact of successful patient outcomes specific to modalities across all burn care domains has not been shown. Nonetheless, as the expansion of technology reaches new heights, the burn care field continues to increase its capabilities to meet new challenges and progress patient outcomes.

When conducting a patient tele-burn rehabilitation visit, it is important for the provider to have access to the medical record and perform a thorough chart review prior to rehabilitative sessions. Relevant documents to review prior to tele-burn appointments include, but are not limited to, surgical, psychology, inpatient and outpatient occupational and physical therapy notes, physiatric, diagnostic testing, and imaging results.[3] The patient's identity should be confirmed at the start of each visit, especially with new patient evaluations. Patient identity can be confirmed by photo ID, more formally by government-issued photo ID, or by verbal confirmation of full name and date of birth.[2] The name and credentials of the clinician should be provided to the patient.[2,12]

There are a variety of platforms currently in use for conducting telehealth sessions. The technology platform being used should comply with and observe the Guidelines for Health Insurance Portability and Accountability Act, institutional regulations, and relevant federal, state, and local laws and regulations.[2,3,13,14] During public health emergencies in many locales, clemency has been given for providers to utilize communication technologies such as FaceTime, Google Chat, or Skype.[3] Outside these times, however, it is of paramount importance to use secure communication, abating third-party risk. It is also important to consider use of a landline versus a mobile device and WiFi versus use of a public network. Sufficient bandwidth to allow for unmistakable visualization and assessment of burn wound and skin graft presentation, range of motion, and compensatory patterns with movement and activity is desirable. Insufficient, unreliable bandwidth may interfere with the ability to effectively conduct telehealth consultations.[12,13]

Licensure is another important consideration for burn clinicians because states vary in privileging, credentialing, licensure, and practice standards. While there may be emergency and enhanced licenses issued to allow clinicians to provide care to patients in differing states from where their licenses have been issued, therapists should ensure that they do not have any licensing restrictions prior to conducting a telerehabilitation session with an out-of-state patient.[12,13] Burn clinicians should also be knowledgeable about their own liability insurance to be in compliance with state licensing and professional board regulations. Additional malpractice insurance should be added if there are restrictions in coverage.[12–14]

Practice

USE OF TELEREHABILITATION FOR INITIAL CONSULTATION PURPOSES

Tele-burn rehabilitation for initial consultations should include clinical reasoning, client occupations, client factors, performance skills, and patterns.[15] Burn clinicians should consider the reliability and applicability of objective measures to the telehealth service delivery model. When utilizing assessment measures, documentations should include modifications and location as these will need to be factored into results.

While the logistics and workflow for telerehabilitation visits vary depending on the software platform utilized, telerehabilitation visits can be broken into three parts: before the visit, during the visit, and after the visit.[3]

Before the Visit

"Before the visit" comprises three elements: (1) identifying or recruiting patients; (2) scheduling the patient; and (3) a test call with the patient.[3]

Identifying Appropriate Patient

Criteria for patient referral to a verified burn center by the American Burn Association should be contemplated when identifying the appropriate patient for telehealth visits. Client factors such as age, physical considerations, context, and environment should be taken into consideration. Moreover, providers need to consider attention span, memory, perception, cognitive levels, and patient temperament, as well as patient vision, hearing, medical history, and current limitations of body structures when evaluating and choosing appropriate patients to utilize tele-burn rehabilitation as a service delivery model.

Scheduling the Patient

Tele-burn rehabilitation visits can be scheduled by a facility scheduling department, by a therapist via phone conversation, or by a web-based scheduling application with synchronous capabilities. Scheduled visits should be confirmed by both parties to maintain consistency. If available, automated appointment reminders 24 hours prior to the visit have been shown to be beneficial in minimizing no show rates. Visits should be conducted during regular work hours and during administrative times allowing for a higher availability of support staff.[3] Considerations should be made for caregiver schedules who would be present to assist with carryover of burn-related medical and rehabilitative interventions.

Test Call With the Patient

Prior to patient's tele-burn rehabilitation visits, instructions should be provided on how to access the virtual platform. Test calls are beneficial in ensuring a successful telehealth visit.[3,16] In addition, these calls determine the patient's understanding of the software, review the process of a telerehabilitation visit, test the digital connection, and establish the optimal environment for the patient's visits. Ideally the visits will be held in a quiet room with minimal distractions and adequate lighting, so both the patient and practitioner can fully visualize the other party and their movements. Test calls within a virtual platform will address any compatibility issues with audio and/or video connections for a chosen device. Furthermore, test calls provide patients with real-time feedback on how to maximize their environment for success.[2]

Confirmation of the patient's information including phone number, email, and address can be obtained during the test call. Details of any caregiver who will be participating in the tele-burn rehabilitation session should be obtained at this time. Support staff can also provide the patient with the contact details of a department representative to call if technical issues arise before, during, or after the visit. If a test call is omitted, there may not be enough time to troubleshoot connectivity issues, especially if patients are lacking in technological proficiency and/or are using outdated devices. A contingency plan should also be established during the test call to ensure the ability to continue visits if technology breakdown arises, for example, loss of telephone access.

During the Visit

The second element of tele-burn rehabilitation consultations happens during the visit. Here the focus is on the virtual connections, delivery of care and interventions, and providing education for optimal carryover of wound care, scar/graft maturation programs, home exercises, and splinting programs.

Patient success relies on acceptability, access, and environmental factors. Ease of use and ability to participate in synchronous video calls increases patient success. Providers and patients should be aware of standard operating procedures that guide responsibilities and expectations of both parties. Sessions should be performed without interruptions and insert no personal information vs. personal information displayed from either party. Both the provider and patient should understand expectations of establishing and assembling the session, therapeutic interventions and participation, and conclusion of the session just as they would an in-person appointment.

Virtual Connections

Successful tele-burn rehabilitation visits are dependent on choosing an appropriate environment in which to conduct synchronous video sessions. Burn clinicians must recognize that not all environmental constraints can be addressed, and many patients will require recommendations to neutralize environmental factors when participating in a tele-burn rehabilitation visit. Subsequent sessions will provide feedback on patients' individualized environmental issues that burn clinicians will encounter when delivering specialized burn services via telehealth.[2, 13]

Location also has a significant influence on the success of tele-burn rehabilitation visits. Burn clinicians should feel comfortable advising patients when choosing a singular location or predetermined locations where sessions will be conducted. If the burn clinician requires the patient to utilize multiple locations during the session, the patient should have a good understanding of the rationale and of what interventions will be conducted where.[13] For example, if working on manual therapies, such as massage and donning pressure garments, the therapist can request the patient be in a bathroom or bedroom setting where the door can be closed and the individual will have privacy. Another example is in the pediatric population where if utilizing running, jumping, sports, or climbing on home playgrounds, you will need to have the session set outside for a predetermined time, taking into consideration body hemostasis and sun exposure.

The location(s) for a teleburn visit should be selected where the level of noise and interruptions can be curtailed. This factor should be foremost in both therapist or physician and patient environments. All parties should have an understanding that the tele-burn session should be free from interruptions by others, door(s) closed if possible, all extraneous noise (TV, phones, alarms) should be placed on mute, and that no other calls should be answered while participating in a telerehabilitation visit. Additionally the burn clinician or facility can educate the patient on the tele-burn rehabilitation suggested settings for sound. When the settings are similar on both the burn clinician and patient's device, clarity of voice and volume are optimized for both parties.[2]

Similarly, all parties involved in tele-burn visits must choose a relevant stable surface on which to place their device. Placing the chosen device on a stable surface will increase picture stabilization and minimize vertigo. Burn clinicians and patients should have all extremities free so that they can fully participate in therapy sessions. Removing distracting items such as jewelry and loose clothing is recommended for easy viewing of the injured areas.[2] Also, when positioning the device on a surface, both parties should ensure that the video frame is focused on the appropriate figure, that is, face, extremities, and trunk.

Another crucial environmental factor is appropriate clothing. Both parties must be aware of acceptable and professional clothing when participating in a tele-burn rehabilitation visit. Facilities can provide information regarding appropriate clothing when engaging in synchronous video sessions. Both parties should be appropriately dressed as if they are meeting in person. Clothing should also be taken into consideration for ease in observing all involved areas during treatment interventions.[3] Burn patients can be directed to wear loose fitting items so that burn clinicians can easily view all affected areas, including areas that have healed by primary intention, grafted sites, donor sites, and any areas that are problematic in the patient's opinion.

Lighting is also a key consideration when conducting a tele-burn rehabilitation visit. Both burn clinician and patient must consider the level of lighting in their space and how it impacts video quality.[13] Platform tests can also address this issue. Effective lighting ensures involved areas and skin integrity including scarring, grafts, and donor sites are clearly displayed within the video frame. Clinicians require effective lighting to assess wounds, scar/graft pigmentation, vascularity and height, and pulling of scars on adjacent cutaneous functional units (CFUs) for development of an indicated treatment plan.

Clear visualization of the patient's face allows for improved communication and rapport building. Being able to thoroughly visualize the patient strengthens the burn clinician's evaluation skills for clinical reasoning and decision-making purposes. It is important to use direct light when available and minimize shadows that have the potential to conceal important diagnostic information.

Lastly, confidential information should never be visible in the burn clinician and patient video frames. Patients should be discouraged from displaying personal information such as account numbers, personal numbers, and potential personal photos. Burn clinicians should refrain from displaying protected health information on screen, even if it is related to the patient participating in the telerehabilitation session. Additionally, burn clinicians should ensure that their chosen environment is in a low-traffic area to protect health information privacy and ensure clinical discussions cannot be overheard by others.[2,3,13]

Intervention—Delivery of Care

Tele-burn rehabilitation sessions give burn survivors access to expert clinicians who specialize in burn care assessments, monitoring, interventions, and treatments. Interventions provided in a tele-burn rehabilitation setting may resemble in-person visits, however, with the distinction of utilizing the home environment and provided equipment. Therapeutic intervention relies on the burn clinician's ability to guide the patient through their program while ensuring maximum benefit. Interventions will require increased communication and activity mirroring throughout the session, as well as potential instructional videos for dressing changes, exercises including stretching and strengthening, and splint and pressure therapy don/doffing.

Identifying or predetermining patient needs and goals will increase the provider's ability to maximize the benefit of synchronous video sessions. Successful service delivery also requires providers and patients to limit the changing of rooms or the scene in the home environment for optimal utilization of time and to prevent interruptions.[15,16] Patients may need frequent education and reorienting regarding their therapeutic progression, as they may feel overwhelmed with their current functioning level. Thus tele-burn rehabilitation clinicians must direct the patient's focus and manage patient expectations as they would in person. Successful communication and mirroring may provide the patient with increased knowledge and confidence to utilize their home and environment on their own to progress their rehabilitation goals and needs independently. Furthermore, it is important for the provider to remain focused and maintain familiar patterns before implementing new changes to the patient's home environment.[2]

Burn patients in the remodeling and maturation stages of healing often experience hypersensitivities, which limit functional abilities. Desensitization techniques are found to be helpful to normalize sensations. When addressing hypersensitivity in a tele-burn rehabilitation session, planning is important. The patient should have three to four household items, prerequested by the clinician, available for the scheduled session as opposed to having the patient find items during the session. Items should include soft materials, coarse material, metal objects, and objects useful for tapping and vibration. Items such as cotton balls, tissues, massage with lotion, face cloth, denim, raw macaroni or rice, paper clips, nuts/bolts, and/or pencil erasers are some examples. In the pediatric population, items can include playdough, kinetic sand, oobleck (a mixture of cornstarch and water), slime, or a soft loofah during bath time, if skin integrity allows. Use of compression sheets and weighted blankets are also items which could be utilized to address the proprioceptive aspect of tactile defectiveness or hypersensitivities.

Many exercises performed in a clinic setting can also be carried out in a tele-burn rehabilitation session. Stretching, strengthening, endurance, and recreational activities are important aspects to incorporate into sessions. Clinicians should discuss what exercise items the patient has access to in order to maximize the utility of tele-burn rehabilitation sessions. For example, resistance bands, weights, therapy balls, foam rollers, and exercise equipment such as treadmills and bikes can be utilized. In the pediatric population, functional examples include animal walks, wheelbarrow walking, or climbing on home playground equipment.

Stretching is of the utmost importance to maintain pliability and flexibility of soft tissues, joints and increase skin excursion. Clinicians should address stretching and range of motion limitations with consideration of CFUs. CFUs are defined as continuous tissues that accommodate with movement in all planes of motion, based on tissue pliability.[17] For example, a burn to the anterior neck is at increased contracture susceptibility because of decreased natural integument pliability following a burn injury. An anterior neck burn may lead to recruitment of integument proximal and distal to the cervical spine leading to a flexion contracture. Integument must be recruited proximally from the cheeks and jaw to a broad range distally from the sternal notch to the pubic bone to achieve full range of motion when forming neck extension. CFUs are regarded as clinical pearls in burn care when reporting range of motion. Successful establishment of a virtual plan of care depends on the clinician's ability to educate patients on the impact of scarring and how scarring affects joint planes of motion in relation to function and movement. Educating burn survivors to recognize the impact of CFUs increases their own visible recognition and enhances self-monitoring of the integument system, therefore making the burn survivor more proficient in reporting limitations and progress, as well as in adequately performing stretching. Stretching by means of active, active assistive, or passive range of motion will elongate inelastic scar tissue and may prevent contractures that ultimately impact function. Burn survivors can be taught how to independently stretch using their contralateral side, making use of resistive bands, stable furniture, walls, and/or doors. Moreover, burn survivors can independently stretch during targeted activity or by utilizing their environment with focus on the contralateral direction.[17]

A common complication of a burn injury is the development of burn contractures that not only cause limitations to range of motion but also interfere with function and cosmesis. Contractures are common at the shoulders, elbows, knees, wrists, digits, hips, ankles, and toes, which can lead to joint subluxation, dislocations, and postural changes such as scoliosis or kyphosis.[18, 19] Monitoring of range of motion, posture, and compensatory movements is imperative to counteract contractures and soft tissue imbalances for reconstructive surgical planning.

Orthoses are regularly utilized in burn settings to protect delicate tissue and grafts, manage joint positioning, and maintain and/or increase range of motion. The clinician should consider utilizing static-progressive, dynamic, or Merritt orthoses when addressing contractures, joint tightness, or decreased pliability of soft tissues. Static-progressive or dynamic splints allow greater ability to influence tissues and joints over time for possible increased range of motion and functional ability. These types of orthoses are versatile at addressing joint tightness, muscle/skin tightness, and joint contractures, without the patient needing to be seen in person for consistent modification as gains are achieved. Small adjustments can be made virtually, such as increasing the line-of-pull of the dynamic component of splints, progressing or decreasing tension, or the angle of positioning of dials or changes in strapping. Still, if a burn survivor requires a new custom fit orthosis or adjustments to a splint within the prescribed splinting routine, an in-person visit should be scheduled. If the burn clinician anticipates issues with the ability to carry over a dynamic or static-progressive splinting program or transportation issues for returning for splint adjustments, prefabricated, static three-dimensional (3D) printed, or soft strapping splints should be used. Examples include but are not limited to prefabricated wrist splints, prefabricated anticontracture/antispasticity splints, hinged knee braces, prefabricated neoprene thumb splints, flexion straps for the digits, facial taping, Benik pediatric prefabricated braces, and Watusi neck collars. The rationale for splint use and tolerance for the splint will determine the wear schedule.

Programs may have to be adjusted by increasing sets and repetitions, if heavier weights or resistive bands are not available. Introducing alternative means of strengthening such as yoga, Tai Chi, or Pilates is another way of strengthening and is easily modified to the tele-burn platform.[20]

Patients can be instructed to complete endurance activities prior to sessions as a warm up or after tele-burn rehabilitative sessions. Having a patient walk outside or on a treadmill, use a bike, or walk up and down stairs in their environment are some examples. Using household tasks to address standing tolerance and balance such as standing to make a light snack or beverage, when on the computer to do work or playing a game, folding laundry at a kitchen table or counter top, or making a bed can be helpful.

Recreational activity is another way to address endurance capability of a burn patient. Participating in sports, using technologies such as an electronic gaming consule dancing, and gardening are suggestions for patients to participate in between tele-burn rehabilitative sessions.[21]

Wound care is another important aspect of burn care. Lighting and picture quality are important for burn care clinicians to accurately assess wounds to determine medically indicated treatment. Digital evaluation of wounds has been found to be comparable to standard evaluation of wounds.[22] Considerations regarding dressings include the knowledge and familiarity of the burn care provider, dressings that allow for shorter healing times, and dressings that require longer intervals between changes. Moreover, increased patient tolerance and comfort for dressing changes within the home environment should be considered.[23] Having enough supplies is critical for carryover of wound care routines by patients and their caregivers via tele-burn visits. Dressings can be soaked off with water in a sink or shower prior to scheduled tele-burn rehabilitation sessions to maximize time of the session and not rush the patient, potentially leading to increased anxiety. In the effort to maximize time, instructing the patient and caregivers to have all dressing supplies laid out for easy access is important.

Skin care is of utmost importance when managing a burn survivor. Traditionally, massage and pressure management programs are initiated to address skin/graft maturation and assist with itch. Measuring for custom garments poses an issue if a patient is unable to be seen in person. Clinicians can use convential compression clothing items such as sports bras, tighter bike shirts, bike shorts, or feminine or masculine shaping products to provide prefabricated pressures without the need to obtain custom measurements. Patients and caregivers can take general measurements with the direction of the clinician for interim pressure therapy garments. Clinicians should contact the preferred vendor for a list of interim garments readily available that can be mailed to the patient. Alternatively, consider using elastic adhesive taping, such as kinesiotape, to provide pressure on raised, red, rigid scars, grafts, and donor sites. Elastic adhesive taping can be easily purchased at local pharmacies, sporting stores, and online vendors.

Special Considerations in Burns

Ethically, burn clinicians should maintain the same level of professionalism and clinical practice in the delivery of telerehabilitation practice as during in-person care. Accordingly, services should be culturally proficient to provide services to all populations, including assessing and incorporating culturally relevant contexts to enhance telerehabilitation interactions.[2,13]

Regular and appropriate communication with other team members involved in the patient's care should continue, especially when the patient's telehealth visits may be conducted individually with each provider. Established communications lend to strong care coordination and planning for further reconstructive/surgical procedures.[13,16]

When treating child and adolescent populations, developmental status should be evaluated with consideration to age, motor functioning, and speech, language, and sensory integration. Further consideration on room size, toys, and planned developmentally appropriate activities will allow the child or adolescent to fully participate in age-appropriate interventions maximizing their skill set. Attention should be paid to how caregiver and/or parent involvement influences the sessions.[13]

Identifying patient needs for interpreters for spoken languages or American Sign Language communication is vital to telerehabilitation success. Coordination with interpreters needs to be established prior to tele-burn visits by providers. Each burn clinician should utilize facility-provided policies and approved services. In the event there is no recognized language service provider, the telerehabilitation provider must identify reputable and secure service agents.[20] Additionally, this information should be easily identifiable in patient records.

Some conditions may necessitate that the tele-burn rehabilitation session include a caregiver or family member to assist with rehabilitative interventions such as stretching, donning splints and pressure therapies, and graft/skin care. Providers should ensure ample time is scheduled to allow for the caregiver or family member to be able to carry out the desired interventions. Additionally, time should allow for both the patient and caregiver or family member to ask questions.[4, 5, 12, 13]

Chronic itch is common after a burn injury, with reports upward of 67% to 73% of patients experiencing this symptom.[24] Itch can be addressed with various medications, pressure therapy, and moisturizing lotions such as aloe vera and lanolin to help skin quality or texture. Massaging is thought to provide itch relief by the gate theory as well as desensitization of the skin.[25] Other topical applications that have been found to have a positive result are colloidal oatmeal, liquid paraffin, and doxepin cream. Effectiveness of itch interventions should be monitored, and adjustment made as medically indicated. Improving or worsening symptoms, the Burning Man Itch Scale, Visual Analog Scale, Numeric Pain Rating Scale, and visualizing the affected areas looking for open skin from scratching are examples of tools the burn care provider can use to monitor the severity of itch.[26]

Heterotopic ossification is another complication of a burn injury. It is typically associated with a greater total body surface area percentage, inhalation injuries, mechanical ventilation, a greater amount of surgical procedures, sepsis, and delayed initiation of active movement.[27] With tele-burn rehabilitation sessions, the burn care provider is unable to palpate and assess the joint end ranges for a firm, hard feel. However, loss of range of motion, inability to tolerate resting splints, increases of pain within the same arch of motion, challenges with loading the joints, decreased functional abilities, and joint appearance can be monitored. A joint with localized pain, erythema, and reports of heat or a palpable firm mass are signs heterotopic ossification or other acute problems could be occurring and should be red flags, indicating the need for a face-to-face visit.

From the provider perspective, burn clinicians can gain proficiency and knowledge from an assortment of resources, continuing education opportunities, tele-burn rehabilitation forums, webinars, research articles, and mentoring relationships.[2, 13] Enhanced understanding will advance practice, participation, and documentation to achieve desired optimal patient outcomes.

Providing Education/Supplies for Patient

Education is a critical component in treatment of burn injuries. Education provides patients with disease-related information, acts as a guide and reference when carrying over therapeutic interventions, provides patients with expectations, and empowers them to have an active role in their recovery continuum.

Traditionally, educational handouts or individualized videos are can be directly provided to the patient during in-person visits. When using tele-burn rehabilitation models, the ability to provide electronic educational handouts and videos is dependent on the virtual platform being utilized. Many electronic medical records have integrated reliable electronic home exercise programs that can be emailed directly to the patient, including individualized instructions and video references. These exercise programs can be incorporated during a telerehabilitation visit so the patient can ask questions to the burn rehabilitation therapist in real-time.

When electronic home exercises programs are not available through virtual platforms, burn therapists should use established written educational handouts. Handouts can be referenced during a session and sent to the patient in the mail. Patients can also be directed to a hospital-established educational websites where materials are readily available for access.

Ample supplies should be provided when the patient is discharged from the hospital in anticipation of home needs and telerehabilitation visits.[2] While recommendations of products change

TABLE 8.1 ■ **Patient Supply Reference.**[a,b]

Item	Description	Price ($)
Resistance Band		
2 to 3 packs	5 ft × 4 in	$10–17
Individual	5 ft × 4 in	$6–7
Elastic Adhesive Tape		
1 roll	16 ft × 2 in	$8–18
Scar Padding		
1 sheet	5 in × 6 in	$20–26
4 to 8 sheets	1.5 in × 3 in	$14–25
Resistive Putty		
Varying resistances: min, mod, heavy	2 oz	$3–4
	4 oz	$9–10
	5 oz	$10–11
Self-Adherent Wrap		
1″	5 yd	$2–14
2″	5 yd	$5–6

[a]The table includes but is not limited to common items used during a tele-burn rehabilitation session. Costs reflect those of 2020. Keep in consideration costs change over time as well as companies may discontinue or not carry items in future years.
[b]All items can be purchased through various online vendors.

as wounds heal, grafts/skin mature, and the patient makes progress in deficit areas, this demands regular reevaluation. Supply chain resources can be provided to the patient for purchase ranging from wound care supplies to pressure therapy and strengthening devices. Table 8.1 is an example of a reference sheet that could be provided to a patient. Items, description, cost, and location of local and/or online companies could be included. (Narrative Citation: Hannah Sherritt, BA [June, 2020]).

After the Visit

Documentation and Billing

Reimbursement for tele-burn rehabilitative services has not kept pace with the rapid expansion of telehealth services.[11] Payment policies are critical to support the prompt growth of telerehabilitation services. Coverage, billing, and payment policies can vary greatly from state to state within the United States, and country to country around the world. While the patient should be aware of their benefit coverage, therapists should have insight into reimbursement of services via telerehabilitation. Burn clinicians should also be knowledgeable of their malpractice coverage for tele-burn rehabilitative services versus traditional in-person visits.[2,3,12]

Reimbursement depends on adequate clinical documentation of improvements in deficit areas, functional abilities, and resolution of adverse symptoms. Tele-burn rehabilitative initial evaluations, treatment notes, progress notes, and discharge evaluations should incorporate all elements of in-person documentation. Components include visit number, diagnosis, date of injury, date of surgeries, current condition, pain scale, objective measures, tele-burn rehabilitative interventions performed, assessment/plan, and a time stamp. Short-term and long-term goals should be outlined in both initial evaluations and progress notes. Virtual visit type should be mentioned (e.g., telephone versus video). Many states require a virtual visit acknowledgment.[2] For example: *This real-time, interactive virtual clinical encounter was conducted using videoconferencing technology from clinic or home office. The patient participated in the visit from home/temporary residence or other location as specified. Consent for virtual care, including informing the patient that insurance will be billed, and that in-person care is available in case of emergencies or as needed otherwise, was discussed at the time of scheduling.* (Example from Massachusetts General Hospital Outpatient Documentation.)

Burn clinicians should consider the reliability and applicability of objective measures to the tele-burn service delivery model. When utilizing assessment measures, documentation should include modifications and location as these will need to be factored into results.[2,4,5] Appendix A provides examples of data collection and recommended documentation verbiage that can be captured and used in the virtual platform (Narrative Citation: Marie T. Figueroa, PT, DPT, ATC and Julie Maggio, PT, DPT, NCS [personal communication, June 2020]).[2,3] The list is not all inclusive, nor are all tests/measures listed for a successful virtual session. Safety of the patient should be taken into consideration when requesting to perform virtual testing.[3] Fig. 8.1 demonstrates an alternative way of obtaining goniometric values via virtual platforms. Any deviation from standard range of motion positioning when using a goniometer should be noted in the burn clinician's documentation.

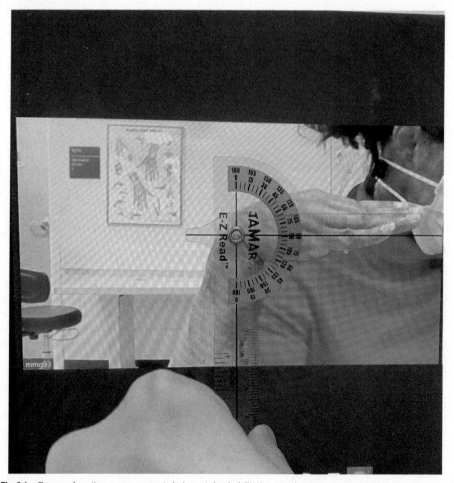

Fig. 8.1 Range of motion measurement during a telerehabilitation session.

CASE REPORT

INITIAL PHYSIATRIST VISIT FOLLOWING HOSPITAL DISCHARGE

Patient is a 33-year-old male who sustained a 57% total body surface area burn from malicious intent with an accelerant. Full thickness burns were sustained to bilateral upper extremities including bilateral hands, the right flank and trunk, as well as superficial partial thickness and deep thickness burns to the face and thighs. Length of stay was 97 days including requiring a tracheostomy. Sedation was required for a total of 64 days. The patient discharged from acute rehabilitation requiring treatment for upper extremity neuropathies, weaknesses, and range-of-motion limitations as well as weaning from medication.

APPLICATION OF TELEBURN REHABILITATION IN THE REHABILITATIVE PROCESS

The patient's initial evaluation was performed in clinic where formal medical assessment of cardiac, respiratory, integument, musculoskeletal, and psychological state was performed. Objective measures and testing included vitals, electromyography, range of motion, sensory testing, strength measurements, and a thorough assessment of skin. Specifically, Semmes Weinstein monofilament test, dynamometer grip, and pinch testing were performed by therapy. Subsequent physician and therapy visits were conducted via teleburn platforms. Virtual examinations included assessment and monitoring of coordination, motor nerve performance, skin integrity, strength, range of motion, and functional abilities versus limitations. In addition the patient required weaning from medications after discharge from the rehabilitation facility.

INTERVENTIONS

Teleburn visits included detailed burn care education, individualized home programs for scar mobilization, nonpharmacological interventions for itch and sleep hygiene, range-of-motion interventions, and activities to maximize function. Teleburn visits also addressed specific pharmacological interventions that focused on weaning of opioids and benzodiazepines, reducing pain and anxiety, and titrating increased gabapentin to better manage neuropathic pain, itch, and sleep. Contractures were monitored for improvements, and a home exercise and stretching program was modified to address evolving goals of care. The patient was referred to outpatient occupational and physical therapy, and psychological services based on findings were noted during telehealth sessions. Education was provided regarding rehabilitation interventions and plans as well as local and national resources for peer support and burn survivor community organizations.

OUTCOME

The patient was able to be weaned from all opioid and benzodiazepine medications with close monitoring of pain, itch, and sleep hygiene over a 6-month period. A healthy sleeping program was established, as well as participation in outpatient occupational and physical therapy for return to their preinjury level of independence with activities of daily living and instrumental activities of daily living. The patient joined a local burn survivor support organization and attended monthly peer support virtual meetings.

CASE REPORT

SPLINTS, EXERCISE, AND SENSORY REEDUCATION

Patient is a 55-year-old male who sustained full thickness burns to his bilateral hands, wrists, and distal forearms when he tripped and fell into the hot coals of a campfire. Surgical procedures include both full thickness and split thickness skin grafts to the dorsum of bilateral hands and digits. Limitations include decreased active range of motion, strength, and hypersensation to both textures and temperatures affecting his ability to independently complete self-care, which in turn affected his ability to perform homemaking tasks and return to work.

APPLICATION OF TELEBURN REHABILITATION IN THE REHABILITATIVE PROCESS

The patient's occupational therapy initial evaluation was in person where formal range of motion, strength, integumentary, and sensation testing were performed. Barriers were documented at this time, realizing the patient would transition to virtual follow-ups. Photographs were taken and uploaded into the electronic medical record. In anticipation of telehealth follow-up sessions, splints were fabricated to maximize stretch to tight soft tissues, joints, and skin. Educational instructions were provided and reviewed. Strengthening products, specifically, progressive resistive therapeutic foams and resistive therapeutic bands, were provided for initiation at a later point in the rehabilitative course.

INTERVENTIONS

Occupational therapy visits were conducted twice a week, lasting 45 minutes in duration. The patient was instructed to warm up prior to scheduled videoconferencing either by heat for 10 minutes to predetermined affected areas or use the static progressive metacarpal flexion splint for 30 minutes. Sessions focused on both active and active-assisted range of motion, proprioception, desensitization, stereognosis, strength, and functional activities utilizing the home environment. Examples of home items include resistive therapeutic bands, resistive therapeutic foam, pasta, rice, bed, sheet, table, and facial tissues. Sessions also monitored static-progressive orthoses for exercise progression and fit as able.

OUTCOMES

Gains were determined by ability to return to preinjury activities of daily living, instrumental activities of daily living, and work tasks. Follow-up visits were decreased to one time per week as the patient made steady gains, then transitioned to every other week. Active range of motion was documented via goniometric measurements by placing a goniometer to the computer screen to measure the angle of motion. Strength was progressed through a range of resistive therapeutic foams, resistive therapeutic bands, and the weight of objects the patient could carry and open. Endurance was measured by length of time able to tolerate activities with limited fatigue, for example, minimal fatigue when making a simple meal versus maximal fatigue when making a simple meal. Sensation was progressed from soft to firm textures and from cold to warmer temperatures per patient tolerance.

CASE REPORT

PRESSURE THERAPY

Patient is a 20-year-old-female who sustained 37% total body surface area full thickness burns to the right dominant upper extremity when a pan of hot grease spilled on her arm. Full thickness burns included the right hand, wrist, forearm, and elbow. Surgical procedures included both full thickness and splint thickness grafts to the dorsum of bilateral hands, digits, wrist, forearm, and elbow. Limitations in this case study were skin and graft integrity as well as scar maturation.

APPLICATION OF TELEBURN REHABILITATION IN THE REHABILITATIVE PROCESS

The patient's occupational therapy initial evaluation was performed via a teleburn platform. The patient was advised to use a computer versus a smaller screen such as a cell phone and be in a well-lit room. The patient had her boyfriend present during therapy sessions to assist with any necessary interventions. Objective measurements for both active and active-assisted range of motion were obtained with a goniometer placed on the screen and the patient displaying pertinent anatomical structures. The modified Vancouver Scar Scale was also utilized. Educational material and instruction on skin care, massage, and pressure therapy products were discussed and demonstrated. A small package of supplies was mailed to the patient after the telehealth appointment. In addition the patient was provided with an electronic supply list and locations to purchase items. All follow-up appointments were via a teleburn platform.

INTERVENTIONS

The initial evaluation lasted 60 minutes. Follow-up visits ranged from 30 to 45 minutes depending on the interventions being performed and the patient's availability. Appointments were scheduled once per week for a month after the initial evaluation. Each session focused on pressure therapy and graft management/maturation. Sessions began with scar massage performed by the patient and by her boyfriend in the areas she was unable to adequately reach. The focus in sessions was directed to areas of pulling when observed with movement. Pressure therapies were initiated, utilizing Coban wrap, beta-pile web spacers, kinesiotaping for web spaces, and nail beds. The patient and her boyfriend applied and donned the above materials with the direction of the OT. Interim gloves were utilized when possible. It was not possible to measure custom garments due to restrictions on the patient coming into the hospital.

OUTCOMES

Gains were determined by the patient's ability to return to preinjury activities of daily living, instrumental activities of daily living, and work tasks. Follow-up visits were decreased to once per week, then transitioned to every other week. Active range of motion was documented by goniometric measurements by placing a goniometer to the computer screen to measure the angles of motion. Strength was progressed through a range of t-foams, progressive t-bands, as well as the weight of objects the patient could carry and open. Endurance was measured by time to cut when cooking. Sensation progressed from soft to firm textures and from cold to warmer temperatures per patient tolerance. Exercises and education were provided by the electronic service MedBridge. Educational handouts specific to the splinting routine were mailed using the US Postal Service.

A/AAROM AND EXERCISE

The patient is a 19-year-old female who sustained 34% total body surface area burns following the explosion of a bonfire after accelerant was added to the flames. The patient sustained both deep partial and full thickness burns to the face, trunk, and circumferential right lower extremity. The posterolateral knee, chin, neck, chest, and bilateral upper extremities including axilla and hands sustained full thickness burns. The patient required multiple surgeries as well as split thickness grafts to all areas with exception to chest and trunk which healed by primary intention.

APPLICATION OF TELEBURN REHABILITATION IN THE REHABILITATIVE PROCESS

The patient's initial evaluation and follow-up physical therapy sessions were performed via a teleburn platform. The patient was advised to use a computer and be in a well-lit room. The patient presented with contractures, as well as terminal ROM limitations within bilateral knee extension, knee flexion, bilateral shoulder flexion, and abduction. The patient reported issues with weight bearing and composite active and active-assisted range of motion of the upper extremities due to adaptive shortening in the CFUs. The patient also reported difficulty ambulating after prolonged sitting, difficulty loading through the upper extremities to push herself out of bed, and limited circumferential grip to hold onto daily objects. The patient was asked to report difficulty performing tasks on a scale of 1 to 10 each session for ease of reporting with a score of 1 being unable to perform and 10 being able to perform without difficulty.

INTERVENTIONS

Sessions began with guided low-load progressive stretch utilizing environmental objects that allowed the patient to grade stretch as directed by the therapist. For example the patient began seated at a table with a focus on wrist extension and graded weight bearing on the upper extremities, and transitioned to standing with loading through upper extremity with extended elbows focusing on downward loading and shifting her weight anteriorly, posteriorly, right, and left. Additionally, therapy sessions focused on standing balance and range of motion while utilizing the home environment. Standing balance and weight-shifting balance were guided and allowed for graded pressures throughout the lower extremities. Standing balance was addressed with the patient standing at her kitchen counter and reaching in all planes to specific targets as well as standing on one leg for brief periods of time. Knee flexion and ankle dorsiflexion limitations were targeted by utilizing an ottoman.

The patient was also guided through body weight exercise to focus on strength and endurance in the quadruped position allowing varying weight on the upper extremities, lower extremities, right side, and left side of the body. Transitional movements from quadruped to quadruped on forearms, child's pose, lifting contralateral extremities, and lowering into prone were included.

OUTCOMES

Strength and mobility routines were initiated and progressed. The therapist and patient established routines that the patient could perform safely and independently. The patient was educated on activity analysis and how to grade exercises appropriately with safety in mind.

Note: *TBSA*, Total body surface area; *FTB*, full thickness burn; *SPT*, splint thickness skin graft; *DTB*, deep thickness burn; *LOS*, Length of stay; *UE*, upper extremities; *ROM*, range of motion; *PT*, physical therapy; *OT*, occupational therapy; *ADLs*, activities of daily living; *IADLs*, instrumental activities of daily living; *FTSG*, full thickness skin graft; *STSG*, split thickness skin graft; *AROM*, active range of motion; *t-foam*, therapeutic foam; *t-band*, therapeutic resistive bands; *AAROM*, active assistive range of motion; *coban*, self-adherent pressure wrap; *kinesiotape*, elastic adhesive tape; *WB*, weight bearing.

Recommendations for Research

Tele-burn rehabilitation is a rapidly evolving service delivery model that can improve access of burn rehabilitation services and specialists. In anticipation of the important role tele-burn rehabilitation will have on burn care services, it is crucial that updated and augmented resources are available to burn rehabilitation clinicians. These include future research and tele-burn-related continuing education. Suggestions include patient satisfaction studies, studies of burn rehabilitation clinicians' competence and feasibility, and impact studies on health-related quality of life and function, clinical safety, and technical feasibility of telerehabilitation. Crossover studies may also provide advantages highlighting optimal timing of tele-burn rehabilitation initiation, determining optimal therapy interventions, and combination of interventions. Development of virtual measurement tools for range of motion and edema is needed.

Given the gaps in current knowledge, there is also a need in development of telerehabilitation burn care practice guidelines and development of adequate clinical documentation and clinical measures and consistent outcome measures need to be researched for reimbursement purposes. Furthermore, quantitative studies are needed to investigate the efficacy of service delivery to specific domains of rehabilitation such as positioning and orthosis management, scar and contracture management, exercise prescription, and education. Lastly, investigation is also needed to examine the delivery of burn care information, communication, and treatment via virtual technologies, as well as which platforms are most relevant to low- and middle-income populations.

APPENDIX A ■ **Tele-burn Visit Documentation and Objective Data Collection Guidance.**

Tests and Measures	Virtual Care	Examples of Documentation
Vitals	• Evaluate for tachypnea, cyanosis, orthostatic symptoms as applicable • If patient has heart rate monitor (wrist or chest) and/or automatic blood pressure cuff, can have them provide values	Normal rate of breathing Appears well oxygenated Denies dizziness or orthostatic changes with position
Pain	• Obtain a history of pain • Exacerbating/alleviating factors • Associated symptoms • Effects of symptoms on activities/function symptoms	Quality Location Intensity Radiation Timing
Itch	• Exacerbating/alleviating factors • Associated symptoms • Strategies that relieve symptom and/or intensity	Rating on a 1 to 10 scale Using an itch scale with pediatrics such as the Burn Man Itch Scale[26]
Posture	• Can be observed in sagittal and front planes easily but transverse plane is more difficult to visualize	Forward head posture Protracted/retracted shoulders Sitting in an anterior/posterior pelvic tilt In standing, rest on the Y ligaments
Gait	• When analyzing gait it is best if the patient has an open area that is sufficient for gait to be assessed • Make sure that the camera is positioned in such a way that the patient can be seen in their entirety throughout the whole gait cycle • Frontal plane observations are the most easily obtained virtually as sagittal plane observations require either a very large space or another person available to film while moving with the patient. Transverse plane observations may be more difficult to visualize depending on the region	Symmetric Nonantalgic Heel-to-toe gait pattern

Continued

APPENDIX A ■ Tele-burn Visit Documentation and Objective Data Collection Guidance—cont'd

Tests and Measures	Virtual Care	Examples of Documentation
AROM	• Can still document quality of motion as able • Ensure you can fully visualize the joint in question • For some joints, if the camera can be positioned appropriately, it may be possible to measure joint angles with a goniometer on the screen • Compare simultaneously to the uninvolved/normal side if possible as the patient's baseline • The examples are in the adjacent column	Percentages: 0%, 25%, 75%, 100% The patient has 75% of right composite flexion The patient is limited by 25% of right composite flexion Approximations via observation +/− degree The patient has +/− 90 degrees of elbow flexion Severity: minimal, moderately, severely, end-range limitation Right elbow flexion is moderately limited Functional ability: Range of motion in relation to function Right shoulder is able to forward flex shoulder to brush hair Comparison to the other side Right ankle dorsiflexion is mildly limited as compared to the left
PROM and muscle length	• Although ideally performed manually in the clinic by the therapist, there may be some limited tests that may be performed virtually either by the patient on themselves or by a caregiver/family member while you observe	PROM ankle dorsiflexion performed with a towel or strap PROM elbow extension performed with a towel or strap Shoulder flexion performed in supine by using either the other arm to assist (must differentiate patients perceived end range vs. limited by pain)
Integument	• Swelling comparative assessment between sides • Skin integrity including wounds, grafts, donor site location	Mild, moderate, severe edema or swelling Clean, dry, erythema, hypopigmentation, hyperpigmentation, blanching on stretch/movement, drainage, percentage of graft take Use a measuring tape to outline the dimensions of the wound, graft, donor site location Example: Right upper extremity graft with 100% take, red appearance, blanching with stretch
Strength	• Although may not necessarily be able to use traditional grading scale in its entirety due to the inability to provide resistance, may consider the following testing/language to indicate ability to move against gravity and control load • In later phases of rehabilitation, with post-ops, for example, in-person visits may be required in order to obtain more specific strength grading for proper progression • Gravity eliminated/against gravity	Due to the constraints of virtual visits, Manuel Muscle Test (MMT) unable to be formally performed. Observations include: – Right shoulder flexion: At least 3/5 – Right shoulder flexion: Able to move through the full AROM with yellow Thera band – Right ankle plantar flexion: In unilateral (or bilateral) stance, able to rise on toes in full range of motion (can also indicate number of times performed)

Continued

APPENDIX A ■ **Tele-burn Visit Documentation and Objective Data Collection Guidance.—cont'd**

Tests and Measures	Virtual Care	Examples of Documentation
Palpation	• Instruct patient to touch areas of tenderness • Document differences in adjacent areas and/or on the contralateral side	Minimal, moderate, maximal tenderness to palpation and the location Warm to touch, no temperature differences as perceived by the patient Trigger points, knots as perceived by the patient
Motor control/tone /proprioception	• Observations can still be made in the frontal and sagittal plane and depending on the joint, much less likely the transverse plane • Observations can include abnormal movements at rest and with activities	Patient able to perform full active movements, no co-contraction No posturing with position changes Tremor, dystonia, clonus
Sensation	• What textures is the patient able to tolerate vs. hypersensitivity • Touch involved dermatomal regions reporting abnormal sensations • Utilize diagram of dermatomes • Use tip of a pencil and eraser for sharp/dull sensation	Sensation to light touch Sharp/dull subjectively intact Able to tolerate clothing, pressure garments on the upper body Hypersensitivity noted in the feet causing the patient not to tolerate socks
Functional tests	• Many functional tests can still be performed with quantitative and qualitative data	Squatting (bilateral, unilateral) Single leg stance (time able to hold, amount of sway, hip drop noted) Hopping (bilateral and unilateral mechanics) Activities of daily living: Don/doffing socks/shoes, brushing hair, donning coats, pull over shirts, pressure garments IADLs: Household tasks such as cutting, making a snack, lifting pots/pans, typing
Coordination	• You can look at some elements of this including Rapid alternating movement (RAM) of UE is defined under the case reports. UE is the upper extremity is defined under the case reports. UE is the upper extremity, foot tapping and finger opposition • If support person present, they could perform finger to nose with that person while you observe quality of movement or from nose to computer screen	Rapid alternating movements intact and symmetric; finger-to-nose and heel-to-shin intact, bilaterally

Continued

APPENDIX A ▪ Tele-burn Visit Documentation and Objective Data Collection Guidance.—cont'd

Tests and Measures	Virtual Care	Examples of Documentation
Functional mobility	• Take advantage of the environment and have patient show you various tasks throughout the home if video will travel and support person present • Virtual visits are an excellent opportunity to see patients performing functional tasks in their home environment rather than simulating them in the clinical environment • Virtual visits to assess functional mobility in the home/office are considered best practice if the patient has the audiovisual capability and can safely perform • This assessment will require a well-placed camera/device or a family member who is willing to film the patient performing the task • Documentation to include safety	Carrying a child Doing household chores Working at a computer Getting out of bed or a favorite chair, couches, floor Navigation of stairs Navigation in the kitchen for homemaking and cooking tasks and/or home office, home gym
Sleep	• Sleep hygiene	Healthy habits to assist in sleep such as exercises and eating well Medication patient may be using such as over–the-counter melatonin
Standardized tests	• The following standardized tests can be done at home provided safety is not an issue and patient has adequate setup: • 6-minute walk (2 minutes is a modified version that may be more amenable to home) • Gait speed and Timed Up and Go test (TUG) require specific distances markers and is likely too much to ask for a patient to set up, however, if you have a particularly motivated person and/or good supports at home they may be willing and able to do this	Five times sit to stand and 30-second chair stand – Ask patient to measure chair they are using so this can be documented – You will be timing while patient performs test – Note in chart that it was done in particular chair in home, so you can recreate throughout virtual treatment sessions

Continued

APPENDIX A ■ **Tele-burn Visit Documentation and Objective Data Collection Guidance.—cont'd**

Tests and Measures	Virtual Care	Examples of Documentation
Special tests/ provocative tests that can be performed virtually: as directed by the clinician, performed by the patient	• Not all special tests will be able to be performed reliably in a virtual environment so perform as able using clinical judgment • Can perform active tests that do not need to be manually done by the therapist • Consider the possibility of utilizing a reliable family member who can be instructed by the therapist under direct supervision to perform correctly along with patient subjective feedback • Make sure to document who performed the testing and that the "test results may be limited due to the constraints of a virtual visit"	Phalen's (carpal tunnel syndrome) Elbow flexion test (ulnar nerve entrapment at elbow) Finkelstein test (De Quervain's tenosynovitis) Tinel test (median/ulnar nerve entrapment at the wrist) Carpometacarpal grind test (carpometacarpal arthritis) Drop arm test (supraspinatus tear) Lift-off test (subscapularis injury) Speed test (biceps tendon injury) Neer sign (subacromial impingement) Sulcus sign test (glenohumeral instability) Single leg squat (knee valgus, patellofemoral syndrome) Noble compression test (iliotibial band syndrome) Patellar grind test (patellofemoral syndrome) Ankle/foot single leg heel raise (posterior tibialis dysfunction) Foot doming (intrinsic foot weakness) Single leg stance/squat (gluteus medius weakness) Thomas test (iliopsoas tightness/ contracture)

AROM, Active range of motion; *IADLs*, instrumental activities of daily living; *PROM*, passive range of motion.

References

1. Serghiou MA, OTT S, Cowan A, et al. Burn rehabilitation along the continuum of care. In: Herndon DN. *Total Burn Care.* 5th ed. Elsevier Science Limited; 2018:476–508.
2. AOTA. Telehealth in occupational therapy (Position Paper). *Am J Occup Ther.* 2018;72(Suppl 2): 7212410059. https://doi.org/10.5014/ajot.2018.72S219.4.
3. Verduzco-Gutierrez M, Bean AC, Tenforde AS, et al. How to conduct an outpatient telemedicine rehabilitation or prehabilitation visit. *PM R.* 2020;12(7):1–7. https://doi.org/10.1002/pmrj.12380.
4. Smith AC, Kimble R, Mill J, et al. Diagnostic accuracy of and patient satisfaction with telemedicine for the follow-up of paediatric burns patients. *J Telemed Telecare.* 2004;10(4):193–198. https://doi.org/10.1258/1357633041424449.
5. Smith AC, Youngberry K, Mill J, et al. A review of three years' experience using email and videoconferencing for the delivery of post-acute burns care to children in Queensland. *Burns.* 2004;30(3):248–252. https://doi.org/10.1016/j.burns.2003.11.003.
6. Liu YM, Mathews K, Vardanian A, et al. Urban telemedicine: the applicability of teleburns in the rehabilitative phase. *J Burn Care Res.* 2017;33(1):e235–e239. https://doi.org/10.1097/BCR.0000000000000360. PMID: 27294853.
7. Redlick FP, Roston B, Gomez M, et al. The role of telemedicine in follow-up burn care. *J Burn Care Res.* 2001;22(Suppl 2):277. https://doi.org/10.1097/00004630-200103002-00260.
8. Nguyen LT, Massman NJ, Franzen BJ, et al. Telemedicine follow-up of burns: lessons learned from the first thousand visits. *J Burn Care Res.* 2004;25(6):485–490. https://doi.org/10.1097/01. BCR.0000144538.82184.19.

9. Saffle JR, Edelman L, Theurer L, et al. Telemedicine evaluation of acute burns is accurate and cost-effective. *J Trauma*. 2009;67(2):358–365. https://doi.org/10.1097/TA.0b013e3181ae9b02.
10. Syed-Abdul S, Scholl J, Chen CC, et al. Telemedicine utilization to support the management of the burns treatment involving patient pathways in both developed and developing countries: a case study. *J Burn Care Res*. 2012;33(4):e207–e212. https://doi.org/10.1097/BCR.0b013e318241b6b7.
11. Hickey S, Gomez J, Meller B, et al. Interactive home telehealth and burns: a pilot study. *Burns*. 2017;43(6):1318–1321. https://doi.org/10.1016/j.burns.2016.11.013.
12. Theurer L, Bashshur R, Bernard J, et al. Policy: American Telemedicine Association Guidelines for tele-burn. *Telemed e-Health*. 2017;23(5):365–375. https://doi.org/10.1089/tmj.2016.0279.
13. American Psychiatric Association. *Best Practices in Videoconferencing-Based Telemental Health*. 2018. file:///C:/Users/kgs1/Downloads/APA-ATA-Best-Practices-in-Videoconferencing-Based-Telemental-Health.pdf.
14. Neville C. Telehealth: a balanced look at incorporating this technology into practice. *SAGE Open Nurs*. 2018;4:1–5. https://doi.org/10.1177/23779608/8786504.
15. Dorsey ER, Topol EJ. State of telehealth. *N Engl J Med*. 2016;375(14):154–159. https://doi.org/10.1056/nejmc1610233.
16. National Rural Health Resource Center. Creating a Framework to Support Measure Development for Telehealth. 2020. www.qualityforum.org. file:///C:/Users/andri/Downloads/Creating%20a%20Framework%20to%20Support%20Measure%20Development%20for%20Telehealth%20(2).pdf. ISBN 978-1-68248-065-6.
17. Richard RL, Lester ME, Miller SF, et al. Identification of cutaneous functional units related to burn scar contracture. *J Burn Care Res*. 2009;30(4):625–631. https://doi.org/10.1097/bcr.0b013e3181ac016c.
18. Schneider JC, Holavanahalli R, Goldstein R, et al. A prospective study of contractures in burn injury: defining the problem. *J Burn Care Res*. 2006;27:508–514.
19. Schneider JC, Holavanahalli R, Helm P, et al. Contractures in burn injury part II: investigating joints of the hand. *J Burn Care Res*. 2008;29:606–613.
20. Model Systems Knowledge Translation Center. *Burn Injury Factsheets*. 2019. https://msktc.org/burn/factsheets; Accessed 09.11.20.
21. Hughes G, Hudgins B, MacDougall J. Using telehealth technology to improve the delivery of health services to people who are deaf. The 26th Annual International Conference of the IEEE Engineering in Medicine and Biology Society. San Francisco, CA; 2004:3084-3087. 10.1109/IEMBS.2004.1403871.
22. Roa L, Gómez-Cía T, Acha B, et al. Digital imaging in remote diagnosis of burns. *Burns*. 1999;25:617–623.
23. Bezuhly M, Fish JS. Acute burn care. *Plast Reconstr Surg*. 2012;130:349e–358e.
24. Van Laarhoven A, Ulrich D, Evers A, et al. Psychophysiological processing of itch in patients with chronic post-burn itch: an exploratory study. *Acta Derm Venereol*. 2016;96(5):613.
25. Baker RA, Zeller RA, Klein RL, et al. Burn wound itch control using H1 and H2 antagonists. *J Burn Care Rehabil*. 2001;22:263–268.
26. Morris V, Murphy LM, Rosenberg M, et al. Itch assessment scale for pediatric burn survivor. *J Burn Care Res*. 2012;33(3):419-424. 10.1097/BCR.0b013e3182372bfa.
27. Orchard G, Paratz J, Blot S, et al. Risk factors in hospitalized patients with burn injuries for developing heterotopic ossification-a retrospective analysis. *J Burn Care Res*. 2015;36(4):465–470.

CHAPTER 9

Multiple Sclerosis and Telerehabilitation

Deborah Backus ■ Dawn Ehde ■ Mitchell Wallin

Introduction to Multiple Sclerosis

Multiple sclerosis (MS) is an unpredictable, potentially disabling disease of the central nervous system (CNS) largely affecting young adults. The mean age at diagnosis is typically between 20 and 49 years; however, the prevalence in children and adolescents (<18 years) and in later adulthood (>50 years) is increasing.[1,2]

In 2020 an estimated 2.8 million people, or 35.9 per 100,000, were affected with MS worldwide, although prevalence increases with increasing latitude.[2] Rates are higher in Europe and North America, estimated at 127.0 to 164.6 per 100,000, respectively, and lower in Africa at only about 2.8 to 3.3 per 100,000 population.[3] The prevalence of MS is two to four times higher in women; however, men experience poorer prognosis and worse disease course.[2]

MS is characterized by focal lesions disseminated throughout the brain and spinal cord. These lesions, or plaques, result from damage to the myelin sheaths caused by the immune system's release of autoreactive lymphocytes that cross the blood-brain barrier to attack the oligodendrocytes, the myelin producing cells in the CNS. Originally it was thought that MS attacks only myelin in the white matter of the CNS, but more recent evidence shows the presence of plaques, neurodegeneration, and gliosis in the gray matter of the brain and spinal cord as well.[4] Demyelination and axonal damage impair or completely block neural transmission between the different regions of the CNS and between the CNS and its effectors (e.g., the skeletal muscle and body organs). In the more progressive stages of the disease there is profound brain tissue loss and atrophy, further compounding the poor neural transmission resulting from MS.

The cause of MS is not known, although environmental and genetic causal factors have been identified and may interact with lifestyle and other modifiable risk factors.

The diagnosis of MS is made through obtaining a complete medical history, a full neurological examination, and clinical and laboratory tests, including blood tests, lumbar puncture and cerebrospinal fluid assessment, magnetic resonance imaging (MRI), and electrophysiological tests, such as measurement of evoked potentials. A diagnosis is made based on the presence of at least two lesions in different areas of the brain, which occur at two different times, and when other causes of the neurological signs and symptoms can be eliminated.

MS is a heterogeneous and unpredictable disease. The clinical signs and symptoms can vary over time and in severity, within and between persons with MS, depending on the location and extent of the lesions in the brain and spinal cord. Symptoms of MS are related to the location and extent of the damage in the CNS and include sensorimotor, cognitive, and emotional symptoms, as detailed in Table 9.1.

TABLE 9.1 ■ Symptoms of Multiple Sclerosis

Symptom	Specific Changes
Fatigue	
Somatosensory	• Paresthesias or dysesthesias • Trigeminal neuralgia • Pain • Lhermitte's sign (electric shock sensation that runs down the spine elicited by neck flexion) • Sensory ataxia

Motor	• Paresis or paralysis
	• Altered muscle recruitment and patterns of activation
	• Dyssynergias
	• Spasticity
	• Balance deficits
	• Walking impairment
	• Movement disorders
	  • Tremors
	  • Dysmetria
	  • Dysdiadochokinesia
	  • Cerebellar ataxia
	• Vestibular dysfunction
	  • Vertigo

Visual disturbance	• Optic neuritis • Diplopia • Central scotoma • Nystagmus
Bowel and bladder disturbance	• Urinary urgency, incontinence, or retention • Bowel incontinence or constipation
Sexual dysfunction	• Impotence • Premature ejaculation • Disturbed intimacy
Cognitive disorders	• Slowed processing speed • Impaired memory and learning • Deficits in attention and concentration • Visuospatial deficits • Executive dysfunction
Emotional disorders	• Mood disorders, including depressive disorder • Euphoria • Emotional dysregulation syndrome • Anxiety and anxiety disorders
Communication disorders	• Slowed, slurred, or low speech volume • Swallowing deficits and dysphagia

The course of MS is also variable, ranging from benign, with mild symptoms and little to no disability, to rapidly progressing, with severe disability and, potentially, death. There are four main clinical courses of MS: clinically isolated syndrome (CIS), relapsing-remitting MS (RRMS), secondary progressive MS (SPMS), and primary progressive MS (PPMS), outlined in Table 9.2. Both SPMS and PPMS can be further classified as active, that is, with relapses or new MRI activity, or not active, and with progression or without progression.

Although, in general, women are two to four times more likely to have MS than men, in RRMS women are more affected than men, and in PPMS women and men are equally represented.

TABLE 9.2 ■ **Clinical Course of Multiple Sclerosis**

Clinical Course	Characteristics
Clinically isolated syndrome (CIS)	The first episode of neurological symptoms due to inflammation in the CNS that lasts at least 24 hours.
Relapsing-remitting MS (RRMS)	Patients experience relapses, or periods of new or worsening MS signs and symptoms not caused by another illness and that last more than 48 hours, interspersed with periods of stability; typically, patients with RRMS will return to functional ability at or at least close to prior to the relapse.
Secondary progressive MS (SPMS)	RRMS can eventually transition to SPMS, wherein a patient's neurological function and disability will progressively worsen over time.
Primary progressive MS (PPMS)	Diagnosed when the onset of symptoms is followed by progressive worsening of neurological function and accumulation of disability, without relapses and remission.

CNS, Central nervous system; *MS*, multiple sclerosis.

Defining the clinical course of MS is critical to determining treatment options and prognosis. Persons with RRMS or SPMS experience more inflammation and disruption of myelin, and more brain lesions than those with PPMS. Persons with PPMS generally have more spinal cord lesions than brain lesions.

COMORBIDITIES AND SECONDARY CONDITIONS IN MS

The experience of MS is complicated by the presence and extent of comorbidities,[5] defined as a total burden of the chronic disease.

Physical comorbidities, such as hypertension, hyperlipidemia, and chronic lung disease, can exacerbate or increase the rate of progression of disability.[6] However, psychiatric comorbidities, such as those related to mood and anxiety, can also have a negative impact and may require intervention.[7] Nearly 25% of adults with MS have a depressive disorder.[8] Chronic pain is also a prevalent comorbidity, affecting more than half of those with MS.[9] Sleep disorders, including primary insomnia and obstructive sleep apnea, are also common.[5]

Several lines of evidence suggest that at least some of the disability that occurs after MS is due to secondary deconditioning, and not just brain and spinal cord damage alone. Furthermore, people with MS are known to be less physically active than those without MS. Therefore exercise is an important component of rehabilitation in MS, critical for combating the progression of disability and deconditioning that occurs due to the symptoms, such as fatigue and pain, and heat sensitivity, environmental barriers, and poor self-efficacy for physical activity and exercise.[10]

Medical Management of MS

MEDICAL ASSESSMENT IN MS

The American Academy of Neurology (AAN) provides recommended performance measures to facilitate optimal quality of MS management.[11] These measures include clinical and laboratory assessments to determine diagnosis, comparison MRI within 24 months of MS diagnosis, and measures of current level of disability, fall risk, bladder dysfunction, level of physical activity, fatigue, cognitive impairment, depression, and quality of life.

Measures of Disability

Measures of disability can include clinically administered tests or patient-reported outcome measures (PROMs). The most widely used clinical measures are the Expanded Disability Status Scale (EDSS) and the MS Functional Composite (MSFC). Originally developed in 1983 by Dr. John Kurtzke,[12] the EDSS provides a scoring system based on the integrity of eight different functional systems to determine a person's level of disability. Functional systems are functional neural networks or regions of the CNS and include pyramidal, cerebellar, brainstem, sensory, bowel and bladder, visual function, and cerebral function. Scores for the EDSS range from 0 (no limitations) to 10 (death) in 0.5 unit increments. EDSS scores below 5.0 refer to people who are able to walk without a walking aid and are determined based on the number of functional systems affected, whereas those above 5.0 are determined largely by mobility impairment.

The MSFC comprises three independent functional measures: timed 25-foot walk test (walking), nine-hole peg test (arm and hand function), and the paced auditory serial addition test (PASAT; cognitive processing speed).[13]

Other less frequently utilized clinical measures include the European Database on MS Grading System,[14] Functional Independence Measure,[15] and the Guy's Neurological Disability Scale.[16]

It is now well recognized that the patient's perspective on their disease status and impact, as well as their health and quality of life, is a critical component of their disease management and rehabilitation. PROMs are those captured directly from patients or their care partners. PROMs of disability can be used to replace or to supplement the clinical assessment, or as a surrogate for clinical assessments when patients are being managed remotely. Measures of disease progression and disability include the patient-determined disease steps (PDDS)[17] and the MS rating scale, revised.[18] PROMs can also be used to collect information related to symptoms, health status, and quality of life. For instance the 12-item MS walking scale has been shown to be correlated with clinical assessments of walking and thus may be a useful tool when it is not possible to safely perform the timed 25-foot walk test or 2- or 6-minute walk tests remotely.

While potentially of great use, especially for telemedicine and telerehabilitation approaches for MS care, the use of PROMs in MS can also be challenging. An important consideration is that many PROMs were designed for pen and paper delivery, and remote use would require a more accessible option, such as through an electronic or internet-delivery mechanism. Furthermore, cognitive impairment or physical limitations may pose barriers to a patient's ability to complete PROMs remotely. Thus strategies are necessary for systematically delivering PROMs remotely. Nonetheless, PROMs may be an important tool for bridging the gap between remote assessments and delivery of care.

DISEASE MANAGEMENT IN MS

There is no known cure for MS; thus medical management of MS is directed at slowing or halting the disease process and ameliorating MS symptoms. Medical management for RRMS and SPMS is different from that for PPMS. Disease-modifying therapies (DMTs) are used to decrease the immune-mediated attacks and inflammation in the CNS, speed the recovery after relapse, slow the progression of the disease, and manage MS symptoms. There are several DMTs for persons with RRMS and SPMS. In contrast, there is only one DMT available to persons with PPMS. DMTs can be delivered using injection, orally, or via infusion. Table 9.3 presents the DMTs currently available to persons with MS.

Regardless of the clinical course, early treatment is essential. Early and aggressive treatment can decrease the relapse rate and the formation of new lesions, reduce brain atrophy, and potentially slow the progression and accumulation of disability due to MS.

TABLE 9.3 ▦ **DMTs for Persons With Multiple Sclerosis**

Agent	Features	Risks/Side Effects
Injectable Treatments		
Interferon beta medications	• Among the most commonly prescribed DMTs to treat MS • Injected under the skin or into muscle • May reduce frequency and severity of relapses	• Possible flu-like symptoms and injection-site reactions • Possible liver damage; requires blood tests to monitor liver enzymes • May develop neutralizing antibodies that can reduce drug effectiveness
Glatiramer acetate (Copaxone, Glatopa)	• Injected beneath the skin • May block immune system's attack on myelin	• Possible skin irritation at the injection site
Ofatumumab (Kesimpta)	• Injected beneath the skin • A humanized monoclonal antibody that binds to CD20 surface antigens on lymphocytes • For RRMS and active SPMS	• Infection risk • Injection-related reaction
Oral Treatments		
Fingolimod (Gilenya)	• Once-daily • Can reduce relapse rate	• Slowed heart rate (HR); monitor HR and blood pressure (BP) for 6 hours after first dose • Possible rare serious infections, headaches, high BP, and blurred vision
Dimethyl fumarate (Tecfidera)	• Twice-daily oral medication • Can reduce relapse rate	• Possible flushing, diarrhea, nausea, and lowered white blood cell count • Requires regular blood test monitoring
Diroximel fumarate (Vumerity)	• Twice-daily capsule • Similar to dimethyl fumarate	• Typically fewer side effects than dimethyl fumarate
Teriflunomide (Aubagio)	• Once-daily • Can reduce relapse rate	• Possible liver damage, hair loss, and other side effects • Associated with birth defects when taken by both men and women; must use contraception when taking this medication and for up to 2 years afterward • Requires regular blood test monitoring
Siponimod (Mayzent)	• Once-daily • May reduce relapse rate • May help slow progression of MS • Also approved for SPMS	• Possible viral infections, liver problems, and low white blood cell count • Possible changes in HR; may require HR and BP monitoring after the first dose • Possible headaches and vision problems • Harmful to a developing fetus; women who may become pregnant should use contraception • Requires blood test monitoring on a regular basis

(Continued)

TABLE 9.3 ■ DMTs for Persons With Multiple Sclerosis—Cont'd

Agent	Features	Risks/Side Effects
Cladribine (Mavenclad)	• Given in two treatment courses, spread over a 2-week period, over 2 years • Generally prescribed as second-line treatment for RRMS • Also approved for SPMS	• Possible upper respiratory infections, headaches, tumors, serious infections, and reduced levels of white blood cells • People who have active chronic infections or cancer should not take this drug • Women who are pregnant or breast-feeding and their partners should use contraception when taking and for the following 6 months • May require monitoring with blood tests
Infusion Treatments		
Ocrelizumab (Ocrevus)	• A humanized monoclonal antibody medication • The only DMT approved by the FDA to treat both RRMS and PPMS • Reduced relapse rate in RRMS • Slowed worsening of disability in both RRMS and PPMS	• Possible irritation at the injection site, low BP, a fever, and nausea, among others • Some people may not be able to take ocrelizumab, including those with a hepatitis B infection • Possible increase in the risk of infections and some types of cancer, particularly breast cancer
Natalizumab (Tysabri)	• To block the movement of potentially damaging immune cells from bloodstream to brain and spinal cord • May be considered a first-line treatment for some people with severe MS or as a second-line treatment in others	• Increases the risk of progressive multifocal leukoencephalopathy (PML) in people who are positive for antibodies to the causative agent of PML, JC virus
Alemtuzumab (Campath, Lemtrada)	• Reduces relapse	• Increases risk of infections and other autoimmune disorders, including thyroid autoimmune diseases and rare immune-mediated kidney disease

DMTs, Disease-modifying therapies; *FDA*, US Food and Drug Administration; *MS*, multiple sclerosis; *PPMS*, primary progressive MS; *RRMS*, relapsing-remitting MS; *SPMS*, secondary progressive MS.

SYMPTOM MANAGEMENT

See Table 9.4.

Rehabilitation Management in MS

Rehabilitation is a critical component of MS care and includes interventions to reduce the impact of symptoms, improve function and maintain independence, prevent deconditioning and secondary conditions, and manage the psychosocial impact of this chronic disease.[19-21] Physical activity and exercise are key elements of rehabilitation for people with MS.[10,22] Evidence-based guidelines for people with MS[23] suggest that people with MS with mild-to-moderate disability should perform

TABLE 9.4 ■ **Management of Signs and Symptoms of Multiple Sclerosis**

Sign or Symptom	Strategies

Spasticity or spasms	• Pharmacological
	  • Baclofen (Lioresal, Gablofen)
	  • Dantrolene (Dantrium)
	  • Diazepam (Valium)
	• Surgical
	  • Posterior rhizotomy
	  • Tendonotomy

Fatigue	• Amantadine (Gocovri, Osmolex) • Modafinil (Provigil) • Methylphenidate (Ritalin) • Physical therapy • Occupational therapy • Behavioral interventions
Walking impairment	• Dalfampridine (Ampyra)

Depression/mood dysregulation	• Pharmacological
	  • Selective serotonin reuptake inhibitors
	  • Tricyclic antidepressants
	• Psychotherapy (cognitive behavioral therapy)
	• Physical activity

Bladder dysfunction	• If spastic
	  • Pharmacological anticholinergic medications
	• If flaccid
	  • Intermittent catheterization
	  • Suprapubic catheterization
	• If infection ensues
	  • Antibiotics
	• Dietary modifications

Pain	• Physical therapy
	• Cognitive behavioral and mindfulness-based interventions
	• Pharmacological
	  • Anticonvulsants
	  • Serotonin-norepinephrine reuptake inhibitors
	  • Antispasticity medications (baclofen, tizanidine)
	  • Cannabinoids

30 minutes each of moderate intensity aerobic and anaerobic (strength training) exercise a minimum of twice weekly to improve health, function, and quality of life. There is some evidence that physical activity and exercise may improve physical functioning,[24] cognitive function and capacity,[25] and even neural measures of disease status.[26] Thus the nature of MS warrants care that is coordinated and delivered by a comprehensive, interdisciplinary team. This team includes neurologists, primary care physicians, advance practice professionals, pharmacists, and mental health, rehabilitation, and wellness professionals. This team needs to work together with the patient and their family to determine a long-range plan for effective management of MS, related comorbidities, and potential secondary conditions and telerehabilitation can be a beneficial component of this care plan.

Telemedicine and Telerehabilitation

MS can produce a variety of neurological deficits, making it difficult for patients to access specialty care (Reich, 2018). In addition, the management of patients with MS (pwMS) has become more complex as more DMTs and specialty care interventions have become available, requiring neurology, medical specialists (e.g., rehabilitation, mental health), and primary care providers to coordinate care.[27] Despite improvements in therapy, at least 31% of pwMS do not have access to specialty care.[28] With the advent of the high-speed internet, inexpensive cameras, and monitoring software, telemedicine and telerehabilitation have shown promise in bridging the gap between providers and their patients who have limited access to MS specialty care.[29-31] A recent survey of over 6000 PwMS in North America found 84% exchange health information electronically with their providers and 46% of those with a smart phone or tablet accessed a health care app.[32] Younger age, having comorbidities, higher income, and education were associated with higher e-health utilization.

STUDIES PERTAINING TO TELEHEALTH AND MS

For understanding the overall neurological deficits in a person with MS, there is no substitute for a live examination. That said, a remote physical examination using telemedicine can be integrated into an initial assessment of person with MS as a way to generate testing decisions and an initial management plan. When possible, the live visit serves as a baseline for the patient and gives context to future telemedicine visits. Having telemedicine templates in the electronic medical record and several clinical video telehealth CVT platforms to choose from when connecting to person with MS through another clinic or into the home environment makes the initial remote visit more efficient.

Four studies found telemedicine approaches to be effective for remote neurological examinations and generating an EDSS score in persons with MS.[33-36] Telephone- (interclass correlation $\alpha = 0.88$),[33] clinic CVT– ($\alpha = 0.96$–0.97),[34] and home CVT–based ($P > 0.05$; Kappa [unweighted]: 0.72 within 0.5 on EDSS)[35,36] EDSS assessments showed high correlations and no significant differences compared with in-person examinations, particularly for those with higher disability (EDSS > 6.0). For remote examinations that utilized a health care aid at the patient site, certain aspects of the remote EDSS showed lower correlations with the live assessment including the brain stem ($\alpha = = 0.79$–0.72),[34] cerebellar ($\alpha = 0.57$–0.56),[34] and sensory ($\alpha = 0.74$–0.72)[34,35] functional systems (FS). For the telemedicine-based EDSS that did not utilize an in-home examination assistant, Pearson correlations between individual FS ranged between modest 0.37 (vision) and high at 0.79 (bowel and bladder). Overall, despite some challenges in specific aspects of the neurological examination, an accurate disability assessment can be achieved using a remote video examination in persons with MS and greater accuracy can be attained within functional systems by the use of a remote examination assistant.

Monitoring MS DMT adherence and untoward effects has been shown to be feasible using telemedicine. Reminders sent via cell phones were successful in improving adherence to DMTs[37] as were telephone counseling and remote monitoring.[38] A more comprehensive program of engagement had mixed results with adherence.[39] There has been a move to implement intravenous DMTs in the home setting.[40] This is more convenient for patients and allows for the use of telemedicine for follow-up assessments.

A recent systematic review and metaanalysis of the efficacy of various telerehabilitation approaches on motor, cognitive, and participation outcomes for persons with MS provides a useful overview and assessment of teleapproaches for delivering rehabilitation and exercise interventions, and suggests that these integrated approaches are feasible and meaningful.[41]

Home-based telerehabilitation with physical therapy has been shown to be similar to or more beneficial than usual rehabilitation care in persons with MS.[42,43] Exergaming platforms have been developed for home use, with individualized modules and monitoring capabilities.[44] Finlayson et al.[45] examined fatigue management using a telephone conference group intervention with a two-group time series design and wait-list controls. This teleoccupational therapy program was more effective than the control condition for reducing fatigue impact but not severity. Changes in fatigue were maintained for 6 months with moderate effect sizes.[45] A more recent trial using a version of this teleconference intervention and combining it with a telephone-delivered physical activity intervention also found that the teleconference fatigue self-management program was efficacious in reducing fatigue impact and promoting physical activity in people with MS.[46]

Motl and colleagues[47] have also demonstrated the utility of telephone and internet delivery of exercise programs combined with behavioral strategies to increase physical activity in people with MS. One recent randomized controlled trial (RCT) examined the feasibility and effectiveness of a 4-month home-based exercise training and coaching program based on physical activity guidelines for MS for persons with mild-to-moderate MS.[48] Participants were randomized into an intervention or wait-list control condition. The intervention comprised a pedometer, elastic resistance bands, DVD, training manual, calendars, log-book, video coaching calls, and newsletters. All participants completed home-based assessments before and after the intervention. Fifty-one participants (n = 57) in the intervention group completed 71% of the exercise sessions. There was a moderate increase in self-reported exercise behavior of the intervention participants as measured by the Godin leisure-time exercise questionnaire scores ($d \geq 0.5$), suggesting the potential benefit of a teleapproach for increasing physical activity in persons with MS as well as the need for further research in this area.

Four studies have investigated the use of telerehabilitation in evaluating cognitive function for persons with MS.[37,49–51] Settle et al. (2015) showed statistical equivalence between persons with MS who completed a remote clinical video telerehabilitation or in-office cognitive assessment using the automated neuropsychological assessment metrics test ($P = 0.124$). However, there was some variability in the scores for the home-based clinical video telerehabilitation symbol digit modalities tests ($P = 0.018$). George et al.[50] found that the Modified Telephone Interview for Cognitive Status, a validated phone assessment for cognitive function in the elderly, distinguished a significant cognitive impairment between persons with MS and a control group (mean difference = $-0.60, P = 0.001$).[50]

In a randomized, double-blind, controlled trial of home-based telerehabilitation in persons with MS, there was a significantly greater improvement in the primary outcome of cognitive functioning in the telerehabilitation group compared with the routine care control group (mean change in composite z-scores: 0.25 vs. 0.09, $P = 0.03$).[51] Another study found that internet-based cognitive therapy was associated with improvements in fatigue severity and impact ($P < 0.001$), anxiety ($P < 0.001$), depression ($P < 0.001$), and quality-adjusted life when compared to only receiving standard care.[49]

Telerehabilitation approaches have also been used to deliver a variety of behavioral treatments addressing mood, chronic pain, and fatigue in adults with MS. One of the earliest applications in MS was the use of telephone-delivered cognitive behavioral therapy (CBT) for treating depression. Several RCTs conducted in MS samples have demonstrated the efficacy of telephone-delivered CBT[52] and telephone-delivered physical activity counseling[53,54] for treating depression. In these studies, sessions were time-limited, generally between 8 and 16, 45- to 60-minute sessions, and were delivered by psychologists or master's level social workers with training in MS.

Studies have also demonstrated the efficacy of telerehabilitation cognitive behavioral interventions for chronic pain[55] and for fatigue[55,56] in persons with MS. The evidence to date suggests that self-management interventions delivered via telerehabilitation have high levels of treatment adherence and satisfaction.[55] Although most of the studies to date have examined 1:1 telerehabilitation interventions, two studies are currently underway examining the use of videoconferencing to deliver mindfulness, cognitive behavioral, and behavioral activation interventions for chronic pain to groups of 8 to 12 pwMS.[57,58] A web-based symptom management program, *My MS Toolkit*, also showed promising evidence for improving symptom management in a pilot trial of persons with MS.[59] However, the extent to which people with MS will engage with and benefit from asynchronous web- and app-based interventions remains to be seen, given the lack of research in this area.

In addition to symptom management, recent evidence suggests that other types of interventions promoting emotional and physical well-being in people with MS may be safely and effectively delivered via telerehabilitation. The National MS Society's Everyday Matters program, a six-session positive psychology intervention delivered to a group of people with MS via teleconferencing, increased resilience and satisfaction with social roles in people with MS.[60]

Telerehabilitation can also be used to support in-person and interdisciplinary care. In one example of this prior to the COVID-19 pandemic, MS patients participating in a 12-session collaborative care clinic-based intervention for pain and depression were allowed to choose whether to have their appointments in person or by telerehabilitation (in this case, telephone).[61] Social workers delivered the intervention, which included coordination of medical and rehabilitation treatments and evidence-based behavioral interventions for pain and mood (e.g., CBT and mindfulness meditation training). Patients showed a preference for receiving at least some of their 45- to 60-minute sessions with the interventionist by telerehabilitation; 40% chose telephone only, 52% chose a combination of in-person and telephone, and only 8% chose to receive all of their sessions in person at their MS care center. Weekly interdisciplinary rounds where the panel of patients being followed were reviewed and care plans modified were also conducted by telerehabilitation to allow experts outside the MS center to participate in the care of the patients (e.g., a psychiatrist). Interdisciplinary rounds can readily be conducted virtually if doing so facilitates participation of providers.

IMPROVING CARE BY CONNECTING PROVIDERS

In addition to facilitating care at the patient level, telerehabilitation has also been used to connect community health care providers, especially from rural or underserved areas, with MS specialists. MS Project Extension for Community Health Outcomes (ECHO) was created in 2014 to improve the quality of MS care in underserved areas and by non-MS specialists.[62,63] In this care model, providers who care for people with MS in the community, typically from rural regions, meet regularly (e.g., weekly) with MS specialists (typically from regional MS centers) via live, interactive videoconferences. During these sessions, the providers and experts participate in a brief (~15 minutes) didactic module followed by case-based discussion and consultation.[62] The didactic modules are drawn from a curriculum of educational topics relevant to caring for pwMS (e.g., DMTs, managing an MS relapse, mobility) and delivered by different members of the interdisciplinary MS Project ECHO team. The goal of the program is to foster a community learning environment that includes both experts and generalists who, in turn, expand their own knowledge, skills, and self-efficacy for managing MS patients in their community settings. Preliminary research from the initial ECHO site (Pacific Northwest) found that participants reported improvements in their knowledge and expertise in caring for MS patients and that the program had broad reach into rural communities.[63] The National MS Society and original investigators have partnered to expand the project to include three sites across the United States ("ECHO MS") using a hub-and-spoke model. After the onset of the COVID-19 pandemic, this group pivoted to conduct ECHO MS COVID-19 Response Clinics to respond to the needs of MS providers and community during the COVID-19 pandemic. This effort reached 199 providers from multiple disciplines from across the United States.[64,65]

CONDUCTING A TELEREHABILITATION VISIT

MS is a chronic, progressive disease, and although DMTs can help manage the MS pathology, and symptom management can control the various symptoms, symptoms often remain, and disability accumulates and can progress over time. Thus having ways to monitor patients remotely may increase the likelihood of identifying problems when they occur, and therefore providing treatment in a more timely manner. This, in turn, may reduce or slow the progression or worsening of disability and decrease unnecessary health care utilization, such as emergency care, hospitalization, and extra physician visits.

Providers new to telerehabilitation often wonder if they will be able to establish a strong bond or collaboration with their patients when using technology to connect. The evidence to date has demonstrated that strong therapeutic alliances—the collaborative relationship between a provider and patient—can result from behavioral or psychotherapeutic interventions delivered via telerehabilitation in persons with MS.[55,66]

Telerehabilitation does, however, hold considerable promise for bridging gaps in MS patients' access to rehabilitation therapies, nonpharmacological treatments, behavioral health interventions, and symptom self-management programs. Even before the COVID-19 pandemic, evidence-based nonpharmacological interventions for many common MS comorbidities, including mood disorders and chronic pain, were underutilized.[67,68] Poor access is multifactorial, with geographic barriers, environmental factors (e.g., lack of transportation or childcare to attend therapies), and an insufficient workforce, with expertise in MS, being commonly cited barriers. Whether the increased access to and payment of telemedicine and telerehabilitation around the United States and the world, which has resulted from the COVID-19 pandemic, will remain post-pandemic is unknown. Knowledge gained from the increased use of virtual care during COVID-19 combined with recent and current research on telerehabilitation interventions in MS will hopefully be used to inform the use of and best practices for telerehabilitation in the future.

Recommendations

As summarized in this chapter, there is a need for telemedicine and telerehabilitation approaches for people with MS, but there is also limited evidence to date that supports the use of telerehabilitation for some aspects of care in people with MS. More and better quality trials are needed.[69] Pragmatic clinical studies are particularly needed to assess the effectiveness of telemedicine and telerehabilitation delivery of care relative to in-person care as well as in real-world settings. Several pragmatic clinical trials are currently underway in the MS population, including two that compare clinic- and home-based telerehabilitation interventions[47,70] and one comparing fatigue interventions delivered via telerehabilitation.[59] Trials of telerehabilitation interventions should include patient satisfaction outcomes and process measures (e.g., treatment adherence, therapeutic alliance) in addition to treatment outcomes.

In addition to monitoring patients for changes in their status, clinical assessments of walking, balance, strength, and somatosensation are often necessary to determine a patient's needs and to define a relevant and effective treatment plan. However, remotely assessing these impairments may not only be difficult but may also pose a safety concern. For instance, persons with MS have been shown to be at risk for falls, and those with balance impairment are at an even greater risk of falling when walking. Thus asking them to perform walking assessments or related interventions alone, while being observed remotely, poses a significant safety concern and is not recommended. Therefore tools that allow providers and clinicians to safely monitor and assess their patients will lead to higher quality of care and potentially improved function, health, and quality of life for people with MS.

Walking impairment is common in MS and may be useful as an indicator of level of disability. Goldman et al. demonstrated that the timed 25-foot walk test may serve as a predictor of overall disability.[71] However, clinical assessments such as the timed 25-foot walk test and the 2- or 6-minute walk tests do not always correctly depict a patient's abilities in their home or community. PROMs of mobility, such as the 12-item MS walking scale, are limited by patient recall as well as their own perception of their abilities, which may be biased. Remote monitoring using wearable devices may provide an objective measure that can be used to track disease progression, determine when function is deteriorating, help to define a patient's goals and treatment plan, and measure response to therapies. For instance, a study by Block et al. found that step counts measured by a Fitbit accelerometer (Fitbit, LLC) correlated with greater disability on the EDSS ($P < 0.001$) and showed important variability in walking activity within individual EDSS categories,[72] information that could be used to monitor patient status remotely. More research is necessary in this area.

Telerehabilitation encompasses a wide array of assessment and intervention services, some of which may be better suited to the telerehabilitation format, for a particular individual. For instance, Plow et al. recently reported on the response heterogeneity of individuals in an RCT of telerehabilitation approaches in persons with MS.[73] Research is needed to determine for whom and under what conditions telerehabilitation approaches are effective in the care of the person with MS. Other research areas worth exploring include strategies for maximizing participation in telerehabilitation therapies, exploring the use of hybrid approaches, and finding ways to best harness technology to engage patients in proactively managing their disease, their symptoms, and functioning, including in between health care visits. The use of telerehabilitation/mobile assessments, mobile health (mHealth), remote patient monitoring, and patient-generated health data (e.g., activity data captured by patient's mobile devices such as a watch or phone) remain relatively unexplored and potential avenues for future research.

CASE STUDY

Ms. Simms is a 41-year-old African American female attorney with relapsing-remitting multiple sclerosis (MS), who lives in Washington, DC. She started a new MS disease-modifying medication in January 2020. She experiences balance problems and difficulty with walking independently. She also expresses that she has some additional difficulty when walking and talking at the same time (dual tasking), and with remembering things. She was referred for a neuropsychology evaluation and to physical therapy and speech therapy for further assessment. Neuropsychology evaluation showed Ms. Simms had normal cognitive function that declined minimally with fatigue. The speech therapist provided her with strategies to help with memory. The physical therapist determined a need for an assistive device while walking, saw Ms. Simms for three in-person visits to help address balance and gait deviations, and provided a home exercise program for strengthening and balance.

Ms. Simms traveled in early March to see her family in New York City. Five days after arriving, Ms. Simms developed a high fever, cough, mild arm skin rash, and increasing right leg weakness. She went to a nearby emergency room and tested positive for COVID-19 with mild right leg weakness. Her vital signs, serum laboratory testing, and chest x-ray were normal. Ms. Simms was told to rest and quarantine herself for 14 days. The patient called her neurology clinic in Washington, DC for advice about her weakness and modifications in her MS treatment.

A number of remote interventions could be used to address this patient's acute neurological symptoms while she was quarantined with COVID-19. A secure televideo-based history and physical examination could be initiated by her neurology providers to assess the patient's current neurological deficits, the skin rash, and consider the need for changes in the patient's MS-directed therapy or symptomatic MS therapy. Additionally, a physical therapy assessment could also be generated to assess for acute changes in gait and changes in the home-based physical therapy and exercise program. The physical therapist could provide remote therapy and an exercise trainer could provide and oversee exercise using a teleconference platform, such as Zoom.

Although this case illustrates how an infectious disease pandemic has forced medical providers to use telemedicine to address acute and chronic disease management,[74] these same approaches can be utilized for patients who are in communities or situations where they cannot access in-person MS care. It must also be noted that health insurance reimbursements and cross-state or country medical provider laws have been modified to accommodate the use of telemedicine and telerehabilitation during the COVID-19 pandemic, and the current status of any care provided must be considered in light of local rules.

References

1. Reich D, Lucchinetti C, Calabresi P. Multiple sclerosis. *N Engl J Med*. 2018;378(2):169–180.
2. Walton C, King R, Rechtman L, et al. Rising prevalence of multiple sclerosis worldwide: insights from the atlas of MS. *Multiple Scler*. 2020;26(14):1816–1821.
3. Wallin MT, Culpepper WJ, Nichols E, et al. Global, regional, and national burden of multiple sclerosis 1990–2016: a systematic analysis for the Global Burden of Disease Study 2016. *Lancet Neurol*. 2019;18(3):269–285.
4. Lassmann H. Multiple sclerosis pathology. *Cold Spring Harb Perspect Med*. 2018;8(3):a028936.
5. Marrie RA, Cohen J, Stuve O, et al. A systematic review of the incidence and prevalence of comorbidity in multiple sclerosis: overview. *Multiple Scler J*. 2015;21(3):263–281.
6. Zhang T, Tremlett H, Zhu F, et al. Effects of physical comorbidities on disability progression in multiple sclerosis. *Neurology*. 2018;90(5):e419–e427.
7. McKay KA, Tremlett H, Fisk JD, et al. Psychiatric comorbidity is associated with disability progression in multiple sclerosis. *Neurology*. 2018;90(15):e1316–e1323.
8. Marrie RA, Reingold S, Cohen J, et al. The incidence and prevalence of psychiatric disorders in multiple sclerosis: a systematic review. *Multiple Scler*. 2015;21(3):305–317.
9. Foley PL, Vesterinen HM, Laird BJ, et al. Prevalence and natural history of pain in adults with multiple sclerosis: systematic review and meta-analysis. *PAIN®*. 2013;154(5):632–642.
10. Backus D. Increasing physical activity and participation in people with multiple sclerosis: a review. *Arch Phys Med Rehabilitation*. 2016;97(9):S210–S217.
11. Rae-Grant A, Bennett A, Sanders AE, et al. Quality improvement in neurology: multiple sclerosis quality measures: executive summary. *Neurology*. 2015;85(21):1904–1908.
12. Kurtzke JF. Rating neurologic impairment in multiple sclerosis: an expanded disability status scale (EDSS). *Neurology*. 1983;33(11). 1444-1444.
13. Fischer JS, Rudick RA, Cutter GR, et al. The Multiple Sclerosis Functional Composite measure (MSFC): an integrated approach to MS clinical outcome assessment. National MS Society Clinical Outcomes Assessment Task Force. *Multiple Scler*. 1999;5(4):244–250.
14. Confavreux C, Compston DA, Hommes OR, et al. EDMUS, a European database for multiple sclerosis. *J Neurol Neurosurg Psychiatry*. 1992;55(8):671–676.
15. Brosseau L, Wolfson C. The inter-rater reliability and construct validity of the functional independence measure for multiple sclerosis subjects. *Clin Rehabilitation*. 1994;8(2):107–115.
16. Sharrack B, Hughes RA. The Guy's Neurological Disability Scale (GNDS): a new disability measure for multiple sclerosis. *Multiple Scler J*. 1999;5(4):223–233.
17. Hohol MJ, Orav EJ, Weiner HL. Disease steps in multiple sclerosis: a simple approach to evaluate disease progression. *Neurology*. 1995;45(2):251–255.
18. Wicks P, Vaughan TE, Massagli MP. The multiple sclerosis rating scale, revised (MSRS-R): development, refinement, and psychometric validation using an online community. *Health Qual Life Outcomes*. 2012;10(1):1–12.
19. Kraft GH. Rehabilitation still the only way to improve function in multiple sclerosis. *Lancet*. 1999; 354:2016–2017.
20. Bennett S.E., Bednarik P., Bobryk P., et al. *A Practical Guide to Rehabilitation in Multiple Sclerosis*. 2015. Available at: http://www.cmeaims.org/rehab-primer-cme.php. Accessed 24.02.16.
21. Sutliff MH, Bennett SE, Bobryk P, et al. Rehabilitation in multiple sclerosis: commentary on the recent AAN systematic review. *Neurology: Clin Pract*. 2016;6(6):475–479.
22. Motl RW, Pilutti LA. The benefits of exercise training in multiple sclerosis. *Nat Rev Neurol*. 2012; 8(9):487–497.
23. Latimer-Cheung AE, Ginis KAM, Hicks AL, et al. Development of evidence-informed physical activity guidelines for adults with multiple sclerosis. *Arch Phys Med Rehabilitation*. 2013;94(9):1829–1836.
24. Dalgas U, Stenager E. Exercise and disease progression in multiple sclerosis: can exercise slow down the progression of multiple sclerosis? *Therapeutic Adv Neurological Disord*. 2012;5(2):81–95.
25. Sandroff BM, Motl RW, Scudder MR, et al. Systematic, evidence-based review of exercise, physical activity, and physical fitness effects on cognition in persons with multiple sclerosis. *Neuropsychol Rev*. 2016;26(3):271–294.

26. Negaresh R, Motl RW, Zimmer P, et al. Effects of exercise training on multiple sclerosis biomarkers of central nervous system and disease status: a systematic review of intervention studies. *Eur J Neurol.* 2019;26(5):711–721.

27. Tornatore C, Phillips JT, Khan O, et al. Consensus opinion of US neurologists on practice patterns in RIS, CIS, and RRMS: evolution of treatment practices. *Neurology: Clin Pract.* 2016;6(4):329–338.

28. Minden S. Access to health care for people with multiple sclerosis. *Mult Scler.* 2007;13:547–558.

29. Mutgi SA, Zha AM, Behrouz R. Emerging subspecialties in neurology: telestroke and teleneurology. *Neurology.* 2015;84(22):e191–e193.

30. Campion EW, Dorsey E, Topol E. State of telehealth. *N Engl J Med.* 2016;375(2):154–161.

31. Department of Veterans Affairs Health Administration. VA Telehealth Services. www.telehealth.va.gov; Accessed 15.10.20.

32. Marrie RA, Leung S, Tyry T, et al. Use of eHealth and mHealth technology by persons with multiple sclerosis. *Mult Scler Relat Disord.* 2019;27:13–19.

33. Huda S, Cavey A, Izat A, et al. Nurse led telephone assessment of expanded disability status scale assessment in MS patients at high levels of disability. *J Neurol Sci.* 2016;362:66–68.

34. Kane RL, Bever CT, Ehrmantraut M, et al. Teleneurology in patients with multiple sclerosis: EDSS ratings derived remotely and from hands-on examination. *J Telemed Telecare.* 2008;14(4):190–194.

35. Wood J, Wallin M, Finkelstein J. Can a low-cost webcam be used for a remote neurological exam? *Stud Health Technol Inform.* 2013;190:30–32.

36. Bove R, Bevan C, Crabtree E, et al. Toward a low-cost, in-home, telemedicine-enabled assessment of disability in multiple sclerosis. *Mult Scler.* 2019;25:1526–1534.

37. Settle JR, Robinson SA, Kane R, et al. Remote cognitive assessments for patients with multiple sclerosis: a feasibility study. *Mult Scler.* 2015;21(8):1072–1079.

38. Turner AP, Sloan AP, Kivlahan DR, et al. Telephone counseling and home telehealth monitoring to improve medication adherence: results of a pilot trial among individuals with multiple sclerosis. *Rehabil Psychol.* 2014;59(2):136.

39. Jongen PJ, Ter Veen G, Lemmens W, et al. The interactive web-based program MSmonitor for self-management and multidisciplinary care in persons with multiple sclerosis: quasi-experimental study of short-term effects on patient empowerment. *J Med Internet Res.* 2020;22(3):e14297.

40. Schultz TJ, Thomas A, Georgiou P, et al. Developing a model of care for home infusions of natalizumab for people with multiple sclerosis. *J Infus Nurs.* 2019;42(6):289.

41. Di Tella S, Pagliari C, Blasi V, et al. Integrated telerehabilitation approach in multiple sclerosis: a systematic review and meta-analysis. *J Telemed Telecare.* 2020;26(7-8):385–399.

42. Huijgen BC, Vollenbroek-Hutten MM, Zampolini M, et al. Feasibility of a home-based telerehabilitation system compared to usual care: arm/hand function in patients with stroke, traumatic brain injury and multiple sclerosis. *J Telemed Telecare.* 2008;14(5):249–256.

43. Ortiz-Gutiérrez R, Cano-de-la-Cuerda R, Galán-del-Río F, et al. A telerehabilitation program improves postural control in multiple sclerosis patients: a Spanish preliminary study. *Int J Environ Res Public Health.* 2013;10(11):5697–5710.

44. Chanpimol S, Benson K, Maloni H, et al. Acceptability and outcomes of an individualized exer-gaming telePT program for veterans with multiple sclerosis: a pilot study. *Archives of Physiotherapy.* 2020;10(1):1–10.

45. Finlayson M, Preissner K, Cho C, et al. Randomized trial of a teleconference-delivered fatigue management program for people with multiple sclerosis. *Multiple Sclerosis Journal.* 2011;17(9):1130–1140.

46. Plow M, Finlayson M, Liu J, et al. Randomized controlled trial of a telephone-delivered physical activity and fatigue self-management interventions in adults with multiple sclerosis. *Arch Phys Med Rehabil.* 2019;100(11):2006–2014.

47. Motl RW, Backus D, Neal WN, et al. Rationale and design of the STEP for MS trial: comparative effectiveness of supervised versus telerehabilitation exercise programs for multiple sclerosis. *Contemp Clin Trials.* 2019;81:110–122.

48. Learmonth YC, Adamson BC, Kinnett-Hopkins D, et al. Results of a feasibility randomised controlled study of the guidelines for exercise in multiple sclerosis project. *Contemp Clin Trials.* 2017;54:84–97.

49. Moss-Morris R, McCrone P, Yardley L, et al. A pilot randomised controlled trial of an Internet-based cognitive behavioural therapy self-management programme (MS Invigor8) for multiple sclerosis fatigue. *Behav Res Ther.* 2012;50(6):415–421.

50. George MF, Holingue CB, Briggs FB, et al. Feasibility study for remote assessment of cognitive function in multiple sclerosis. *J Neurol Neuromedicine*. 2016;1(8):10.
51. Charvet LE, Yang J, Shaw MT, et al. Cognitive function in multiple sclerosis improves with telerehabilitation: results from a randomized controlled trial. *PLoS One*. 2017;12(5):e0177177.
52. Mohr DC, Hart SL, Julian L, et al. Telephone-administered psychotherapy for depression. *Arch Gen Psychiatry*. 2005;62(9):1007–1014.
53. Bombardier CH, Ehde DM, Gibbons LE, et al. Telephone-based physical activity counseling for major depression in people with multiple sclerosis. *J Consult Clin Psychol*. 2013;81(1):89.
54. Turner AP, Hartoonian N, Sloan AP, et al. Improving fatigue and depression in individuals with multiple sclerosis using telephone-administered physical activity counseling. *J Consult Clin Psychol*. 2016;84(4):297.
55. Ehde DM, Elzea JL, Verrall AM, et al. Efficacy of a telephone-delivered self-management intervention for persons with multiple sclerosis: a randomized controlled trial with a one-year follow-up. *Arch Phys Med Rehabil*. 2015;96(11):1945–1958.
56. Pöttgen J, Moss-Morris R, Wendebourg JM, et al. Randomised controlled trial of a self-guided online fatigue intervention in multiple sclerosis. *J Neurol Neurosurg Psychiatry*. 2018;89(9):970–976.
57. Day MA, Ehde DM, Burns J, et al. A randomized trial to examine the mechanisms of cognitive, behavioral and mindfulness-based psychosocial treatments for chronic pain: study protocol. *Contemp Clin Trials*. 2020;93:106000.
58. Ehde DM, Alschuler KN, Day MA, et al. Mindfulness-based cognitive therapy and cognitive behavioral therapy for chronic pain in multiple sclerosis: a randomized controlled trial protocol. *Trials*. 2019;20(1):1–12.
59. Kratz AL, Alschuler KN, Williams DA, et al. Development and pilot testing of a web-based symptom management program for multiple sclerosis: My MS toolkit. *Rehabil Psychol*. 2021;66(2):224–232.
60. Alschuler KN, Arewasikporn A, Nelson IK, et al. Promoting resilience in individuals aging with multiple sclerosis: results from a pilot randomized controlled trial. *Rehabil Psychol*. 2018;63(3):338.
61. Ehde DM, Alschuler KN, Sullivan MD, et al. Improving the quality of depression and pain care in multiple sclerosis using collaborative care: the MS-care trial protocol. *Contemp Clin Trials*. 2018;64:219–229.
62. Johnson KL, Hertz D, Stobbe G, et al. Project Extension for Community Healthcare Outcomes (ECHO) in multiple sclerosis: increasing clinician capacity. *Int J MS Care*. 2017;19(6):283–289.
63. Alschuler KN, Stobbe GA, Hertz DP, et al. Impact of multiple sclerosis project ECHO (Extension for Community Healthcare Outcomes) on provider confidence and clinical practice. *Int J MS Care*. 2019;21(4):143–150.
64. Alschuler KN, Altman JK, Ehde DM. Feasibility and acceptability of a single-session, videoconference-delivered group intervention for pain in multiple sclerosis. *Rehabil Psychol*. 2021;66(1):22–30.
65. Alschuler KN, von Geldern G, Ball D, et al. Rapid transfer of knowledge for multiple sclerosis clinical care during COVID-19: ECHO MS. *Mult Scler Relat Disord*. 2020;46:102600.
66. Beckner V, Vella L, Howard I, et al. Alliance in two telephone-administered treatments: relationship with depression and health outcomes. *J Consult Clin Psychol*. 2007;75(3):508.
67. Ehde DM, Dillworth TM, Turner JA. Cognitive-behavioral therapy for individuals with chronic pain: efficacy, innovations, and directions for research. *Am Psychol*. 2014;69(2):153–166.
68. Minden SL, Feinstein A, Kalb RC, et al. Evidence-based guideline: assessment and management of psychiatric disorders in individuals with MS. Report of the Guideline Development Subcommittee of the American Academy of Neurology. *Neurology*. 2014;82(2):174–181.
69. Proctor BJ, Moghaddam N, Vogt W, et al. Telephone psychotherapy in multiple sclerosis: a systematic review and meta-analysis. *Rehabil Psychol*. 2018;63(1):16.
70. Rimmer JH, Thirumalai M, Young HJ, et al. Rationale and design of the tele-exercise and multiple sclerosis (TEAMS) study: a comparative effectiveness trial between a clinic-and home-based telerehabilitation intervention for adults with multiple sclerosis (MS) living in the deep south. *Contemp Clin Trials*. 2018;71:186–193.
71. Goldman MD, Motl RW, Scagnelli J, et al. Clinically meaningful performance benchmarks in MS: timed 25-foot walk and the real world. *Neurology*. 2013;81(21):1856–1863.
72. Block VJ, Lizee A, Crabtree-Hartman E, et al. Continuous daily assessment of multiple sclerosis disability using remote step count monitoring. *J Neurol*. 2017;264(2):316–326.

73. Plow M, Motl RW, Finlayson M, Bethoux F. R Response heterogeneity in a randomized controlled trial of telerehabilitation interventions among adults with multiple sclerosis. *J Telemed Telecare*. 2020: 1357633X20964693. http://dx.doi.org/10.1177/1357633X20964693. Epub ahead of print. PMID: 33100184.
74. Grossman SN, Han SC, Balcer LJ, et al. Rapid implementation of virtual neurology in response to the COVID-19 pandemic. *Neurology*. 2020;94(24):1077–1087.

Telerehabilitation in Amyotrophic Lateral Sclerosis

Colleen O'Connell ▓ Suzanne Salsman

Introduction

Amyotrophic lateral sclerosis (ALS) is a progressive neurodegenerative disease characterized by loss of motor neurons in the motor cortex, brainstem, and spinal cord.[1] ALS is manifested by upper (UMN) and lower motor neuron (LMN) signs and symptoms affecting bulbar, limb, and respiratory musculature, usually with focal disease onset and eventual spread to other body regions.[2] It is a terminal disease with no curative treatment, with respiratory failure leading to death typically 3 to 5 years following symptom onset.[1,2] Clinical findings of UMN and LMN disease, in conjunction with electromyography, can help confirm the diagnosis and extent of denervation, but ALS is otherwise a diagnosis of exclusion, with normal imaging and laboratory testing ruling out reversible disorders with similar features.[1] Treatment options, such as riluzole or edaravone, can improve survival or slow decline, but the benefit is measured in months. Therefore the focus of care for ALS patients is most often symptom management, as well as optimizing day-to-day function and quality of life through various rehabilitation interventions.[2,3]

ALS is the most frequent neurodegenerative disorder of midlife, and the global incidence of ALS has remained at one or two new cases per year per 100,000 people.[1] Prevalence increases with age, with the median age of onset at 65 years for sporadic cases of European ancestry[2] and males more often affected than females, at a ratio approaching 2:1.[1] Clinical presentations of ALS are often grouped into classifications of inheritance (familial or sporadic), phenotype (bulbar- or limb onset), and sub-phenotypes (ALS-FTD, pseudobulbar palsy, progressive spinal muscle atrophy, and primary lateral sclerosis). Further classification can be made by genetic features as evolving technologies for gene mapping have identified multiple ALS genes.[1] Among these, a unifying cause for motor neuron degeneration in ALS remains unclear. Familial forms and bulbar onset have poorer prognosis with regard to speed of disease progression. Overall the heterogeneity of ALS with respect to clinical presentation, disease progression, potential disease pathophysiology, and genetic features has led clinicians and researchers to recognize ALS as a syndrome affecting multiple systems.[4]

Clinically, ALS patients present with impairments as related to progressive weakness, fasciculations, muscle atrophy, spasticity, speech and swallowing difficulty, respiratory compromise, and in some cases neuropsychological impairments. Limb onset is the most common presentation, seen in about two-thirds of ALS patients, with weakness impacting mobility and upper extremity function.[2] Bulbar onset accounts for about one-third of cases, with impairments in swallowing and speech affecting nutrition and communication.[2] In addition, about 5% to 15% of ALS patients may fulfill criteria for frontotemporal dementia (ALS-FTD),[2] and, more widely, cognitive or behavioral impairment occurs in up to 50% of ALS patients within the spectrum of FTD.[5] Rates of decline are predicted by the ALS functional rating scale (FRS), forced vital capacity (FVC), and manual muscle test; however, cognition, psychosocial factors, nutritional status, and respiratory function have also been shown to be related to outcome.

Two disease-modifying pharmacological therapies can be offered to ALS patients. In some studies, riluzole has been shown to have a modest benefit on survival between 3 and 12 months.[6] Edaravone may be effective in slowing functional decline in a select group of ALS patients over 6 months.[7] Early referral to a specialized ALS multidisciplinary clinic (MDC) is recommended.[6,7] Involvement in an MDC has been shown to be an independent predictor of survival, with patients living 7.5 months longer.[8–10] Various studies have shown that multidisciplinary care is associated with better outcomes, including increased utilization of riluzole, noninvasive positive pressure ventilation (NIPPV), percutaneous feeding tubes, and adaptive equipment along with, most importantly, improved quality of life.[7–10] Evidence suggests that NIPPV lengthens survival and if initiated early can slow the rate of FVC decline.[6,11–13] Use of percutaneous endoscopic gastrostomy (PEG) feeding tube has also been shown to prolong survival.[6,7] Regular moderate-intensity exercise is probably beneficial for function and quality of life.[7]

In a specialized ALS MDC, rehabilitation needs can be assessed and coordinated to ensure early and appropriate timing of care based on best practice guidelines (see Table 10.1). Multidisciplinary care involves a team-based approach, which most often includes a physician,

TABLE 10.1 ■ Published Clinical Practice Guidelines in Amyotrophic Lateral Sclerosis

Guideline	Year Published	URL
Canadian best practice recommendations for the management of amyotrophic lateral sclerosis	2020	http://doi.org/10.1503/cmaj.191721
Home mechanical ventilation for patients with amyotrophic lateral sclerosis: a Canadian Thoracic Society clinical practice guideline	2019	http://doi.org/10.1080/24745332.2018.1559644
Motor neurone disease: assessment and management **NICE** guideline (UK)	2016 (updated 2020)	http://nice.org.uk/guidance/ng42/
EFNS Task Force on diagnosis and management of amyotrophic lateral sclerosis (Europe)	2012	http://doi.org/10.1111/j.1468-1331.2011.03501.x
Practice parameter update—the care of the patient with amyotrophic lateral sclerosis: drug, nutritional, and respiratory therapies (an evidence-based review). Report of the Quality Standards Subcommittee of the American Academy of Neurology	2009 (reaffirmed 2020)	http://aan.com/Guidelines/home/GuidelineDetail/370
Practice parameter update—the care of the patient with amyotrophic lateral sclerosis: multidisciplinary care, symptom management, and cognitive/behavioral impairment (an evidence-based review): report of the Quality Standards Subcommittee of the American Academy of Neurology	2009 (reaffirmed 2020)	http://aan.com/Guidelines/home/GuidelineDetail/371

NICE, National Institute for Health and Care Excellence.

physiotherapist, occupational therapist, speech-language pathologist, dietician, respiratory therapist, and registered nurse.[3,7] In order to address specific medical complications of this progressive disease, additional physician specialists, such as respiratory therapy or respirology, gastroenterology, and interventional radiology, and health professions, such as orthotics, assistive technology, social work, and psychology, may be linked to the clinic.[3,7] As the disease progresses, end-of-life care is often coordinated through consultation with palliative care. In addition, in Canada, information about medical assistance in dying is provided when requested.[7]

MDCs provide prospective care, with early introduction of rehabilitation interventions in the anticipation of and planning for disease progression. Studies indicate that for people with ALS to maintain their quality of life, it is important that rehabilitation providers help maintain the person's independence for as long as possible so that they feel empowered and in control of their lives.[14] Rehabilitation expertise in interventions such as mobility and communication aids, swallowing and nutrition, exercise, management of pain and spasticity, respiratory care and secretion management, fatigue and sleep disorders, as well as cognition and psychosocial issues, is used to maximize patient independence, function, safety, and quality of life and to minimize disease-related symptoms.

Management of patients with ALS should be a collaboration between the family physician and the multidisciplinary ALS clinic, with the ALS clinic staff and a dedicated nurse available for remote consultation between patient visits.[7] The frequency of MDC visits will be dictated by the patient's needs and rate of progression, as well as the patient's ability to attend. Physical impairments, fatigue, and geography can limit an ALS patient from attending in-person visits to the MDC. When these challenges are present, telerehabilitation and telehealth monitoring are feasible and may be able to supplement clinic-based multidisciplinary care.[15]

Telerehabilitation in Amyotrophic Lateral Sclerosis

Best practice and evidence-based guidelines recommend that persons with ALS (PALS) should be managed by specialized MDCs (Table 10.1). Benefits of such care include improved survival, reduced hospitalizations, greater use of adaptive equipment, increased use of interventions such as feeding tubes and noninvasive ventilation, and better quality of life.[7,16] Barriers to accessing such clinics are well recognized and include time and distance to travel, economic and family burdens, stress/anxiety, and fatigue associated with the effort, particularly as the disease progresses and mobility, swallowing, breathing become more difficult. Additionally, such specialized care is typically centered in larger urban areas and academic centers, potentially huge distances for some families. Emerging evidence supports that telerehabilitation can allow for timely and cost-effective care for PALS, including access to multidisciplinary care, with outcomes similar to those followed by in-person clinics.[17] With technology advances and greater access to mobile services, there has been a marked upswing in the study and reporting of telerehabilitation and telehealth experience in ALS care (Table 10.2). Research and practice have been recently accelerated by the global COVID-19 pandemic, with in-person visit restrictions necessitating a shift to virtual solutions.[18,19] Ongoing management and monitoring are particularly critical in this population whose care needs steadily change with the unrelenting disease progression. A recent systematic review captures that telehealth in ALS is well received by patients and caregivers while highlighting the importance of training and support.[20] Recognizing this important strategy for ALS care, in the recently published Canadian best practice recommendations, delivery of multidisciplinary care through telerehabilitation and telehealth monitoring was recommended as "feasible and may be able to supplement clinic-based multidisciplinary care."[7] Three broad categories of telerehabilitation approaches have been described.

TABLE 10.2 ■ **Selected Published Research on Telehealth, Telemedicine, and Telerehabilitation in Persons With Amyotrophic Lateral Sclerosis (PALS)**

Study/Year/Country	Sample Description	Method/Intervention	Outcomes	Key Findings
Capozzo et al. Telemedicine is a useful tool to deliver care to patients with amyotrophic lateral sclerosis during COVID-19 pandemic: results from Southern Italy 2020 Italy	n = 31 PALS already diagnosed and followed at the MDC	Emergency use of telemedicine visit by telephone with neurologist	Satisfaction with intervention	All participants refused video and opted for phone; 85% were satisfied with the phone consultation and 90% were willing to continue with the program
Helleman et al. Telehealth as part of specialized ALS care; feasibility and user experiences with "ALS home-monitoring and coaching" 2020 Netherlands	n = 50 PALS app users Survey n = 23 PALS 9 HCP Interview n = 12 PALS	ALS app for self-monitoring and alerts with nurse practitioner follow-up	Adherence rates to self-reporting User surveys and interviews	87% adherence for reporting monthly ALSFRS-R; majority were satisfied with and HCP endorsed as added value
Ando et al. Incorporating self-reported questions for telemonitoring to optimize care of patients with MND on noninvasive ventilation (MND OptNIVent) 2019 UK	n = 13 on NIV 7 survived to study completion (5 male)	Self-report questionnaire submitted via weekly telemonitoring	ALSFRS-R Ventilator settings SpO₂	The question set together with weekly ventilator and oximetry monitoring facilitated the maintenance of ventilation and SpO₂ levels despite illness progression
Ando et al. Experience of telehealth in people with motor neurone disease using noninvasive ventilation 2019 UK	n = 13 on NIV 7 survived to study completion (5 male)	Participants used a telemonitoring device for 24 weeks, reporting weekly ventilator and oximetry data through a tablet-based application	Thematic analysis of semi-structured interviews ALSFRS-R	Telemonitoring was positive experience; participants endorsed could reduce costs and burden and promoted physical and psychological well-being
Hobson et al. Process evaluation and exploration of telehealth in motor neuron disease in a UK specialist centre 2019 UK	n = 40 PALS and 37 primary informal caregivers	Usual care in-person visits with telemedicine tablet-based application as an add-on service, compared to usual care alone	Interviews on outcomes and experiences, descriptive analysis of implementation, and use of the application	Adherence was 70% among PALS; technology barriers were overcome by face-to-face training. Changes to alert system algorithms were recommended to address mismatch between patient and nurse expectations

TABLE 10.2 ■ Selected Published Research on Telehealth, Telemedicine, and Telerehabilitation in Persons With Amyotrophic Lateral Sclerosis (PALS)—Cont'd

Study/Year/Country	Sample Description	Method/Intervention	Outcomes	Key Findings
Pulley et al. Multidisciplinary amyotrophic lateral sclerosis telemedicine care: the store and forward method 2019 United States	n = 18 PALS completed 27 visits	Trained nurse performed home visits and video-recorded assessments that were later reviewed by the MDC team	Survey of satisfaction	Patients were all satisfied with the telemedicine visits
Braga et al. Telemonitoring of a home-based exercise program in amyotrophic lateral sclerosis: a feasibility study 2018 Portugal	n = 10 patients with ALS onset 6 to 24 months ALSFRS-R ≥ 30 FVC > 70%	Assessment of a telemonitoring system (TMS) for home exercise program	Compliance as captured by the TMS	Telemonitoring over 6 months was feasible and safe for monitoring a home aerobic (15 min of under 75% max HR) exercise program
James et al. Patients' perspectives of multidisciplinary home-based e-Health service delivery for motor neurone disease 2018 Australia	n = 12 PALS and 1 MND support association	Assessment of information technology use and home-based telehealth	Descriptive analysis of survey and interview	Patients are willing and able to participate in telehealth, particularly videoconferencing
Van De Rijn et al. Experience with telemedicine in a multidisciplinary ALS clinic 2018 United States	n = 97 PALS	Retrospective chart review of PALS using video televisits	Descriptive analysis of intervention	Most commonly addressed issues were medication management, goals of care, research, and equipment
Selkirk et al. Delivering tertiary center specialty care to ALS patients via telemedicine: a retrospective cohort analysis 2017 United States	n = 32 telehealth and 36 in-person clinic; no significant differences between groups other than telehealth lived further distance	Comparison of patients who chose videoconference to those followed through in-person clinics	Survival ALSFRS-R Quality of care indicators (adherence to select AAN best practices)	No difference in survival Patients receiving telemedicine had lower rates of disease progression; overall concluded quality of care and outcomes were similar

(Continued)

TABLE 10.2 ■ Selected Published Research on Telehealth, Telemedicine, and Telerehabilitation in Persons With Amyotrophic Lateral Sclerosis (PALS) —Cont'd

Study/Year/Country	Sample Description	Method/Intervention	Outcomes	Key Findings
Geronimo et al. Incorporation of telehealth into a multidisciplinary ALS Clinic: feasibility and acceptability 2017 United States	n = 11 PALS, 12 caregivers, 15 HCP ALSFRS-R (0–37)	Videoconference ALS MDC with patient at home, held every 3 months in place of in-person clinic	Qualitative assessment of survey feedback	Telehealth experiences were rated highly, and deemed to be feasible and acceptable. Participants endorsed positives of no travel and less time required, noting challenges with technology and missing the physical examination as dislikes
Maier et al. Online assessment of ALS functional rating scale compares well to in-clinic evaluation: a prospective trial 2012 Germany	n = 127 (n = 81 completed)	Online portal for self-administration of the ALSFRS-R	Comparison of onsite and online assessments at baseline and 3.5 months	Correlation between onsite evaluation and online testing of ALSFRS-R was highly significant ($r = 0.96$; $P < 0.001$)
Nijeweme-d'Hollosy et al. Teletreatment of patients with amyotrophic lateral sclerosis 2006 Netherlands	n = 4 (three male) Computer savvy Mean age 42.3	Add-on teletreatment sessions with ALS rehabilitation physicians	Survey and interview of satisfaction and experiences with teletreatment	Participants were satisfied and positive about sessions; symptom management and disease progression were acceptable topics for teletreatment, while acceptance of diagnosis and end-of-life preference discussions were preferred to be held face to face

AAN, American Academy of Neurology; *ALS*, amyotrophic lateral sclerosis; *ALSFRS-R*, ALS functional rating scale-revised; *HCP*, health care profession; *MDC*, multidisciplinary clinic; *NIV*, noninvasive ventilation.

SYNCHRONOUS MULTIPARTICIPANT CONSULTATION, CLINIC, OR THERAPY SESSION FORMAT

Ranging from simple two-way telephone conversations to multisite, multiparticipant, video-enabled conferencing (Fig. 10.1), this format most commonly supports a more traditional consultation, facilitating discussion of symptoms management and disease progression. A small (n = 4) computer-savvy PALS prospective study from the Netherlands evaluated participants' satisfaction with secure web-based teletreatments with their ALS rehabilitation physician.[21] Patients could schedule their sessions from a general website that included ALS information along with the login link. Treatment sessions were hosted on a virtual private network, and satisfaction and experience were evaluated through participant questionnaires and interviews. Session topics including symptoms, rehabilitation, and other treatments and monitoring disease progress were suitable for teletreatment, whereas discussions on acceptance of the diagnosis and end-of-life care preferences were preferred to take place in face-to-face sessions. As noted, it is well recognized that PALS should be followed by MDCs that specialize in ALS every 3 to 4 months. Geographically and environmentally, this creates an obvious challenge for access, particularly for those at greater distances, and/or as disease progresses and travel (even short distances) becomes difficult.[20,22] In Australia, a monthly telerehabilitation clinic facilitated MDC access every 3 to 4 months for 38 PALS who would have otherwise traveled upward of 1800 km or would not have been able to attend due to

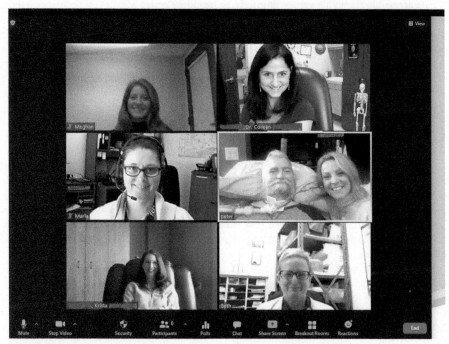

Fig. 10.1 ALS multidisciplinary clinic health via a secure Zoom Health videoconference. Sessions in this clinic are approximately 1 hour and can include several disciplines along with the patient and family and/or caregiver. Patients are seen every 3 to 4 months and may choose an in-person visit or a telerehabilitation clinic visit. This team pictured from New Brunswick, Canada has been providing ALS telerehabilitation clinics for over 15 years; the patient and his wife have participated in the multidisciplinary telerehabilitation clinics for over 7 years. *ALS*, Amyotrophic lateral sclerosis.

disease state. Patients attended the sessions hosted at local hospitals or community health centers, and multiple participants could log on, allowing a team approach, including support and guidance for local care providers. Symptom management predominated sessions.[23] A feasibility study evaluated feedback from participants in multidisciplinary videoconference ALS clinics, where patients and their caregiver used their home devices to attend clinics remotely with their ALS team instead of in-person visits. The researchers found the synchronous video clinics to be highly effective, allowing communication with staff while minimizing travel and time and stress.[15] Another author suggested patients preferred face-to-face visits, but videoconferencing is "the next best thing," and that initial face-to-face visits would facilitate later transition to telehealth.[24]

Direct therapy can also be supported through telerehabilitation. For instance, moderate-intensity exercise is recommended for maintaining function and for positive influence on quality of life.[7] Such programs should be personalized to the PALS abilities, home supports, and disease state. Published evidence suggests that home exercise programs are feasible and safe, and that telemonitoring of home exercise is an effective option.[25]

TELEREHABILITATION MONITORING THROUGH REMOTE DEVICES

Telemonitoring devices have enjoyed popularity in general society mainly as fitness tracking tools; step counters, sleep quality evaluators, and nutrition monitors have become commonplace and are accessible through a variety of interfaces including smart watches and other wearables. Telerehabilitation home monitoring equipment is commercially available for several conditions, with upload features that can allow data sharing with health professionals, who can then act on the data. Download data from home ventilators including bi-level devices can provide details on compliance, utilization, pressures, oxygen saturations, volumes, and mask leaks. Medical alert service devices now have fall detection technology options that can initiate a call for help if a fall is detected. Wearable motion devices can provide enriched mobility data captured through accelerometers and gyroscopes. Devices for measuring respiratory muscle function including peak cough flow and slow vital capacity are available for home use. Digital diaries can be used by patients and carers to submit survey data or validated patient-reported outcome measures as means of monitoring disease symptoms, progression, outcomes, and experiences. Ando et al. reported in a series of articles on the positive outcomes of a home telemonitoring system for management of noninvasive ventilation among PALS.[26,27] Participants submitted weekly responses to a respiratory-focused questionnaire, along with ventilator and oximetry reports, through a tablet-based application. In addition to facilitating timely respiratory interventions, the interviewed participants endorsed that the timely interventions contributed positively to their physical and psychological well-being reassured that their data were being monitored and could be acted upon.

In a prospective study of PALS using a web-based portal to complete several ALS outcome assessments, participants reported none to low time burden, emotional, or physical strain with the tasks.[28] One of the most widely used patient-reported outcome measure in ALS is the ALS Functional Rating Scale Revised (ALSFRS-R); typically administered at every 3- to 4-month clinic visit, the scale has been validated for self-administration and for telephone use.[28] A recent study from the Netherlands demonstrated high adherence to PALS self-reporting of monthly ALSFRS-R through an ALS app[29] and a UK exploration study found PALS reported a greater awareness of their condition using a telerehabilitation application.[30-32] Coupled with additional home monitoring devices, such tools are also improving patients' access to clinical drug trials by reducing the need for frequent in-person visits, which could otherwise preclude some PALS participation.

STORE-FORWARD EDUCATION OR TRAINING RESOURCES

Web-based hosting of educational materials is a common practice, with many advocacy associations and national specialty organizations providing patient/family and health care professional resources. Materials include practical tips for symptom management, exercise, health system navigation tools, and information about the disease, research, and support services. Stored and asynchronous options of web-hosted presentations such as "ask the expert" forum, information sessions, or podcasts are common media. Specific training on therapy techniques or treatments is available for health care professionals as well as care providers and patients; for instance, noninvasive ventilation and respiratory management techniques are provided at no charge through online video modules from CANVent, a respiratory service at the Ottawa Hospital Rehabilitation Center (www.canventottawa.ca). A unique study reported on the outcome of a store and forward strategy for delivering multidisciplinary care, in which a trained nurse conducted assessments and evaluations in home visits with PALS, which were video recorded for team members who followed up with a live teleconference.[33]

Practice

SYMPTOM MANAGEMENT

The ongoing management of problematic symptoms is a key focus of rehabilitation in ALS and is a major role of telerehabilitation. Dedicated MDC team visits can occur either in a large group format with all team members present with the PALS and family/caregiver or the team member(s) can "enter" the room singly or in pairs for more private sessions. Follow-up visits for specific needs identified can be coordinated for a future date between the PALS and relevant team members; for instance, a PALS reports increased hand weakness and difficulties feeding themselves and accessing their computer, then a dedicated visit with the occupational therapist and assistive technologies team member can be arranged either in person or through another telerehabilitation visit. During visits, it is usually preferable to have caregivers or family members present with the PALS to assist if needed with technology setup, positioning, or communication particularly if the PALS is in a more advanced stage of the disease. Symptoms that should be routinely addressed include pain, mood, sleep, fatigue, secretions, saliva, cramps, spasticity, and pseudobulbar effect.[7,16,34,35]

FUNCTIONAL ASSESSMENT

Anchored by the ALSFRS-R, domains of mobility, activities of daily living, respiratory and nutritional status, communication, and cognition are evaluated at every clinic visit. Rehabilitation in ALS aims to proactively optimize function and maintain quality of life throughout the course of the disease. Assessment of electronic aids to daily living, augmentative and alternative communication, and assistive technologies to improve or maintain independence, communication, and safety can also include consideration and training to allow for telerehabilitation participation.

DIRECTED THERAPY

Guided instruction on specific exercise, positioning, or use of a device can be provided through both synchronous and asynchronous telerehabilitation options. A range of motion and stretching program or teaching of airway clearance techniques can be demonstrated and practiced "live," with store and forward handouts or videos of the program for reference. Pharmaceutical and nonpharmaceutical treatments recommended for disease and/or symptom management can also be prescribed and outcomes monitored.[36]

EDUCATION AND SUPPORT

Quality of life maintenance is a vital aspect of the PALS and family support and care; engagement of social workers, psychologists, spiritual care, and counseling can be facilitated by telerehabilitation intervention and support. Family members who may live at a distance, but who are integral to the PALS support network, can participate in educational sessions or attend clinic visits. Case conferencing options with multiple stakeholders can more efficiently address navigation and planning issues, thus reducing stressful tasks for the PALS and family.

Special Considerations

The diagnosis of ALS is clinical-based and requires a hands-on physical examination of the patient to identify the UMN and LMN findings essential to making the diagnosis. Electrodiagnostic studies, brain, and spinal cord imaging are complementary to the physical examination and assist in ruling out other potential diagnoses. Currently, no biomarkers for the disease have been identified that could otherwise confirm or reject the diagnosis. Hence, a thorough physical examination as part of diagnostic evaluation should not be performed remotely. Individuals who cannot travel to a specialized ALS clinic could potentially be evaluated by community neurologists with telesupport from ALS experts.

An individual suspected of having a disease like ALS, along with their family, can understandably experience intense worry and fear while being investigated. Best practice guidelines have recommended a comprehensive approach to communicating the diagnosis.[6,7,16] Breaking the news by confirming a diagnosis of ALS should be done face to face with a specialist with expertise in ALS and who knows the patient during a dedicated appointment time and in an appropriate environment that is quiet, comfortable, and private.[16] The approach should be highly individualized to the particular patient's needs.

Telerehabilitation can provide meaningful and needed management support throughout the disease course after a patient has received the diagnosis of ALS (Fig. 10.1). Discussions on advanced care planning and decisions around end-of-life care are particularly personal and difficult, yet essential, and require a patient-centered individualized approach, similar to delivering the diagnosis. Such conversations may not be always appropriate through telerehabilitation, and as such should be addressed earlier in the course of the disease when face-to-face visits are possible.

Recommendations

Telerehabilitation is a viable and effective strategy to complement and enhance the care and management of persons and their families affected by ALS. Such approaches should be considered when:[15]

1. Diagnosed PALS lack resources to travel to ALS clinics or cannot travel due to distance, weather, or other circumstance.
2. Disease progression has made travel difficult or uncomfortable.
3. PALS can still attend face-to-face clinics, but not for a duration that allows visits with all team members.
4. Emergent or urgent issues that need to be addressed between clinic visits.
5. Inclusion of family members and/or local care providers is needed as part of the care and support team but are unable to attend an in-person clinic.
6. The patient and practitioners feel this is an appropriate option.

In facilitating telerehabilitation within an ALS clinic services, strategies and considerations include:

- Technology to enable telecare is included among the devices evaluated and prescribed by the care team.

- Computer and/or telecommunications access options should be explored early in disease course; allowing time to source reliable, appropriate equipment and ensure training is offered to optimize access and participation.
- Avoid a "one-size-fits-all" approach; the ALS team must take a personalized approach, mindful of the ALS practice parameter of high priority on self-determination.
- As the disease can cause relentless physical, as well as emotional, social, and economic, deterioration, the rehabilitation team must be proactive, flexible, and creative and anticipate the diverse needs of PALS and their families/caregivers.

Further research efforts to develop and validate outcome measures for remote assessment will assist in prospective evaluation of telerehabilitation interventions, as well as facilitate clinical trials in ALS.[37] The COVID-19 pandemic has heightened the urgency and drive to optimize digital tools for remote monitoring of progressives diseases like ALS,[38] in addition to assistive technologies in general.[39] Finally, identification and evaluation of barriers and facilitators to telerehabilitation will help with implementation strategies.[20]

Telerehabilitation can optimize access and allow for efficient and timely person-centered care throughout the ALS disease trajectory, while addressing the well-recognized gaps in access to care.[22,40] Whether serving as a bridge between clinic visits or extending access to MDC teams after the patient is no longer able to travel, there is a valuable role and important need for telerehabilitation in the care of PALS. There is tremendous potential for dedicated and well-resourced telerehabilitation services to significantly improve the overall experience, support and outcomes for PALS and their family and carers, and health systems should enact to implement such services as standard in ALS care.

CASE STUDY

WB is a 79-year-old male retired artist who is admitted to his local hospital for an acute episode of dyspnea, functional decline, and other complications of ALS. The hospital is located 100 km away from where the ALS clinic is located. Since the time of his diagnosis 3 years ago, Mr. Byrne has declined referral to the ALS clinic by his family doctor.

His local hospital was set up for telehealth and, on the recommendation of his inpatient team, he agreed to meet with members of the ALS clinic via telerehabilitation to discuss his concerns and obtain some guidance on symptom management and transition into long-term care. A multidisciplinary team of a physiatrist, clinical nurse, speech-language pathologist, dietician, physiotherapist, and occupational therapist was available to meet with WB's team, which included the attending physician, a continuing care coordinator, inpatient nursing, the hospital health director, and WB's partner, L. A Polycom video conferencing system using RealPresence software and a dedicated server with encrypted secure connections was used for the telehealth visit.

Over the past year, WB had experienced a rapid progression of his disease, with increasing leg weakness, dysarthria, and dysphagia. Hand clawing began to impair any independence with activities of daily living and precluded use of his manual wheelchair. He became fully dependent on home nursing care and a mechanical lift for all transfers. In the 2 weeks prior to admission, he was increasingly agitated and frustrated with his partner and caregivers. Complications from comorbid diabetes furthered his frustrations, with painful diabetic peripheral neuropathy affecting transfers and being legally blind from retinopathy and cataracts impacting communication. He had been keeping in contact with friends using email but could no longer type or see the words on the tablet screen. His agitation and anxiety increased when he was no longer able to paint.

On examination via telerehabilitation, WB was positioned upright in a geriatrics chair with pillows supporting either side of his trunk. He was of good body weight and did not appear frail. His speech was dysarthric due to low volume and projection. He demonstrated a very weak cough. One of his nurses assisted in extending out the fingers of his clawed hands to a functional position without discomfort. There was intrinsic muscle wasting. He was able to get his arms overhead and extend at the elbows against gravity. He did not have any active movement in his legs. He was able to flex and extend his neck against gravity with control.

CASE STUDY —cont'd

A recent swallowing study with modified barium by the dietician at his hospital recommended modified diet, avoiding dry foods and ensuring foods were well moistened. PEG tube placement was discussed and declined by WB. Pulmonary function tests were not available as WB had declined transfer to another local hospital where they were carried out.

Based on this assessment, the ALS team was able to make several recommendations that helped address WB's concerns. Some were completed via telerehabilitation by the ALS team members.

WB had noted that decreased level of communication was greatly impacting his care and level of frustration. A local speech-language pathologist was contacted to meet with WB to trial a voice amplifier and introduce alternative communication strategies in anticipation of further decline in speech. His inpatient team was encouraged to contact the Canadian National Institute for the Blind and they completed a successful trial of a tablet with a larger screen, larger font, and varying brightness to help with his visual impairment. Given his relatively preserved upper extremity function, he was able to use a communication board at bedside to communicate his discomfort with transfers more easily.

Occupational therapy provided nighttime hand wrist splints to address his hand clawing and he learned to use a universal cuff and stylus for typing, some painting, and later a text to speech app. A trial of power wheelchair mobility was successful with use of joystick primarily due to preserved arm movement proximally. He is now exploring head array control systems.

WB and his partner also completed a respiratory health class via telemedicine with the ALS team physiotherapist, where he learned breathing exercises, assisted cough technique, and was introduced to use of a cough assist machine. When WB was transferred to long-term care, the physiotherapist provided instruction on use of a cough assist machine to his care workers at the facility via telerehabilitation.

Prior to transfer to long-term care, WB met with the palliative care team at his local hospital to determine and document his goals of care. Although he elected not to schedule future follow-up with the multidisciplinary ALS team, the team did provide further information around PEG tube placement and acknowledged that they would be happy to provide follow-up by telerehabilitation for him and his care workers in long-term care settings.

References

1. Brown RH, Al-Chalabi A. Amyotrophic lateral sclerosis. *N Engl J Med*. 2017;377:162–172. https://doi.org/10.1056/NEJMra1603471.
2. van Es MA, Hardiman O, Chio A, et al. Amyotrophic lateral sclerosis. *Lancet*. 2017;390:2084–2098. https://doi.org/10.1016/S0140-6736(17)31287-4.
3. Majmudar S, Wu J, Paganoni S. Rehabilitation in amyotrophic lateral sclerosis: why it matters. *Muscle Nerve*. 2014;50(1):4–13. https://doi.org/10.1002/mus.24202.
4. Swinnen B, Robberecht W. The phenotypic variability of amyotrophic lateral sclerosis. *Nat Rev Neurol*. 2014;10(11):661–670. https://doi.org/10.1038/nrneurol.2014.184.
5. Strong MJ, Abrahams S, Goldstein LH, et al. Amyotrophic lateral sclerosis—frontotemporal spectrum disorder (ALS-FTSD): revised diagnostic criteria. *Amyotroph Lateral Scler Frontotemporal Degener*. 2017;18:153–174. https://doi.org/10.1080/21678421.2016.1267768.
6. Miller RG, Jackson CE, Kasarskis EJ, et al. Practice parameter update: the care of the patient with amyotrophic lateral sclerosis: drug, nutritional, and respiratory therapies (an evidence-based review): report of the Quality Standards Subcommittee of the American Academy of Neurology [published correction appears in Neurology. 2009 Dec 15;73(24):2134] [published correction appears in Neurology. 2010 Mar 2;74(9):781]. *Neurology*. 2009;73(15):1218–1226. https://doi.org/10.1212/WNL.0b013e3181bc0141.
7. Shoesmith C, Abrahao A, Benstead T, et al. Canadian best practice recommendations for the management of amyotrophic lateral sclerosis. *CMAJ*. 2016;192(46):E1453–E1468. https://doi.org/10.1503/cmaj.191721.
8. Rooney J, Byrne S, Heverin M, et al. A multidisciplinary clinic approach improves survival in ALS: a comparative study of ALS in Ireland and Northern Ireland. *J Neurol Neurosurg Psychiatry*. 2015;86:496–501. https://doi.org/10.1136/jnnp-2014-309601.
9. Traynor BJ, Alexander M, Corr B, et al. Effect of a multidisciplinary amyotrophic lateral sclerosis (ALS) clinic on ALS survival: a population-based study, 1996-2000. *J Neurol Neurosurg Psychiatry*. 2003;74:1258–1261. https://doi.org/10.1136/jnnp.74.9.1258.

10. Van den Berg JP, Kalmijn S, Lindeman E, et al. Multidisciplinary ALS care improves quality of life in patients with ALS. *Neurology*. 2005;65:1264–1267. https://doi.org/10.1212/01.wnl.0000 180717.29273.12.

11. Gonzalez Calzada N, Prats Soro E, Mateu Gomez L, et al. Factors predicting survival in amyotrophic lateral sclerosis patients on non-invasive ventilation. *Amyotroph Lateral Scler Frontotemporal Degener*. 2016;17:337–342. https://doi.org/10.3109/21678421.2016.1165256.

12. McKim DA, Road J, Avendano M, et al. Canadian Thoracic Society Home Mechanical Ventilation Committee. Home mechanical ventilation: a Canadian Thoracic Society clinical practice guideline. *Can Respir J*. 2011;18(4):197–215. https://doi.org/10.1155/2011/139769.

13. Rimmer KP, Kaminska M, Nonoyama M, et al. Home mechanical ventilation for patients with amyotrophic lateral sclerosis: a Canadian Thoracic Society clinical practice guideline. *Can Journal of Respiratory, Critical Care, and Sleep Med*. 2019;3(1):9–27. https://doi.org/10.1080/24745332.2018.155 9644.

14. Soofi AY, Dal Bello-Haas V, Kho ME, et al. The impact of rehabilitative interventions on quality of life: a qualitative evidence synthesis of personal experiences of individuals with amyotrophic lateral sclerosis. *Qual Life Res*. 2018;27:845–856. https://doi.org/10.1007/s11136-017-1754-7.

15. Geronimo A, Wright C, Morris A, et al. Incorporation of telehealth into a multidisciplinary ALS clinic: feasibility and acceptability. *Amyotroph Lateral Scler Frontotemporal Degener*. 2017;18:555–561. https://doi.org/10.1080/21678421.2017.1338298.

16. EFNS Task Force on Diagnosis and Management of Amyotrophic Lateral Sclerosis: Andersen PM, Abrahams S, et al. EFNS guidelines on the clinical management of amyotrophic lateral sclerosis (MALS)--revised report of an EFNS task force. *Eur J Neurol*. 2012;19(3):360-375. http://dx.doi.org/10.1111/j.1468-1331.2011.03501.x

17. Selkirk SM, Washington MO, McClellan F, et al. Delivering tertiary centre specialty care to ALS patients via telemedicine: a retrospective cohort analysis. *Amyotroph Lateral Scler Frontotemporal Degener*. 2017;18(5-6):324–332. https://doi.org/10.1080/21678421.2017.1313867.

18. De Marchi F, Cantello R, Ambrosini S, Mazzini L. CANPALS Study Group. Telemedicine and technological devices for amyotrophic lateral sclerosis in the era of COVID-19. *Neurol Sci*. 2020;41(6):1365–1367. https://doi.org/10.1007/s10072-020-04457-8.

19. Capozzo R, Zoccolella S, Musio M, et al. Telemedicine is a useful tool to deliver care to patients with Amyotrophic Lateral Sclerosis during COVID-19 pandemic: results from Southern Italy. *Amyotroph Lateral Scler Frontotemporal Degener*. 2020;21(7-8):542–548. https://doi.org/10.1080/21678421.2020.1773502.

20. Helleman J, Kruitwagen ET, van den Berg LH, et al. The current use of telehealth in ALS care and the barriers to and facilitators of implementation: a systematic review. *Amyotroph Lateral Scler Frontotemporal Degener*. 2020;21(3-4):167–182. https://doi.org/10.1080/21678421.2019.1706581.

21. Nijeweme-d'Hollosy WO, Janssen EP, Huis in 't Veld RM, et al. Tele-treatment of patients with amyotrophic lateral sclerosis (ALS). *J Telemed Telecare*. 2006;12(suppl 1):31–34. https://doi.org/10.1258/135763306777978434.

22. Paganoni S, Simmons Z. Telemedicine to innovate amyotrophic lateral sclerosis multidisciplinary care: the time has come. *Muscle Nerve*. 59(1):3-5. https://doi.org/10.1002/mus.26311

23. Henderson R, Hutchinson N, Douglas J, et al. Telehealth for motor neurone disease. *Med J Aust*. 2014;201:31. https://doi.org/10.5694/mja14.00170.

24. James N, Power E, Hogden A, et al. Patients' perspectives of multidisciplinary home-based e-Health service delivery for motor neurone disease. *Disabil Rehabil Assist Technol*. 2019;14(7):737–743. https://doi.org/10.1080/17483107.2018.1499139.

25. Braga AC, Pinto A, Pinto S, et al. Tele-monitoring of a home-based exercise program in amyotrophic lateral sclerosis: a feasibility study. *Eur J Phys Rehabil Med*. 2018;54(3):501–503. https://doi.org/10.23736/S1973-9087.18.05129-8.

26. Ando H, Ashcroft-Kelso H, Halhead R, et al. Experience of telehealth in people with motor neurone disease using noninvasive ventilation [published online ahead of print, 2019 Sep 12]. *Disabil Rehabil Assist Technol*. 2021;16(5):490–496. https://doi.org/10.1080/17483107.2019.1659864.

27. Ando H, Ashcroft-Kelso H, Halhead R, et al. Incorporating self-reported questions for telemonitoring to optimize care of patients with MND on noninvasive ventilation (MND OptNIVent). *Amyotroph Lateral Scler Frontotemporal Degener*. 2019;20(5–6):336–347. https://doi.org/10.1080/21678421.2019.1587630.

28. Maier A, Holm T, Wicks P, et al. Online assessment of ALS functional rating scale compares well to in-clinic evaluation: a prospective trial. *Amyotroph Lateral Scler.* 2012;13(2):210–216. https://doi.org/10.310 9/17482968.2011.633268.

29. Helleman J, Van Eenennaam R, Kruitwagen ET, et al. Telehealth as part of specialized ALS care: feasibility and user experiences with "ALS home-monitoring and coaching". *Amyotroph Lateral Scler Frontotemporal Degener.* 2020;21(3-4):183–192. https://doi.org/10.1080/21678421.2020.1718712.

30. Hobson EV, Baird WO, Partridge R, et al. The TiM system: developing a novel telehealth service to improve access to specialist care in motor neurone disease using user-centered design. *Amyotroph Lateral Scler Frontotemporal Degener.* 2018;19(5-6):351–361. https://doi.org/10.1080/21678421.2018.1440408.

31. Hobson EV, Baird WO, Bradburn M, et al. Using telehealth in motor neuron disease to increase access to specialist multidisciplinary care: a UK-based pilot and feasibility study. *BMJ Open.* 2019;9(10):e028525. https://doi.org/10.1136/bmjopen-2018-028525. [Published 2019 Oct 22].

32. Hobson E, Baird W, Bradburn M, et al. Process evaluation and exploration of telehealth in motor neuron disease in a UK specialist centre. *BMJ Open.* 2019;9(10):e028526. https://doi.org/10.1136/bmjopen-2018-028526. [Published 2019 Oct 22].

33. Pulley MT, Brittain R, Hodges W, et al. Multidisciplinary amyotrophic lateral sclerosis telemedicine care: the store and forward method. *Muscle Nerve.* 2019;59(1):34–39. https://doi.org/10.1002/mus.26170.

34. Miller RG, Jackson CE, Kasarskis EJ, et al. Practice parameter update: the care of the patient with amyotrophic lateral sclerosis: multidisciplinary care, symptom management, and cognitive/behavioral impairment (an evidence-based review): report of the Quality Standards Subcommittee of the American Academy of Neurology. *Neurology.* 2009;73(15):1227–1233. https://doi.org/10.1212/WNL.0b013e3181bc01a4.

35. National Clinical Guideline Centre (UK). *Motor Neurone Disease: Assessment and Management.* London: National Institute for Health and Care Excellence (UK); February 2016.

36. Van De Rijn M, Paganoni S, Levine-Weinberg M, et al. Experience with telemedicine in a multi-disciplinary ALS clinic. *Amyotroph Lateral Scler Frontotemporal Degener.* 2018;19(1-2):143–148. https://doi.org/10.1080/21678421.2017.1392577.

37. Govindarajan R, Berry JD, Paganoni S, et al. Optimizing telemedicine to facilitate amyotrophic lateral sclerosis clinical trials. *Muscle & Nerve.* 2020;62:321–326. https://doi.org/10.1002/mus.26921.

38. Bombaci A, Abbadessa G, Trojsi F, et al. Telemedicine for management of patients with amyotrophic lateral sclerosis through COVID-19 tail. *Neurol Sci.* 2021;42(1):9–13. https://doi.org/10.1007/s10072-020-04783-x.

39. Pinto S, Quintarelli S, Silani V. New technologies and Amyotrophic Lateral Sclerosis - Which step forward rushed by the COVID-19 pandemic? *J Neurol Sci.* 2020;418:117081. https://doi.org/10.1016/j.jns.2020.11708.

40. Haulman A, Geronimo A, Chahwala A, et al. The use of telehealth to enhance care in ALS and other neuromuscular disorders. *Muscle Nerve.* 2020;61:682–691. https://doi.org/10.1002/mus.26838.

CHAPTER 11

Telerehabilitation in Geriatrics

Yannis E. Dionysiotis

Introduction

The worldwide population over 60 is expected to increase by 2 billion between 2000 and 2050. Interestingly, people in some economically privileged countries, such as the United States and other high-income countries, do not have the same life expectancy as those in countries such as Norway. However, life expectancy does not equate with quality of life and it is important to realize that quality of life varies with age and may be better or worse for elderly people than younger people, depending on their place of residence. Moreover, the elderly in some low- and middle-income countries report a higher quality of life as compared with the elderly in wealthier countries.[1,2]

The United Nations principles for the elderly include independence, participation, dignity, care, and fulfillment of personal expectations and ambitions. According to these principles the World Health Organization defines "active aging" as "the process of developing and maintaining the functional ability that enables well-being in older age." Taking into consideration the variability of experience and capability in the elderly, a lifelong approach to healthy living is appropriate to preserve and defend the principles mentioned earlier.[3]

In 1909 Ignatz Nascher proposed the term "geriatrics" for care of the elderly from the Greek words geras (Γῆρας), old age, and iatrikos (Ιατρικός), relating to the physician. He believed using the term geriatrics would help facilitate the same focus on the elderly as the word pediatrics provides to childhood. His goal was to emphasize the necessity of considering senility and its associated disorders apart from maturity and to assign it a separate place in medicine.[4,5] Accordingly, geriatric rehabilitation is defined as a multidisciplinary set of evaluative, diagnostic, and therapeutic interventions whose purpose is to restore functional ability or enhance residual functional capacity in elderly people with disabling impairments.[6] Elderly individuals with diseases such as stroke or traumatic fractures (e.g., hip fractures) and frail elderly with other primary diagnoses (e.g., chronic obstructive pulmonary disease [COPD], heart failure, and cancer) benefit from geriatric rehabilitation.

Importantly, a gradual or acute functional decline in the community may not always mandate hospitalization but may indicate a need for multidisciplinary rehabilitation.[7] Rehabilitation can reverse functional deterioration due to organic disorders and improve quality of life for older people with or without disability; however, there are many challenges to maintenance of health for aging individuals. Chronic illnesses and disorders such as cardiovascular disease, frailty, osteoporosis, and bladder and bowel incontinence have a higher incidence in the elderly. There is a greater use of health care, medical, and community services, which increases expense.[2] Most elderly individuals suffer from at least one chronic illness and a high percentage have comorbidities requiring regular support from physicians. Additionally, they also must develop their own systems for self-management, remaining healthy through the recognition and interpretation of their own bodily changes, determining how they respond to treatments and when to seek professional health care for new or worsening issues. Some elderly individuals are not able to self-manage, which leads to frequent hospitalizations.[8] Thus it is important to find ways to ensure independence of the elderly and allow them to remain in their homes instead of being institutionalized or hospitalized.[9]

Telerehabilitation in Geriatrics

We live in a knowledgeable society with vast sources of information and communication available in our world.[10,11] Technology has advanced rapidly and includes many tools to improve the health of the elderly; however, the needs of the elderly in using technology are different than those of the young.[12] Use of the internet in the elderly is associated with better maintenance of physical health, lower rates of mental illness, and higher integration and participation compared to non-use.[13,14] Furthermore, elderly individuals may benefit from technologies designed for those with movement disorders, memory, hearing, or visual problems associated with aging.[2]

Home monitoring systems can also allow health care professionals to monitor the elderly and recommend specific therapies.[8] Telemonitoring is especially beneficial for patients with chronic diseases that require care coordination or who reside significant distances from their providers. The goal of telemonitoring is to identify and manage disorders, functional decline, and other key changes in medical status and to prevent the need for acute care services in the emergency department or hospital, or long-term care in a nursing facility. Physicians, nursing personnel, or therapists receive a collection of clinical data from the patient that are transmitted, processed, and managed by another health care provider through an interface system.[15,16] Thus the patient has a constant, albeit indirect, connection to their own provider.

In addition to using telerehabilitation to monitor the vital signs of the elderly at home, it can be used to send and receive information via phone calls, short message service, media message service, internet, and so on, in remote areas (e.g., islands or for people who live hundreds of kilometers from a health care facility). Initial teleconsultations and follow-up appointments with specialists can also help the elderly, particularly in such areas as geriatric psychiatry and psychology, and are being used substantially in long-term care facilities. For the integration of comprehensive system-based telerehabilitation services for the elderly, administrative, clinical, technical, and ethical principles must be taken into consideration; services should include evaluation, assessment, monitoring, prevention, intervention, supervision, education, consultation, and coaching.[17,18]

There are many ways that telerehabilitation can help the elderly. In addition to other purposes, telerehabilitation can be used for remote clinical assessment of the individual's functional abilities in their environment and for clinical therapy. Telerehabilitation can help solve issues that impact elderly people with mobility disorders, lack of transportation to rehabilitation facilities and services, and a mismatch of provider availability with patient numbers. Telerehabilitation allows the provision of rehabilitation services to clients residing long distances from a rehabilitation center or a health center, overcoming a lack of trained clinicians in a specific region.[19] This is especially important for remote, underserved populations and may improve health conditions and quality of life and prevent complications due to lack of care. Closer interaction of patients and caregivers and/or families with physicians and therapists and improved follow-up can also be facilitated.[20] Mobility impairments lead to social isolation and telerehabilitation has been shown to help elderly, disabled persons who usually stay at home to engage with other persons via groups or therapy.[21] The elderly are also prone to falling from balance disorders related to neurological diseases, such as stroke or vestibular problems causing dizziness with standing. Medications can also cause problems with orthostasis and dizziness and telerehabilitation has proved effective in preventing falls.[22]

Telerehabilitation can be utilized to monitor individuals with disorders such as chronic pain, spinal stenosis, stroke, amputation, Parkinson's disease, and dementia.[23] Additionally, there is evidence about the beneficial use of telerehabilitation for pain reduction in chronic nonmalignant musculoskeletal pain, low back pain, lumbar stenosis, neck pain, and osteoarthritis.[24]

Promising results for enhancing outcomes beyond those from face-to-face interventions in the natural environment include increased patient participation, providing care in the patient's own environment, and increasing patient satisfaction. For some individuals, rehabilitation service delivery at home is at least as effective as delivery of this service in hospital, and in some cases adds contextual factors that enhance rehabilitation and outcomes.[25,26] For example, due to shortened lengths of stay in acute inpatient rehabilitation, shifting care to a lower-cost health setting with the addition of videoconferencing is often possible. Videoconferencing has also been used in the elderly with chronic diseases to provide specialty care at home. Moreover, with expectations for the aging population and health care expenditures to grow in the future, telehealth may assist in solving the looming health care crisis by allowing for services at home, decreasing costs, and the need for travel and saving time.[22,27]

Telerehabilitation can be used to improve quality of life and people's overall ability for social-ization.[28] Aging, with or without a disability, can lead to social isolation at home. Interaction through telerehabilitation with a therapist may be challenging for those with severe disabilities; however, interactive e-communication may result in some patients feeling as if the therapist was in their room and thereby support the elderly individual.[29,30] Group therapy has also been uti-lized to provide the elderly an opportunity to meet and interact while performing activities, thus allowing the participants to get to know each other and begin to develop friendships.[31] Fig. 11.1 presents the group program "Online Fellowship" organized from Médecins du Monde Greece and supported by TIMA—Charitable Foundation (Vaduz, Liechtenstein). Through the "Online Fellowship," isolated elderly people of the Greek population were joined in virtual teams to pro-vide companionship and discussion groups. Group members perform simple activities, such as drinking coffee online at a specific time of day. The technology used is simple, suitable for the elderly, and it is hoped that this may be a permanent solution to assist this population. A web application for "Online Fellowship" was created and a tablet device was given to each participant to connect via video call. The team includes psychologists and nurses, as well as the specialized physicians of Médecins du Monde Greece staff. In addition to group video chat, each elderly individual may have one-on-one counseling sessions with the physician or psychologist. Of note, the application also provides the ability to listen to recorded books. Another benefit of telereha-bilitation is providing support to the caregivers of the elderly, since being a caregiver is a physically and emotionally draining job[32] and a virtual team of telerehabilitation specialists can decrease a caregiver's sense of isolation and insecurity.[33]

Telerehabilitation in the elderly has benefits in many clinical areas. Studies investigating the use of telerehabilitation for elderly people in various clinical areas were presented in a compre-hensive review.[34] In cardiology, telehealth may be successful in prevention programs to decrease cardiac risk factors, increasing exercise levels for heart failure patients and reducing anxiety levels after cardiac surgery.[35-37] In neurology, telehealth has a positive effect on caregivers of persons with ischemic stroke in problem-solving skills and preparedness, mental health and social func-tioning.[38] In breast cancer patients, improved physical activity and decreased fatigue have been reported[39] and in urological conditions improved continence of post-prostatectomy patients and older women was documented, with results equivalent to those from face-to-face care.[40,41] Physical and functional improvements have been documented in knee arthroplasty rehabilitation[42] and an individualized intervention promoted greater physical activity versus a general training interven-tion in persons with fibromyalgia or rheumatoid arthritis.[43,44]

Telerehabilitation studies on chronic pain reported a significant beneficial long-term effect on work capacity, considered an important outcome for individuals with complex, long-term problems.[45,46] In COPD patients with a risk of hospital readmission, the use of telehealth resulted in fewer emergency admissions and primary care visits along with improvements in health-related qual-ity of life.[47,48] A case control study provided evidence suggesting that home telerehabilitation, linked to care coordination, could improve the functional and cognitive status of frail older individuals.[49]

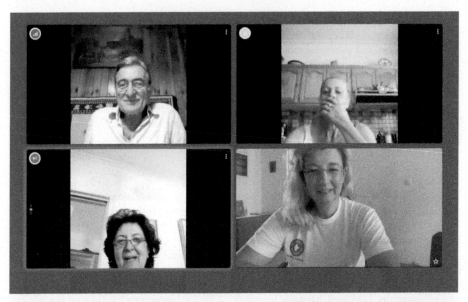

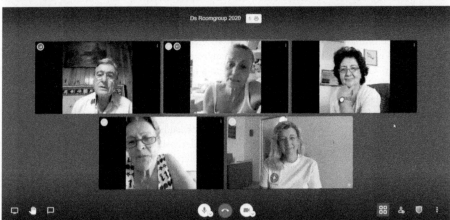

Fig. 11.1 Group program "Online Fellowship" in zoom platform, Dr. Greka A (picture on the bottom right), on behalf of Médecins du Monde Greece, coordinates the discussion (published with permission).

Another review on telerehabilitation in community-based patients with various diseases found improved outcomes similar or better than traditional interventions.[50] Reviews of telehealth studies in the elderly are summarized in Table 11.1.

Studies of telerehabilitation related to musculoskeletal concerns have demonstrated comparable outcomes and patient satisfaction with physical visits.[51] Feasibility of measurement of pain, swelling, range of motion (ROM), muscle strength, balance, gait, and functional outcomes has been demonstrated with overall good concurrent validity. Interrater and intrarater reliability showed good to excellent levels for telerehabilitation for low back pain, ankle disorders, elbow disorders, total knee replacement, and nonarticular lower limb disorders.[52] Effectiveness of telerehabilitation was documented in improving function after total knee replacement; moreover, there was good patient satisfaction.[53-55] A recent metaanalysis assessed the efficacy of telerehabilitation

TABLE 11.1 ■ Notable Reviews Conducted in Telerehabilitation for Elderly

Study, Country	N	Intervention	Type of Study	Findings
Frederix (2015)[61] Belgium	N/A	Telerehabilitation program for cardiac patients	Review of 37 studies	Feasible and effective additional and/ or alternative form of rehabilitation vs. conventional in-hospital CR
Jiang (2018)[56] China	442	Assessed the efficacy of telerehabilitation for patients after TKA compared with FTF rehabilitation	Metaanalysis of 4 RCTs	Improved WOMAC, extension range and quadriceps strength compared to FTF rehabilitation
Gokalp (2013)[74] UK	224	To identify and summarize ADL telemonitoring, and review the effects of ADL telemonitoring systems on telecare of the elderly	Review of 25 studies	Most ADL telemonitoring studies reported benefits for care
Vitacca (2018)[63] Italy	11324	The effects of various telemanagement programs for patients with COPD	Review of 46 RCTs	Telemonitoring in COPD is difficult; other services received by patients (GP network, home care, access to hospital, social care) need to be considered
Laver (2013)[60] Australia	933	To determine whether the use of telerehabilitation leads to improved ability to perform activities of daily living amongst stroke survivors	Cochrane review of 10 trials	Evidence was insufficient to draw conclusions on the effects of the intervention on mobility, HRQoL, or participant satisfaction. No studies evaluated the cost-effectiveness of telerehabilitation

ADL, Activities of daily living; COPD, chronic obstructive pulmonary disease; CR, cardiac rehabilitation; FTF, face-to-face; HRQoL, health-related quality of life; RCT, randomized controlled trial; TKA, total knee arthroplasty; WOMAC, Western Ontario and McMaster Universities Osteoarthritis Index.

for patients after total knee arthroplasty compared with face-to-face rehabilitation. In four randomized controlled trials involving 442 patients comparable pain relief, improvement in the Western Ontario and McMaster Universities Osteoarthritis Index (WOMAC), and significantly higher extension ROM and quadriceps strength were noted and they recommended telerehabilitation for patients after total knee arthroplasty.[56]

Telerehabilitation has also been studied for overall wellness in aging. A 24-week telerehabilitation program significantly decreased the risk of emergency hospital admissions and GP visits and improved quality of life in a cohort of 128 (64 intervention, 64 control) cognitively intact older persons who were independent in ambulation but had known risk factors for deconditioning and readmission. The care plan included: (1) an individually tailored exercise program of stretching and strengthening, balance training, and walking; (2) a nursing intervention to facilitate the exercise program and develop a transitional care plan emphasizing functional ability and need for assistance with activities of daily living (ADL); and (3) postdischarge follow-up consisting of nurse home visits, weekly phone calls for 1 month, followed by monthly follow-up for the next 5 months.[57] Another case control study evaluated the extent to which 111 frail elderly men (primary diagnoses of hypertension, diabetes, respiratory disease, or heart disease) receiving home-telehealth technology had improved functional and cognitive outcomes compared to 115 similar age-matched controls, who did not receive home-telehealth.[49] After 1 year, improvements in both instrumental activities of daily living (IADL) tasks (using the telephone, getting to a place out of walking distance, shopping for groceries or clothes, preparing meals, doing housework, taking medicine, and handling money) and ADL independence were found in the intervention group. Moreover, over the same time the home-telehealth group experienced significantly greater improvements in measures of cognitive status (cognitive subscale of the Functional Independence Measure); however, no significant effect in cognition (measured by Mini Mental State Examination) was found.[49]

A systematic review of telerehabilitation interventions found that home-based telerehabilitation is promising in improving the health of stroke patients and in supporting caregivers. Health professionals and participants reported high levels of satisfaction and acceptance of telerehabilitation interventions.[58] A metaanalysis revealed no significant differences between telerehabilitation and control groups in the Barthel index, Berg balance scale, Fugl-Meyer upper extremity scale, and stroke impact scale scores; however, more studies were necessary to evaluate health-related quality of life and cost-effectiveness.[59] Similarly, a recent Cochrane review of telerehabilitation after stroke concluded that short-term posthospital discharge telerehabilitation programs have not documented reduced depressive symptoms, improved quality of life, or independence in ADL in comparison to usual care. No serious adverse events were related to telerehabilitation; however, this remains an area where more studies are needed.[60]

Cardiac telerehabilitation (CR) appears feasible and effective in addition or alternatively to conventional in-hospital cardiac rehabilitation; however, studies of safety and cost-effectiveness are lacking.[61] A program for veterans showed that a nurse-directed home telerehabilitation management program for veterans with chronic systolic heart failure resulted in a significant reduction in hospitalization rates, improvement in symptoms, and medication compliance, despite a high incidence of comorbidities.[62]

Whilst few pulmonary rehabilitation programs are currently offering telerehabilitation, this is likely to grow as telehealth applications become increasingly accessible to patients and clinicians. In COPD patients, teleconsultations have been shown to be an effective means to assess patients' disease prior to the initiation of pulmonary rehabilitation, and telehealth pulmonary rehabilitation has been shown to be as effective as institution-based pulmonary rehabilitation at improving functional exercise capacity and health-related quality of life.[63,64]

TELEMONITORING STUDIES

A rehabilitation plan may need adjustments during therapy and remote telemonitoring can provide information on selected physiological parameters. Telerehabilitation may be used for geriatric patients with neurological conditions such as stroke or spinal cord injury to monitor symptoms like pain and spasticity.[65,66] Technology may be used diagnostically by monitoring elderly patients' health parameters and vital signs in their homes. With home equipment, heart rate, ECG, blood pressure, pulse oxygenation, glucose, temperature, and other parameters can be monitored. Having the ability to monitor specific parameters supports diagnostic efforts and can facilitate rapid access to urgent consultation and triage. Identification of worsening heart failure in an elderly population produced a similar outcome to "usual" and decreased clinic and emergency room visits and unplanned rehospitalizations for heart failure.[67] Another study examined the feasibility and acceptability of monitoring hypertension in the elderly by transmitting blood pressure and bodyweight data to a server that was monitored remotely by nurses. Around 92% of participants indicated improvements in their health due to the system and providers noted ease in monitoring health and preventing hospital readmissions.[68] Studies have also found improvements in glycemic control, increased awareness of diabetes mellitus, and improved quality of life in persons with diabetes.[69-72] A feedback system for patients with type 2 diabetes initiating insulin therapy is also useful. Patients self-monitor their blood glucose levels, transmit their readings by telephone or internet, and the provider evaluates results and recommends dose titration via telephone or internet.[73]

In contrast, Bashshur et al. reported that the use of telemonitoring is superior to office visits in terms of emergency visits, hospitalizations, complications, and quality of life for diabetes, hypertension, pain, congestive heart failure, cancer care, rehabilitation after stroke, and dementia. They documented better results compared with office visits in all the aforementioned chronic diseases, emergency situations, and hospitalizations, providing key findings regarding the effects of telemonitoring in cardiac heart failure (CHF), stroke, and COPD. Data strongly support that telemonitoring of patients with CHF is likely to reduce mortality and morbidity and is cost-effective for these chronic illnesses.[16] Importantly, this review was used by US Congressional Committees in policy decisions and telemonitoring is a covered service in the US Medicare program.[16,33]

Technical improvements have been documented in methods for detecting changes in ADL; however, few clinical benefits have been documented through these systems.[74]

Telerehabilitation can be used to provide seniors in long-term facilities or hospice programs access to rehabilitation specialists and palliative care providers without leaving their home or a facility. Remote health monitoring and management seems exceptionally promising for individuals with terminal illness because follow-up of patients with chronic conditions is often difficult.[75-77] In summary, telerehabilitation can facilitate follow-up for elderly persons in many different scenarios by eliminating a need for travel.

Performing a Geriatric Telerehabilitation Visit

Performance of a telerehabilitation visit involves unique preparation when working with the elderly. Clinicians performing virtual visits must be aware of the difficulties older adults may have using technology. The elderly are a heterogenic group and visual and auditory impairments, anxiety, lack of privacy, lack of dexterity, and cognitive issues may impede the patient's use of telehealth devices. Thus the potential for the use of telerehabilitation must be individually assessed.[78] Having knowledge of the patient's health condition, capabilities, and history is important in virtual visits. Additionally, the presence of a family person or carer to help in case of technical problems or difficulties is also important for persons with severe disabilities.

Informed consent should be taken prior to a telehealth visit and an emergency phone number should be available. Patients must be educated to choose a comfortable, quiet place for their visit. It may be beneficial to take vital signs—temperature, heart rate, blood pressure, weight, and blood sugar—using home equipment. It is helpful to have patients write their questions prior to visits and keep their medication available and it may be appropriate to ask for a log of the patient's vitals or pain levels. Visits may be private or grouped. Group sessions for therapy purposes can be beneficial to maximize the use of highly skilled resources.[79] At the end of the visit, it is especially important to have elderly patients repeat instructions and confirm that they are properly informed about the need for laboratory studies or for a follow-up visit.[80,81]

Each patient and provider must overcome any personal hesitation to embrace telerehabilitation, concerns about security, user friendliness, and the possible need for specialized training.[82,83] Barriers to the use of telehealth can include font size and difficulty in reading, the need to use devices with widgets and mice, and difficulties in using and handling smartphones. Moreover,

TABLE 11.2 ■ Criteria for Participant Selection for Geriatric Telerehabilitation Sessions

Inclusion Criteria	Exclusion Criteria
No cognitive impairment	Heart rate at rest <40 or >120 beats/min
Stable respiratory and circulation status	Systolic blood pressure <70 mmHg at rest
Ability to communicate	Poorly controlled arrhythmia
Ability to walk (walking aids included)	Chest pain at rest; effort angina pectoris; shortness of breath
Ability to exercise following directions	Blood oxygen saturation (SaO2) at rest <90%
Consent by the participant	Body temperature <38°C
In case of caregiver not familiar with rehabilitation ability to exercise with his help	No nystagmus, cold sweat, or nausea

Adapted and modified from Moriichi et al. (2020).[84]

cultural and religious issues may be a barrier. The elderly can have delayed responses, and a lack of immediate feedback and technical problems may lead to frustration and reduce motivation (Table 11.2).[84]

Live video creates a telepresence experience and provides visible and nonverbal information about the behavior of an older person in their environment. However, some believe that it is difficult for the provider to interpret a user's fine movements in a telerehabilitation session. As such, the combined use of audio/video conferencing with wearable sensors has been assessed and shown to improve the quality of measurements.[85,86]

Recommendations for Research

As can be seen by the earlier discussion, there are many areas where research in geriatric telerehabilitation is necessary. There are opportunities to expand physical therapy, occupational therapy, and speech therapy services via telerehabilitation. Psychological services, educational services, addiction management, and pain management services need to be developed. Availability of both synchronous and asynchronous visits needs to be expanded with physical medicine and rehabilitation physicians, and the benefits of home monitoring for elderly individuals with disabilities must be explored. Furthermore, future expansion of telehealth services in palliative care programs and geriatric specialty clinics is appropriate.[16,33,79]

Use of simple technologies combined with technological support, clear instructions, and tailored technological developments (such as adjustable stands and high visibility controls) could further increase ease of use and diminish safety risks. Future research should focus on these insights and should examine the conditions and populations in which telerehabilitation is most beneficial[87] because telerehabilitation visits are convenient, reduce costs of traveling, save time, and are environmentally friendly.[88]

Future research needs to support feasibility and benefits of various rehabilitation types provided by telerehabilitation systems. This is paramount for people with limited access to therapy due to geographical distance, transport difficulties, and a lack of local services. The COVID-19 pandemic has emphasized the importance of remote delivery of telerehabilitation services to support ongoing rehabilitation services and guarantee continuity of care to people requiring rehabilitation.

CASE STUDY

EH is an 82-year-old female living 50 miles away from the nearest hospital with a history of hypertension, CHF, and mild dementia who fell and sustained an intertrochanteric hip fracture. She was transported to the hospital by her family, where she was treated with an intramedullary nail and was offered the opportunity for rehabilitation in a skilled nursing facility or in her home. The decision was made for her to be rehabilitated in her home where she resided with her daughter and son-in-law and their three children rather than go to a skilled facility where she would be away from her family. After 2 days in acute care where she had a walker, bedside commode, wheelchair, and hospital bed ordered, she returned home. She underwent telephysical therapy and occupational therapy daily with the assistance of her daughter. She was able to resume short distance ambulation and became independent in transfers and self-care in the comfort of her home. Moreover, she was able to see her orthopedist and physiatrist virtually twice per week and provide updates on the appearance of her wound, her lower extremity swelling, pain levels, and the impact of the oxycodone she had been prescribed on her bowel habits.

References

1. HelpAge. *Global AgeWatch Index 2013.* http://www.helpage.org/globalagewatch/reports/global-agewatch-index-2013-insight-report-summary-andmethodology/.
2. Bujnowska-Fedak MM, Grata-Borkowska U. Use of telemedicine-based care for the aging and elderly: promises and pitfalls. *Smart Homecare Technol TeleHealth.* 2015;3:91–105.
3. World Health Organization *Active Ageing: A Policy Framework.* 59. Geneva: World Health Organization; 2009. http://whqlibdoc.who.int/hq/2002/WHO_NMH_NPH_02.8.pdf.
4. Nascher JL. Geriatrics. *NY Med J.* 1909;90:358–359.
5. Forciea MA. Geriatric medicine: history of a young specialty. *Virtual Mentor.* 2014;16(5):385–389.
6. Boston Working Group on Improving Health Care Outcomes Through Geriatric Rehabilitation. *Med Care.* 1997;35(suppl 6):JS4–JS20.
7. Van Balen R. *What is Geriatric Rehabilitation? Towards a Unifying Concept.* British Geriatrics Society; 2017. https://www.bgs.org.uk/blog.
8. Foster MV, Sethares KA. Facilitators and barriers to the adoption of telehealth in older adults: an integrative review. *Comput Inform Nurs.* 2014;32(11):523–533.
9. Narasimha S, Agnisarman S, Chalil Madathil K, et al. Designing home-based telemedicine systems for the geriatric population: an empirical study. *Telemed J E Health.* 2018;24(2):94–110.
10. Casado-Muñoz R, Lezcano-Barbero F, Rodríguez-Conde MJ. Active ageing and access to technology: an evolving empirical study. *Comunicar.* 2015;23:37–46.
11. UNESCO *Reflection and Analysis by UNESCO on the Internet (186 EX/37).* Paris: Author; 2011. https://unesdoc.unesco.org/ark:/48223/pf0000192096.
12. Wagner N, Hassanein K, Head M. Computer use by older adults: a multi-disciplinary review. *Comput Hum Behav.* 2010;26(5):870–882.
13. Gracia E, Herrero J. *Brecha Digital y Calidad de Vida de las Personas Mayores.* Madrid: IMSERSO; 2008. http://goo.gl/MYfNZg.
14. Dionyssiotis Y. Active ageing. *J Frailty Sarcopenia Falls.* 2018;3(3):125–127.
15. Paré G, Jaana M, Sicotte C. Systematic review of home telemonitoring for chronic diseases: the evidence base. *J Am Med Inform Assoc.* 2007;14(3):269–277.
16. Bashshur RL, Shannon GW, Smith BR, et al. The empirical foundations of telemedicine interventions for chronic disease management. *Telemed J E Health.* 2014;20(9):769–800.
17. Exum E, Hull BL, Lee A, et al. Applying telehealth technologies and strategies to provide acute care consultation and treatment of patients with confirmed or possible COVID-19. *J Acute Care Phys Ther.* 2020;11(3):103–112.
18. Richmond T, Peterson C, Cason J, et al. American Telemedicine Association's principles for delivering telerehabilitation services. *Int J Telerehabil.* 2017;9(2):63–68.
19. Theodoros DG. Telerehabilitation for service delivery in speech-language pathology. *Journal of Telemedicine and Telecare.* 2008;14(5):221–224.

20. Russell TG. Telerehabilitation: a coming of age. *Aust J Physiother.* 2009;55(1):5–6.
21. Hill A. Telerehabilitation in Scotland: current initiatives and recommendations for future development. *Int J Telerehabil.* 2010;2(1):7–14.
22. Deutsch JE, Maidan I, Dickstein R. Patient-centered integrated motor imagery delivered in the home with telerehabilitation to improve walking after stroke. *Phys Ther.* 2012;92(8):1065–1077.
23. Cooper R, Fitzgerald S, Boninger M, et al. Telerehabilitation: expanding access to rehabilitation expertise. *Proceedings of the IEEE.* 2001;89(8):1174–1191.
24. Fiani B, Siddiqi I, Lee SC, et al. Telerehabilitation: development, application, and need for increased usage in the COVID-19 era for patients with spinal pathology. *Cureus.* 2020;12(9):e10563 21.
25. McCue M, Fairman A, Pramuka M. Enhancing quality of life through telerehabilitation. *Phys Med Rehabil Clin N Am.* 2010;21(1):195–205.
26. Brennan DM, Mawson S, Brownsell S. Telerehabilitation: enabling the remote delivery of healthcare, rehabilitation, and self-management. *Stud Health Technol Inform.* 2009;145:231–248.
27. Holden MK, Dyar TA, Dayan-Cimadoro L. Telerehabilitation using a virtual environment improves upper extremity function in patients with stroke. *IEEE Trans Neural Syst Rehabil Eng.* 2007;15(1):36–42.
28. Betty N. *Telerehabilitation as Means to Improve Elderlys' Independence while Living at Home.* Degree thesis Human Ageing and Elderly Service: Arcada University of Applied Sciences; 2013.
29. Taylor DM, Stone SD, Huijbregts MP. Remote participants' experiences with a group-based stroke self-management program using videoconference technology. *Rural Remote Health.* 1947;2012:12.
30. Hoenig H, Sanford JA, Butterfield T, et al. Development of a teletechnology protocol for in-home rehabilitation. *J Rehabil Res Dev.* 2006;43(2):287–298.
31. Sveistrup H, McComas J, Thornton M, et al. Experimental studies of virtual reality-delivered compared to conventional exercise programs for rehabilitation. *Cyberpsychol Behav.* 2003;6(3):245–249.
32. Dionyssiotis Y, Vellidou E, Konstantinidis ST, et al. Education Program for Carers in Facilities with Neuro Disabled Subjects EPoCFiNDS. *J Frailty Sarcopenia Falls.* 2019;4(2):45–50.
33. Merrell RC. Geriatric telemedicine: background and evidence for telemedicine as a way to address the challenges of geriatrics. *Healthc Inform Res.* 2015;21(4):223–229.
34. Hailey D, Roine R, Ohinmaa A, et al. Evidence on the effectiveness of telerehabilitation applications. *Health Technology Assessments/Systematic Reviews.* 2010 978-1-897443-87-3.
35. Mittag O, China C, Hoberg E, et al. Outcomes of cardiac rehabilitation with versus without a follow-up intervention rendered by telephone (Luebeck follow-up trial): overall and gender-specific effects. *Int J Rehabil Res.* 2006;29:295–302.
36. Tomita MR, Tsai BM, Fisher NM, et al. Improving adherence to exercise in patients with heart failure through internet-based self-management. *J Am Geriatr Soc.* 2008;56:1981–1983.
37. Beckie T. A supportive-educative telephone program: impact on knowledge and anxiety after coronary artery bypass graft surgery. *Heart Lung.* 1989;18:46–55.
38. Grant JS, Elliott TR, Weaver M, et al. Telephone intervention with family caregivers of stroke survivors after rehabilitation. *Stroke.* 2002;33:2060–2065.
39. Pinto BM, Frierson GM, Rabin C, et al. Home-based physical activity intervention for breast cancer patients. *J Clin Oncol.* 2005;23:3577–3587.
40. Moore KN, Valiquette L, Chetner MP, et al. Return to continence after radical retropubic prostatectomy: a randomized trial of verbal and written instructions versus therapist-directed pelvic floor muscle therapy. *Urology.* 2008;72:1280–1286.
41. Hui E, Lee PS, Woo J. Management of urinary incontinence in older women using videoconferencing versus conventional management: a randomized controlled trial. *J Telemed and Telecare.* 2006;12:343–347.
42. Russell TG, Buttrum P, Wootton R, et al. Low-bandwidth telerehabilitation for patients who have undergone total knee replacement: preliminary results. *J Telemed and Telecare.* 2003;9(suppl 2):S44–S47.
43. Lorig KR, Ritter PL, Laurent DD, et al. The internet-based arthritis self-management program: a one-year randomized trial for patients with arthritis or fibromyalgia. *Arthritis Rheum.* 2008;59:1009–1017.
44. van den Berg MH, Ronday HK, Peeters AJ, et al. Using internet technology to deliver a home-based physical activity intervention for patients with rheumatoid arthritis: a randomized controlled trial. *Arthritis Rheum.* 2006;55:935–945.

45. Brattberg G. Internet-based rehabilitation for individuals with chronic pain and burnout II: a long-term follow-up. *Int J Rehabil Res.* 2007;30:231–234.
46. Brattberg G. Internet-based rehabilitation for individuals with chronic pain and burnout: a randomized trial. *Int J Rehabil Res.* 2006;29:221–227.
47. Nguyen HQ, Donesky-Cuenco D, Wolpin S, et al. Randomized controlled trial of an internet-based versus face-to-face dyspnea self-management program for patients with chronic obstructive pulmonary disease: pilot study. *J Med Internet Res.* 2008;10:e9.
48. Wewel AR, Gellermann I, Schwertfeger I, et al. Intervention by phone calls raises domiciliary activity and exercise capacity in patients with severe COPD. *Respir Med.* 2008;102:20–26.
49. Chumbler NR, Mann WC, Wu S, et al. The association of home-telehealth use and care coordination with improvement of functional and cognitive functioning in frail elderly men. *Telemed J E Health.* 2004;10:129–137.
50. Kairy D, Lehoux P, Vincent C, et al. A systematic review of clinical outcomes, clinical process, healthcare utilization and costs associated with telerehabilitation. *J Disabil Rehabil.* 2009;31:427–447.
51. Lee AC, Davenport TE, Randall K. Telehealth physical therapy in musculoskeletal practice. *J Orthop Sports Phys Ther.* 2018;48(10):736–739.
52. Mani S, Sharma S, Omar B, et al. Validity and reliability of Internet-based physiotherapy assessment for musculoskeletal disorders: a systematic review. *J Telemed Telecare.* 2017;23(3):379–391.
53. Marion K. Telerehabilitation—a future opportunity in the field of rehabilitation. In: Marion Karppi, Heidi Tuominen, Anne Eskelinen, Regina Santamäki Fischer, Anneli Rasu, eds. *Active Ageing Online. Interactive Distance Services for the Elderly on Baltic Islands. VIRTU Project 2010–2013.* Turku University of Applied Sciences Turku; 2013. ISBN 978-952-216-357-8.
54. Tousignant M, Boissy P, Moffet H, et al. Patients' satisfaction of healthcare services and perception with in-home telerehabilitation and physiotherapists' satisfaction toward technology for post-knee arthroplasty: an embedded study in a randomized trial. *Telemed J E Health.* 2011; 17(5):376–382.
55. Russell TG, Blumke R, Richardson B, et al. Telerehabilitation mediated physiotherapy assessment of ankle disorders. *Physiother Res Int.* 2010;15(3):167–175.
56. Jiang S, Xiang J, Gao X, et al. The comparison of telerehabilitation and face-to-face rehabilitation after total knee arthroplasty: a systematic review and meta-analysis. *J Telemed Telecare.* 2018;24(4):257–262.
57. Courtney M, Edwards H, Chang A, et al. Fewer emergency readmissions and better quality of life for older adults at risk of hospital readmission: a randomized controlled trial to determine the effectiveness of a 24-week exercise and telephone follow-up program. *J Am Geriatr Soc.* 2009;57:395–402.
58. Johansson T, Wild C. Telerehabilitation in stroke care—a systematic review. *J Telemed Telecare.* 2011;17(1):1–6.
59. Tchero H, Tabue Teguo M, Lannuzel A, et al. Telerehabilitation for stroke survivors: systematic review and meta-analysis. *J Med Internet Res.* 2018;20(10):e10867.
60. Laver KE, Adey-Wakeling Z, Crotty M, et al. Telerehabilitation services for stroke. *Cochrane Database Syst Rev.* 2020;1(1):CD010255.
61. Frederix I, Vanhees L, Dendale P, et al. A review of telerehabilitation for cardiac patients. *J Telemed Telecare.* 2015;21(1):45–53.
62. Schofield RS, Kline SE, Schmalfuss CM, et al. Early outcomes of a care coordination-enhanced telehome care program for elderly veterans with chronic heart failure. *Telemed J E Health.* 2005;11(1):20–27.
63. Vitacca M, Montini A, Comini L. How will telemedicine change clinical practice in chronic obstructive pulmonary disease? *Ther Adv Respir Dis.* 2018;12 1753465818754778.
64. Selzler AM, Wald J, Sedeno M, et al. Telehealth pulmonary rehabilitation: a review of the literature and an example of a nationwide initiative to improve the accessibility of pulmonary rehabilitation. *Chron Respir Dis.* 2018;15(1):41–47.
65. Tenforde AS, Hefner JE, Kodish-Wachs JE, et al. Telehealth in physical medicine and rehabilitation: a narrative review. *PM R.* 2017;9(5S):S51–S58.
66. Yozbatiran N, Harness ET, Le V, et al. A tele-assessment system for monitoring treatment effects in subjects with spinal cord injury. *J Telemed Telecare.* 2010;16:152–157.
67. Dar O, Riley J, Chapman C. A randomized trial of home telemonitoring in a typical elderly heart failure in North West London: results of the Home-HF study. *Eur J Heart Fail.* 2009;11:319–325.

68. Czaja SJ, Lee CC, Arana N, et al. Use of a telehealth system by older adults with hypertension. *J Telemed Telecare*. 2014;20(4):184–191.

69. Trief PM, Teresi JA, Eimicke JP, et al. Improvement in diabetes self-efficacy and glycemic control using telemedicine in a sample of older, ethnically diverse individuals who have diabetes: the IDEATel project. *Age Ageing*. 2009;38:219–225.

70. Jaana M, Parè G. Home telemonitoring of patients with diabetes: a systematic assessment of observed effects. *J Eval Clin Pract*. 2007;13:242–253.

71. Verhoeven F, van Gemert-Pijnen L, Dijkstra K, et al. The contribution of teleconsultation and videoconferencing to diabetes care: a systematic literature review. *J Med Internet Res*. 2007;9:e37.

72. Bujnowska-Fedak MM, Puchała E, Steciwko A. The impact of telehome care on health status and quality of life among patients with diabetes in a primary care setting in Poland. *Telemed J E Health*. 2011;17:153–160.

73. Del Prato S, Nicolucci A, Lovagnini-Scher AC, et al. Telecare provides comparable efficacy to conventional self-monitored blood glucose in patients with type 2 diabetes titrating one injection of insulin glulisine-the ELEONOR study. *Diabetes Technol Ther*. 2012;14(2):175–182.

74. Gokalp H, Clarke M. Monitoring activities of daily living of the elderly and the potential for its use in telecare and telehealth: a review. *Telemed J E Health*. 2013;19(12):910–923.

75. Shah MN, Gillespie SM, Wood N, et al. High-intensity telemedicine-enhanced acute care for older adults: an innovative healthcare delivery model. *J Am Geriatr Soc*. 2013;61(11):2000–2007.

76. Make B, Dutro MP, Paulose-Ram R, et al. Undertreatment of COPD: a retrospective analysis of US managed care and medicare patients. *Int J Chron Obstruct Pulmon Dis*. 2012;7:1–9.

77. Dhamane AD, Moretz C, Zhou Y, et al. COPD exacerbation frequency and its association with health care resource utilization and costs. *Int J Chron Obstruct Pulmon Dis*. 2015;10:2609–2618.

78. Peel NM, Russell TG, Gray LC. Feasibility of using an in-home video conferencing system in geriatric rehabilitation. *J Rehabil Med*. 2011;43(4):364–366.

79. Amanda O. *Telerehabilitation and Geriatrics – Expanding Access and Care Services to Prevent Frailty and Falls. Course Code: LMS-1019-3*. American Physical Therapy Association (APTA); 2020. https://apta-apps.apta.org/Login/SSO.aspx?RedirectTo=https://learningcenter.apta.org/Login/CustomLogin/APTASSO1.aspx.

80. AgingInPlace. *Telehealth and Seniors*. AgingInPlace; 2021. https://aginginplace.org/telehealth-and-seniors/.

81. Lin FR, Yaffe K, Xia J, et al. Hearing loss and cognitive decline in older adults. *JAMA Intern Med*. 2013;173(4):293–299.

82. Call VRA, Erickson LD, Dailey NK, et al. Attitudes toward telemedicine in urban, rural, and highly rural communities. *Telemed J E Health*. 2015;21(8):644–651.

83. Demiris G, Rantz M, Aud M, et al. Older adults' attitudes towards and perceptions of "smart home" technologies: a pilot study. *Med Inform Internet Med*. 2004;29(2):87–94.

84. Moriichi K, Fujiya M, Ro T, et al. A novel telerehabilitation with educational program for caregivers using telelecture is a feasible procedure for fall prevention in elderly people – a pilot study, 21 August 2020, PREPRINT (Version 1) available at Research Square. https://doi.org/10.21203/rs.3.rs-49205/v1.

85. Winters JM, Wang Y. Wearable sensors and telerehabilitation. *IEEE Eng Med Biol Mag*. 2003;22(3):56–65.

86. Zheng H, Black ND, Harris ND. Position-sensing technologies for movement analysis in stroke rehabilitation. *Med Biol Eng Comput*. 2005;43(4):413–420.

87. Shulver W, Killington M, Morris C, et al. "Well, if the kids can do it, I can do it": older rehabilitation patients' experiences of telerehabilitation. *Health Expect*. 2017;20(1):120–129.

88. Alexander M. It's corona calling: time for telerehabilitation! *J Frailty Sarcopenia Falls*. 2020;5(4):86–88.

Telerehabilitation Subspecialties

CHAPTER 12

Telerehabilitation for Pressure Injury

Ingebjørg Irgens

Introduction

The goals of rehabilitation are to improve function, decrease secondary morbidity, and enhance health-related quality of life.[1, 2] Unfortunately, many individuals with disorders requiring rehabilitation are affected by pressure injuries (PIs), which can have a significant negative impact on quality of life. The goal of this chapter is to describe the benefits of utilizing telerehabilitation in the treatment of PIs.

Pressure wound, pressure ulcer, pressure sore, pressure injury, or decubitus are interchangeable terms. Many different descriptions cover this condition, but the optimal description to use is pressure injury (PI), defined as *"A pressure injury is a localized injury to the skin and/or underlying tissue usually over a bony prominence, as a result of pressure, or pressure in combination with shear and/ or friction."*[3] In this chapter, the term PI will be used, because this covers all aspects of skin and tissue damage.[4]

CATEGORIZATION OF PRESSURE INJURY

A PI appearing as intact skin with nonblanchable redness of a localized area or as partial thickness loss of dermis presenting as a shallow open ulcer with a red pink wound bed, without slough, is termed category 1 and 2 pressure ulcer, respectively.[4] In a more severe PI, there will be a full thickness skin loss, with visible subcutaneous fat, termed category 3, or even exposed bone, tendon, and muscle, termed category 4.[4] Finally, there is the full thickness tissue loss PI, in which the base of the ulcer is covered by slough and/or eschar, termed unstageable PI, and the suspected deep tissue PI, with unknown depth, purple or maroon localized area of discolored intact skin, or blood-filled blister due to damage of underlying soft tissue from pressure and/or shear.[4] Table 12.1 shows the different categorizations of PIs.

Amongst people with PIs, those who suffer from spinal cord injury (SCI) are at particular risk due to paralysis, reduced skin sensitivity, and skin that is exposed to moisture for extended periods of time.[5] Individuals with SCI and PI are often hospitalized for long periods of time and need frequent outpatient care for both treatment and monitoring.[5] Traveling can also cause more difficulties for persons who have to travel long distances to get to a hospital. Traveling can worsen the condition or cause new PIs to develop.[5-9] It is therefore important to have follow-up options for this group, without the need to travel to outpatient clinics. These issues, while not as well researched, are similar with individuals with other diagnoses who are at risk for PI such as people who are at bed rest for long periods, people in the intensive care unit (ICU), people who recently underwent hip surgery, and people suffering from neurodegenerative neuromuscular diseases such as multiple sclerosis and amyotrophic lateral sclerosis, as well as stroke and brain injury. Due to changes in body mass index, reduced activity, and function in general, as well as skin losing its elasticity, the elderly are also at a particular risk of developing a PI.

TABLE 12.1 ■ **Categorization of PIs, according to the European Pressure Ulcer Advisory Panel (EPUAP), National Pressure Injury Advisory Panel (NPIAP), and Pan Pacific Pressure Injury Alliance (PPPIA) (2019).**

Categorization	Description	Illustration
1	Intact skin with non-blanchable redness of a localized area. Darkly pigmented skin may not have visible blanching, but its color may differ from the surrounding skin.	
2	Partial thickness loss of dermis, presenting as a shallow open wound with a red/pink wound bed, without slough. It may also present as an intact or open/ruptured serum-filled or serosanguineous blister.	
3	Full thickness tissue loss. Subcutaneous fat may be visible, but bone, tendon or muscle are not exposed. Some slough may be present. Undermining and tunnelling may be included.	
4	Full thickness tissue loss with exposed bone, tendon or muscle. Slough or eschar may be present. Undermining and tunnelling are often included.	
Unstageable	Full thickness tissue loss in which actual depth of the wound is completely obscured by slough and/or eschar in the wound bed.	
Suspected Deep Tissue Injury	Purple or maroon localized area of discolored, intact skin, or blood-filled blister due to damage of underlying tissue due to pressure and/or shear.	

PI, Pressure injury. Table by the author, illustrations with permission from National Pressure Injury Advisory Panel (NPIAP), 2021.

The prevalence of PI among persons with SCI varies between 35% and 80%,[8,10,11] depending on how different studies define PI, and depending on the time since the SCI when the PI occurrences were measured. The occurrence of PIs in people with and without SCIs also depends on underlying health conditions. The overall prevalence of PI in acute care hospitals varies between 6.7% and 15%.[12] However, the total percentage of those who develop such ulcers is most likely higher, especially in high-risk groups, such as patients with hip fracture and patients in the ICU.[9–12]

Health-reported quality of life (HRQoL) is reduced in persons with long-standing SCI and especially in persons with comorbidities.[13] Australians with SCI have rated their physical health status as worse than the general population, and PI has caused an adverse impact on the HRQoL and self-esteem of patients with SCI.[14,15] PIs most often occur when one or more known risk factors are present, such as impaired nutritional status, reduced or impaired general condition, reduced mobility and activity, and moisture, shear and friction, as well as reduced ability to perceive stimuli. People with spinal cord lesions and other forms of paralysis that lead to reduced sensorimotor function and use of wheelchairs are particularly vulnerable. PI can also cause serious complications, with consequences for the individual consumer as well as for the capacity of the health care service. PIs occur at home, in institutions, and in hospitals. All care providers must have basic knowledge in preventing PIs in their care receivers, due to the fact that people with disabilities have an increased risk of incurring PI, and that PI can be difficult to treat. There is a need to monitor the occurrence of PI, both as part of quality improvement measures and as a basis for management and leadership in hospitals and in the community. Red marks and damage to the skin can be signs that something has changed, for example, weight gain or weight reduction, changed surface pressure, changed transfer techniques, a new life situation, and so on.

When pressure damage has occurred, measures must be taken to limit the scope and encourage healing of the PI. Having the necessary knowledge and competency will make the care providers available to take care of the consumer's needs, treat them, and guide colleagues. All professional groups that see bare skin must be able to recognize red marks that indicate that a PI is developing, and relevant professional groups must be familiar with general procedures for evaluating and treating PIs.

Telerehabilitation in Pressure Injury Follow-Up

Telerehabilitation[16] has changed our options for offering medical services to patients.[17] Moreover, telerehabilitation has also changed our possibilities for sharing knowledge to health care providers, and knowledge transfer can be performed through peer mentoring, courses, and training, both virtual and on-site. Changing weather conditions, climate change, and pandemics with the need to reduce the risk of infection[18] have led to new possibilities for reaching out to patients in hospitals and outpatient clinics. Telerehabilitation is a way to overcome the barriers of distance,[19] and several different services are available to patients in need of long-term rehabilitation.[20,21] Telerehabilitation makes PI rehabilitation services more accessible and results in a more coordinated and secured transfer of knowledge between the patient, regional, or local services and other necessary providers throughout the course of treatment.[19] If consumers and residents receive proper PI treatment at the right place and time, through comprehensive and coordinated health care services that are adapted to the individual's specific needs, healing of PIs will be optimized and there can be a rapid return to the individual's premorbid functional level.

Care for PIs should be offered at a local level, where consumers live, so they can remain functional and have their lives disrupted as little as possible by the PI. Thus rehabilitation professionals have a responsibility to educate, support, and mentor local health care providers about treatment of PI. It is also important that the organization of health care services includes and secures the provision of rehabilitation services, no matter the geographical location of the care provider or care receiver.

A telerehabilitation model should aim to take advantage of active involvement and feedback based on experience and evaluation from consumers, their families, and local health care services.[19,22-26] Studies have reported that when rehabilitation services are carried out in a consumer's familiar surroundings they are more pertinent to everyday life.[23] This is important for consumers with

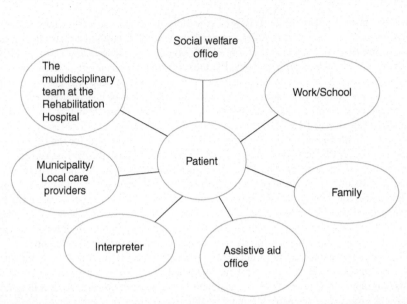

Fig. 12.1 The different participants cooperating together with the consumer in the rehabilitation process. Videoconference collaboration can be performed with specialized health care providers (the rehabilitation hospital) located on one side, while the care receivers and/or local care providers and other collaborators are located on the other.

complex needs and in need of long-term follow-up such as individuals with SCI and PI.[21, 23, 24] Thus providing informed care at a local level contributes to proper use of the health resources with reduced consumption of travel costs and in-hospital services.

Videoconferencing is a way of offering communication directly to consumer and provider simultaneously,[21] and videoconference collaboration can be performed with specialized health care providers (the rehabilitation hospital) located in one area, while the care receivers and/or local care providers and other collaborators are located in another. Other collaborators can include health care professionals at other hospitals, representatives for employers, school, the assistive aids office, the social welfare benefit office, and an interpreting service, as shown in Fig. 12.1.

Using telerehabilitation makes it easier to provide PI care using a modern means of communication, which in turn simplifies provider-to-provider communication and improves the consumer's accessibility to health care providers and other collaborators.[22, 27] These communication channels are also an effective way to perform PI follow-up regarding education, knowledge transfer, prevention, and treatment.[28] Good health care services are characterized by effective, coordinated, safe, and secure services and include the care receivers. Telerehabilitation ensures continuity and utilization of resources in a proper way, as well as accessibility and regional distribution of services, and puts the consumer in the center of the service.[29, 30] Thus a proper PI service should include knowledge translation, competence, and quality in the field of support and education not only to patients and relatives, but also to local care providers, taking care of everyday health care services. Accordingly cooperation between local authorities, consumer organizations, and other relevant partners is strengthened in ways that benefit society socioeconomically.[31, 32]

Telerehabilitation for PI follow-up can be performed in several ways. Sometimes it is necessary for the providers to communicate directly to other care providers or to other caregivers, and direct communication to the consumer is often useful. However, store and forward communication,

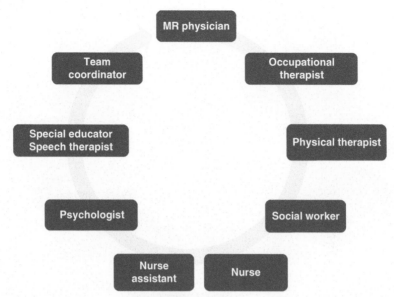

Fig. 12.2 The basic members of the multidisciplinary team. The members should attend based on present issues. Extended team members include urologist, neurologist, hand surgeon, plastic surgeon, orthopedist, psychiatrist, pediatrician, nutritionist, sexual adviser, orthopedic engineer, peer consultant, activity consultant, leisure consultant, driving school consultant, hospital chaplain, and hospital pharmacist.

where still photos or videos are sent to health care receivers or users, can also be a suitable solution where the consumers or local care providers need general information.

Different means of web-based treatment or online education are also solutions that can give both care receivers and care providers evidence-based knowledge and guidance regarding prevention and treatment.

THE MULTIDISCIPLINARY TEAM AND TELEREHABILITATION IN PRESSURE INJURY FOLLOW-UP

The multidisciplinary rehabilitation team includes a large number of different health care professionals (Fig. 12.2), and a smaller selection of necessary team members can participate in meetings, depending on the issue.

All participants in the PI treatment team must know the risk factors for PI development. These risk factors affect healing and therefore affect planning of further rehabilitation. Fig. 12.3 provides an overview of overall risk factors that must be known by members of the care team, regardless of where rehabilitation takes place.

MULTIDISCIPLINARY APPROACH

Determination of whether aids, like a wheelchair, are dangerous to a consumer or the environment must be performed, for example, if the cognitive function is reduced. The physician and psychologist are important in clarifying this issue.

Is a wheelchair suitable for multiple purposes such as wheelchair racing and general community mobility or is it best suited indoors? Here, it is important that the physiotherapist clarify what the patient is able to do in terms of exercise. The occupational therapist is important

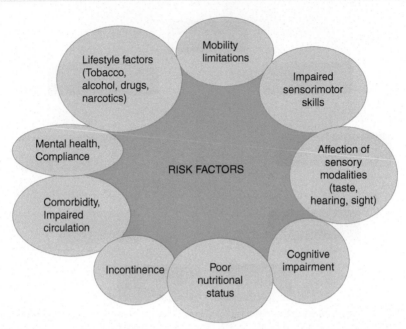

Fig. 12.3 The figure provides overall risk factors for development of PI, as well as risk factors affecting the healing. *PI*, Pressure injury. (Adapted from Stephens and Bartley, JTV [2018] and adjusted for people with disabilities.)

in relation to facilitation of necessary pressure-relieving measures, as well as the acquisition of aids, including wheelchair cushions and mattresses.[28] It is important that the wheelchair fit the intended use, for example, what happens if the back of the chair is folded? Is folding possible? What does the patient need? Is it impossible to get hold of a wheelchair or cushion? Is it possible to make a cushion of foam rubber? A needs assessment should be conducted by team members. It is also important to check the possibility of receiving new assessments on a regular basis, for example, assess age and how well the assistive device works in relation to the use it was intended for, and whether the consumer is comfortable with the use. How easy is it to repair damage and when should the assistive device be replaced? Seating pressure measurement is recommended to ensure that the correct cushion is selected in the wheelchair and that the cushion has the best pressure distribution, and seating comfort.[28] The same should be applied when choosing a mattress. Observation of the skin in relation to morning and evening care should be conducted either by nurses at the hospital or local care providers. Any incontinence issues must also be addressed by the physician, nurse, or other personnel with necessary competency.

Adjusting rehabilitation services is also important, for example, if a consumer is ambulatory; it can be difficult to work on ambulation with shoes or bracing that are the cause of the ongoing PI, or if the shoes exacerbate PIs that are already present. Shoes with straps over the back of the foot are an example of footwear that is unsuitable if there is ongoing PI or risk of PI in this area. Shoes with stiff heel caps can also cause pressure to the heels and be a risk factor for PI development. An orthotist or orthopedic technician is a good resource for clarifying issues regarding what shoes to wear. A physiotherapist should contribute with training and treatment of body areas that are particularly exposed to stress, for example, shoulder strain if the consumer uses a manual wheelchair. Seat balance and positioning can cause pressure in several body areas, in addition to friction if the

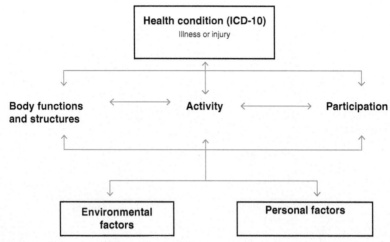

Fig. 12.4 The International Classification of Functioning (ICF) model. The ICF is a good tool to map health and disability.

seat slides forward in the chair. All care providers must observe whether seating comfort, balance, and positioning are appropriate.[28]

If the consumer suffers from lower extremity edema, it is important to focus on pressure prevention alongside treatment of the swelling. Elevation of the legs while the person is in a sitting position will cause the seat to slide forward and the individual may be exposed to pressure and friction. The result is increased risk of pressure damage. All care providers must ensure that the consumer sits in a good and pressure-relieving manner. Compression stockings and tilt of the wheelchair to elevate the legs are recommended solutions for lower extremity edema, as well as appropriate medical therapies.

Chronic or periodic pain can cause difficulties in finding comfortable sitting and lying positions. This can result in restless sitting and lying, which in turn can result in friction and an increased risk of PI. Pain-relieving medication and treatment are appropriate. The same goes for mental health, mood swings, and depression. Mental health issues can have a negative effect on self-care, which in turn will increase the risk of PIs. A psychologist or psychiatrist should be involved if an individual with disability has mental health issues and a social worker is important to follow-up income and social welfare benefits. Telerehabilitation can be also used together with on-site consultations to offer multidisciplinary assessments of the patient's state of health, body functions and structures, environmental factors, and ongoing activity.

USE OF TELEREHABILITATION IN PRESSURE INJURY MANAGEMENT, PREVENTION, AND TREATMENT WITH THE INTERNATIONAL CLASSIFICATION OF FUNCTIONING, DISABILITY, AND HEALTH FRAMEWORK

PI is a complex condition that requires close cooperation between the health care providers and the consumer to be able to identify and map problem areas and set treatment goals. The International Classification of Functioning, Disability and Health, known more commonly as ICF (Fig. 12.4), is the World Health Organization's (WHO) framework for measuring health and disability at both individual and population levels.[33] The ICF model is a framework for describing function and disability in relation to a state of health and is a good starting point for conducting a comprehensive, multidisciplinary identification of the risk of PI in consumers. The model gives

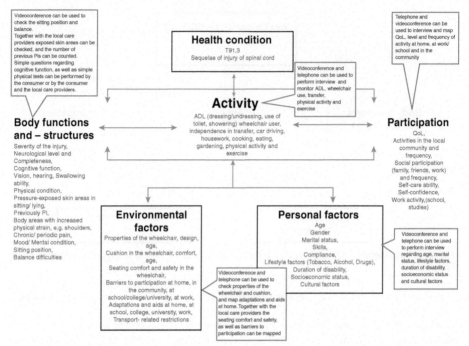

Fig. 12.5 This figure shows where and how in the ICF model telerehabilitation can be implemented for mapping, and for educational purposes. *ICF*, International Classification of Functioning.

a description of the level of function within environmental factors affecting a person's ability for activity and participation.[33] Telerehabilitation is a well-suited modality to include in the ICF framework regarding follow-up of PIs.

PIs affect opportunities for activity and participation. While the consumer is in the rehabilitation hospital/ward, the PI may affect the possibilities for optimal rehabilitation. At home, the PI may affect the person's opportunity for work/school and physical activity. The PI can also cause isolation, and in some cases stigma, especially if the PI smells unpleasant. It is therefore important to have updated knowledge and competence to be able to map the risk of having a PI, as well as to have the competence to treat the PI according to updated, evidence-based guidelines, as this will affect the person's ability and opportunities for participation. However, access to this information and to guidelines may often be limited. Telerehabilitation and provision of education and mentoring from experienced health care professionals will help these individuals.

The health and personal factors shown in Fig. 12.4 are usually mapped during inpatient rehabilitation. By also including social and environmental factors, the ICF model[33] will assist care providers in conducting a good, comprehensive mapping and assessment of most factors that affect the person's function and opportunity for activity and participation in their local environment. This applies to both positive and limiting factors. In addition, any cultural factors must also be mapped if these are perceived as limiting in participation. Most of the mentioned factors can be mapped via, for example, videoconference or telephone consultations to the consumer's home, with or without collaboration from the local care providers, as shown in Fig. 12.5. This will provide insight into potential risk factors for PI and can be carried out regularly by the multidisciplinary team in cooperation with local health care providers after discharge from rehabilitation. By using videoconferencing care providers at the rehabilitation center can perform remote visits to the consumer's home and check for

---

LIFE SITUATION
Family life, work/ school and leisure activities.

ROUTINES FOR POSITION CHANGE AND PRESSURE RELIEF IN SITTING AND LYING
Key points are the time you sit and how often you change position.
Position change usually occurs unconsciously, but when you lack sensitivity and/ or are unable to change position yourself, the routines must take over for missing signals.
The mapping must focus on how the person relates to the need for relief measures, and how this is integrated into daily life at home, at work/ school and in leisure activities.

ASSISTIVE AIDS
Assess all surfaces for the need for pressure-distributing adjustments. The most important areas are in the wheelchair(s), in the bed, on the toilet, in the shower and in the car seat. Pressure-distributing surface adjustments at work or in leisure activities may be necessary. Map the age of the aids to identify any need for replacement.

TRANSFER TECHNIQUE
Observe transfer techniques to detect any inappropriate technique, which causes stretching of the skin or bump to the surface.

SITTING POSITION
Observe the person sitting on a bench to identify risk areas. Skew positions in the pelvis and back, as well as length differences in the thighs/ calves give asymmetry that can increase the risk of PI.
The vertebral column may also be exposed.

CLOTHING AND SHOES
Check seams, buttons, pockets, shoe size, etc.

Fig. 12.6 Checklist of risk factors regarding development of PI. *PI*, Pressure injury.

preventative factors, as preventative factors, as well as educate the consumer and the local care providers in PI prevention.

A checklist of potential PI risk factors to be aware of during follow-up should be made, no matter whether the consultation is being performed via videoconference, telephone, or on-site at the hospital. Fig. 12.6 gives an example of such a checklist. The checklist should be used at every consultation to be able to register any positive or limiting changes in body function and structures, environmental and personal factors, as well as activity and participation. Action should be taken regarding any limiting changes, while positive changes should be facilitated.

To achieve improvement of public health, and more sustainable health services, a number of strategies should be highlighted—better prevention, earlier treatment, and better interaction between health care providers. Furthermore, consumers should have their proper treatment at the right place and time through comprehensive and coordinated health care services that are adapted to the individual. It is particularly important to ensure good coordination when the responsibility for a patient is transferred between hospitals and municipalities, and between departments and units within hospitals and municipalities. An important task is to ensure the best possible services to consumers. This requires coordination of services from a vast number of collaborators, as shown in Fig. 12.1.

Telerehabilitation is the perfect way to ensure interaction between all levels of care providers, and it enables the consumer to be in the center of the collaboration, because videoconference solutions make it possible to interact provider-to-consumer or providers-to-consumer, as well as provider-to-consumers if the service does not affect privacy of the consumers.

Provider-to-consumer or a smaller group of providers-to-consumer will be useful if the tele-rehabilitation concerns treatment of one specific consumer. For instance, if a physician and wound nurse at a spinal cord unit need to consult a plastic surgeon at another department or at another hospital, the consultation can include participants at three different locations. The consumer will not have to travel to the spinal cord unit and then be transferred to the plastic surgeon and then back home again. Thus time and expenses can be decreased using videoconference instead of traveling to on-site consultations. This type of consultation will also take care of privacy rights for the consumer.

If the goal is to meet the consumer's needs regarding community services, it is possible to have a meeting as shown in Fig. 12.1, where a lot of different care providers participate.

On the other hand, if the goal is to educate and prevent pressure injury on a more general basis, it is possible to hold a videoconference with a group of consumers or care providers. This way of interaction will also favor peer work, because the participants will have the opportunity to discuss and exchange experiences in a group, without having to travel.

For educational purposes, webinars, e-learning programs, and store and forward programs of particular focus are good solutions for the participants, because these will allow the possibility of education and knowledge transfer according to the recipient's immediate needs and wishes.

Special Considerations

PIs often occur near intimate body areas, which may be visible on the screen. This is an ethical issue that needs to be emphasized; in particular if performing videoconference with the consumer. Guidelines and checklists regarding how to secure privacy and dignity need to be set and all participants need to know the recommendations regarding ethical concerns. Videoconference communication should take place through encrypted channels to prevent uninvited participants from being a part of the consultation. The videoconference connection should be initiated by the health care providers and should be approved by the consumer, or local care providers at the consumer's home, before log on. All videoconferencing should take place in real-time, and neither sound nor images should be recorded or archived outside the consumer's medical record. The telerehabilitation process must meet the standards and rules set by the data protection authority in each country and state.

There is a need for PI documentation to take place in a consistent manner. Therefore it is necessary to have guidelines on what and how to register. By using common measurement tools and a common wound language, the quality of prevention, registration, and treatment of PIs will be ensured and thus contribute to the best possible quality of wound care, both in terms of multidisciplinary approach and in terms of knowledge transfer and training. The following will focus on PI treatment, no matter the location of the follow-up, but with the aim of giving advice and proper rehabilitation at the right time and place.

MAPPING THE RISK

It is important to have good tools for mapping risk factors and treatment. The consumer's ability to follow recommended measures (compliance) will be important in the assessment, in addition to clarifying the consumer's independence in self-care, and/or the need for a helping hand from assistants.

Vision Zero is for no PI to occur during hospitalization or municipality follow-up. However, PI can occur in all situations that involve pressure over time on exposed body areas. To prevent damage from pressure or shear, the consumer's risk of incurring such damage must be examined. Therefore a risk assessment is warranted as soon as possible after admission to the hospital or transfer to the municipality health care service. Three simple risk assessment questions to ask are:

1. Does the consumer have any PI?
2. Does the consumer need help to change position in the chair or bed?
3. Do you consider it likely that the consumer may suffer a PI?

The consumers should also ask themselves the same questions:

1. Do I have a PI?
2. Do I need help to change position in the chair or bed?
3. Do I consider it likely that I will suffer a PI?

If yes on any of the questions, action should be taken to prevent occurrence of PI and/or treat any PI present.

There are several valid and reliable forms to use in PI risk mapping, and whatever form is chosen should at least contain questions regarding:

- Sensory function
- Humidity/moisture/bowel and bladder incontinence
- Activity level
- Mobility
- Nutrition
- Friction and shear forces
- Cognitive function

The degree of paralysis and sensory loss, the occurrence of extensive spasticity, use of tobacco/smoking, hygiene, and skin care should be identified, along with any comorbidities for example, cardiovascular disease, lung disease, autonomic dysreflexia, neurogenic bladder and bowel, diabetes mellitus, and kidney disease. If hospitalized or in a nursing home, the level of albumin, prealbumin, and hematocrit, along with the level of vitamin C and zinc, should be measured. Supplements should be considered if intake is insufficient and deficiency is present.

Relevant risk assessment forms are Braden scale,[34] Norton scale,[35] and Spinal Cord Injury Pressure Ulcer Scale (SCIPUS).[36]

Mobility and level of function are also important measurements regarding risk evaluation. When mapping the level of function, the choice of tool is important with regard to what form provides useful information for assessing the current function, and for targeting and improving the rehabilitation measures. The ICF model in Fig. 12.4[33] includes three levels of function: the whole or parts of the body, the whole individual, and the individual in a given social context. These three parts are summarized as body functions and structures, activities, and participation. When injured or acquiring an illness, all three levels of functioning can be affected. Several data sets and forms have been developed with the aim to map the impact of injury or disease on the functional levels.

Functional Independence Measure (FIM)

FIM (formerly short for Functional Independence Measure)[37] is a multidisciplinary mapping tool used in rehabilitation. FIM is a measurement of the ability to perform daily tasks. The FIM tool can be managed face-to-face, as well as via, for example, videoconference, and is used to collect data individually and to present data to large groups. The degree of activity limitation will change during the rehabilitation. The changes that appear in the FIM mapping can be used to capture improvements in performance in activity in daily living. Mapping of personal factors, including additional illnesses, physical fitness, compliance, motivation, self-drive, and psychological aspects, must also be carried out because these will affect the degree of function, activity, and participation. The grade of function, activity, and participation could in turn affect the development of risk factors such as depression, which then could affect the risk of developing PI, or affect the healing of a present PI. FIM maps motor and cognitive function in individuals with complex needs. It shows changes in function and measures any progress in rehabilitation[37] and is a good tool to use in the PI risk mapping.

Spinal Cord Independence Measure (SCIM III)

The Spinal Cord Independence Measure, version III (SCIM III)[38] is an adapted measuring tool intended for people with SCI, and it measures various activities of daily living. SCIM III[38] is a widely used research tool for mapping treatment effect in the population of SCI. It is considered specific and sensitive enough to be able to measure change in function over time. It helps describe the level of function and hence the indirect risk of PI development.

JOINT MOBILITY ASSESSMENT

Knowledge-based guidelines recommend relieving the wound area as much as possible, once a PI has occurred. For many consumers, this results in prolonged immobilization in bed. This in turn increases the risk of new PIs due to pressure and lack of position variation while bedridden. In addition, the risk of reduced joint mobility increases, for example, stiffness and/or contracture. This is unfortunate and can be painful. Contractures also increase the risk of moisture and skin-to-skin friction, which in turn increases the risk of ulceration. Joint mobility should be mapped for passive and possibly active movements.

ICF[33] makes it easier to clarify where it is important to make an effort to reduce the risk, and what action should be done to facilitate healing if a PI has occurred. When a PI has occurred, it is important that the multidisciplinary team or the local health care providers make a comprehensive assessment of which rehabilitation measures should be implemented, which should continue, and which may be delayed. It is also important to evaluate whether initiated and ongoing measures actually work satisfactorily, and whether the patient utilizes the measures and aids. The entire team around the individual consumer must participate in this assessment, on-site and/or via, for example, videoconference. Nonfunctioning measures must be quickly adjusted and readjusted. All assessments must be documented in the medical record.

MAPPING THE TREATMENT

If all health care personnel use the same structure for the assessment, it is possible to compare the assessments with previous documentation and determine whether initiated treatment has an effect.[3, 29, 39–41] Length, width, and depth must be measured to assess the size of the PI, and the measurements should be performed at the first consultation and then regularly.[42]

A structured, but simple assessment tool to detect changes in the PI is TIMES.[29]

TIMES is an acronym for:

T Tissue
I Infection/inflammation
M Moisture
E Edge
S Surrounding skin

TIMES[29] is easy to use as a collaborative assessment tool in a videoconference consultation to the patient's home. Health care providers will be able to assess tissue, edges, and surrounding skin by performing remote visual examination of the PI. In collaboration with the local care providers, any smell and color of the PI can be assessed, together with an assessment of the amount and consistency of the moisture. Such a consultation will also give the patient or their next of kin the opportunity to inform providers of any changes in mood, pain, spasticity, autonomic dysreflexia, sleep pattern, or new limitations and barriers in everyday life.

An assessment with TIMES[29] is recommended to be used at each dressing change, and measurement of the PI size can be performed every week.[42] A reduction in the size of the wound is an indication that the wound is healing.[43]

Other similar models, such as the Pressure Ulcer Scale for Healing (PUSH) tool,[44] are also reliable for collaboration between care providers in measuring changes in PI development over time.

Recommendations for Research

Geographical locations can be a barrier to receiving PI care because long-distance travel can result in adverse consequences for the consumer.[45] The expenses associated with transportation are large, in both monetary and environmental costs.[45] Communication via telerehabilitation ensures consumers receive care and makes it possible for consumers and local health care providers to interact digitally.[31] This allows for remote collaboration between health care workers and consumers, something consumers and their family members have desired.[22, 23]

Studies highlight current issues in the performance of telerehabilitation. Yuen et al.[32] discuss the lack of high-speed internet services reducing participation rate, as well as lack of computer literacy and incompatibility of participants' computers using videoconferencing programs. Further research should be performed on this topic.

Woo et al.[46] emphasize the need for provider assistance regarding the use of at-home monitoring programs. Successful provision of services has shown high consumer satisfaction[30] and services were found to be cost-effective.[45] Research on technical issues, satisfaction, cost-benefit, and environmental savings in the follow-up is warranted.

Telerehabilitation is still a "new" way of thinking, but also a very good way to provide cooperation and collaboration. Telerehabilitation follow-up of PI could be transferred to many aspects of health care in all parts of the world, giving the opportunity to support and educate at local level on a regular basis or during times of disaster and worsening climate change.

CASE STUDY

Peter W has a cervical SCI. He uses an electric wheelchair as a means of transport. Peter has a PI on the foot. Peter is not careful and crashes the wheelchair, and the foot with the PI, against random objects in the room. This means the PI worsens, in addition to the fact that there is a great risk of new PIs on feet, legs, hands, and arms caused by the accidents. There is also an increased risk of injuring family members and care providers. Peter's ability to cooperate regarding appointments and insight into his own condition is reduced. Thus the multidisciplinary team/local care providers must assess which measures should be adjusted in relation to Peter still maintaining the opportunity for rehabilitation, PI healing, and prevention, without limiting the possibility for activity and participation as described in Fig. 12.7.

Many factors are involved in PI healing. Knowledge and competence among the therapists will be important. However, it is also important to focus on Peter's understanding of his disease or condition, his ability to understand the necessity of the recommended measures, and his ability to follow the advice given (compliance); that is, Peter's ability to actively participate and cooperate in a positive way, in terms of rehabilitation.

Some factors are difficult for Peter to take responsibility for, such as mental or cognitive illness, depression, vision, and hearing. Here, the multidisciplinary team and the local care providers have an important role in the rehabilitation. Peter must be made aware and gain knowledge so he can take responsibility for his own body and health within the possibilities of his condition. Prevention of PI should be a topic at all rehabilitation units. However, it is known that people who have never had a PI are unable to associate themselves with the severity of such an injury. The education must therefore be easily understandable, repeated several times, and supplemented with written materials such as booklets and e-learning courses, electronic store and forward tools, and webinars. Peter must also understand that changing his daily routines in connection with travel and leisure activities entails an increased risk of incurring pressure damage. Thus he must have suitable aids and strategies to be able to continue preventative care, even in such circumstances.

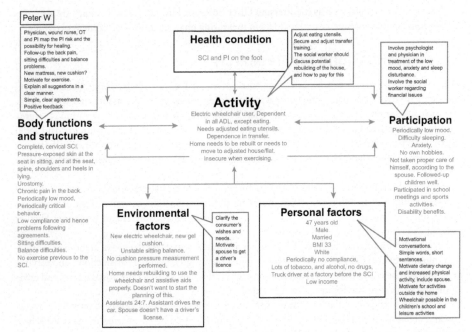

Fig. 12.7 The ICF model used as tool for mapping and identifying the level of activity and participation in the rehabilitation process of a consumer with SCI where PI on the foot was recently discovered. Most of the suggested actions are possible to perform via videoconference if the consumer and spouse are safe with this method of collaboration. *ICF,* International Classification of Functioning; *OT,* occupational therapist; *PI,* pressure injury; *PT,* physiotherapist; *SCI,* spinal cord injury.

References

1. United Nations Convention on the Rights of Persons with Disabilities (CRPD), Rule 3, article 25-26. https://www.un.org/disabilities/documents/convention/convention_accessible_pdf.pdf; Accessed 07.09.20.
2. ISCoS. The International Spinal Cord Society. https://www.iscos.org.uk/. Accessed October 7th 2020.
3. National Pressure Injury Advisory Panel. https://npiap.com/; Accessed 09.26.21.
4. European Pressure Ulcer Advisory Panel, National Pressure Injury Advisory Panel and Pan Pacific Pressure Injury Alliance. Prevention and Treatment of Pressure Ulcers/Injuries: Quick Reference Guide. Emily Haesler (Ed.). EPUAP/NPIAP/PPPIA: 2019. https://www.internationalguideline.com/static/pdfs/Quick_Reference_Guide-10Mar2019.pdf; Accessed 09.26.21.
5. Houghton PE, Campbell KE, CPG Panel. *Canadian Best Practice Guidelines for the Prevention and Management of Pressure Ulcers in People with Spinal Cord Injury. A Resource Handbook for Clinicians.* 2013. https://onf.org/wp-content/uploads/2019/04/Pressure_Ulcers_Best_Practice_Guideline_Final_web4.pdf. Accessed September 25th 2021.
6. Lidal IB, Snekkevik H, Aamodt G, et al. Mortality after spinal cord injury in Norway. *J Rehabil Med.* 2007;39:145–151.
7. Dejong G, Tian W, Hsueh CH, et al. Rehospitalization in the first year after traumatic spinal cord injury after discharge from medical rehabilitation. *Arch Phys Med Rehabil.* 2013;94:S87–S97.
8. Hoff JM, Bjerke LW, Gravem PE, et al. Pressure ulcers after spinal cord injury. *Norwegian Medical Association.* 2012;132:838–839.
9. Sezer N, Akkuş S, Uğurlu FG. Chronic complications of spinal cord injury. *World J Orthop..* 2015;6(1):24–33. https://doi.org/10.5312/wjo.v6.i1.24. eCollection 2015.
10. Chen Y, Devivo MJ, Jackson AB. Pressure ulcer prevalence in people with spinal cord injury: age-period-duration effects. *Arch Phys Med Rehabil.* 2005;86(6):1208–1213.
11. Vanderwee K. Pressure ulcer prevalence in Europe: a pilot study. *J Eval Clin Pract.* 2007;13(2):227.

12. Bjørlo K, Ribu L. Pilotstudie av trykksårprevalens I et norsk sykehus. (Pilot study of the PI prevalence in a Norwegian hospital). *Sykepleien Forskning.* 2009;4(4):299–305.
13. Lidal IB, Veenstra M, Hjeltnes N, et al. Health-related quality of life in persons with long-standing spinal cord injury. *Spinal Cord.* 2008;46(11):710–715.
14. Lala D, Dumont FS, Leblond J, et al. Impact of pressure ulcers on individuals living with a spinal cord injury. *Arch Phys Med Rehabil.* 2014;95(12):2312–2319. https://doi.org/10.1016/j.apmr.2014.08.003. 2014 Aug 25.
15. Lourenco L, Blanes L, Salomé GM, et al. Quality of life and self-esteem in patients with paraplegia and pressure ulcers: a controlled cross-sectional study. *J Wound Care.* 2014;23(6):331–334. 336-337.
16. Center for Connected Health Policy. What is Telehealth? http://www.cchpca.org/what-is-telehealth; Accessed 07.10.20.
17. Demiris G. Integration of telemedicine in graduate medical informatics education. *J Am Med Inform Assoc.* 2003;10(4):310–314. https://doi.org/10.1197/jamia.M1280.
18. Centers for Disease Control and Prevention. Using Telehealth to Expand Access to Essential Health Services During the COVID-19 Pandemic. National Center for Immunization and Respiratory Diseases (NCIRD), division of viral diseases. 2020. https://www.cdc.gov/coronavirus/2019-ncov/hcp/telehealth. html; Accessed 07.10.20.
19. Irgens I, Bach B, Rekand T, et al. Optimal management of health care for persons with disability related to spinal cord injury: learning from the Sunnaas model of telerehabilitation. *Spinal Cord Ser Cases.* 2020;6:88. https://doi.org/10.1038/s41394-020-00338-6.
20. Banbury A, Nancarrow S, Dart J, et al. Telehealth interventions delivering home-based support group videoconferencing: systematic review. *J Med Internet Res.* 2018;20(2):e25. https://doi.org/10.2196/jmir.8090.
21. Irgens I, Rekand T, Arora M, et al. Telehealth for people with spinal cord injury: a narrative review. *Spinal Cord.* 2018;56:643–655. https://doi.org/10.1038/s41393-017-0033-3.
22. Aanestad M, Driveklepp AM, Sørli H, et al. Participatory continuing design: "Living with" video-conferencing in rehabilitation. In: Kanstrup AM, Bygholm A, Bertelsen P, Nøhr C, eds. *Participatory Design & Health Information Technology.* 1st edn. Amsterdam: IOS Press BV; 2017:45–59. https://doi.org/10.3233/978-1-61499-740-5-45.
23. Moser I. Chapter 3. *Velferdsteknologi. En ressursbok (Welfare technology. A resource manual).* Oslo: Cappelen Damm; 2019:69–84. ISBN: 978820253648.
24. Irgens I, Kleven L, Sørli H, et al. Telemedicine brings specialist healthcare services to patients' homes. *Tidsskr Nor Legeforen.* 2015;135:1716–1717. https://doi.org/10.4045/tidsskr.15.0770.
25. Øra Hege P, Kirmess M, Brady MC, et al. The effect of augmented speech-language therapy delivered by telerehabilitation on poststroke aphasia - a pilot randomized controlled trial. *Clin Rehabil.* 2020;34(3):369–381. https://doi.org/10.1177/0269215519896616.
26. Høye H, Jahnsen RB, Løvstad M, et al. A mindfulness-based stress reduction program via group video conferencing for adults with cerebral palsy – a pilot study. *Frontiers in Neurology.* 2020;11:195. https://doi.org/10.3389/fneur.2020.00195.
27. Dàvalos ME, French MT, Burdick AE, et al. Economic evaluation of telemedicine: review of the literature and research guidelines for benefit-cost analysis. *Telemed J E Health.* 2009;15(10):933–948. https://doi.org/10.1089/tmj.2009.0067.
28. Stephens M, Bartley C. Understanding the association between pressure ulcers and sitting in adults what does it mean for me and my carers? Seating guidelines for people, carers and health & social care professionals. *Journal of Tissue Viability.* 2018;27(1):59–73. https://doi.org/10.1016/j.jtv.2017.09.004.
29. Johansen E, Leren L, Bredesen IM, et al. Bruk verktøyet TIMES til å vurdere sår strukturert. [Use of TIMES as tool for a structured assessment of ulcers]. *Sykepleien.* 2019. https://doi.org/10.4220/Sykepleiens.2019.75698.
30. Yuen HK. Effect of a home telecare program on oral health among adults with tetraplegia: a pilot study. *Spinal Cord.* 2013;51(6):477–481. https://doi.org/10.1038/sc.2012.176.
31. Aanestad M, Jensen TB. Collective mindfulness in post-implementation IS adaptation processes. *Inf Organ.* 2016;26:3–27. https://doi.org/10.1016/j.infoandorg.2016.02.001.
32. Yuen J, Thiyagarajan CA, Belci M. Patient experience survey in telemedicine for spinal cord injury patients. *Spinal Cord.* 2015;53(4):320–323. https://doi.org/10.1038/sc.2014.247.

33. International Classification of Functioning, Disability and Health (ICF). https://www.who.int/classifications/icf/en/; Accessed 07.10.20.
34. Braden Scale – For Predicting Pressure Sore Risk. https://www.in.gov/isdh/files/Braden_Scale.pdf; Accessed 07.10.20.
35. The Norton Pressure Sore Risk-Assessment Scale Scoring System. https://shrtn.on.ca/norton_pressure_sore_risk_assessment; Accessed 07.10.20.
36. Delparte JJ, Scovil CY, Flett HM, et al. Psychometric properties of the spinal cord injury pressure ulcer scale (SCIPUS) for pressure ulcer risk assessment during inpatient rehabilitation. *Arch Phys Med Rehabil.* 2015;96(11):1980–1985. http://www.ncbi.nlm.nih.gov/pubmed/26205694.
37. Linacre JM, Heinemann AW, Wright BD, et al. The structure and stability of the functional independence measure. *Arch Phys Med Rehabil.* 1994;75(2):127–132. https://doi.org/10.1016/0003-9993(94)90384-0.
38. Itzkovich M, Shefler H, Front L, et al. SCIM III (Spinal Cord Independence Measure version III): reliability of assessment by interview and comparison with assessment by observation. *Spinal Cord.* 2018;56:46–51. https://doi.org/10.1038/sc.2017.97.
39. Delparte JJ, Scovil CY, Flett HM, et al. Psychometric properties of the spinal cord injury pressure ulcer scale (SCIPUS) for pressure ulcer risk assessment during inpatient rehabilitation. *Arch Phys Med Rehabil.* 2015;96(11):1980–1985.
40. Salzberg CA, Byrne DW, Cayten CG, et al. A new pressure ulcer risk assessment scale for individuals with spinal cord injury. *Am J Phys Med Rehabil.* 1996;75:96–104.
41. Salzberg CA, Byrne DW, Kabir R, et al. Predicting pressure ulcers during initial hospitalization for acute spinal cord injury. *Wounds.* 1999;11:45–57.
42. Nichols E. Wound assessment Part 1: How to measure a wound. *Wound Essentials.* 2015;10(2):51–55.
43. Keast DH, Bowering CK, Evans AW, et al. Measure: a proposed assessment framework for developing best practice recommendations for wound assessment. *Wound Repair Regen.* 2004;12(suppl 3):1–17.
44. NPUAP. Pressure Ulcer Scale for Healing (PUSH). https://npuap.org/page/PUSHTool; Accessed 10.10.20.
45. Irgens I, Hoff JM, Sørli H, et al. Hospital based care at home; study protocol for a mixed epidemiological and randomized controlled trial. *Trials.* 2019;20:1–12. https://doi.org/10.1186/s13063-019-3185-y.
46. Woo C, Seton JM, Washington M, et al. Increasing specialty care access through use of an innovative home telehealth-based spinal cord injury disease management protocol. (SCI DMP). *J Spinal Cord Med.* 2016;39(1):3–12. https://doi.org/10.1179/2045772314Y.0000000202.

CHAPTER 13

Telerehabilitation for Pain Management

Jennifer Kurz ■ Daniel Hussey

Introduction

Telemedicine (the use of telecommunication and information technologies [ITs] to deliver patient care at a distance) has great potential to play a practical, cost-effective, and meaningful role in chronic pain management. Chronic pain is one of the highest impact problems in health care, with more than 100 million American adults affected, which is more than those affected by heart disease, cancer, and diabetes combined. Pain care, as a whole, costs the United States upward of $635 billion each year in specialty visits, interventional procedures, surgery, and lost productivity.[1] Chronic pain is the number one cause of long-term disability in the United States, with indirect costs (reduced or missed work productivity) accounting for more than 50% of this burden.[2] In 2016 approximately 20% of US adults had chronic pain, and 8% had high-impact chronic pain limiting at least one major life activity.[3] Furthermore, up to 80% of postoperative patients do not have adequate pain management.[4] Persistent pain syndromes destroy an individual's quality of life—including engagement in physical activity and with society—as well as increase risks for other serious noncommunicable diseases, such as obesity, cardiovascular disease, and mental health disorders, including addiction. Inappropriate and dangerous opioid prescribing and misuse of opioids has been associated with 130 US deaths per day from opioid overdose, and an economic burden of $78.5 billion per year.[5] There are approximately 2.3 million people with opioid use disorder in the United States, and 5 to 8 million medical opioid users still suffering with chronic pain. Globally, chronic pain is one of the leading causes of disability. Low back pain is the leading cause of years lost to disability in high-income, high-middle-income, and middle-income countries, and a top cause of years lost to disability in all quintiles of the sociodemographic index.[6] Neck pain, osteoarthritis, opioid use disorder, and tension headaches are chronic pain–related disorders within the top 30 global culprits of years lost to disability.[6]

To identify why in-person nonpharmacological treatments are poorly implemented in chronic pain practices, Becker et al.[7] determined barriers as seen from pain patients, nurses, and primary care providers' perspectives. For patients, high costs, low motivation, and transportation issues were the main barriers to care. For providers, the main barriers included inability to promote nonpharmacological therapy once opioid therapy was initiated, and patients' skepticism about efficacy of these approaches. It will take a seismic shift in mindset to overcome these barriers, on the part of both chronic pain patients and the many providers who treat them. With the use of telerehabilitation for pain management, however, at least some of these barriers, including transportation, motivation, and cost, may be overcome. According to Pew Research Center data, 81% of American adults now own a smartphone, making the internet a ubiquitous tool to deliver cognitive behavioral and other nonpharmacological, integrative pain management therapies directly to patients.

With burgeoning telerehabilitation options, such as pain apps and trackers, virtual pain programs, and internet-based tools, patients may be empowered to participate more in lifestyle and behavior changes, as well as access behavioral-psychological, nonpharmacological pain therapies not often found in conventional pain care clinics. Patient engagement in Zoom multidisciplinary pain programs and other telerehabilitation platforms can enable these mobility-impaired, often isolated individuals to find evidence-based self-management therapeutic options as well as social connection—a key ingredient to successful pain management programs and long-term patient engagement. There is an extremely high prevalence of serious comorbid mood disorders with chronic pain, with as much as 50% to 70% of chronic pain patients showing signs of significant depression or anxiety. In fact, the presence of a persistent pain syndrome is a leading risk factor for suicide in these patients.[3] With remote access to providers who offer helpful psychological and even pharmacological (i.e., medication-assisted therapy [MAT], for addiction therapy) support via telerehabilitation, patients with comorbid chronic pain, mental health, and opioid use disorders no longer need their access to care be limited by location, time constraints, or physical handicaps. The field of telerehabilitation for pain management is still emerging, however, and there is much work to be done.

The National Pain Strategy recommends a comprehensive, biopsychosocial approach to pain care, tailored to individual patient needs.[4] This requires providers treating the same patient to have a consistent message: after red flags and treatable medical causes for pain are ruled out or addressed, the emphasis should be on education and pain coping strategies, which can be delivered via telerehabilitation. Multidisciplinary, functional restoration pain rehabilitation models that encourage activity engagement despite pain, improve cognitive coping strategies, and address underlying mental health issues are the gold standard approach to chronic pain care.[8, 9] Unfortunately, due to health care systems' incentivization of pharmacological care and procedures over self-care and education,[10] and because access to multidisciplinary pain programs has been historically limited for the majority of chronic pain patients, including the most vulnerable, low-income patients with few resources, the problem of chronic pain and its cost is not going away any time soon. With the COVID-19 pandemic, which forced isolation and restrictions on helpful resources such as live group therapies, physical treatments, and access to pain management providers, this problem is further highlighted. However the pandemic also brings hope for the newly expanded role of telerehabilitation[11] to improve access to evidence-based cognitive behavioral and integrative pain management therapies.

Telerehabilitation in Pain Management

Pain management providers may be better positioned than ever to deliver the most significant part of multidisciplinary pain care directly to patients' homes, with the ease and flexibility offered by technology. Telerehabilitation, with multiple platforms available for chronic pain management, provides global access to internet-based pain programs, mobile health pain apps for symptom tracking and stress management, and even new pain therapies, such as virtual reality (VR) programs. Virtual consultations with pain doctors, psychologists, and other mental and behavioral health experts are encouraged, particularly during the age of COVID-19. Mobile app and internet-delivered psychological therapies with the most evidence, such as cognitive behavioral therapy (CBT), acceptance and commitment therapy (ACT), mindfulness meditation, and stress management, have already shown great promise with telerehabilitation.[12-18] Individual consultations or group sessions, interdisciplinary team conferences, support groups, pain education workshops and programs, pain apps and software, and integrative mind-body treatments can all be offered virtually via the internet.

OVERCOMING GEOGRAPHY/PHYSICAL LIMITATIONS TO PAIN CARE

Pain rehabilitation programs inclusive of psychological and behavioral pain treatments are often confined to big cities and academic centers or small community centers invested in integrative or alternative pain care, so their influence cannot extend to the masses of chronic pain sufferers globally. With only 8000 to 9000 pain medicine specialists in the United States, who are mainly congregated in large cities, there is the added obstacle of geography in providing pain management expertise to remote areas. Clearly, patients residing in more remote regions may take advantage of telerehabilitation to access pain care. Boston's MGH SCOPE (Safer/Competent Opioid Prescribing Education) telemedicine study[19] involved a 13-month study of 238 virtual evaluations of pain patients from Martha's Vineyard, a small island off the Massachusetts mainland only accessible by ferry. This study demonstrated that it is possible and feasible to maintain a telerehabilitation pain program with acceptable patient satisfaction. The inability to travel to pain clinics and pain care providers due to illness, inclement weather, or other external factors can be overcome by telerehabilitation. There is also access for the pain patients with debilitating physical impairments who previously required a support network or insurance coverage for transportation to and from numerous specialty appointments and treatments. This is pertinent for the most disabled, mobility-impaired patients with cumulative medical problems.

EVOLUTION OF TELEREHABILITATION FOR PAIN MANAGEMENT

Telehealth delivery of pain care, including internet and mobile app pain programs, has been appreciated and studied since the 1990s, but many online programs are not standardized or evidence-based, and many are undergoing active development. Prior to COVID-19, telerehabilitation was not implemented in most outpatient pain clinics. There was not enough incentive to provide telerehabilitation routinely, as it was not covered by insurance in the same way in-person visits were in the United States. With the March 2020 Medicare ruling opening access to virtual visits in almost every field of nonessential specialty care, this suddenly changed. Telemedicine as a platform for health care delivery has been rapidly transformed during the public health crisis, from a poorly utilized intervention into a mainstream form of health care delivery.

In this chapter, some of the more recent programs and reviews that can be found in the expansive, burgeoning field of telerehabilitation for pain management will be highlighted. With implementation already underway, the wider vision of a more comprehensive, integrative pain care model—a model in which elements of pain psychology, mind-body strategies, and lifestyle medicine can be delivered remotely through platforms such as Zoom, online pain programs, pain apps, and VR—may become the norm rather than the exception. The level of participation, engagement, and expectation on the part of patients, as well as providers, must change for this to be successfully accomplished, which cannot happen overnight. We have included numerous international studies in this chapter, which is perhaps a reflection of how the role of telemedicine has been appreciated outside the United States for many years. Virtual pain care has great potential to change the way we think about and treat chronic pain, but there are also real practical obstacles and inherent inequities in this type of care delivery that must not be overlooked.

Chronic pain management should involve evidence-based pain psychology,[20, 21] which can be delivered virtually. Treating the person as an individual, influenced by unique biopsychosocial determinants of pain, rather than only structural pathologies to be targeted by external physical interventions, is consistent with evidence-based pain psychology strategies such as CBT and the more recent "third wave" psychological therapy, ACT. CBT encourages cognitive and behavioral change techniques, focusing on changing maladaptive thoughts and behaviors with a goal-oriented, problem-solving approach. ACT focuses on the role of acceptance and mindfulness rather than cognitive change, increasing psychological flexibility to foster moment-to-moment awareness, acceptance, and a commitment to values and direction. Both pain interventions can improve quality of life, pain acceptance, function, and self-efficacy, and reduce pain, emotional burden, and distress.[22-26] Unfortunately, these interventions are not always offered. Perhaps access to interdisciplinary, psychologically informed pain care is still limited, in part, because not all insurers or stakeholders have been assured of the economic success of such models.[10] Evidence for long-term successful outcomes is also not assured. Results from a 13-year follow-up study from Mayo Clinic on patients who finished extended pain rehabilitation programs with multidisciplinary therapies showed that 68% still had functional impairments and difficulty returning to daily life, and 53% of the patients had deteriorated 3 years after a multidisciplinary pain management program.[27] The attrition rates are likely related to multiple factors, such as absence of long-term provider-patient engagement, worsening chronic illness, and decreased patient motivation over time. In a study on an internet-based booster program to support patients after discharge from interdisciplinary pain centers, findings suggested there could be small but real benefits.

Telerehabilitation for chronic pain is a promising and cost-effective method of delivering psychological care. With telerehabilitation, direct access to evidence-based pain education and pain psychology, counseling, and pain coping strategies can be delivered by providers on an ongoing, long-term basis without the requirement of physical face-to-face encounters. Allowing patients the flexibility to access care at their own pace and from the comfort of their home is a huge perk of this technology. For the past decade, researchers from around the world have been investigating delivery of internet-based chronic pain prevention and treatment programs based on pain psychology.[28] In a systemic review of three technology-enhanced psychological treatment modalities, including telephone, interactive voice response, and internet (n = 9890), evidence suggested that across modalities, technology-assisted psychological interventions are efficacious for improving self-management of chronic pain in adults.[29]

A large number of trials for various mental health and physical conditions have been developed, with internet-delivered CBT taking the early lead.[14] In the Cooperative Pain Education and Self-management (COPES) trial,[30] 125 VA patients with chronic back pain were treated with either interactive voice response-based-CBT (IVR-CBT) or individual CBT sessions. IVR is the use of a phone's touch-tone keypad to provide responses to automated scripts. The pain intensity scale measured by the numeric rating scale (NRS) showed a reduction with IVR (−0.77) similar to in-person care (−0.84), with a 95% confidence interval (CI) for the difference between groups, indicating noninferiority for the IVR form of delivery. There were improvements in physical function, sleep quality, and physical quality of life at 3 months relative to baseline, with no advantage for either treatment, and treatment dropout was a little lower in IVR-CBT (patients completed on average 2.3% more sessions).

For the past two decades, a range of health domains, including chronic pain and mood disorders, have been targeted with eHealth interventions based on CBT principles. These programs are currently seeing wider applications for children and adults, with the type of available help ranging from text-based, educational websites to custom-built software applications. In several systematic reviews of internet-based interventions for chronic pain,[31] small but significant improvements in pain experience and reductions in functional disability were reported. Online programs for pain have progressed from uncontrolled case studies and feasibility trials to many randomized clinical trials. While early applications of "self-management" tools focused on biofeedback, more recent approaches attempt to teach patients a variety of pain coping skills and strategies, including self-monitoring, goal setting, relaxation training, physical exercise, attention and emotional control, belief reappraisal, and self-efficacy (planning, coping, and pacing). In an online Chronic Pain Management Program studied in 2012,[32] self-directed, web-based pain education, CBT skills, and social networking were incorporated into an interactive learning environment. Of 305 adult participants, 162 chronic pain patients were randomly assigned unsupervised access to the program for approximately 6 weeks, while 143 were assigned to the wait-listed control group with treatment as usual. A comprehensive assessment was administered before the study and approximately 7 and 14 weeks thereafter. All recruitment, data collection, and participant involvement took place online. The program resulted in increased pain knowledge and decreased perceived pain magnitude (severity, interference, and emotional burden), disability, and catastrophizing.

Internet delivery of ACT for chronic pain is an area of growing interest, with expanding evidence for long-term benefit and cost-effectiveness.[33] Telerehabilitation may be used to enhance delivery of ACT, either in isolation or as a complement to traditional face-to-face delivery. Telerehabilitation interventions can provide opportunities for tracking, forming, and reinforcing through reminders and feedback, which is a cornerstone process in ACT: psychological flexibility. Participants are encouraged to engage in experiential exercises and metaphors that may be particularly relevant to their in-the-moment perception of pain. Willingness to experience pain with a moment-to-moment awareness, consistent with mindfulness, is another key feature of ACT. Perhaps there is no one better to ask about the experience of providing ACT concepts online than Dr. Joe Tatta, founder of the *Healing Pain Podcast* and the Integrative Pain Science Institute, who has built a career treating chronic pain and educating providers who treat chronic pain via Zoom. He has a worldwide following with well-received provider training programs featuring ACT, functional nutrition, and other internet-based educational programs for chronic pain.

Herbert et al.[34] showed, in a noninferiority trial of US veterans with chronic pain (n = 128), that ACT delivered via video teleconferencing was noninferior to in-person delivery of ACT for the primary outcome of pain interference and several secondary measures at posttreatment and at 6-month follow-up. A three-arm randomized controlled trial (RCT) compared an internet-guided self-help ACT intervention ("Living with Pain") with an internet-based control arm (i.e., expressive writing) and a wait-list group.[35] Results showed that participants in the ACT arm improved on several domains of chronic pain disability, including psychological flexibility and pain catastrophizing, compared to both control groups. In another three-arm German RCT (n = 302), a guided online ACT-based program ("ACTonPain"), which included e-coaches (psychologists) providing feedback 2 days after each module, showed significantly less pain interference and higher pain acceptance at posttreatment and at 6-month-follow-up compared with the other groups.[36] Patient guidance involved regular feedback, explanations, motivation, and reminders to adhere to treatment. Guidance seems to improve treatment effects and can be cost-effective, but more evidence is needed. This general consensus is in line with a 2014 systemic review on the impact of guidance on internet-delivered mental health interventions.[37] In theory, blended therapies, which include technology-enhanced booster sessions or evidence-based apps with in-person therapy, are ideal.

In a 2015 metaanalysis involving 22 RTCs of internet interventions for chronic pain, there were overall small-to-moderate effect sizes, with these sizes comparable with those seen for reviews of psychological pain care strategies in general.[38] In general, systemic reviews of internet-delivered CBT, ACT, and mind-body pain therapies suggest beneficial and comparable outcomes to their in-person delivery counterparts, with good patient satisfaction. In Andersson's metaanalysis[39] of 13 controlled trials (n = 1053) comparing in-person to internet-delivered CBT, participants consented to being randomized to either ICBT or conventional face-to-face CBT (n = 6 individual format, n = 7 group format) for a variety of mental health conditions, including depression, anxiety, panic disorder, and phobias. The two treatment formats were equally effective in addressing many of these conditions. This metaanalysis mirrored findings by Cuijpers et al.[40] who found no differences between guided self-help and face-to-face therapies.

As Dr. Kurt Kroenke, a leader of opioid reduction risk strategies, aptly states:

Telehealth is not only useful for monitoring and adjusting analgesics but also for the delivery of nonpharmacological therapies such as pain self-management, cognitive-behavioral therapy, mindfulness-based therapy, and motivational interviewing for exercise. Also, pain is frequently comorbid with other symptoms such as depression, insomnia and fatigue. Several studies in patients with cancer have documented the effectiveness of telecare management of pain along with other symptoms. This multisymptom approach might not only improve outcomes in individual patients with pain who suffer from other comorbid symptoms but also increase the cost-effectiveness of a telehealth service designed to cover multiple symptoms.

Pain Apps/Trackers

Technology-assisted self-management treatments have shown significant benefits in the chronic pain population. In the first large Cochrane review of technological interventions for pain, there were 15 studies involving 2000 participants.[33] Reviews identify small-to-moderate reductions in pain, disability, and distress in intervention groups compared with any control,[38] including active, standard care, or wait-list control, with little difference between remote and in-person therapies (see Fig. 13.1).[40, 44] A 2019 network metaanalysis review of 30 RCTs (5394 participants) involving "eHealth" modalities aimed to determine which were most effective for reducing pain interference in chronic pain patients.[41] These included internet-based and telephone-supported interventions, interactive voice response, VR (a three-dimensional [3D] computer-generated environment an individual may explore, interact with, and manipulate), videoconferencing (the use of high-quality real-time video and audio connection via online internet networks), and mobile phone apps (mobile-based or mobile-enhanced programs). This review found that that mobile apps and VR for pain were two of the most effective interventions; however, there was a bias of underrepresentation of many modalities.

There has been significant work in the field of pain apps and trackers, along with telephone, interactive voice response, and website interventions. There is a growing number of pain apps,

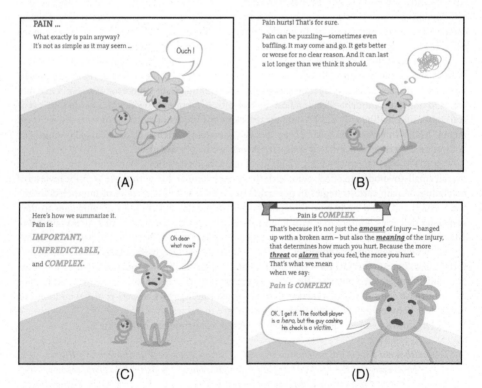

Fig. 13.1 Example screens of module 1 in PTSM. *PTSM,* Pain Tracker Self-Manager.

and, although many are not evidence-based, there is a push from industry and other stakeholders to advance these technologies further, with gamification and other motivators to improve patient adherence.

There is a growing market for pain apps that can deliver pain symptom tracking and monitoring, as well as self-management coping strategies, including relaxation therapy, yoga, and guided imagery. From a New Zealand systemic review of 939 pain apps available through 2018, using the search term, "pain management," in both Google Play and App stores, 19 apps met the review's inclusion criteria, with meditation and guided relaxation most frequently included in self-management strategies. Only three apps (*Curable, PainScale-Pain Diary and Coach,* and *SuperBetter*) met the largest number of criteria to foster self-management of pain, according to the review, with self-monitoring of symptoms (n = 11) and self-tailoring of strategies (n = 9) frequently featured. Although two apps (*Headspace* and *SuperBetter*) have been shown to improve health outcomes, none of the included apps have been evaluated in people with persistent pain.[42] Another notable app is "WebMAP Mobile," created by Dr. Tonya Palermo and her team at Seattle Children's Research Institute for adolescents with chronic pain, which includes CBT skills for coping and activity engagement. "Solution for Kids in Pain" (SKIP) is a self-proclaimed "knowledge mobilization network" based at Dalhousie University and co-led by Children's Healthcare Canada. The web-based program includes some of the evidence-based pain apps available commercially, including "Symple," "Liv," CareClinic," "Migraine Buddy," and "Pain Coach." The more one searches, the more apps there seem to be, not to mention the innumerable websites and webpages available for chronic pain. These can be loosely organized into the following subsets: mindfulness/meditation (e.g., "Calm," "Headspace," or "Yoga for Beginners"), stress and mental health, distraction, biofeedback, and pain education.

Another randomized trial of an internet-delivered Pain Tracker Self-Manager (PTSM), utilizing Butler and Moseley's pain model, ACT metaphors, and verbal/visual cues, showed significant reductions of pain intensity and interference, perceived disability, catastrophizing and fear.[45]

With digital medicine constantly evolving into an ever more user-friendly, accessible platform, along with the ubiquity of mobile phones and internet culture, there is a growing potential to educate patients, provide more counseling on nonpharmacological, noninterventional pain therapies, and promote self-management for chronic pain. Providers have access to evidence-based electronic health record systems that already allow for electronic administration of pain assessments and outcome measures, as well as email and telerehabilitation virtual visit communication with patients. Several web-based systems, such as Collaborative Health Outcomes Information Registry (CHOIR),[43] deliver multidisciplinary pain history intakes, which may help providers with their evaluations.

However, as the industry of eHealth becomes more commercialized in the private sector, a concern is raised regarding the loss of quality in the heterogeneity. Quantity does not mean quality, and there in turn may be a lack of standardized, evidence-based resources that health care providers will be confident enough in to start prescribing routinely to patients. Furthermore, adherence and compliance issues are existing challenges. Will telerehabilitation self-management apps and educational websites be able to engage patients consistently enough and in a personalized manner in order to foster sustainable practice?

Digital therapies have already shown to be effective for outcomes associated with some of the most common, noncommunicable, high-morbidity disease states in the Western world, including diabetes type 2, hypertension, and insomnia. In a recent, large-scale longitudinal cohort study by Baily et al.[46], 10, 264 adult participants with chronic knee and back pain used a 12-week digital care mobile app program for pain education, sensor-guided exercise therapy, and behavioral health support with one-on-one remote health coaching. Participants experienced a 68.45% improvement in visual analogue scale (VAS) pain between baseline and 12 weeks, and although 78.6% of completers achieved minimally important changes in pain, the level of engagement correlated with improvement in pain, and secondary depression and anxiety scores decreased by 57.9% and

58.3%, respectively. Furthermore, work productivity increased by 61.5%. This bodes well for the applicability and feasibility of further pain app development for self-management strategies, including self-monitoring and relaxation therapies.

Virtual Reality in Pain Management

In the past few decades, VR technology has emerged from science fiction to become a multibillion-dollar industry with promising applications in entertainment, business, and medicine. VR is most commonly composed of a simulated 3D image or environment, visualized by equipment such as a head-mounted display, sometimes with a screen for each eye to create the perception of depth of field. The environment can be interacted with by using electronic equipment such as gloves or a handheld controller or joystick with or without additional motion sensors. Other forms of VR may include a camera capturing the user and using software to integrate them into a virtually rendered environment displayed on a screen where they can see themselves in a simulated environment and, by tracking their movements, they may interact with rendered objects onscreen. The underlying technology behind VR hardware has been a perpetually limiting factor in the realism and fidelity of the simulated environments. Recent advances, however, have led to an exponential growth in the adaption of the technology within the gaming entertainment industry over the last several years.[47] In the future, the user interface and experience may be achieved directly via neural implants. Many major technology companies, including Apple, Facebook, Google, Nintendo, and Sony, are actively innovating in this rapidly growing sector of the entertainment industry.

The promise of VR has long been recognized by the medical community as a potential means to improve patient experience and outcomes. By the year 2000, VR was found to reduce pain scores for burn patients during physical therapy (PT) and was hypothesized to serve as an effective distraction from pain.[48] For example, David Patterson and Hunter Hoffman's "Snow World" VR program (Fig. 13.2) has been shown to reduce the acute pain in pediatric burn victims by 35%

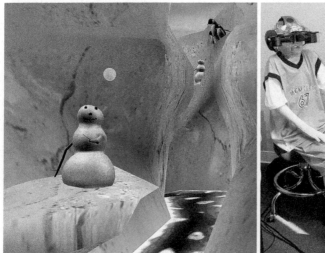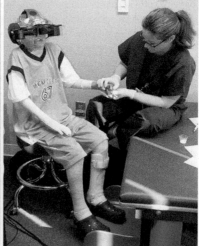

Fig. 13.2 SnowWorld image by Ari Hollander and Howard Rose. Right photo shows a child with a severe burn using VR pain distraction during physical therapy skin stretching range of motion exercises at Shriners Hospitals for Children Galveston TX. Left photo shows SnowWorld, the first VR world designed for pain reduction. (With permission from Hunter Hoffman, Director of the Virtual Reality Research Center at the Human Photonics Lab, University of Washington, Seattle, WA, www.vrpain.com).

to 50%.[49] There is a growing body of evidence supporting the use of VR as an adjunct therapy for reducing acute pain in pediatric and adult patients during medical procedures and in the inpatient setting.[50-54] There may also be a role for VR in patients with chronic pain. Studies with fibromyalgia and complex regional pain syndrome patients have shown reduction in pain scores.[55-57] Studies investigating chronic musculoskeletal pain, such as assessing and improving reduced neck range of motion in chronic neck pain, and pain relief through distraction in the chronic pain population, are promising.[58-61]

Unfortunately, the existing evidence base for the use of VR in the chronic pain population is limited by small sample size, lack of comparison to a non-VR group, or conduction in experimental or clinical settings rather than as a form of telerehabilitation. As the understanding of the effects of VR on pain perception have advanced, it has been suggested that it may serve as more than a distraction from pain and produce neurophysiological changes related to conditioning and exposure therapies, with potential for longer lasting efficacy in chronic pain control.[62] There is also emerging evidence of efficacy for home-based VR programs teaching methods of behavioral medicine self-management skills and techniques for chronic pain patients with low back pain and fibromyalgia.[63] Unfortunately a lack of high-quality long-term studies leaves the question of what lasting or durable effect VR therapy has on chronic pain unanswered.

More large, high-quality studies would help to clarify the efficacy for VR as a viable modality for chronic pain management. Not all patients are able to tolerate VR interventions, especially head-mounted displays, with nausea and motion sickness as commonly cited adverse effects that may limit exposure time or prevent use of this intervention for some individuals. Further investigation into the cost-effectiveness and practical feasibility of equipping patients with VR capable technology at home would help clarify if the potential of VR can translate into meaningful adoption in clinical practice. Currently, VR is an emerging, rapidly improving technology with intriguing potential as a nonpharmacological modality for management of chronic pain.

Addiction Medicine/Opioid Weaning

One of the most patent benefits of telemedicine is its ability to reach more rural or remote patients who are in need of medical care. This is most pertinent for the opioid use disorder population trying to access MAT therapy. There have been several retrospective reviews of MAT therapy delivered through telemedicine, which show not only feasibility but also good retention in treatment.

For example, there is a 2015 retrospective review of 177 patients enrolled in a telemedicine buprenorphine program, which provided treatment to patients at a drug treatment center in rural Maryland. Chart reviews to examine retention in treatment and rates of continued opioid use revealed 98% retention at 1 week, 91% at 1 month, 73% at 2 months, and 57% at 3 months. Of patients still engaged in treatment at 3 months, 86% had opioid-negative urine toxicology. This program showed that telemedicine delivery of buprenorphine for remote patients is feasible and a potential tool to expand MAT therapy.[64] Another retrospective review of medical records of 100 patients participating in telepsychiatry versus in-person group-based outpatient buprenorphine MAT programs showed no significant difference in terms of additional substance use, time to 30 days ($P = 0.09$) and 90 days of abstinence ($P = 0.22$), or retention rates at 90 and 365 days ($P = 0.99$).[65]

In a recent small Australian chronic pain pilot study (n=20) a "Pain ROADMAP" *(Rediscover Occupation Achieve & Develop Through a Monitoring App for Pain)* mobile phone app and an MD-accessible internet portal provided patient self-monitoring information such as activity data (collected via an activity tracker watch-like device), pain intensity, opioid intake, and daily participation data in the form of a diary. Five of seven patients taking as-needed opioids for chronic pain were able to stop taking opioids completely, and, on average, patients decreased their oral morphine equivalent daily dose (MEDD) by 20% during the study period. Consumer feedback was excellent, with all participants indicating satisfaction.[66]

There are growing web-based programs and trainings for providers and patients, including an online CBT program for substance abuse, "CBT4CBT.com," which offers evidence-based information and support for providers as well as patients.

Special Considerations

There are cons as well as pros to telemedicine pain care delivery, which should also be reviewed. The practice of pain care clearly cannot only take the form of virtual "talk therapy" or pain education. The innate value of a comprehensive, hands-on physical examination cannot be understated. As pain management physicians, physical therapists, and other hands-on providers all know, the most clinically significant soft tissue musculoskeletal pathologies are picked up best not by advanced imaging, but by physical contact with patients—observing the surface anatomy, assessing true joint ranges and neurological deficits, and palpating pain regions. More than anything, the connection we make from human face-to-face encounters—from the first eye contact with another individual, to the observation of subtle body cues such as pain behaviors and expressions, to the essential benefits of human touch—is incomparable in many ways. As a pain management provider who has had to transition rapidly between in-person visits to virtual visits during the COVID-19 crisis, the inherent obstacles and difficulties that arise from the less tech-savvy, the poor audiovisual connections, the mutual lack of telehealth visit preparation, and the often slow and nonideal elements of screen communication are felt in every visit.

For most internet and app-based pain programs, chronic pain patients and other stakeholders are rarely involved in the early development process of eHealth interventions (Fig. 13.3).[67] There is a lack of guidance from health care providers and intended users in their development, which results in a large divide between the commercial and scientific interests in eHealth and telemedicine, with product development often based on demand for technological innovations rather than evidence-based knowledge and/or user needs. There is a real need to study how to translate existing face-to-face psychological and integrative interventions into electronic formats, while focusing on the real needs of patients with pain.[68] According to a preliminary qualitative study of chronic pain patients interviewed about eHealth attitudes and needs, patients' needs could be summarized into three components: (1) the need for reliable knowledge about pain and pain management; (2) support in finding lifestyle balance, physically and mentally, through increased

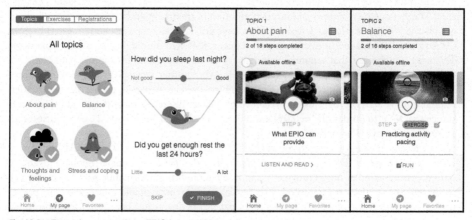

Fig. 13.3   Example screens from EPIO intervention application.

awareness and tracking of factors such as sleep, mood, physical activity, and pain; and (3) social support, including peer support and advice on how to communicate with others, such as family, friends, and health care providers.[69] There is more work to be done in telemedicine to show that these needs can be reliably met.

Another serious challenge of telemedicine for pain management, particularly with the unguided internet-based interventions for pain, is low adherence and high attrition rates.[70, 71] There may be low uptake and adherence depending upon patients' acceptance of internet and mobile-based interventions, anxiety concerning data security, discomfort with use of these interventions and psychological interventions in general, and social influence by friends, family, and health professionals, as well as a lack of trust in the effectiveness.[72] The problem of adherence may be further compounded by the inherent difficulties faced by chronic pain populations, such as limited health care information retention and poor ability to concentrate.[73] To overcome this major barrier, it is important that telemedicine interventions, perhaps, be guided by the actual providers involved in patient care, with a promise for long-term follow-up of ideas and practices promoted by these interventions. It has been shown by previous work that unguided or recorded telemedicine interventions are much less successful that those that involve active engagement and immediate feedback with providers.

For eHealth interventions and processes to be successful, a focus on the entire person (i.e., a holistic view), including context, social supports, and intervention setting, is necessary.[74] For development of pain apps that are user-friendly and pertinent, there should clearly be input from all stakeholders. If a more integrative, interdisciplinary process is used in software and content development of pain interventions, perhaps more user-friendly, meaningful interventions will be developed for patients living with chronic pain.

To try to meet some of these telemedicine shortcomings, researchers of one particular pain app, "EPIO" (named after the Greek goddess for soothing pain, *Epio*), developed a user-centered design approach by obtaining feedback from a broad range of stakeholders, including patients, their spouses, health care providers, eHealth experts, researchers, editors, and IT software developers.[68] The result was a comprehensive pain app, still under research, including nine modules on relevant pain education topics, such as CBT, ACT, balanced lifestyle and stress management, pacing, coping, improving social networks/communication, and others.

Other than the obvious fact that there is a definite learning curve for telerehabilitation and eHealth adaptation and adherence, there is also the deeper, more insidious problem of socioeconomic inequities faced by the populations who have limited access to telehealth. According to one study by Dr. Roberts and Dr. Ateev, 41% of nationwide Medicare patients do not have an internet-capable computer or smartphone at home.[75] It was also found that elderly, Black and Latinx patients, those of lower income, enrolled in Medicaid, or with a disability were less likely to have access to the internet. These are the very same patients who, along with suffering from other health problems, are perhaps most vulnerable to chronic, disabling pain conditions, yet they have the least access to good health care in general.

Recommendations

The field of telerehabilitation for pain management is on the rise. More research is needed in terms of how telerehabilitation can serve various pain populations, including developing further user-friendly, effective pain management apps, VR programs, and other technology-assisted treatments in the management of chronic pain. There is great potential for mobile health app and internet-based program technology to allow providers evidence-based pain intake and outcome measures and access to available online resources for CBT, ACT, and other pain psychology therapies. Self-monitoring apps and pain trackers, stress management and mindfulness meditation programs, pain psychology programs, opioid weaning programs, and even interdisciplinary pain programs may be delivered more readily via telerehabilitation. Already established pain programs, such as Beth Darnall's "Empowered Relief," or Butler and Moseley's "Explain Pain," may be delivered virtually. Chronic pain patients, isolated by their conditions and withdrawn from normal engagement in society and physical activity (the latter a necessary part of recovery), may have more opportunities with telerehabilitation to learn and sustain self-management pain coping skills and healthier behaviors.

Further research is needed in terms of what exact programs and apps can be implemented successfully via telerehabilitation. We still need to determine the most appropriate patient selection: who may adapt best to telerehabilitation applications, and how. Patient adherence and dropout is a pertinent issue in this population, as it is even for in-person multidisciplinary and pain psychology programs, but with guided internet-based interventions that include real-time feedback and meaningful, long-term patient-provider connections, compliance and adherence may be improved. We still do not even completely know exactly what form of pain psychology works best, for whom, and in what format—one-on-one with a pain psychologist, multidisciplinary/interdisciplinary programs, or mobile apps and internet-based pain programs. A recent Delphi panel of pain experts sought to create a consensus statement about which pain psychological methods are most helpful and effective. According to this study, the three necessary components include: pain education, including education about the role of thoughts in pain; activity engagement, including pacing, goal setting and graded exposure; and cognitive approaches.[76] Whether the latter included CBT, a third wave strategy, such as ACT or mindfulness based stress reduction (MBSR), or another psychological therapy approach was not specified. Relaxation training and relapse prevention were also deemed necessary components. All of these components, however, can be delivered via telerehabilitation.

There is still much to be learned in terms of patient selection and outcomes of virtual interdisciplinary pain programs. There is growing consensus that program participation and app usage is feasible, but patient selection (including selection bias), effect sizes, and long-term outcomes are variable. In a metaanalysis of research quality of telemedicine trials in pain management, only 9 studies were included in a search of 155 publications on this topic. Most were not RCTs, pain conditions were too heterogeneous to make an overall conclusion, and outcomes were primarily based on subjective criteria such as reduction of pain intensity. More trials need to be included to involve functional outcomes, including health care utilization reduction and cost-effectiveness in a time of "pay-for-performance" reimbursement and cost containment pressures.

Conclusion

It has long been understood that chronic pain and suffering is a complex, long-term, biopsychosocial condition that requires mental and behavioral health management as much as, if not more than, conventional physical treatments. In our current model of health care specialization, we are often accustomed to breaking down human pathology into the minutia of tissue pathology, with the provider's lens focused on the particular body part in which they have chosen to specialize—scientifically explaining, targeting, and treating each target with the reliable tools of pharmacology, procedures, or surgery. Conventional pain care typically involves specialty visits, advanced imaging and interpretation, PT referrals, pharmacological treatments, procedures, and sometimes surgery for the indicated, refractory cases. But for many living with chronic pain, these treatments are still not enough. Despite ever complex diagnostic capability in modern medicine, including even the possibility of identification of biomarkers and genes that predispose individuals to chronic pain, this has yet to result in any measurable improvement in the function or quality of life of a chronic pain patient. For decades, the gold standard approach to comprehensive pain care is multimodal, including interdisciplinary programs that can truly integrate behavioral-psychological approaches, such as patient engagement in healthy activity, mindfulness, and cognitive reappraisal.

Telerehabilitation-delivered pain psychology and self-management programs for chronic pain, which are cost-effective compared to multiple specialty visits and physical interventions, may be more beneficial for this population than interventional procedures and surgery. For one, there is the clear potential to reach a wider patient population than in-person alternatives. Pain management and behavioral health providers can now connect with chronic pain patients in remote regions. Mobility-impaired, resource scarce, or acutely ill patients in pain have serious barriers to travel, which limit access to pain management providers and outpatient therapists, let alone multidisciplinary pain care centers. With internet connections linked directly to personal mobile devices, consultations and individual and group therapies may be delivered on a regular, consistent basis, and at the patient's own pace. Another advantage is that providers can see how people potentially behave and perform in real time, in their actual home environments. Pain app technology, and even more direct treatment applications such as VR, comprise a growing industry for development.

It is a new age for telemedicine, which has seen exponential expansion attributable to COVID-19 pressures to expand coverage of these services, as well as ongoing development worldwide from various stakeholders in these technologies. As different and difficult as telemedicine is compared to what most pre-COVID-19 pain practices were about (which, in my own outpatient pain physiatry practice, is still predominantly about human touch and physical procedures), by adapting and learning to use the expanding technology and pain care tools and delivery systems supported by telemedicine, this may become an ever more utilized and integrated, permanent part of our pain care delivery model.

CASE STUDY

Ms. Smith is a 52-year-old female with a past medical history of anxiety, depression, obesity, diabetes mellitus type 2, and hypertension. She has suffered from chronic back pain for over a decade, which has been managed by her primary care physician with trials of acetaminophen, NSAIDs, muscle relaxants, and a brief course of oxycodone for a severe flare-up 1 year ago. She has had difficulty engaging with physical therapy due to poor follow-up. She has also struggled to maintain a home exercise routine over the past several years. Her symptoms have progressed over the past year and her current medication regimen is becoming progressively ineffective. One month ago, a lumbar spine magnetic resonance imaging (MRI) showed evidence of moderate-to-severe degenerative disc disease and zygapophyseal arthropathy and severe stenosis at the L4-L5 and L5-S1 levels. Her PCP has referred her to the pain medicine clinic, and her first appointment is subsequently scheduled as a telerehabilitation visit.

QUESTION

What special considerations might be important for a successful encounter with a new patient using audio-video technology?

ANSWER

Prior to the patient encounter (ideally, at the time of booking the appointment), ensure that your clinical staff has confirmed that your patient has the appropriate technology and internet connection in their home to support a virtual medicine visit. The patient should have a smartphone/tablet or home PC/laptop with a webcam and microphone that will be available to them and an internet connection with sufficient bandwidth to support a videoconference call.

The health care provider should consider their own environment before starting the virtual appointment. Some providers mix in-person clinical encounters with virtual ones in their schedule. Under these circumstances there should be adequate technology, such as a webcam with microphone connected to their workstation computer to support videoconferencing technology. The environment should be appropriately quiet and private to support a confidential patient encounter. This may be achieved by hosting the appointment in the provider's private office or in a clinic's patient room.

The videoconferencing platform used should be HIPAA (or internationally equivalent) compliant. The platform should use end-to-end encryption of audio, video, and screen sharing data. Some examples of telerehabilitation platforms that support HIPAA compliant patient encounters may include Zoom and Doximity. Please refer to local rules and regulations when identifying whether any technology platform will meet the local standards for safe and confidential patient encounters.

CASE STUDY —cont'd

QUESTION

At the time of the encounter with Ms. Smith, what strategies may be employed to optimize the space, camera angle, and lighting?

ANSWER

During the initial history taking, we recommend the patient find a space where they can position the camera in a stable place. Optimizing the visit during the physical examination can be more challenging. We can expect that the space available for each patient will be variable, but when possible, having enough space for a full-body view is ideal.

Variable factors include the size of the patient's available space, their height, functional status, background noise, and lighting. Placing the camera on the floor tilted upward and having the patient position themselves several feet away (sometimes up to 8–9 feet away) usually results in a full view of the patient's body. If the patient is using a smartphone or tablet, they can try to tilt the device between the floor and wall with the camera facing outward. If they are using a laptop, they can tilt the monitor beyond 90 degrees to achieve a similar effect. Other options include propping the device on a chair, stepping stool, table, or even bed.

If natural lighting is insufficient or unavailable, lamps or other lighting behind the camera is best, and avoid lighting behind the patient if possible.

While taking Ms. Smith's history, it becomes clear that her poor compliance with PT follow-up is due to a lack of easy access to therapists. She lives in a rural area and the nearest PT office is over a 45-minute drive away. Furthermore, she was afraid of exercising because she was worried the movements would "make my pain worse and cause more damage." She looked up some of the terminology in her MRI report on the internet and was afraid it meant she was going to have to undergo spine surgery. Furthermore, she is the primary caretaker for her husband, who has been disabled and unable to work for several years. She stated that it would be extremely challenging to care for her husband and recover from major surgery. She was equally hesitant to try any invasive injections. She expressed concern that she would never return to her previous level of activity and that eventually she may not be able to sufficiently care for her husband.

QUESTION

After taking a thorough history of Ms. Smith's pain, what are some expectations for performing an examination?

ANSWER

Due to the nature of telerehabilitation, without the ability to palpate, assess passive range of motion, and complete a comprehensive neurological and musculoskeletal examination, a comprehensive examination of the patient is impossible. The patient should be educated about these limitations. However, much insight can be gained during a telerehabilitation visit. The goal of the examination should be to assess the patient's posture, gait, active range of motion, functional strength, and provocative movements. For example, if a patient is able to walk on their toes for several steps and perform bilateral single leg squats, their lower extremity strength is grossly intact. Clinical judgement should be used to assess how safe the environment is and the level patient's stability and balance, if they are ambulatory, before requesting they perform activities that increase the risk of a fall.

Other elements of the examination can also aid in the refinement of the differential diagnosis. Ask the patient to demonstrate reproducible painful movements, if they are able. Finally, some special tests can be approximated. For example, with Ms. Smith, one might have her sit slumped over in a chair and ask her to gently bring her leg into extension.

After your virtual examination of Ms. Smith, she asks you what you recommend as next steps to help with her increasingly painful back.

QUESTION

What are some ways to leverage telerehabilitation to provide comprehensive pain management care for Ms. Smith given her limited access to local health care resources?

ANSWER

Ms. Smith would benefit greatly from virtual PT sessions where the therapist could lead and supervise a home exercise plan that would simultaneously increase the probability of her maintaining compliance with follow-up and likely decrease her fear associated with the potential for pain with movement. Additionally the plan could account for her home environment including insight from the layout of the patient's home.

CASE STUDY —cont'd

Ms. Smith might also benefit from telerehabilitation-based interdisciplinary group sessions where groups of patients can have virtual sessions with pain physicians, psychologists, behavioral health experts, and/or physical therapists who can provide education and lead sessions focused on CBT, ACT, mindfulness meditation, and/or stress management strategies. Offering resources to attend virtual support group sessions may also provide benefit as Ms. Smith is both suffering from chronic pain and serves as the primary caregiver for a loved one.

After providing education about her pain syndrome and how to optimize her pain management strategies by discussing the options available to her virtually, Ms. Smith is eager to try virtual sessions with a PT and to attend some virtual group meetings. You agree to follow up in 3 months to track her progress and address the next steps pending her clinical course at that time.

QUESTION

What special considerations should be taken into account with documenting a telerehabilitation encounter?

ANSWER

Documentation should include reference to the virtual nature of the encounter. We recommend documenting if the encounter was performed with audio only or audiovisual technology including the technology platform (e.g., Zoom), if applicable. We recommend documenting that consent was given by the patient to use telerehabilitation technology for the encounter. We also recommend documenting where the patient was at the time of examination, for example, their home.

For the physical examination, we recommend describing the findings without specifically referencing special test names. For example, in this we would describe Ms. Smith's pain with leg extension while slumped in her chair as follows: "When seated, with curved flexion of the spine, patient endorsed pain radiating from her back down her posterior leg to the level of the knee with left leg extension" in place of "Positive Slump test."

References

1. Institute of Medicine. *Relieving Pain in America: A Blueprint for Transforming Prevention, Care, Education, and Research.* Washington DC: The National Academies Press; 2011.
2. Phillips CJ, Harper C. The economics associated with persistent pain. *Curr Opin Support Pall Care.* 2011;5:127–130.
3. Edwards RR, et al. Pain-related catastrophizing as a risk factor for suicidal ideation in chronic pain. *Pain.* 2006;126:272–279.
4. Mackey S. Future directions for pain management: lessons from the Institute of Medicine Pain Report and the National Pain Strategy. *Hand Clin.* 2016;32(1):91–98.
5. Florence CS, et al. The economic burden of prescriptions opioid overdose, abuse, and dependence in the U.S. *Med Care.* 2016;54(10):901–906.
6. GBD 2016 Disease and Injury Incidence and Prevalence Collaborators. Global, regional, and national incidence, prevalence, and years lived with disability for 328 diseases and injuries for 195 countries, 1990-2016: a systematic analysis for the Global Burden of Disease Study 2016 [published correction appears in Lancet. 2017 Oct 28;390(10106):e38]. *Lancet.* 2017;390(10100):1211–1259. https://doi.org/10.1016/S0140-6736(17)32154-2.
7. Becker WC, Dorflinger L, Edmond SN, et al. Barriers and facilitators to use of non-pharmacological treatments in chronic pain. *BMC Fam Pract.* 2017;18(1):41.
8. Friedly J, Standaert C, Chan L. Epidemiology of spine care: the back pain dilemma. *Phys Med Rehab Clin N Am.* 2010;21(4):659–677. https://doi.org/10.1016/j.pmr.2010.08.002.
9. Gatchel RJ, Okifugi A. Evidence-based scientific data documenting the treatment and cost-effectiveness of comprehensive pain programs for chronic nonmalignant pain. *J Pain.* 2006;7:779–793.
10. Kress HG, Aldington D, Alon E, et al. A holistic approach to chronic pain management that involves all stakeholders: change is needed. *Curr Med Res Opin.* 2015;31(9):1743–1754.
11. Centers for Medicare & Medicaid Services. Medicare Telemedicine Health Care Provider Fact Sheet. Centers for Medicare & Medicaid Services. 2020; cms.gov/newsroom/fact-sheets/medicare-telemedicine-health-care-provider-fact-sheet.

12. Andersson G. *The Internet and CBT: A Clinical Guide*. Florida FL: CRC Press; 2015.

13. Andersson G, Ljótsson B, Weise C. Internet-delivered treatment to promote health. *Curr Opin Psychiatry*. 2011;24(2):168–172.

14. Buhrman M, Gordh T, Andersson G. Internet interventions for chronic pain including headache: a systematic review. *Internet Interv*. 2016;4:17–34.

15. Hedman E, et al. Cognitive behavior therapy via the internet: a systematic review of applications, clinical efficacy and cost-effectiveness. *Expert Rev Pharmacoecon Outcomes Res*. 2012;12(6):745–764.

16. Mehta S, et al. Internet-delivered cognitive behaviour therapy for chronic health conditions: a systematic review and meta-analysis. *J Behav Med*. 2019;42(2):169–187.

17. Thurnheer SE, et al. Benefits of mobile apps in pain management: systematic review. *JMIR Mhealth Uhealth*. 2018;6(10):e11231.

18. Trompetter HR, et al. Internet-based guided self-help intervention for chronic pain based on acceptance and commitment therapy: a randomized controlled trial. *J Behav Med*. 2015;38(1):66–80.

19. Hanna G, et al. Development and patient satisfaction of a new telemedicine service for pain management at Massachusetts General Hospital to the island of Martha's Vineyard. *Pain Med*. 2016;17(9):1658–1663.

20. Eccleston C, et al. Psychological therapies (Internet-delivered) for the management of chronic pain in adults. *Cochrane Database Syst Rev*. 2014;2014(2):CD010152.

21. Rosser BA, Vowles KE, Keogh E, et al. Technologically-assisted behaviour change: a systematic review of studies of novel technologies for the management of chronic illness. *J Telemed Telecare*. 2009;15(7):327–338.

22. Eccleston C, Morley SJ, Williams AC. Psychological approaches to chronic pain management: evidence and challenges. *Br J Anaesth*. 2013;111(1):59–63.

23. Mann EG, et al. Self-management interventions for chronic pain. *Pain Manag*. 2013;3(3):211–222.

24. McCracken LM, Turk DC. Behavioral and cognitive-behavioral treatment for chronic pain: outcome, predictors of outcome, and treatment process. *Spine (Phila Pa 1976)*. 2002;27(22):2564–2573.

25. McCracken LM, Vowles KE. Acceptance and commitment therapy and mindfulness for chronic pain: model, process, and progress. *Am Psychol*. 2014;69(2):178–187.

26. Morley S, Eccleston C, Williams A. Systematic review and meta-analysis of randomized controlled trials of cognitive behaviour therapy and behaviour therapy for chronic pain in adults, excluding headache. *Pain*. 1999;80(1-2):1–13.

27. Maruta T, et al. Status of patients with chronic pain 13 years after treatment in a pain management center. *Pain*. 1998;74(2):199–204.

28. Andersson G. Using the Internet to provide cognitive behaviour therapy. *Behav Res Ther*. 2009; 47(3):175–180.

29. Heapy AA, et al. A systematic review of technology-assisted self-management interventions for chronic pain: looking across treatment modalities. *Clin J Pain*. 2015;31(6):470–492.

30. Heapy AA, et al. Interactive voice response-based self-management for chronic back pain. The COPES noninferiority randomized trial. *JAMA Intern Med*. 2017;177(6):765–773. https://doi.org/10.1001/jamainternmed.2017.0223.

31. Bender JL, et al. Can pain be managed through the Internet? A systematic review of randomized controlled trials. *Pain*. 2011;152:1740–1750.

32. Ruehlman L, et al. A randomized controlled evaluation of an online chronic pain self management program. *Pain*. 2012;153:319–330. https://doi.org/10.1016/j.pain.2011.10.02.

33. Eccleston C, et al. Psychological therapies (internet-delivered) for the management of chronic pain in adults. *Cochrane Database Syst Rev*. 2014;2(2):CD010152.

34. Herbert MS, et al. Telehealth versus in-person acceptance and commitment therapy for chronic pain: a randomized noninferiority trial. *J Pain*. 2017;18(2):200–211.

35. Trompetter HR, et al. Internet-based guided self-help intervention for chronic pain based on Acceptance and Commitment Therapy: a randomized controlled trial. *J Behav Med*. 2015;38(1):66–80.

36. Lin J, et al. An internet-based intervention for chronic pain. *Dtsch Arztebl Int*. 2017;114(41):681–688. https://doi.org/10.3238/arztebl.2017.0681.

37. Baumeister H, et al. The impact of guidance on Internet-based mental health interventions—a systematic review. *Internet Interv*. 2014;1:205–215.

38. Buhrman M, Gordh T, Andersson G. Internet interventions for chronic pain including headache: a systematic review. *Internet Interv*. 2016;4:17–34.

39. Andersson G, et al. Guided Internet-based vs. face-to-face cognitive behavior therapy for psychiatric and somatic disorders: a systematic review and meta-analysis. *World Psychiatry.* 2014;13(3):288–295. https://doi.org/10.1002/wps.20151.

40. Cuijpers P, et al. Is guided self-help as effective as face-to-face psychotherapy for depression and anxiety disorders? A meta-analysis of comparative outcome studies. *Psychol Med.* 2010;40:1943–1957.

41. Slattery B, et al. An evaluation of the effectiveness of the modalities used to deliver electronic health interventions for chronic pain: a systematic review with network meta-analysis. *J Med Internet Res.* 2019;21(7):e11086.

42. Devan H, Farmery D, Peebles L, et al. Evaluation of self-management support functions in apps for people with persistent pain: systematic review. *JMIR Mhealth Uhealth.* 2019;7(2):e13080.

43. CHOIR. https://choir-stanford-edu.treadwell.idm.oclc.org/; Accessed September 2020.

44. Martorella G, et al. Tailored web-based interventions for pain: systematic review and meta-analysis. *JIMR.* 2017;19:e385.

45. Viladarga R, et al. Theoretical grounds of Pain Tracker Self Manager: an Acceptance and Commitment Therapy digital intervention for patients with chronic pain. *J Contextual Behav Sci.* 2020;15:172–180.

46. Bailey J, et al. Digital care for chronic musculoskeletal pain: 10,000 participant longitudinal cohort study. *J Med Internet Research.* 2020;22(5):e18250. https://doi.org/10.2196/18250.

47. Rogers S. The Year Virtual Reality Gets Real. *Forbes Magazine.* 2019. www.forbes.com/sites/solrogers/2019/06/21/2019-the-year-virtual-reality-gets-real/#35021ba76ba9.

48. Hoffman HG, Patterson DR, Carrougher GJ. Use of virtual reality for adjunctive treatment of adult burn pain during physical therapy: a controlled study. *Clin J Pain.* 2000;16(3):244–250.

49. Hoffman HG, et al. Virtual reality as an adjunctive non-pharmacologic analgesic for acute burn pain during medical procedures. *Ann Behav Med.* 2011;41(2):183–191.

50. Gold JI, Kim SH, Kant AJ, et al. Effectiveness of virtual reality for pediatric pain distraction during IV placement. *Cyberpsychol Behav.* 2006;9(2):207–212.

51. Atzori B, Grotto RL, Giugni A, et al. Virtual reality analgesia for pediatric dental patients. *Front Psychol.* 2018;9:2265.

52. Gold JI, Mahrer NE. Is virtual reality ready for prime time in the medical space? A randomized control trial of pediatric virtual reality for acute procedural pain management. *J Pediatr Psychol.* 2018;43(3):266–275.

53. Haisley KR, Straw OJ, Müller DT, et al. Feasibility of implementing a virtual reality program as an adjuvant tool for peri-operative pain control; results of a randomized controlled trial in minimally invasive foregut surgery. *Complement Ther Med.* 2020;49:102356.

54. Dascal J, Reid M, IsHak WW, et al. Virtual reality and medical inpatients: a systematic review of randomized, controlled trials. *Innov Clin Neurosci.* 2017;14(1-2):14–21.

55. Botella C, Garcia-Palacios A, Vizcaíno Y, et al. Virtual reality in the treatment of fibromyalgia: a pilot study. *Cyberpsychol Behav Soc Netw.* 2013;16(3):215–223.

56. Garcia-Palacios S, Herrero R, Vizcaíno Y, et al. Integrating virtual reality with activity management for the treatment of fibromyalgia: acceptability and preliminary efficacy. *Clin J Pain.* 2015;31(6):564–572.

57. Sato K, Fukumori S, Matsusaki T, et al. Nonimmersive virtual reality mirror visual feedback therapy and its application for the treatment of complex regional pain syndrome: an open-label pilot study. *Pain Med.* 2010;11(4):622–629.

58. Sarig-Bahat H, Weiss PL, Laufer Y. Neck pain assessment in a virtual environment. *Spine (Phila Pa 1976).* 2010;35(4):E105–E112.

59. Harvie DS, Broecker M, Smith RT, et al. Bogus visual feedback alters onset of movement-evoked pain in people with neck pain. *Psychol Sci.* 2015;26(4):385–392.

60. Wiederhold BK, Gao K, Sulea C, et al. Virtual reality as a distraction technique in chronic pain patients. *Cyberpsychol Behav Soc Netw.* 2014;17(6):346–352.

61. Jones T, Moore T, Choo J. The impact of virtual reality on chronic pain. *PLoS One.* 2016;11(12):e0167523.

62. Gupta A, Scott K, Dukewich M. Innovative technology using virtual reality in the treatment of pain: does it reduce pain via distraction, or is there more to it? *Pain Med.* 2018;19(1):151–159.

63. Darnall BD, Krishnamurthy P, Tsuei J, et al. Self-administered skills-based virtual reality intervention for chronic pain: randomized controlled pilot study. *JMIR Form Res.* 2020;4(7):e17293.

64. Weintraub E, Greenblatt AD, Chang J, et al. Expanding access to buprenorphine treatment in rural areas with the use of telemedicine. *Am J Addict*. 2018;27(8):612–617. https://doi.org/10.1111/ajad.12805. Epub 2018 Sep 28.
65. Zheng W, et al. Treatment outcome comparison between telepsychiatry and face-to-face buprenorphine medication-assisted treatment for opioid use disorder: a 2-year retrospective data analysis. *J Addict Med*. 2017;11(2):138–144.
66. Ireland D, Andrews N. Pain ROADMAP: a mobile platform to support activity pacing for chronic pain. *Stud Health Technol Inform*. 2019;266:89–94.
67. Cranen K, et al. Toward patient-centered telerehabilitation design: understanding chronic pain patients' preferences for web-based exercise telerehabilitation using a discrete choice experiment. *J Med Internet Res*. 2017;19(1):e26.
68. Solem L, et al. A user-centered approach to an evidence-based electronic health pain management intervention for people with chronic pain: design and development of EPIO. *J Med Internet Res*. 2020;22(1):e15889.
69. Solem L, et al. Patients' needs and requirements for eHealth pain management interventions: qualitative study. *J Med Internet Res*. 2019;21(4):e13205.
70. Kelders SM, Kok RN, Ossebaard HC, et al. Persuasive system design does matter: a systematic review of adherence to web-based interventions. *J Med Internet Res*. 2012;14(6):e152.
71. Ludden GD, van Rompay TJ, Kelders SM, et al. How to increase reach and adherence of web-based interventions: a design research viewpoint. *J Med Internet Res*. 2015;17(7):e172.
72. Lin J, et al. A web-based acceptance-facilitating intervention for identifying patients' acceptance, uptake, and adherence of internet- and mobile-based pain interventions: randomized controlled trial. *J Med Internet Res*. 2018;20(8):e244.
73. Friis K, Lasgaard M, Osborne RH, et al. Gaps in understanding health and engagement with healthcare providers across common long-term conditions: a population survey of health literacy in 29,473 Danish citizens. *BMJ Open*. 2016;6(1):e009627.
74. Van Gemert-Pijnen JE, et al. A holistic framework to improve the uptake and impact of eHealth technologies. *J Med Internet Res*. 2011;13(4):e111.
75. Roberts ET, Mehrotra A. Assessment of disparities in digital access among Medicare beneficiaries and implications for telemedicine. *JAMA Intern Med*. 2020;180(10):1386–1389. https://doi.org/10.1001/jamainternmed.2020.2666.
76. Sharpe L, Jones E, Ashton-James CE, et al. Necessary components of psychological treatment in pain management programs: a Delphi study. *Eur J Pain*. 2020;24(6):1160–1168.

CHAPTER 14

Telerehabilitation for Musculoskeletal Injuries

Nicole B. Katz ■ Adam S. Tenforde

Introduction

The musculoskeletal (MSK) system, composed of the bones, muscles, tendons, and ligaments in the body, provides structural support and enables movement. An injury to this intricate system may result in decreased strength, immobility, and/or pain. Therefore when a patient presents with an MSK injury, performing a thorough physical examination and prescribing therapeutic exercises are pillars of clinical care.

As the implementation of telemedicine has increased, so has telerehabilitation. Through information and communication technologies, the conventional practices of patient interviews, consultations, and physical therapy (PT) can be provided remotely.[1,2] Since the 1990s, the use of different modalities to provide synchronous (real-time communication) and asynchronous (communication with a time lag) telerehabilitation has been explored. Initially implemented as a means for providing care to patients unable to attend in-person appointments due to access or resource limitations, the need for remote care increased drastically in the wake of the COVID-19 global pandemic. This development highlighted the lack of widespread understanding of how to implement telemedicine—a vulnerability within the health care system. For these reasons, it is essential to understand the previously assessed methodologies for providing telerehabilitation for MSK injuries, as well as the current suggestions for implementation, in order to provide optimal MSK care.

Telerehabilitation in Treating MSK Conditions

Telerehabilitation may be most applicable to the diagnosis of MSK injuries that do not require extensive physical examination for diagnosis, or for management of previously diagnosed conditions.[3] Studies reported that 36% to 67% of diagnoses were in agreement, and 73% to 89% were similar to the diagnoses made in-person when utilizing synchronous telerehabilitation, with the lower range reported for telerehabilitation guiding a remote practitioner, and the upper range representing telerehabilitation provided to patients in their own homes.[4,5] Moreover the pain generator identified was found to be in agreement in 94% of cases for patients with knee pain who participated in telerehabilitation from home compared with those who received traditional in-person assessments.[4] A systematic review and metaanalysis on synchronous telerehabilitation for MSK conditions by Cottrell et al.[6] concluded that when compared with conventional care, telerehabilitation may yield superior outcomes for improvement on physical function, reduced disability, and similar improvement of pain. Specifically, there is strong evidence in support of the diagnosis and management of conditions including osteoarthritis (OA) of the hand, knee, and hip[7–14] as well as pathologies of the shoulder[15,16] and spine[13,15,17] through telerehabilitation provided to patients at home[8–11,14–17] and remote facilities.[7,12,13]

OA is the leading cause of disability in the United States, and it is estimated that four million people in the United States have symptomatic knee OA.[18, 19] Management of OA is largely focused on optimizing patients' quality of life,[20] and telerehabilitation designed for this pathology has been shown to result in a greater improvement in quality of life compared with clinic-based treatment.[9] Patient education on lifestyle factors including regular exercise, weight loss, and the role of interventions can be easily communicated through the use of telehealth. Moreover, telerehabilitation programs are as effective as office-based PT in improving the function of patients with knee OA.[14] In fact, a review on telerehabilitation for OA by Pietrak et al.[21] indicated that, besides patients reporting high satisfaction and perceived improved communication with their health care professionals both virtually and in person, telerehabilitation for OA successfully improved health distress, activity limitation, self-reported global health, fatigue, and pain in report of patient numbers that ranged from 121 to 855.[10–12, 21–23]

Shoulder pain (e.g., rotator cuff injuries) has also been shown to improve through virtual care, with outcomes similar to conventional in-person care (sample sizes of patient populations n = 11–145).[13, 15, 16] For patients with rotator cuff injuries, telerehabilitation allowed for significantly decreased pain and improved movement, function, and muscular strength. Equally important to the clinical improvement is the perception of the treatment modality, and in a study conducted by Macías-Hernández et al.,[16] all participating patients stated that they would recommend this platform to others. Moreover, for patients with nonspecific shoulder or spine pain, the incorporation of telerehabilitation with virtually provided myofeedback-based treatment resulted in decreased pain intensity and disability after 4 weeks, and remained after 3 months.[15]

Similar to OA, low back pain and neck pain are highly prevalent and are among the leading contributors to years lived with disability in the United States.[24] Nonspecific neck and low back pain have also been shown to improve through the use of telerehabilitation. Previous studies assessing telerehabilitation conducted by physical therapists and orthopedic surgeons to a patient's home or general health clinic, respectively, have illustrated outcomes at least comparable to conventional in-person care.[13, 15, 17] A study by Iles et al.[17] reported that patients with nonchronic low back pain who received telerehabilitation in addition to in-person care improved significantly more than those receiving in-person care alone when assessing activity and recovery expectation.

Without adequate management, acute MSK injuries may become chronic conditions. Globally, chronic MSK injuries affect over 25% of the population, are the leading cause of pain and disability, and account for 21.3% of morbidity.[25] Similar to acute MSK conditions, the evaluation of telerehabilitation for chronic MSK pain revealed promising results.[26, 27] For patients with chronic MSK pain, the addition of telerehabilitation appointments to a prescribed home exercise program reduced chronic neck pain symptoms and disability at 6 months, and increased compliance with their home exercise program.[27] Telecare may also play an important role in the pharmaceutical management of chronic MSK pain. Kroenke et al.[26] illustrated that the addition of automated symptom monitoring and as-needed telephone calls with a pain-specialist nurse resulted in improved pain scores by 12 months for patients with chronic MSK pain. As evidenced by the literature, appropriate implementation of telerehabilitation may bring benefits to patients otherwise inaccessible.

Practice

In practice, rehabilitation for MSK injuries often requires a collaborative approach that involves a variety of specialized therapists and health care professionals. Beyond enabling clinical care, telerehabilitation has the benefit of supporting multidisciplinary care and communication amongst care team members.[28] This aspect of telerehabilitation is evidenced through a study by Careau et al.[29] that found videoconferences dedicated to interprofessional care plan development have a mean productivity level of 96% with the most common advantage noted being good eye-contact.

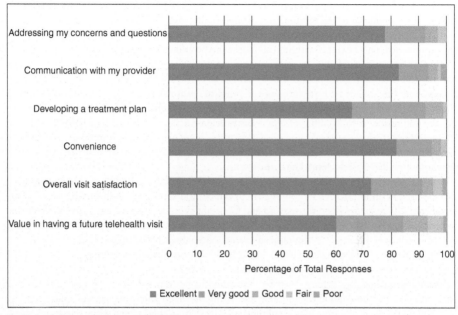

Fig. 14.1 Patient-centered outcomes following completion of telemedicine visit.

CLINICAL ROLE IN OUTPATIENT MSK CARE

For outpatient care, telemedicine for MSK injuries may be used for initial evaluation, to monitor response to treatment, or a combination of both. The initial outpatient MSK encounter tradition-ally begins with a visit to evaluate the injury and continues with follow-up appointments to assess treatment efficacy and recovery progress. Telemedicine may be used as an alternative to any of these interactions. Synchronous teleconferencing is the form of telerehabilitation that most resembles the traditional clinic interaction, and a study evaluating this type of telerehabilitation for an outpatient PM&R-based MSK and Sports Medicine clinic found that overall, 91.6% to 95.0% patients (in the various measures, (Fig. 14.1[3]) and 92% of physicians rated their experiences as "excellent" or "very good". Synchronous videoconferencing has been shown to be a valid alternative to traditional outpatient MSK care,[5, 13, 30] but where it is best incorporated may vary by MSK condition.

As an accurate diagnosis is essential for proper care and often requires an extensive physical examination, the initial evaluation should be conducted in person if possible. Additionally, patients and physicians prefer this initial in-person appointment to aid in establishing a strong physician-patient relationship.[3] However, for patients in remote areas with limited access to specialized MSK care or with conditions requiring less extensive physical examinations for diagnosis, telemedicine may be a valid alternative to the initial consultation and used to determine if an in-person appoint-ment is needed.[31,32] Once a diagnosis has been made, telerehabilitation may also be incorporated into conventional care with proven benefit of decreasing need for in-person visits.[33, 34]

CLINICAL EVALUATION

When evaluating a patient remotely, the physical examination relies on the clear transmission of visual, audio, and/or haptic data (data obtained from patient contact with technology).[28] To enable effective communication, a patient participating in video-based telerehabilitation should be instructed to be in a well-lit, private area with room to perform full-body movements and dressed in a manner conducive to the examination of their injury (e.g., for a knee injury, shorts should be worn and socks and shoes removed). Patients should also be told ahead of their appointments that the camera used must be stable without being held and positioned so that the physician can view the body part being evaluated.[35] In synchronous telemedicine, the physician may demonstrate the physical examination maneuver for the patient to perform on himself or herself, or may have others assist the patient with performing the physical examination testing.[36] In accordance with the standards of in-person medicine, a clear understanding of which examinations should be performed and how best to document them is key in telemedicine (Tables 14.1 and 14.2).[36]

In addition to specific physical examination tests, range of motion is commonly assessed and can be accomplished using telemedicine. Verduzco-Gutierrez et al.[36] suggested that while using synchronous video-based telemedicine, the practitioner can guide the patient through movements to observe active range of motion (Table 14.1).[36] Good et al.[37] illustrated that videoconferencing may be used as an alternative to goniometry in the clinical setting through finding no clinically significant difference between the Oxford and Constant shoulder scores conducted on Skype and in person. However, there are also internet-based and teleconference-based goniometers available, if the practitioner prefers.[38-42] The clinical evaluation enabled by telerehabilitation can be used to determine if and what radiological imaging is needed for further assessment, as well as what medications, therapies, and/or procedures should be prescribed.[3]

Radiological imaging studies must be performed in person, but the review of these studies with patients may be conducted remotely and is important in achieving patient understanding and empowerment. Physicians may accomplish this by sharing their screen while teleconferencing or by utilizing a document camera to provide patients their own copy.[31, 36] Most video teleconferencing systems have a feature that allows a participant to share their screen, which results in both parties seeing whatever is visible on the sharer's computer monitor. This feature allows for providing a detailed discussion of relevance of imaging results, laboratory tests, and other aspects of the physical examination that allow for developing a clinical impression and treatment plan. Notably, Vuolio et al.[13] found no significant differences in the implementation of the management plans between patients who were teleconferencing versus attending in-person appointments for MSK complaints, consistent with earlier reports suggesting adaptation of telemedicine can be accomplished with high patient and provider satisfaction.[3, 43]

CLINICAL MANAGEMENT

Clinical care extends beyond making a diagnosis or prescribing a treatment and largely involves following the patient's progress and adjusting the treatment protocol accordingly. Notably, practitioners must also recognize the limitations of providing care remotely and be prepared to advise patients seek traditional or emergent medical care when found to have alarming symptoms. Whereas a patient suffering from foot pain consistent with the illness script of plantar fasciitis would be suitable for continued telerehabilitation, a patient noting saddle anesthesia and fecal incontinence suggestive of cauda equina syndrome should be advised to seek immediate care at the nearest emergency department if the practitioner cannot see them in clinic immediately. Informing patients at the initial visit that an in-person assessment may be needed based on progression and symptomology would prepare patients for this possibility and likely strengthen the patient-practitioner relationship.

Though follow-up appointments may include the aforementioned clinical telecare techniques for evaluation, additional routes for assessing and addressing progress are available with this virtual medium. Practitioners may opt for patients to send recorded videos of certain movements for their detailed review.[44] Alternatively, internet-based guides that include relevant assessment and treatment items as well as education and goals on which to focus may be utilized.[22] For example,

TABLE 14.1 ■ **A System-Based Approach to Performing and Documenting a Physical Examination via Telemedicine.**

System	System Sub-Area	Adaptation to Virtual Care	Suggested Documentation for Normal Examination
Vital signs		Evaluate for tachypnea, cyanosis, orthostatic symptoms as applicable. May ask patient for height/weight. If patient has heart rate monitor (wrist or chest) and/or automatic blood pressure cuff, can have them provide values	Normal rate of breathing, appears well oxygenated without cyanosis, reports no dizziness or orthostatic changes when asked to stand for 5 minutes after sitting
General		Practitioner's observation, including alertness, general appearance	Alert, cooperative, well-appearing, no acute distress
Respiratory		Practitioner's observation, including labor of breathing, presence of cough, or wheezing	Non-labored breathing, no cough or wheezing
Skin		Practitioner's observation of patient's skin for masses, lesions, or ulcers. Inspect and comment on any skin changes at anatomical site(s) postinjection	No lesions or ulcers visualized on exposed skin. No discharge, drainage, or redness at site(s) of prior Injection
Psychiatric		Practitioner's observation of patient's mood and affect	Normal mood, congruent affect, answers questions appropriately
Neurologic	Mental status	Level of alertness, orientation to visit, able to identify objects, and maintain attention to tasks	Alert and oriented to person, time and reason for visit. Able to identify objects including items of clothing, electronic devices in use, and ability to perform serial 7 s (or spell WORLD backward if fluent in English or more appropriate for education)
	Speech	Rate of speech, word choice, and volume	Fluent and normal rate of speech, no word finding difficulties
	CN I	If patient accompanied, patient may be presented with familiar smell (coffee, bread) to identify with eyes closed	CN 1 confirmed intact as patient able to accurately identify presented odor
	CN II	Practitioner's observation of pupils	Pupils equal and round
	CN III, IV, VI	Ask patient to gaze in different directions	Extraocular movements intact, no nystagmus, no ptosis

Continued

TABLE 14.1 ■ A System-Based Approach to Performing and Documenting a Physical Examination via Telemedicine.—cont'd

System	System Sub-Area	Adaptation to Virtual Care	Suggested Documentation for Normal Examination
	CN V	Ask patient to clench and release jaw	Jaw movements intact and symmetric
	CN VII	Ask patient to smile, raise eyebrows	Symmetric facial movement and smile
	CN VIII	Practitioner's observation of patient's hearing ability	Hearing intact to normal voice
	CN IX/X	Practitioner's observation of vocal quality	Normal vocal quality, no hoarseness
	CN XI	Ask patient to shrug shoulders, rotate neck	Symmetric shoulder shrug and neck rotation
	CN XII	Ask patient to stick out tongue	Tongue protrudes midline
	Motor	Practitioner's observation of abnormal movement at rest including tremor, dystonia, clonus; instruct patient on rapid finger tapping, pronator	No tremor, dystonia, clonus observed. Rapid finger tapping intact. No pronator drift
	Tone	Practitioner's observation on voluntary movement, co-contraction, posturing with position changes	Patient able to perform full active movements, no co-contraction, no posturing with position changes
	Coordination	Practitioner instructs patient on performing rapid alternating movements, finger-to-nose with alternating movements, finger-to-nose with available targets (e.g., edge of computer screen), heel-to-shin	Rapid alternating movements intact and symmetric; finger-to-nose and heel-to-shin intact bilaterally
	Proprioception	Practitioner instructs patient on performing Romberg and tandem walking tests	Negative Romberg; normal tandem walking
	Sensation	Practitioner asks patient or accompanying individual to gently touch appropriate dermatomal regions, simultaneously if possible and report any abnormal sensation. May also provide diagram of dermatomes to further instruct patient. Practitioner can also ask patient to use tip of pencil and eraser to test sharp/dull sensation	Sensation to light touch and sharp/dull subjectively intact

Continued

TABLE 14.1 ■ A System-Based Approach to Performing and Documenting a Physical Examination via Telemedicine. —cont'd

System	System Sub-Area	Adaptation to Virtual Care	Suggested Documentation for Normal Examination
	Strength	Practitioner's observation of whether patient can performing appropriate movements such as antigravity; heel and toe walking can provide additional information about dorsiflexion/plantarflexion strength	Strength at least antigravity in all four limbs. Able to walk on heels and toes without difficulty
Musculoskeletal	Gait	Practitioner's observation of patient's gait	Symmetric, nonantalgic, heel-to-toe gait
	Inspection	Practitioner's observation of relevant body regions as directed by patient and clinical suspicion	No asymmetry; no discoloration, erythema, or swelling; no obvious deformity
	Palpation	Practitioner instructs patient to find area(s) of tenderness and guides patient to palpate relevant associated areas, sense temperature differences in adjacent region or contralateral side, and describes crepitus	No tenderness to palpation; no crepitus reported, equal warmth
	Range of motion	Practitioner guides patient in performing movements to observe active range of motion	Full symmetric, active range of motion in bilateral shoulders, elbows and knees
	Special testing	Practitioner guides patient as appropriate for patient's chief complaint (see Table 14.2)	

CN, Cranial nerve.

this could include a premade protocol available online for patients with a specific condition that details exercises patients may perform at home for better range of motion, mobility, and swelling management.[22]

Therapeutic Intervention

As general practice, PT is a primary intervention prescribed for treating MSK injuries and focuses on the performance of therapeutic exercises to restore function often through improving movement mechanics and increasing strength and flexibility. Traditionally, patients participate in this treatment by attending in-person appointments where they are coached through a progression of exercises and instructed to continue performing these exercises at home independently. However,

TABLE 14.2 ■ **Examples of Special Tests That May Be Performed During Telemedicine Physical Examination.**

	Performed Without Assistance	Performed With Assistance From Nonclinician
Cervical spine	Spurling test (cervical radiculopathy) Roos test (thoracic outlet syndrome)	
Lumbar Spine		Straight leg raise (lumbar radiculopathy) Slump test (lumbar radiculopathy)
Hip/SI joint	Single-leg stance/squat (gluteus medius weakness) Thomas test (iliopsoas tightness/ contracture)	FABER (hip, SI joint, lumbar spine dysfunction) FADIR (femoroacetabular impingement, piriformis) Ely test (rectus femoris tightness/contracture) Stinchfield test (intraarticular hip pathology)
Knee	Thessaly test (meniscal injury) Duck walk (meniscal injury) Single-leg squat (knee valgus, patellofemoral syndrome)	Noble compression test (iliotibial band syndrome) Patellar grind test (patellofemoral syndrome)
Ankle/Foot	Single-leg heel raise (triceps surae, posterior tibialis dysfunction) Foot doming (intrinsic foot weakness) Metatarsal/Morton squeeze test (Morton's neuroma)	Syndesmosis squeeze test (high ankle sprain) Thompson test (Achilles tendon injury
Shoulder	Drop arm test (supraspinatus tear) Yocum test (subacromial impingement) Lift-off test (subscapularis injury) Apley scarf test (acromioclavicular joint pain)	Speed test (biceps tendon injury) Neer sign (subacromial impingement) O'Brien test (AC joint, glenoid labrum injury) Sulcus sign test (glenohumeral instability)
Elbow	Tinel test over ulnar groove (ulnar neuropathy at the elbow)	Cozen test (lateral epicondylosis) Maudsley test (lateral epicondylosis)
Wrist/Hand	Finkelstein test (de Quervain's tenosynovitis) Tinel test (median/ulnar nerve entrapment at the wrist) Phalen test (carpal tunnel syndrome) Carpometacarpal grind test (carpometacarpal osteoarthritis)	
Bone (General)	Palpation, direct and indirect percussion, hop test (bone stress injury)	

Tests are divided into those likely able to be performed by the patient without assistance and those which are most readily performed with another person assisting. These are examples, and this table is not intended to be a complete list; furthermore, these tests may not be reliable virtually. Clinicians should consider safety when asking patients and to perform the tests virtually.

FABER, Flexion, abduction, external rotation test; *FADIR*, flexion, adduction, internal rotation test; *SI*, Sacroiliac joint.

patient education and monitoring for compliance to home exercise program are also important aspects to telerehabilitation and can be accomplished effectively using a telemedicine platform.[43]

SYNCHRONOUS THERAPY

Synchronous teleconferencing closely resembles conventional care, as a patient can learn and execute therapeutic exercises and receive corrections "face-to-face" with a therapist despite being in different locations.[36] This live teleconferencing also enables therapists to measure joint angles with the aforementioned internet- or teleconference-based goniometer.[40-42] An added benefit of this telecare is that therapists may utilize motion analysis tools that allow them to capture still images or video sequences from the live teleconference that they may then review in slow motion for greater assessment.[22] Similar to the synchronous telerehabilitation with a physician previously described, this type of therapy may be incorporated into conventional care or utilized alone.

Patients may attend an initial in-person session to learn specific exercises with hands-on instruction before transitioning to synchronous teleconferencing with their therapist. To aid in the transition to telerehabilitation, therapists can create patient handouts depicting the exercises through photographs of the patients themselves demonstrating them. This type of instruction coupled with synchronous teleconferencing has shown clinically significant improvements in patients with shoulder pain and immobility.[45] Teletherapy may also be integrated into conventional care by simply adding synchronous therapy sessions to a patient's already established in-person appointment schedule to increase frequency of sessions, which favors recovery.[6, 17, 46] Notably, in-person treatment may be required in situations where patients require treatment with modalities (e.g., ultrasound, iontophoresis) or other hands-on aspects of care such as joint mobilizations or massage.[43]

For patients unable to attend any conventional therapy, completely virtually-based care remains a valid option. Despite being unable to provide manual adjustments or corrections, Wong et al.[12] illustrated that 3 months of PT delivered to patients with OA-related knee pain entirely through synchronous teleconferencing resulted in a significant improvement in pain, stiffness, and physical function. This methodology has been shown to be at least as effective as conventional in-person PT.[22, 23, 47]

Whereas some patients may prefer videoconferencing, others may choose to have their telerehabilitation provided through audio-only conversations using a telephone. In fact, this medium has been shown to have a moderate-to-large positive effect on clinical outcomes.[6, 17, 46, 48] Therapists can explain the importance of PT, review exercise programs, and provide real-time coaching at regularly scheduled times, just as would be done with traditional therapy.[27, 48-50] Moreover the accessibility of telephone conversations enables therapists to, with the patients' permission, teach families how best to support the patients during recovery.[46]

ASYNCHRONOUS THERAPY

Asynchronous telerehabilitation may consist of the same components as PT delivered through synchronous teleconferencing—but as recorded videos sent between the practitioner and the patient—or stray further from conventional care. With this modality, patients may utilize telerehabilitation systems in which recorded videos are largely incorporated.[16, 51]

Following an initial synchronous teleconference evaluation with a physician, the therapist can provide recorded videos reviewing the proper execution of therapeutic exercises. These videos may include automated coaching to aid in proper execution.[51] The patient should provide the therapist with recordings of their performance of these therapeutic movements to receive feedback on technique and progression.[16] Through this type of virtual experience, patients with rotator cuff injuries reported a significant decrease in pain, and improved movement, functioning, and muscular strength.[16] As the natural history of rotator cuff injuries is to progress in severity, these findings of improvement after 6 months illustrate the utility of asynchronous PT.[52–54] Moreover all participants noted that they would recommend this platform of care to others.[16]

Alternatively, patients may learn therapeutic exercises not by observing videos of physical therapists, but three-dimensional (3D) avatars.[44] Patients can subsequently perform these exercises while wearing sensors, so movement trajectories could be calculated. These measurements, along with video recordings of the patients performing the exercises, may then be reviewed by the therapist to aid in evaluation and progression of treatment.[44, 55] These biometric data can be used to further customize the PT regimen to enable optimal rehabilitation.[55]

Furthermore a component of virtual reality may be added to allow patients already equipped with sensors and following 3D avatars to experience a manipulated environment similar to one that would be created in an in-person appointment.[1, 56] With specific programming, the software can also assist in injury prevention by identifying when an exercise is being performed improperly, alerting the therapist, and providing an avatar to actually guide the patient accordingly.[56]

Similar to synchronous telerehabilitation, the telephone may also be used in this type of therapy. Text messages can provide education, reminders, and encouragement related to the prescribed therapeutic exercise program as well as identify barriers to adherence. The utility of these measures has been confirmed and shown to result in functional improvement as well as compliance.[57, 58]

WEBSITE-BASED THERAPY

Website-based telerehabilitation is less similar to conventional therapy than the previously described synchronous or asynchronous therapy, but given that searching for health information is the third most popular online activity following emailing and researching a product or service before purchasing, the interest is clear.[59] In fact, as determined in 2003, 80% of American adult internet users have searched online for at least one major health topic, and 54% of US adults have searched online for any health-related information.[59] Taking this into consideration, utilizing the internet to provide therapeutic exercises may be advantageous.

Though this type of telerehabilitation can take many forms, Lorig et al.[10] suggest using a comprehensive password-protected interactive website. Through this medium, patients can conveniently have secure access to education, exercise logs, medication diaries, group bulletin boards, and exercise programs complete with professional instruction at any time. The utility of this platform was assessed on patients with OA and found to have improved health distress, self-reported global health, activity limitation, disability, fatigue, and pain compared with patients participating in usual in-person care at 1 year.[10] Given the endless possibilities of website content and formatting, sites may be tailored to meet specific pathology and population needs through a variety of options.

MULTIMEDIA THERAPY

Practitioners may also choose to integrate synchronous, asynchronous, and/or website-based care to provide a multimedia approach to recovery. For example, a website-based PT program with simultaneous telephone assistance and a synchronous teleconferencing PT program with supplemental written weekly guides have been shown to provide clinically significant results.[22, 50] This ability to combine various telerehabilitation technologies enables the practitioners to individualize treatment plans even further to better address patients' needs.

TYPE OF THERAPY

Equally important to how the therapy is delivered are the type of therapy and the environment in which it is performed. The type of therapy—be it strengthening, conditioning, stretching, biofeedback, or any combination thereof—should be chosen strictly based on the pathology of the patient. Therefore the mode of delivery (virtual or in person) should not impact this aspect and every effort should be made to integrate the proper therapy with telerehabilitation through one of the aforementioned delivery methods (synchronous, asynchronous, website-based).

Similar to conventional clinic-based therapy sessions, through telerehabilitation technologies, therapists have the ability to treat patients individually or as a group. Group sessions can involve a therapist providing therapy to multiple individuals in different locations using a multiuser system or coaching multiple patients who are together themselves while the therapist is remote. For a multiuser interface, all patients may participate from their respective homes, but group sessions may also involve the patients congregating at a central location, such as a gym or community center. With the proper setup (adequate space, internet, screen, audio, and appropriate software), patients may participate together in person in group therapy sessions no matter the location of the therapist. Group sessions with the patients in person or connected virtually provide the added benefits of reducing social isolation and utilizing social support to enhance their recovery.[12] This group dynamic may also be cultivated through the use of website-based bulletin boards, email listservs, and/or group text messaging.[10]

Special Considerations

POSTOPERATIVE MANAGEMENT

The prevalence of joint replacement surgery is expected to rise as a result of growing risk factors (age, obesity, injury), increasing expectations for improved quality of life, and advancements in surgical and anesthetic techniques.[60] Moreover, patients undergoing any orthopedic surgery often require PT postoperatively to recover full MSK function. The same principles discussed in this chapter apply to the telerehabilitation management of these patients and have specifically been explored in patients following anterior cruciate ligament (ACL) reconstructions,[61] lumbar spinal surgeries,[48] as well as shoulder,[62,63] knee,[22,23,33,44,47,64] and hip[33,34,46] joint replacements, with results showing favorability and noninferiority to conventional PT. Patients also reported a preference for postoperative telerehabilitation compared to in-person therapy.[33]

The importance in providing telerehabilitation for postoperative care and ensuring continuity of management illustrates value for the patient and potential to optimize surgical outcomes.[36] This aspect is especially important following surgical interventions that require a greater duration of rehabilitation. For example, following an ACL reconstruction, on average, rehabilitation takes 12 months to complete.[61] Therefore Dunphy et al.[61] evaluated the use of a web-based rehabilitation system that provides videos of individualized therapeutic exercises, instructions, progress logs, educational materials, and the option to directly contact a physical therapist concurrently with scheduled in-person PT. This website-based therapy, Taxonomy for the Rehabilitation of Knee Conditions (TRAK), was found to increase patients' knowledge, confidence, and motivation in regard to their rehabilitation (n = 17). Similarly, Skolasky et al.[48] explored the impact of telephone-based synchronous conversations focused on increasing patients' confidence in and understanding of the importance of PT postoperatively. This study revealed this intervention to significantly increase participation, attendance, and functional outcomes at 3 and 6 months postoperatively (n = 63).

Telerehabilitation following a shoulder joint replacement has also been shown to be beneficial in a variety of measures. Eriksson et al.[63] evaluated synchronous video-based telerehabilitation with a physical therapist to patients at home following shoulder joint replacements and found that patients participating in telerehabilitation received a greater number of treatment sessions, and had significantly greater improvements in pain (visual analogue scale) and shoulder functional ability (constant score and Shoulder Rating Questionnaire (SRQ-S)), as well as improved pain and vitality from baseline compared to the control group that received conventional in-person PT (n = 22).

A subsequent assessment by Eriksson et al.[62] revealed that this intervention also resulted in patients' increased health knowledge, motivation to participate in PT, and independence (n = 10). Moreover, participants noted that despite the distance, they felt a strong rapport with their therapists.[62]

The role of telerehabilitation following lower extremity total joint replacements has also been explored in the literature. In regard to the hip and knee joint, postoperative supplemental synchronous video telerehabilitation with the surgeon was shown to increase postoperative patient satisfaction as well as decrease unscheduled visits and "medical advice" calls to the clinic (n = 78).[33] In patients having undergone total hip replacements, postoperative synchronous telephone calls with a specialist nurse significantly increased physical function, general health, and mental health 3 months following the surgery. Notably, no difference was found in these measures at 9 months (n = 161).[34] An additional implication of this measure is the ability to speak with the patients' families in regard to therapeutic exercises, precautions, and health, which has been shown to significantly increase compliance and functional hip mobility at 6 months postoperatively (n = 249).[46] Following total knee replacements, synchronous video-based telerehabilitation with a physical therapist at the patient's home or home-equivalent environment has been found to achieve outcomes comparable to patients receiving conventional in-person PT with regard to range of motion, strength, balance, limb girth, pain intensity, quality of life, gait assessment (GARS), Patient Specific Functional Scale (PSFS), and Western Ontario and McMaster Universities Osteoarthritis Index (WOMAC) scores (n = 21–205).[22,23,47,64] However, statistically significantly better outcomes were observed when assessing PSFS and the stiffness subscale of the WOMAC (n = 65).[22] Asynchronous video-based telerehabilitation with a physical therapist to the patient's home for this same patient population has also been shown to be at least as effective as traditional in-person PT (n = 142).[44]

COMPLIANCE

Compliance is often a barrier to functional recovery through PT, as a lack of adherence to a home-based exercise program can reduce the benefit of the treatment.[65,66] Because telerehabilitation relies more strongly on the dialogue between the practitioner and the patient, given the barrier to hands-on examinations, education is inherently a larger component in each visit.[36] An advantage of this is that increased education has been linked with a greater locus of control and, subsequently, greater adherence to the recommended treatment.[67,68] Telerehabilitation also has the implicit benefit of motivating patients to perform therapeutic measures in their home environments.[1,69] The literature has shown that asynchronous PT through prerecorded educational videos increases patient confidence and motivation in their rehabilitation,[61] and synchronous PT (alone or as a supplement to conventional PT) increases adherence with therapy.[27,46,49] Logically, eliminating travel time may also help patients participate in follow-up treatment and could be beneficial to reduce situations, such as driving, that can provoke pain in certain conditions, such as back pain or proximal hamstring injuries.

ACCESSIBILITY

Telerehabilitation eliminates barriers that may otherwise prevent patients from obtaining care. These limitations may be derived from a paucity of nearby MSK specialists and therapists or from the patient's mobility status, as well as socioeconomic factors such as financial and scheduling means. Specifically, patients suffering from MSK conditions may be reliant on others for transportation or completely unable to travel to in-person appointments secondary to their immobility or pain.[33] Beyond utilizing telerehabilitation to receive a diagnosis, it is important that patients are able to perform their therapy in accordance with the standard of care. Unsupervised home programs are only prescribed once the patient has established their routine with the therapist. Until then, supervised therapy is important to improve self-efficacy, fear of movement or reinjury, pain, disability, and analgesic consumption.[70] By enabling patients to secure appointments remotely, the medical community is helping to promote personal autonomy and provide equitable health services—especially as access to internet increases.[28,32,36,71,72]

Recommendations

In response to the COVID-19 global pandemic, the literature working to both educate practitioners and standardize the performance and documentation of telerehabilitation has expanded. This includes documenting quality, value, and satisfaction for patients and providers. However, there remains a scarcity of studies evaluating the utility of this care on specific pathologies and different age groups. Additionally, though extensive research has been done to assess the validity and reliability of MSK examination maneuvers performed by practitioners in person, this has yet to be done for these maneuvers when self-performed by the patient. Comparing the sensitivity and specificity of physical examination tests self-conducted by a patient with those performed by a practitioner could provide a greater understanding of the utility of MSK telerehabilitation for diagnostic purposes, and guide future use. Moreover, for which patient populations participating in home PT is safe should be assessed to provide optimal care without increased health and safety risks. Further research should focus on filling these voids to provide practitioners greater support and instruction when using telerehabilitation to treat MSK injuries.

CASE STUDY

A 32-year-old female patient requests an appointment to discuss a 3-month history of right knee pain. As she is an established patient with barriers to attending an in-person appointment, a telemedicine appointment is arranged. When this appointment is scheduled, the patient is advised to secure a well-lit, private area for the appointment and position her hands-free camera to allow her entire body to be visualized. She is also asked to wear shorts, so that her knees may be seen clearly by the physician.

The telemedicine appointment begins with the physician obtaining a history of her knee pain, which reveals a 3-month history of intermittent dull, aching right knee pain that is worse after running, prolonged periods of sitting, and descending stairs. She rates the pain 7/10 at its worst. She is a runner and reports increasing her weekly mileage 4 months ago. She has not tried any modalities to reduce the pain and feels it has been increasing since onset. The physician asks the patient to identify where she feels pain; the patient stands up so that her entire body is visible on the screen, and points to her right patella.

To assess this pathology further, the physician asks the patient to continue standing, so he can visually inspect her knees with special attention to the kinetic chain. She is instructed to rotate to provide a 360-degree view of her anatomy. The physician then demonstrates palpation of the knee, asking the patient to do the same bilaterally and note when any tenderness, crepitus, or warmth is felt; the patient reports no tenderness to palpation, crepitus, or warmth. The physician then explains to the patient that, to better assess her alignment when running, he would like to see her perform a single-leg squat on each side and demonstrates one himself for clarity. The patient performs a single-leg squat on the left side maintaining proper alignment of her hip, knee, and ankle; she notes no pain. Next, she executes a single-leg squat on the right side and significant knee valgus is seen; she notes that the pain felt at the patella is precisely the pain she has been experiencing. The physician subsequently requests the patient to show the bottom of her running shoes to assess the tread wear pattern, which suggests pronation of the right foot greater than the left.

Given this patient's history and physical examination, the physician explains the diagnosis of patellofemoral pain. He counsels the patient to utilize nonsteroidal antiinflammatory drugs (NSAIDs) and ice to control the pain as needed. Activity modification is recommended, including decreasing her total running to the point of not experiencing pain with activity, and improving her alignment to reduce the stress on her patella by performing single-leg squats in the mirror with attention to maintaining her knee in line with a neutral ankle. She is provided a prescription for PT and recommended a virtual follow-up visit in 6 weeks to assess progress and determine the next steps to increase activity. If pain continues or becomes worse, the necessity of an in-person appointment and/or imaging will be considered.

References

1. Russell TG. Telerehabilitation: a coming of age. *Aust J Physiother*. 2009;55(1):5–6.
2. Piron L, Turolla A, Agostini M, et al. Exercises for paretic upper limb after stroke: a combined virtual-reality and telemedicine approach. *J Rehabil Med*. 2009;41:1016–1102.
3. Tenforde AS, Iaccarino MA, Borgstrom H, et al. Telemedicine During COVID-19 for Outpatient Sports and Musculoskeletal Medicine Physicians. *PM R*. 2020 Sep;12(9):926–932.
4. Richardson BR, Truter P, Blumke R, et al. Physiotherapy assessment and diagnosis of musculoskeletal disorders of the knee via telerehabilitation. *J Telemed Telecare*. 2017;23(1):88–95.
5. Lade H, McKenzie S, Steele L, et al. Validity and reliability of the assessment and diagnosis of musculoskeletal elbow disorders using telerehabilitation. *J Telemed Telecare*. 2012;18(7):413–418.
6. Cottrell MA, Galea OA, O'Leary SP, et al. Real-time telerehabilitation for the treatment of musculoskeletal conditions is effective and comparable to standard practice: a systematic review and meta-analysis. *Clin Rehabil*. 2017;31(5):625–638.
7. Allen KD, Oddone EZ, Coffman CJ, et al. Telephone-based self-management of osteoarthritis: a randomized trial. *Ann Intern Med*. 2010;153(9):570–579.
8. Pariser D, O'Hanlon A. Effects of telephone intervention on arthritis self-efficacy, depression, pain, and fatigue in older adults with arthritis. *J Geriatr Phys Ther*. 2005;28(3):67–73.
9. Odole AC, Ojo OD. Is telephysiotherapy an option for improved quality of life in patients with osteoarthritis of the knee? *Int J Telemed Appl*. 2014;2014:903816.
10. Lorig KR, Ritter PL, Laurent DD, et al. The internet-based arthritis self-management program: a one-year randomized trial for patients with arthritis or fibromyalgia. *Arthritis Rheum*. 2008;59(7):1009–1017.
11. Sciamanna CN, Harrold LR, Manocchia M, et al. The effect of web-based, personalized, osteoarthritis quality improvement feedback on patient satisfaction with osteoarthritis care. *Am J Med Qual*. 2005;20(3):127–137.
12. Wong YK, Hui E, Woo J. A community-based exercise programme for older persons with knee pain using telemedicine. *J Telemed Telecare*. 2005;11(6):310–315.
13. Vuolio S, Winblad I, Ohinmaa A, et al. Videoconferencing for orthopaedic outpatients: one-year follow-up. *J Telemed Telecare*. 2003;9(1):8–11.
14. Azma K, RezaSoltani Z, Rezaeimoghaddam F, et al. Telemedicine during COVID-19 for outpatient sports and musculoskeletal medicine physicians. *PM R*. 2020;12(9):926–932.
15. Kosterink SM, Huis 't Veld RM, Cagnie B, et al. The clinical effectiveness of a myofeedback-based teletreatment service in patients with non-specific neck and shoulder pain: a randomized controlled trial. *J Telemed Telecare*. 2010;16(6):316–321.
16. Macías-Hernández SI, Vásquez-Sotelo DS, F-N MV, et al. Proposal and evaluation of a telerehabilitation platform designed for patients with partial rotator cuff tears: a preliminary study. *Ann Rehabil Med*. 2016;40(4):710–717.
17. Iles R, Taylor NF, Davidson M, et al. Telephone coaching can increase activity levels for people with non-chronic low back pain: a randomised trial. *J Physiother*. 2011;57(4):231–238.
18. Vina ER, Kwoh CK. Epidemiology of osteoarthritis: literature update. *Curr Opin Rheumatol*. 2018;30(2):160–167.
19. Deshpande BR, Katz JN, Solomon DH, et al. Number of persons with symptomatic knee osteoarthritis in the US: impact of race and ethnicity, age, sex, and obesity. *Arthritis Care Res (Hoboken)*. 2016;68(12):1743–1750.
20. Hunter DJ, Felson DT. Osteoarthritis. *BMJ*. 2006;332(7542):639–642.
21. Pietrzak E, Cotea C, Pullman S, et al. Self-management and rehabilitation in osteoarthritis: is there a place for internet-based interventions? *Telemed J E Health*. 2013;19(10):800–805.
22. Russell TG, Buttrum P, Wootton R, et al. Internet-based outpatient telerehabilitation for patients following total knee arthroplasty: a randomized controlled trial. *J Bone Joint Surg Am*. 2011;93(2):113–120.
23. Tousignant M, Moffet H, Boissy P, et al. A randomized controlled trial of home telerehabilitation for post-knee arthroplasty. *J Telemed Telecare*. 2011;17(4):195–198.
24. Murray CJ, Atkinson C, Bhalla K, et al. The state of US health, 1990-2010: burden of diseases, injuries, and risk factors. *JAMA*. 2013;310(6):591–608.
25. Vos T, Flaxman AD, Naghavi M, et al. Years lived with disability (YLDs) for 1160 sequelae of 289 diseases and injuries 1990-2010: a systematic analysis for the Global Burden of Disease Study 2010. *Lancet*. 2012;380(9859):2163–2196.

26. Kroenke K, Krebs EE, Wu J, et al. Telecare collaborative management of chronic pain in primary care: a randomized clinical trial. *JAMA*. 2014;312(3):240–248.

27. Gialanella B, Ettori T, Faustini S, et al. Home-based telemedicine in patients with chronic neck pain. *Am J Phys Med Rehab*. 2017;96(5):327–332.

28. Tenforde AS, Hefner JE, Kodish-Wachs JE, et al. Telehealth in physical medicine and rehabilitation: a narrative review. *PM R*. 2017;9(5S):S51–S58.

29. Careau E, Vincent C, Noreau L. Assessing interprofessional teamwork in a videoconference-based telerehabilitation setting. *J Telemed Telecare*. 2008;14(8):427–434.

30. Goldstein Y, Schermann H, Dolkart O, et al. Video examination via the smartphone: a reliable tool for shoulder function assessment using the constant score. *J Orthop Sci*. 2019;24(5):812–816.

31. Aarnio P, Lamminen H, Lepistö J, et al. A prospective study of teleconferencing for orthopaedic consultations. *J Telemed Telecare*. 1999;5(1):62–66.

32. Brennan DM, Mawson S, Brownsell S. Telerehabilitation: enabling the remote delivery of healthcare, rehabilitation, and self management. *Stud Health Technol Inform*. 2009;145:231–248.

33. Sharareh B, Schwarzkopf R. Effectiveness of telemedical applications in postoperative follow-up after total joint arthroplasty. *J Arthroplasty*. 2014;29(5):918–922.

34. Hørdam B, Sabroe S, Pedersen PU, et al. Nursing intervention by telephone interviews of patients aged over 65 years after total hip replacement improves health status: a randomised clinical trial. *Scand J Caring Sci*. 2010;24(1):94–100.

35. Tanaka MJ, Oh LS, Martin SD, et al. Telemedicine in the era of COVID-19: the virtual orthopaedic examination. *J Bone Joint Surg Am*. 2020;102(12):e57.

36. Verduzco-Gutierrez M, Bean AC, Tenforde AS, et al. How to conduct an outpatient telemedicine rehabilitation or prehabilitation visit. *PM R*. 2020;12(7):714–720.

37. Good DW, Lui DF, Leonard M, et al. Skype: a tool for functional assessment in orthopaedic research. *J Telemed Telecare*. 2012;18(2):94–98.

38. Chanlalit C, Kongmalai P. Validation of the telemedicine-based goniometry for measuring elbow range of motion. *J Med Assoc Thai*. 2012;95(suppl 12):S113–117.

39. Dent PA, Wilke B, Terkonda S, et al. Validation of teleconference-based goniometry for measuring elbow joint range of motion. *Cureus*. 2020;12(2):e6925.

40. Russell T. Goniometry via the internet. *Aust J Physiother*. 2007;53(2):136.

41. Russell TG, Jull GA, Wootton R. Can the Internet be used as a medium to evaluate knee angle? *Man Ther*. 2003;8(4):242–246.

42. Russell TG, Wootton R, Jull GA. Physical outcome measurements via the Internet: reliability at two Internet speeds. *J Telemed Telecare*. 2002;8(suppl 3):S50–S52.

43. Tenforde AS, Borgstrom H, Polich G, et al. Outpatient physical, occupational, and speech therapy synchronous telemedicine: a survey study of patient satisfaction with virtual visits during the COVID-19 pandemic. *Am J Phys Med Rehabil*. 2020;99(11):977–981.

44. Piqueras M, Marco E, Coll M, et al. Effectiveness of an interactive virtual telerehabilitation system in patients after total knee arthoplasty: a randomized controlled trial. *J Rehabil Med*. 2013;45(4):392–396.

45. Van Straaten MG, Cloud BA, Morrow MM, et al. Effectiveness of home exercise on pain, function, and strength of manual wheelchair users with spinal cord injury: a high-dose shoulder program with telerehabilitation. *Arch Phys Med Rehabil*. 2014;95(10):1810–1817.

46. Li LL, Gan YY, Zhang LN, et al. The effect of post-discharge telephone intervention on rehabilitation following total hip replacement surgery. *Int J Nurs Sci*. 2014;1:207–211.

47. Moffet H, Tousignant M, Nadeau S, et al. In-home telerehabilitation compared with face-to-face rehabilitation after total knee arthroplasty: a noninferiority randomized controlled trial. *J Bone Joint Surg Am*. 2015;97(14):1129–1141.

48. Skolasky RL, Maggard AM, Li D, et al. Health behavior change counseling in surgery for degenerative lumbar spinal stenosis. Part I: improvement in rehabilitation engagement and functional outcomes. *Arch Phys Med Rehabil*. 2015;96(7):1200–1207.

49. Bennell KL, Campbell PK, Egerton T, et al. Telephone coaching to enhance a home-based physical activity program for knee osteoarthritis: a randomized clinical trial. *Arthritis Care Res (Hoboken)*. 2017;69(1):84–94.

50. Sparrow D, Gottlieb DJ, Demolles D, et al. Increases in muscle strength and balance using a resistance training program administered via a telecommunications system in older adults. *J Gerontol A Biol Sci Med Sci.* 2011;66(11):1251–1257.

51. Obdržálek S, Kurillo G, Seto E, et al. Architecture of an automated coaching system for elderly population. *Stud Health Technol Inform.* 2013;184:309–311.

52. Safran O, Schroeder J, Bloom R, et al. Natural history of nonoperatively treated symptomatic rotator cuff tears in patients 60 years old or younger. *Am J Sports Med.* 2011;39:710–714.

53. Yamanaka K, Matsumoto T. The joint side tear of the rotator cuff: a followup study by arthrography. *Clin Orthop Relat Res.* 1994;304:68–73.

54. Eljabu W, Klinger HM, von Knoch M. The natural history of rotator cuff tears: a systematic review. *Arch Orthop Trauma Surg.* 2015;135:1055–1061.

55. Chughtai M, Kelly JJ, Newman JM, et al. The role of virtual rehabilitation in total and unicompartmental knee arthroplasty. *J Knee Surg.* 2019;32(1):105–110.

56. Rizzo AA, Strickland D, Bouchard S. The challenge of using virtual reality in telerehabilitation. *Telemed J E Health.* 2004;10(2):184–195.

57. Nelligan RK, Hinman RS, Kasza J, et al. Effectiveness of internet-delivered education and home exercise supported by behaviour change SMS on pain and function for people with knee osteoarthritis: a randomised controlled trial protocol. *BMC Musculoskelet Disord.* 2019;20(1):342.

58. Chen HC, Chuang TY, Lin PC, et al. Effects of messages delivered by mobile phone on increasing compliance with shoulder exercises among patients with a frozen shoulder. *J Nurs Scholarsh.* 2017;49(4):429–437.

59. Fox S, Fallows D. *Internet Health Resources: Health Searches and Email Have Become More Commonplace, But There Is Room for Improvement in Searches and Overall Internet Access.* Washington, DC: Pew Research Center; 2003.

60. March LM, Bagga H. Epidemiology of osteoarthritis in Australia. *Med J Aust.* 2004;180(S5):S6–S10.

61. Dunphy E, Hamilton FL, Spasić I, et al. Acceptability of a digital health intervention alongside physiotherapy to support patients following anterior cruciate ligament reconstruction. *BMC Musculoskelet Disord.* 2017;18(1):471.

62. Eriksson L, Lindström B, Ekenberg L. Patients' experiences of telerehabilitation at home after shoulder joint replacement. *J Telemed Telecare.* 2011;17(1):25–30.

63. Eriksson L, Lindström B, Gard G, et al. Physiotherapy at a distance: a controlled study of rehabilitation at home after a shoulder joint operation. *J Telemed Telecare.* 2009;15(5):215–220.

64. Russell TG, Buttrum P, Wootton R, et al. Low-bandwidth telerehabilitation for patients who have undergone total knee replacement: preliminary results. *J Telemed Telecare.* 2003;9(suppl 2):S44–S47.

65. Hayden JA, van Tulder MW, Tomlinson G. Systematic review: strategies for using exercise therapy to improve outcomes in chronic low back pain. *Ann Intern Med.* 2005;142(9):776–785.

66. Kolt GS, McEvoy JF. Adherence to rehabilitation in patients with low back pain. *Man Ther.* 2003;8(2):110–116.

67. Ferguson K, Bole GG. Family support, health beliefs, and therapeutic compliance in patients with rheumatoid arthritis. *Patient Couns Health Educ.* 1979;1(3):101–105.

68. Heiby EM, Carlson JG. The health compliance model. *J Compliance Health Care.* 1986;1(2):135–152.

69. Agostini M, Moja L, Banzi R, et al. Telerehabilitation and recovery of motor function: a systematic review and meta-analysis. *J Telemed Telecare.* 2015;21(4):202–213.

70. Bunketorp L, Lindh M, Carlsson J, et al. The effectiveness of a supervised physical training model tailored to the individual needs of patients with whiplash-associated disorders--a randomized controlled trial. *Clin Rehabil.* 2006;20(3):201–217.

71. International Telecommunication Union. *Individuals Using the Internet, 2005–2019.* 2019. http://www.itu.int/en/ITU-D/Statistics/Pages/stat/default.aspx; Accessed 02.07.20.

72. Theodoros D, Russell T. Telerehabilitation: current perspectives. *Stud Health Technol Inform.* 2008;131:191–209.

CHAPTER 15

Telerehabilitation for Integrative Health

Chelsea G. Ratcliff ◼ Savitha Bonthala ◼ Debbie Torres ◼ Radha Korupolu

Introduction

Integrative therapies have been used for centuries in a variety of cultures to promote health and well-being. The National Center for Complementary and Integrative Health distinguishes two types of integrative approaches: natural products (e.g., dietary supplements) and mind-body practices (e.g., meditation, yoga, and Tai Chi, as well as body-manipulative methods, such as chiropracty, massage, or acupuncture).[1] Interest in mind-body therapies among rehabilitation patients has grown considerably in recent years. Data from the 2002 National Health Interview Survey (NHIS) indicate that roughly one in five individuals with a physical disability, including persons with multiple sclerosis (MS), cerebral palsy, spinal cord injury (SCI),[2] arthritis,[3] and stroke,[4] reported engaging in at least one mind-body therapy (i.e., meditation, yoga, or Tai Chi). NHIS data from 2007 indicate that the use of mind-body therapies nearly doubled for all populations,[5] including those with functional limitations.[6] Recent studies suggest that 40% to 80% of patients with physical disabilities engage in some form of mind-body therapy.[7, 8] This chapter will: (1) review the evidence for in-person and telerehabilitation meditation, yoga, and Tai Chi for persons participating in rehabilitation; (2) highlight areas for future research; (3) present practical strategies to deliver these telerehabilitation mind-body therapies; and (4) present a case study of the delivery of a telerehabilitation meditation program for neurorehabilitation patients.

In-Person Mind-Body Therapies for Rehabilitation Populations

As the use of mind-body therapies has grown, so too has its empirical study. In 2020 over 2800 publications contained the term "mindfulness," over 600 contained the term "yoga," and over 300 contained the term "Tai Chi" in the title, which is 15 times greater than the number of publications related to these therapies 20 years before. Evidence of the impact of these therapies for rehabilitation populations, in particular, continues to mount.

MINDFULNESS-BASED MEDITATION PROGRAMS

Mindfulness-based meditation, the most extensively studied type of meditation, refers to the practice of purposefully turning one's attention to the present moment with a sense of openness, curiosity, and nonjudgment.[9] It can be practiced anywhere in a seated position (preferred) or lying down for any duration. Patients engaging in a mindfulness-based meditation program (MBP) are typically asked to practice daily, with practice lengths ranging from as little as 5 minutes up to 90 minutes. Most MBPs last 4 to 8 weeks, and evidence suggests that at least 4 weeks of practice is needed to impact clinical outcomes.[10] As mindfulness-based meditation involves cultivating a sense of nonjudgment toward the present moment, it may be especially well suited to patients adjusting to a physical disability. In fact, MBPs can lead to increased adaptation to illness, acceptance of physical symptoms, and quality of life (QOL).[11] Unfortunately, research examining MBPs has been plagued by low rigor, resulting in some studies that may seem promising but whose low quality prevents firm conclusions from being drawn. Nevertheless, many studies show the promise of MBPs for improving disease and QOL-related outcomes among individuals with physical disabilities. Specifically, current literature suggests low- to moderate-quality evidence for the effectiveness of MBPs on psychological outcomes (e.g., depression, anxiety, self-efficacy) among individuals with heart failure,[12] stroke,[13, 14] rheumatoid arthritis,[15] SCI,[16] MS,[17] and cancer.[18, 19] There is also some evidence that MBPs are associated with improvement in pain outcomes in individuals with chronic pain[20-25] and various other rehabilitation populations.[15, 16]

YOGA

Yoga combines physical movements and mindful pauses in particular positions (e.g., standing, seated, squatting, lying) with a mental focus on the breath and body.[26] Yoga programs typically last between 4 and 12 weeks, and participants are encouraged to practice at least three times per week. Poses' difficulty levels can range from low to very intense, and as participants increase their strength and flexibility, they may opt to take on more challenging poses. When working with individuals with physical disabilities, yoga instructors must be experienced and capable of suggesting safe modifications to various poses to allow participation and prevent injuries. Given the importance of physical movement among individuals requiring rehabilitation, yoga is often an ideal complement to traditional rehabilitation therapies. Like MBP research, studies on the effects of yoga have varied quality. Currently, evidence suggests that yoga may improve pain and functional outcomes for individuals with musculoskeletal conditions, including chronic low back pain.[27, 28] Yoga practice has also improved psychological outcomes, sleep, and fatigue for cancer survivors,[29] and cognitive functioning for individuals with mild cognitive impairment or dementia.[30] Yoga has also been found to improve a variety of outcomes among cardiac and stroke patients, including biological cardiovascular risk factors (e.g., blood pressure [BP] and cholesterol), QOL, and functional abilities.[31-35] In fact, Medicare funds a lifestyle program involving yoga for individuals with heart disease.[36] In individuals with MS, yoga practice was associated with improvement in mood and fatigue.[37] Though yoga for persons with SCI requires considerable individualized modifications from experienced teachers, one small randomized controlled trial (RCT, n=23) found that a 6-week yoga intervention was feasible and associated with reduced depression and increased self-compassion among individuals with SCI.[38]

TAI CHI

Similar to yoga, Tai Chi combines physical movements with attention to the breath and body, but unlike yoga, Tai Chi involves constant movement from one position to the next.[39] Tai Chi is typically done in a standing position, but some programs have been adapted to a sitting position. Programs usually last 4 to 16 weeks, and evidence suggests at least 5 weeks of practice may be necessary to impact clinical outcomes.[40, 41] Given that Tai Chi is a gentle, contemplative exercise that encourages patients to focus on their body's movement, it can complement traditional rehabilitation therapies. As with MBP and yoga research, studies on the effect of Tai Chi often suffer from low methodological rigor. Nevertheless, current evidence suggests that practicing Tai Chi may significantly improve musculoskeletal pain among individuals with chronic pain,[40,41] and pain, fatigue, sleep, depression, and QOL among cancer survivors.[42] In individuals with neurological disorders such as MS, stroke, and SCI, Tai Chi practice may improve QOL, balance, functional abilities, and pain.[43–46] Additionally, Tai Chi modified for wheelchair use among individuals with SCI demonstrated improvement in sitting balance and handgrip strength,[47] enhanced vagal activity, and decreased sympathetic activity.[48]

Physical disabilities are associated with a host of "secondary" effects, including depression, pain, and fatigue, which can, in turn, lead to reduced engagement in activities of daily living and essential rehabilitation therapies.[49, 50] In fact, patients diagnosed with depression are three times more likely to be noncompliant with medical recommendations.[51] Additionally, stress can exacerbate many conditions such as MS and neurocognitive disorders.[17] These mind-body therapies show promise in improving these secondary effects. In particular, mindfulness-based meditation appears to have reasonably robust moderate effects on psychological outcomes and small effects on pain, whereas yoga and Tai Chi may improve pain, QOL, and functional outcomes in a variety of rehabilitation populations. Importantly, these therapies are acceptable and low risk among rehabilitation populations.

Telerehabilitation Mind-Body Therapies

Given the growing interest in and developing evidence supporting the benefits of mind-body therapies for rehabilitation populations, it is important to examine ways to increase access to these therapies. People with physical disabilities face many barriers to accessing health care, especially rehabilitation and integrative therapies.[52] For example, persons requiring rehabilitation are more likely to be unable to drive, and evidence suggests that finding transportation to in-person mind-body classes is a barrier to adherence.[53, 54] Persons needing rehabilitation often juggle many different medical appointments, preventing them from engaging in in-person integrative therapies.[55] Many health care clinics do not have mind-body therapists on staff, making such therapies inaccessible for patients even if they could attend sessions in person.[55–57] Further, some medical conditions are associated with a high risk of infection (e.g., individuals with cystic fibrosis or posttransplant), preventing these individuals from engaging in in-person group mind-body therapies.[58] The COVID-19 pandemic, which put all patients and providers at risk of infection, dramatically changed the health care landscape, necessitating the move of many therapies to telerehabilitation.[59] Offering telerehabilitation mind-body therapies in the comfort of a person's own home could increase access and adherence, reduce risk of infection, and potentially result in substantial cost savings. However, more cost-effectiveness research is needed to verify this assertion.[60, 61] Here, we review the existing evidence for and lessons learned from telerehabilitation meditation, yoga, and Tai Chi.

MEDITATION

Several studies have examined telerehabilitation MBPs for rehabilitation populations, including individuals diagnosed with cancer, MS, SCI, prehypertension, and osteoarthritis.

Cancer

Telerehabilitation MBPs have been most extensively studied in individuals with cancer. A systematic review of telerehabilitation MBPs for cancer survivors found that these programs were associated with small-to-medium effects on anxiety, depression, and pain,[62] which is generally consistent with in-person studies of MBP.[63, 64] This review also pointed out that delivery methods varied considerably: about one-third of the MBPs reviewed were delivered via a website, one-third via mobile app, and one-third via videoconference or telephone. Typically, patients were provided with audio- and/or video-recordings of mindfulness exercises to support practice in between sessions. Interestingly, few reviewed studies used reminder systems (e.g., email, text messages), which is surprising given that reminder messages may increase adherence to MBPs by eight times.[65]

Though attrition seems to be higher in telerehabilitation MBP (13%–48% for telerehabilitation compared with <25% for in-person),[10, 66] participants tend to complete at least four sessions, which is consistent with the adherence to in-person MBPs.[10] Thus reminder systems may be critical to keep participants engaged, but evidence generally suggests it is feasible, acceptable, and effective for cancer survivors.

Multiple Sclerosis

One study found that individuals diagnosed with MS who were randomly assigned to an 8-week group mindfulness-based stress reduction (MBSR) program led by a trained MBSR facilitator via Skype video chat reported a higher QOL and lower depression, anxiety, and sleep disturbance at the end of intervention compared with those randomly assigned to an 8-week asynchronous online psychoeducation program (n = 139).[67] The effect sizes observed in this study were smaller than those observed in a similar study examining an in-person MBSR intervention for patients with MS.[68] Thus more research is needed to discern if the effects of telerehabilitation MBPs may be weaker than in-person approaches among MS patients and if sustained support (e.g., "booster sessions") is necessary for long-term change. Regarding feasibility, this study noted that at least one participant experienced difficulty with their internet connection each session. However, participants were able to reconnect quickly. Additionally the vast majority of participants (98%) completed the intervention, and dropout rates were similar in both conditions, suggesting that this intervention is acceptable and feasible. Minor adaptations to traditional MBSR were made to meet the needs of individuals with MS in this study (e.g., sessions included a discussion of acceptance of MS-related symptoms), and home exercises were supported by a study-specific website that contained guided meditations instead of physical CDs, which have often been provided to patients in MBSR. Thus telerehabilitation MBPs may need to be adapted to the needs of the particular rehabilitation populations and the online environment.

Spinal Cord Injury

Preliminary evidence also supports the use of telerehabilitation MBPs among persons with SCIs. Individuals with SCI and chronic pain who were randomly assigned to an 8-week individual, asynchronous online mindfulness course reported reduced depression, anxiety, and pain catastrophizing at the end of the intervention and 3 months later compared with those randomly assigned to an 8-week psychoeducation program (n = 67).[69] Specifically, the mindfulness course involved listening to two 10-minute guided meditations available on the study's website for 6 out of 7 days a week for 8 weeks. The guided meditations were adapted to an SCI population (e.g., encouraging participants to consider head tilts or wrist rotations in a mindful movement exercise), again highlighting the need to adapt interventions to the target population. Though the majority (72%) of participants completed the intervention, dropout rates were higher in the intervention group than in the psychoeducational program group, particularly among older, more depressed individuals. Thus strategies to retain older and more severely depressed individuals may be necessary for telerehabilitation MBPs.

Prehypertension

Even relatively low-intensity interventions, such as having an individual use a mobile app, may impact physical health outcomes. One study examined the effect of using the publicly available app, TensionTamer, on BP among patients diagnosed with prehypertension (systolic blood pressure [SBP]: 121–139; n = 64).[70] Participants attended an in-person orientation session to download the app and were randomly assigned to use the Breathing Awareness Meditation sessions for 5-, 10-, or 15-minute intervals twice daily over 6 months. A greater dose (i.e., the 15-minute condition) was associated with reduced adherence, particularly as the program continued. Nevertheless the 15-minute condition was also associated with the greatest reduction in SBP at the 3- and 6-month follow-up. However, all conditions were associated with a significant drop in SBP from baseline, and the effect sizes observed were similar to or greater than in-person meditation studies.[71] Thus app-based MBPs may be an effective alternative to in-person MBPs for prehypertensive individuals. Additionally, longer mobile app–guided meditation (i.e., 15 minutes twice daily) may be ideal during the initial weeks of an MBP and shorter and/or less frequent meditation sessions may be ideal in the following months, which is consistent with preferences reported by stroke survivors enrolled in an at-home MBP.[72] Interestingly, this study measured adherence using built-in photoplethysmography in the TensionTamer app, which collected heart rate throughout each meditation session as the participant placed their index finger on the rear-facing camera on their smartphone. This illustrates just one of the many ways that existing technology can be used to assess adherence to and effects of telerehabilitation mind-body interventions.

Osteoarthritis

Remotely delivered MBPs may also enhance the effectiveness of other rehabilitation therapies. Participants with knee osteoarthritis who were randomly assigned to self-administer transcranial direct current stimulation (tDCS) and listen to a CD of guided mindfulness-based meditation for 20 minutes per day for 10 days reported less pain compared with those assigned to a sham tDCS and sham mindfulness condition (i.e., listening to a CD instructing them to breathe in and out) (n = 30).[73] Though it is not possible to disentangle the effects of mindfulness from those of tDCS in this study, it does suggest that MBPs may be used to augment other telerehabilitation practices.

Summary

Telerehabilitation MBPs lasting at least 4 weeks and involving daily practice for 5 to 15 minutes may lead to improved psychological outcomes, which can have important implications for health and QOL among rehabilitation populations. Unfortunately, much like the in-person research on MBPs for rehabilitation populations, little is known about the direct impacts of telerehabilitation MBPs on functional outcomes. Nevertheless, telerehabilitation MBPs are safe, seem to be feasible even in the face of some technology challenges (e.g., inconsistent internet connection), and may be incorporated with other rehabilitation therapies.

YOGA

Fewer studies have examined telerehabilitation yoga interventions, but initial evidence suggests it is safe and potentially beneficial for individuals diagnosed with heart failure/chronic obstructive pulmonary disease (COPD) and cancer.

Heart Failure/COPD

One nonrandomized trial examined qualitative feedback from six participants with dual heart failure/COPD who participated in a yoga program adapted for heart failure/COPD patients[53] delivered twice weekly for 8 weeks via multipoint videoconference technology (i.e., DocBox).[74] Results suggested the intervention was feasible, as all six participants who began the yoga program attended at least 13 sessions of 18 possible sessions. Qualitative feedback indicated that it was acceptable and motivating, and may be particularly helpful in decreasing breathlessness.[75] Interestingly the technology used in this study (DocBox) allowed participants to livestream yoga classes to their televisions, which had the benefits of presenting the instructor on a relatively large screen, did not require participants to own a tablet or computer, and allowed participants to interact with their instructor, but not other participants. However a member of the research team was required to come to each participant's home to install the videoconference technology (i.e., camera and software), which may not be practical for all rehabilitation settings. Additionally, half of the participants reported having difficulty with their internet connection during classes that prevented them from following the instructor. Participants were divided on their impressions of the group dynamics; half preferred to be able to interact with others and half appreciated the privacy. Thus providing patients with stable internet access and options of attending group or individual yoga classes may be ideal.

Cancer

Another open pilot study collected qualitative feedback from four women undergoing radiation or chemotherapy for breast cancer who participated in a cancer-adapted yoga program[76] twice weekly for 6 weeks using multipoint videoconference software (GoToMeeting), which allowed participants to see and interact with the instructor and other participants.[77] Participants were provided with printed instructions on using the software, and staff were available to provide technical assistance during each class. Recruitment and retention for this study was difficult; a third of those screened did not have internet access, and only half of those who consented attended more than 4 of the 12 possible classes. Thus telerehabilitation programs may need to provide additional support to patients in the form of assistance with internet access and synchronous (i.e., live) orientation to the technology (either in person or via video chat). Additionally, providing telerehabilitation yoga during active chemotherapy/radiotherapy may not be feasible. Indeed, participants suggested the program be offered after active treatment was completed. Qualitative feedback indicated several other areas for improvement, including a more streamlined/user-friendly videoconferencing technology, more class times to accommodate busy schedules, and reduced survey lengths. Thus a user-friendly interface (such as an app) that contains all program content, some of which can be viewed asynchronously in the absence of an internet connection, may be ideal.

Multiple Sclerosis

One ongoing study will examine the effectiveness of a 12-week yoga, Pilates, and neurorehabilitation intervention via 20 prerecorded videos on an app for participants with MS.[57] Though the results of this RCT have not yet been published, the protocol provides several ideas for ways that a yoga intervention may be provided via telerehabilitation. For example, participants are asked to attend an in-person orientation meeting in the clinic with a family or friend present so that they may have assistance in using the app at home. Additionally, participants are classified into four exercise levels, based on their performance on the Timed 25-Foot Walk Test, and are only provided with videos containing exercises/poses appropriate for their functional abilities. As was recommended in previous studies,[77] participants are provided with a tablet, on which the app with appropriate videos is already available, to allow participants to use the program in the absence of internet connection. Additionally, participants will receive regular automated phone calls to encourage adherence. One limitation of this study is the absence of any synchronous yoga instruction, which may be important for sustained interest and adherence.[78]

Heart Disease

Telerehabilitation may also be used to enhance adherence to a home practice of mind-body therapies delivered in person. For example, one study found that cardiac patients discharged from an inpatient rehabilitation program that included yoga training who received four motivational phone calls over the course of 6 months were twice as likely to continue their yoga practice at home postdischarge compared to usual care (n = 228).[79] Participants receiving the motivational phone calls also reported higher mental health-related QOL and had lower SBP compared with usual care 6 months postdischarge. Thus even a very low-intensity telerehabilitation intervention can lead to increased use of rehabilitation techniques, which may in turn lead to improved mental and physical health-related outcomes.

Summary

Telerehabilitation of yoga is novel but shows promise. Reminder phone calls, provision of technological resources (e.g., tablets and/or internet access), and hands-on orientation to technology may increase the feasibility of remotely-delivered yoga.

TAI CHI

Similar to yoga, few studies have examined telerehabilitation Tai Chi interventions for rehabilitation populations, but initial evidence suggests it is safe and potentially beneficial for individuals with cystic fibrosis and elevated fall risk.

Cystic Fibrosis

One RCT compared a Tai Chi program consisting of eight sessions delivered over 3 months via videoconferencing software (Skype) to in-person delivery of the same program for adults and children with cystic fibrosis (n = 40).[58] Both programs had very good engagement and retention rates and both resulted in improved sleep, cough, breathing, and gastrointestinal symptoms. No differences between the telerehabilitation and in-person delivery were observed. Though most participants reported being surprised at how much they benefited from the telerehabilitation, a few reported difficulty with inconsistent internet connection as well as difficulty seeing their instructor clearly on the small screen of their device.[80] Thus assistance with technology (i.e., providing internet access or larger screens) may help increase accessibility for participants.

Increased Fall Risk

Another RCT compared a thrice weekly 15-week group Tai Chi program for older adults at risk for falls delivered in three different ways: synchronously via telerehabilitation (DocBox installed in their home by the research team), synchronously in person at a community center (local YMCA), or asynchronously via prerecorded videos to view at home (n=64).[78] Close to half of participants in the asynchronous condition discontinued the program due to loss of interest, suggesting some synchronous contact with the instructor is important. Both the telerehabilitation and community center Tai Chi programs were associated with significant reduction in falls, improved balance, and increased health-related QOL. This suggests that telerehabilitation Tai Chi may be a feasible, acceptable, and effective intervention for older adults. However, it is important to note that the study team set up DocBox in participants' homes and the instructor viewed participants from three large screens, which may be a challenge for rehabilitation providers in the absence of research funding.

Stroke

Finally, one ongoing study will compare a twice weekly 8-week Tai Chi program for poststroke patients delivered via telerehabilitation versus in person.[54] Though results of this study are not yet available, it is noteworthy that patients are being recruited before they are discharged from an inpatient stay, highlighting the importance of integrating telerehabilitation mind-body programs into patients' larger rehabilitation care.

Summary

Telerehabilitation Tai Chi is novel, but preliminary evidence suggests it may be as effective as in-person Tai Chi at improving health and QOL-related outcomes. Participants may prefer synchronous instruction and may benefit from technological assistance (i.e., sufficiently sized screens and reliable internet connections).

Research Recommendations

Preliminary research suggests that delivering mind-body therapies via telerehabilitation is feasible and acceptable to rehabilitation populations. Though relatively more evidence supports the effectiveness of telerehabilitation MBPs compared to yoga or Tai Chi, more rigorous investigation of each of these integrative approaches is needed.[41] Specifically, high-quality RCTs comparing telerehabilitation mind-body therapies with active control conditions, including in-person mind-body therapies, are essential to determining the effects of these interventions. Additionally, due to the impact of expectancy on outcomes, single-, double-, or triple-blind RCTs are needed. Research is also needed to compare the effects of different program elements (e.g., synchronous vs. asynchronous; individual vs. group; app vs. website platform; text message vs. email vs. automated phone call reminders) on adherence, satisfaction, and clinical outcomes. Additionally, future research should consider including common adherence measures (i.e., logins to the program, time spent viewing the app, etc.)[81] and common outcome measures that include functional limitations, QOL, and disease severity.

Practical Considerations

Ideally, telerehabilitation for integrative health should be integrated as part of the individual's inpatient or outpatient rehabilitation program. This allows for communication among the treatment team, increases trust and safety on the part of the participant,[62] and may also lead to higher patient engagement.[67] However, if a clinic does not have a mind-body therapist on staff, telerehabilitation allows the clinic to partner with a trained individual in any location who can offer these therapies. Providers must also consider whether content will be delivered synchronously (i.e., live sessions that allow for interaction), asynchronously (i.e., prerecorded audio or videos), or both ways (e.g., synchronous weekly sessions with asynchronous content to support daily practice). Previous studies suggest that commonly available videoconferencing programs such as Zoom, GoToMeeting, Webex, or DocBox can be effective methods to providing synchronous sessions. Though DocBox requires equipment be installed in patients' homes, it does allow patients to view the instructor on a larger screen (television). Asynchronous sessions may best be delivered via user-friendly program-specific apps or websites.

Previous research also highlights the importance of live orientation to the chosen technology, so an initial meeting in-person or over video chat, possibly even involving family members who can provide additional assistance, may be particularly useful. If delivering content synchronously, providers will also need to consider whether they prefer their therapy to be delivered in a group or individual format. Evidence suggests both may be beneficial, though a group format may provide much-needed social support to patients who are open to meeting others and may be more cost-effective for providers. Mind-body therapy content should also be adapted to the particular patient population, as evidenced by in-person studies of mind-body therapies. Practice between sessions is essential for any rehabilitation therapy. Telerehabilitation provides patients with reminders via phone call, text message, or smart messaging (i.e., a notification pushed to a device from an app). These types of reminders appear quite effective at increasing home practice[65] and may even increase therapeutic alliance.[82] Thus providers may want to build in reminders to their patients.

CASE STUDY

GROUP TELEREHABILITATION FOR MEDITATION FOR PATIENTS WITH TRAUMATIC BRAIN INJURY

Three patients with traumatic brain injury (TBI) following motor vehicle accidents were provided telerehabilitation meditation sessions as a part of their rehabilitation treatment plan. They were admitted to a postacute brain injury residential rehabilitation center once they were medically stable, where they completed acute intensive rehabilitation 6 to 8 weeks postinjury. Patients A and B presented with moderate expressive aphasia, difficulty with attention to tasks, anxiety, insomnia, and required minimal assistance for activities of daily living and ambulation. Patient C presented with severe expressive aphasia, poor concentration, difficulty initiating and following tasks, and required assistance with activities of daily living and ambulation.

All three individuals were asked to participate in live group meditation sessions delivered via Webex by a rehabilitation physician trained in meditation twice weekly for 6 weeks in the late afternoons, as patients were not engaged in other rehabilitation therapies at that time. Sessions lasted approximately 45 minutes. Each session began with a 10-minute explanation of the proposed meditation exercises, followed by 20 minutes of guided deep breathing exercises, each with 10 repetitions.

- Exercise 1: Guided inhalation and exhalation
- Exercise 2: Guided breathing through alternate nostrils
- Exercise 3: Holding breath after full inhalation (guided), followed by a slow exhalation.

Participants were told that if they could follow the instructions exactly, they simply needed to follow their inhale and exhale. After the breathing exercises, participants were then guided in a 10-minute meditation, in which the provider played soft music and read a meditation script from UCLA's Mindfulness Awareness Resource Center.[83] Finally, participants were encouraged to express their experiences and share one aspect of their life that they were grateful for in this moment.

During the first two sessions, one individual became increasingly agitated and was escorted by a sitter to walk the campus, after which the individual subsequently rejoined the session. None of the participants experienced any adverse effects during the sessions. The participants shared that it was easier to follow the instructions as the sessions continued. Each individual mentioned the meditation sessions as something for which they were grateful, and also reported perceiving a reduction in anxiety, agitation, and sleep disturbance. This remotely-delivered group meditation program suggests the feasibility of participation by persons with cognitive and functional deficits.

References

1. National Center for Complementary and Integrative Health. Complementary, Alternative, or Integrative Health: What's in a Name? https://www.nccih.nih.gov/health/complementary-alternative-or-integrative-health-whats-in-a-name; Updated April 2021. Accessed September 17, 2021.
2. Carlson MJ, Krahn G. Use of complementary and alternative medicine practitioners by people with physical disabilities: estimates from a National US Survey. *Disabil Rehabil*. 2006;28(8):505–513.
3. Quandt SA, Chen H, Grzywacz JG, et al. Use of complementary and alternative medicine by persons with arthritis: results of the National Health Interview Survey. *Arthritis Rheum*. 2005;53(5):748–755.
4. Shah SH, Engelhardt R, Ovbiagele B. Patterns of complementary and alternative medicine use among United States stroke survivors. *J Neurol Sci*. 2008;271(1-2):180–185.
5. Barnes PM, Bloom B, Nahin RL. Complementary and alternative medicine use among adults and children: United States, 2007. *Natl Health Stat Report*. 2008;12:1–23.
6. Okoro CA, Zhao G, Li C, et al. Use of complementary and alternative medicine among US adults with and without functional limitations. *Disabil Rehabil*. 2012;34(2):128–135.
7. Rudra RT, Farkas GJ, Haidar S, et al. Complementary alternative medicine practices and beliefs in spinal cord injury and non-spinal cord injured individuals. *J Spinal Cord Med*. 2018;41(6):659–666.
8. Silbermann E, Senders A, Wooliscroft L, et al. Cross-sectional survey of complementary and alternative medicine used in Oregon and Southwest Washington to treat multiple sclerosis: a 17-year update. *Mult Scler Relat Disord*. 2020;41:102041.
9. Kabat-Zinn J. Mindfulness-based interventions in context: past, present, and future. *Clin Psychol*. 2003;10(2):144–156.
10. Compen F, Bisseling E, Schellekens M, et al. Face-to-face and internet-based mindfulness-based cognitive therapy compared with treatment as usual in reducing psychological distress in patients with cancer: a multicenter randomized controlled trial. *J Clin Oncol*. 2018;36(23):2413–2421.
11. Hardison ME, Roll SC. Mindfulness interventions in physical rehabilitation: a scoping review. *Am J Occup Ther*. 2016;70(3). 7003290030p1-7003290030p9.
12. Zou H, Cao X, Geng J, et al. Effects of mindfulness-based interventions on health-related outcomes for patients with heart failure: a systematic review. *Eur J Cardiovasc Nurs*. 2020;19(1):44–54.
13. Zou L, Sasaki JE, Zeng N, et al. A systematic review with meta-analysis of mindful exercises on rehabilitative outcomes among poststroke patients. *Arch Phys Med Rehabil*. 2018;99(11):2355–2364.
14. Gray LA. Living the full catastrophe: a mindfulness-based program to support recovery from stroke. *Healthcare (Basel)*. 2020;8(4):498.

15. DiRenzo D, Crespo-Bosque M, Gould N, et al. Systematic review and meta-analysis: mindfulness-based interventions for rheumatoid arthritis. *Curr Rheumatol Rep.* 2018;20(12):1–11.

16. Hearn JH, Cross A. Mindfulness for pain, depression, anxiety, and quality of life in people with spinal cord injury: a systematic review. *BMC Neurol.* 2020;20(1):32. https://doi.org/10.1186/s12883-020-1619-5.

17. Levin AB, Hadgkiss EJ, Weiland TJ, et al. Meditation as an adjunct to the management of multiple sclerosis. *Neurol Res Int.* 2014;2014:704691.

18. Carlson LE. Mindfulness-based interventions for coping with cancer. *Ann NY Acad Sci.* 2016;1373(1): 5–12.

19. Xunlin N, Lau Y, Klainin-Yobas P. The effectiveness of mindfulness-based interventions among cancer patients and survivors: a systematic review and meta-analysis. *Support Care Cancer.* 2020; 28(4):1563–1578.

20. Hilton L, Hempel S, Ewing BA, et al. Mindfulness meditation for chronic pain: systematic review and meta-analysis. *Ann Behav Med.* 2017;51(2):199–213. https://doi.org/10.1007/s12160-016-9844-2.

21. Zgierska AE, Burzinski CA, Cox J, et al. Mindfulness meditation and cognitive behavioral therapy intervention reduces pain severity and sensitivity in opioid-treated chronic low back pain: pilot findings from a randomized controlled trial. *Pain Med.* 2016;17(10):1865–1881. https://doi.org/10.1093/pm/pnw006.

22. Zeidan F, Vago DR. Mindfulness meditation-based pain relief: a mechanistic account. *Ann N Y Acad Sci.* 2016;1373(1):114–127. https://doi.org/10.1111/nyas.13153.

23. Zeidan F, Martucci KT, Kraft RA, et al. Brain mechanisms supporting the modulation of pain by mindfulness meditation. *J Neurosci.* 2011;31(14):5540–5548. https://doi.org/10.1523/JNEUROSCI. 5791-10.2011.

24. Omidi A, Zargar F. Effect of mindfulness-based stress reduction on pain severity and mindful awareness in patients with tension headache: a randomized controlled clinical trial. *Nurs Midwifery Stud.* 2014;3(3):e21136. https://doi.org/10.17795/nmsjournal21136.

25. Miller-Matero LR, Coleman JP, Smith-Mason CE, et al. A brief mindfulness intervention for medically hospitalized patients with acute pain: a pilot randomized clinical trial. *Pain Med.* 2019;20(11):2149–2154.

26. Feuerstein G. *The Deeper Dimension of Yoga: Theory and Practice.* United States: Shambhala Publications; 2003.

27. Wieland LS, Skoetz N, Pilkington K, et al. Yoga treatment for chronic non-specific low back pain. *Cochrane Database Syst Rev.* 2017;1:CD010671. https://doi.org/10.1002/14651858.CD010671.pub2.

28. Ward L, Stebbings S, Cherkin D, et al. Yoga for functional ability, pain and psychosocial outcomes in musculoskeletal conditions: a systematic review and meta-analysis. *Musculoskeletal Care.* 2013;11(4):203–217.

29. Danhauer SC, Addington EL, Sohl SJ, et al. Review of yoga therapy during cancer treatment. *Support Care.* 2017;25(4):1357–1372.

30. Brenes GA, Sohl S, Wells RE, et al. The effects of yoga on patients with mild cognitive impairment and dementia: a scoping review. *Am J Geriatr Psychiatry.* 2019;27(2):188–197.

31. Cramer H, Lauche R, Haller H, et al. Effects of yoga on cardiovascular disease risk factors: a systematic review and meta-analysis. *Int J Cardiol.* 2014;173(2):170–183.

32. Amaravathi E, Ramarao NH, Raghuram N, et al. Yoga-based postoperative cardiac rehabilitation program for improving quality of life and stress levels: fifth-year follow-up through a randomized controlled trial. *Int J Yoga.* 2018;11(1):44.

33. Prabhakaran D, Chandrasekaran AM, Singh K, et al. Yoga-based cardiac rehabilitation after acute myocardial infarction: a randomized trial. *J Am Coll Cardiol.* 2020;75(13):1551–1561.

34. Desveaux L, Lee A, Goldstein R, et al. Yoga in the management of chronic disease. *Medical Care.* 2015;53(7):653–661.

35. Lawrence M, Junior FTC, Matozinho HH, et al. Yoga for stroke rehabilitation. *Cochrane Database Syst Rev.* 2017;12(12).

36. Koertge J, Weidner G, Elliott-Eller M, et al. Improvement in medical risk factors and quality of life in women and men with coronary artery disease in the Multicenter Lifestyle Demonstration Project. *Am J Cardiol.* 2003;91(11):1316–1322.

37. Cramer H, Lauche R, Azizi H, et al. Yoga for multiple sclerosis: a systematic review and meta-analysis. *PLoS One.* 2014;9(11):e112414.

38. Curtis K, Hitzig SL, Bechsgaard G, et al. Evaluation of a specialized yoga program for persons with a spinal cord injury: a pilot randomized controlled trial. *J Pain Res.* 2017;10:999–1017. https://doi. org/10.2147/JPR.S130530.

39. Wayne PM, Kaptchuk TJ. Challenges inherent to t'ai chi research: part I—t'ai chi as a complex multi-component intervention. *J Altern Complement Med*. 2008;14(1):95–102.
40. Kong LJ, Lauche R, Klose P, et al. Tai chi for chronic pain conditions: a systematic review and meta-analysis of randomized controlled trials. *Sci Rep*. 2016;6(1):1–9.
41. Hall A, Copsey B, Richmond H, et al. Effectiveness of tai chi for chronic musculoskeletal pain conditions: updated systematic review and meta-analysis. *Phys Ther*. 2017;97(2):227–238. https://doi.org/10.2522/ptj.20160246.
42. Wayne PM, Lee M, Novakowski J, et al. Tai chi and qigong for cancer-related symptoms and quality of life: a systematic review and meta-analysis. *J Cancer Surviv*. 2018;12(2):256–267.
43. Zou L, Wang H, Xiao Z, et al. Tai chi for health benefits in patients with multiple sclerosis: a systematic review. *PloS One*. 2017;12(2):e0170212.
44. Lauche R, Peng W, Ferguson C, et al. Efficacy of tai chi and qigong for the prevention of stroke and stroke risk factors: a systematic review with meta-analysis. *Medicine (Baltimore)*. 2017;96(45):e8517.
45. Lyu D, Lyu X, Zhang Y, et al. Tai chi for stroke rehabilitation: a systematic review and meta-analysis of randomized controlled trials. *Front Physiol*. 2018;9:983.
46. Shem K, Karasik D, Carufel P, et al. Seated tai chi to alleviate pain and improve quality of life in individuals with spinal cord disorder. *J Spinal Cord Med*. 2016;39(3):353–358. https://doi.org/10.1080/10790268.2016.1148895.
47. Tsang WW, Gao KL, Chan KM, et al. Sitting tai chi improves the balance control and muscle strength of community-dwelling persons with spinal cord injuries: a pilot study. *Evid Based Complement Alternat Med*. 2015;2015:523852. https://doi.org/10.1155/2015/523852.
48. Qi Y, Xie H, Shang Y, et al. Effects of 16-form wheelchair tai chi on the autonomic nervous system among patients with spinal cord injury. *Evid Based Complement Alternat Med*. 2020;2020:6626603. https://doi.org/10.1155/2020/6626603.
49. Rao A, Zecchin R, Newton PJ, et al. The prevalence and impact of depression and anxiety in cardiac rehabilitation: a longitudinal cohort study. *Eur J Prev Cardiol*. 2020;27(5):478–489.
50. Rimmer JH, Chen M-D, Hsieh K. A conceptual model for identifying, preventing, and managing secondary conditions in people with disabilities. *Phys Ther*. 2011;91(12):1728–1739.
51. DiMatteo MR, Lepper HS, Croghan TW. Depression is a risk factor for noncompliance with medical treatment: meta-analysis of the effects of anxiety and depression on patient adherence. *Arch Intern Med*. 2000;160(14):2101–2107.
52. Tenforde AS, Hefner JE, Kodish-Wachs JE, et al. Telehealth in physical medicine and rehabilitation: a narrative review. *PM&R*. 2017;9(5):S51–S58.
53. Donesky-Cuenco D, Nguyen HQ, Paul S, et al. Yoga therapy decreases dyspnea-related distress and improves functional performance in people with chronic obstructive pulmonary disease: a pilot study. *J Altern Complement Med*. 2009;15(3):225–234.
54. Tousignant M, Corriveau H, Kairy D, et al. Tai chi-based exercise program provided via telerehabilitation compared to home visits in a post-stroke population who have returned home without intensive rehabilitation: study protocol for a randomized, non-inferiority clinical trial. *Trials*. 2014;15(1):1–9.
55. McCall M, Thorne S, Ward A, et al. Yoga in adult cancer: an exploratory, qualitative analysis of the patient experience. *BMC Complement Altern Med*. 2015;15(1):1–9.
56. Danhauer SC, Griffin LP, Avis NE, et al. Feasibility of implementing a community-based randomized trial of yoga for women undergoing chemotherapy for breast cancer. *J Community Support Oncol*. 2015;13(4):139.
57. Rimmer JH, Thirumalai M, Young H-J, et al. Rationale and design of the tele-exercise and multiple sclerosis (TEAMS) study: a comparative effectiveness trial between a clinic- and home-based telerehabilitation intervention for adults with multiple sclerosis (MS) living in the deep south. *Contemp Clin Trials*. 2018;71:186–193.
58. Carr SB, Ronan P, Lorenc A, et al. Children and Adults Tai Chi Study (CF-CATS2): a randomised controlled feasibility study comparing internet-delivered with face-to-face Tai Chi lessons in cystic fibrosis. *ERJ Open Res*. 2018;4(4). 00042-2018.
59. Koonin LM, Hoots B, Tsang CA, et al. Trends in the use of telehealth during the emergence of the COVID-19 pandemic—United States, January–March 2020. *MMWR Morb Mortal Wkly Rep*. 2020;69(43):1595.

60. Wade VA, Karnon J, Elshaug AG, et al. A systematic review of economic analyses of telehealth services using real time video communication. *BMC Health Serv Res.* 2010;10(1):1–13.
61. Snoswell CL, Taylor ML, Comans TA, et al. Determining if telehealth can reduce health system costs: scoping review. *J Med Internet Res.* 2020;22(10):e17298.
62. Matis J, Svetlak M, Slezackova A, et al. Mindfulness-based programs for patients with cancer via eHealth and mobile health: systematic review and synthesis of quantitative research. *J Med Internet Res.* 2020;22(11):e20709.
63. Cillessen L, Johannsen M, Speckens AE, et al. Mindfulness-based interventions for psychological and physical health outcomes in cancer patients and survivors: a systematic review and meta-analysis of randomized controlled trials. *Psychooncology.* 2019;28(12):2257–2269.
64. Warth M, Zöller J, Köhler F, et al. Psychosocial interventions for pain management in advanced cancer patients: a systematic review and meta-analysis. *Curr Oncol Rep.* 2020;22(1):1–9.
65. Wells C, Malins S, Clarke S, et al. Using smart-messaging to enhance mindfulness-based cognitive therapy for cancer patients: a mixed methods proof of concept evaluation. *Psychooncology.* 2020;29(1):212–219.
66. Bohlmeijer E, Prenger R, Taal E, et al. The effects of mindfulness-based stress reduction therapy on mental health of adults with a chronic medical disease: a meta-analysis. *J Psychosom Res.* 2010;68(6):539–544.
67. Cavalera C, Rovaris M, Mendozzi L, et al. Online meditation training for people with multiple sclerosis: a randomized controlled trial. *Mult Scler.* 2019;25(4):610–617.
68. Grossman P, Kappos L, Gensicke H, et al. MS quality of life, depression, and fatigue improve after mindfulness training: a randomized trial. *Neurology.* 2010;75(13):1141–1149.
69. Hearn JH, Finlay KA. Internet-delivered mindfulness for people with depression and chronic pain following spinal cord injury: a randomized, controlled feasibility trial. *Spinal Cord.* 2018;56(8):750.
70. Adams ZW, Sieverdes JC, Brunner-Jackson B, et al. Meditation smartphone application effects on prehypertensive adults' blood pressure: dose-response feasibility trial. *Health Psychol.* 2018;37(9):850.
71. Dickinson H, Campbell F, Beyer F, et al. Relaxation therapies for the management of primary hypertension in adults: a Cochrane review. *J Hum Hypertens.* 2008;22(12):809–820.
72. Wang X, Smith C, Ashley L, et al. Tailoring self-help mindfulness and relaxation techniques for stroke survivors: examining preferences, feasibility and acceptability. *Front Psychol.* 2019;10:391.
73. Ahn H, Zhong C, Miao H, et al. Efficacy of combining home-based transcranial direct current stimulation with mindfulness-based meditation for pain in older adults with knee osteoarthritis: a randomized controlled pilot study. *J Clin Neurosci.* 2019;70:140–145.
74. Selman L, McDermott K, Donesky D, et al. Appropriateness and acceptability of a tele-yoga intervention for people with heart failure and chronic obstructive pulmonary disease: qualitative findings from a controlled pilot study. *BMC Complement Altern Med.* 2015;15(1):1–13.
75. Donesky D, Selman L, McDermott K, et al. Evaluation of the feasibility of a home-based TeleYoga intervention in participants with both chronic obstructive pulmonary disease and heart failure. *J Altern Complement Med.* 2017;23(9):713–721.
76. Danhauer SC, Mihalko SL, Russell GB, et al. Restorative yoga for women with breast cancer: findings from a randomized pilot study. *Psychooncology.* 2009;18(4):360–368.
77. Addington EL, Sohl SJ, Tooze JA, et al. Convenient and Live Movement (CALM) for women undergoing breast cancer treatment: challenges and recommendations for internet-based yoga research. *Complement Ther Med.* 2018;37:77–79.
78. Wu G, Keyes L, Callas P, et al. Comparison of telecommunication, community, and home-based Tai Chi exercise programs on compliance and effectiveness in elders at risk for falls. *Arch Phys Med Rehabil.* 2010;91(6):849–856.
79. Schröer S, Mayer-Berger W, Pieper C. Effect of telerehabilitation on long-term adherence to yoga as an antihypertensive lifestyle intervention: results of a randomized controlled trial. *Complement Ther Clin Pract.* 2019;35:148–153.
80. Ronan P, Mian A, Carr SB, et al. Learning to breathe with Tai Chi online-qualitative data from a randomized controlled feasibility study of patients with cystic fibrosis. *Eur J Integr Med.* 2020;40:101229.
81. Donkin L, Christensen H, Naismith SL, et al. A systematic review of the impact of adherence on the effectiveness of e-therapies. *J Med Internet Res.* 2011;13(3):e52.
82. Clough BA, Casey LM. Technological adjuncts to increase adherence to therapy: a review. *Clin Psychol Res.* 2011;31(5):697–710.
83. UCLA. Mindful Awareness Research Center. https://www.uclahealth.org/marc/.

CHAPTER 16

Telerehabilitation in Neurogenic Bladder and Bowel Dysfunction

Christina-Anastasia Rapidi ■ Giulio Del Popolo ■ Michele Spinelli
■ Antonis Kontaxakis ■ Renatos Vasilakis ■ Gianluca Sampogna

Introduction

NEUROGENIC BOWEL AND BLADDER DYSFUNCTION

The lower abdominal area includes organs carrying out essential functions, like urination, defecation, sexual activity, and fertility. The lower urinary tract (LUT), distal gastrointestinal (GI) tract, and genital system interact under both physiological and pathological conditions.[1] Pelvic physiological function depends on coordinated communication among all organs of the sacral area. The LUT and distal GI tract share a common embryological origin, innervation, and functions of storage and excretion phases of urine and feces, respectively. Pelvic cross-sensitization among pelvic organs is conveyed by neural, endocrine, paracrine, and immune mechanisms. Diseases in one of the pelvic organs may provoke alterations in their cross-talk, subsequently causing clinical comorbidities within a single anatomical structure. Experimental data, from both human and animal studies, suggest different cause-and-effect interactions; for example, chronic intestinal inflammation may provoke changes in detrusor activity with increased frequency of micturition, while neurogenic cystitis may be associated with abdominal hyperalgesia.[2] The understanding of these altered cross-reflexes is mandatory to identify potential targets to plan and perform effective treatments in patients with comorbid disorders like neurogenic bladder and bowel dysfunction.

Neurogenic bladder and bowel dysfunction occur as a consequence of many different diseases or traumatic injuries of the central or peripheral nervous system, for example, spinal cord injury (SCI), spina bifida (SB), multiple sclerosis (MS), Parkinson's disease (PD), stroke, and traumatic brain injury (TBI).[3] Neurogenic sexual dysfunction is a common comorbidity, but it will be discussed in another chapter.

Neurogenic bladder dysfunction may present with different symptoms. The physiological bladder cycle encompasses two phases.[4] During the filling phase, bladder distention takes place under low pressures and the inner urinary sphincter remains closed due to the influence of the sympathetic nervous system (SNS), via the T10–L2 nerve roots, while the external urinary sphincter remains closed via the pudendal nerves originating from the S2–S4 nerve roots. During the voiding phase, the bladder contracts under the influence of the parasympathetic nervous system (PNS), via the S2–S4 nerve roots, and the urinary sphincter relaxes to allow emptying.

LUT symptoms (LUTS) may be classified into two categories: obstructive LUTS, such as weak and/or intermittent stream, straining, hesitancy, terminal dribbling, incomplete voiding, urinary retention, and overflow incontinence; and voiding or irritative LUTS, such as polyuria, urge incontinence, painful urination, and nocturia.[5]

When the bladder contracts involuntarily before complete filling, the condition is called detrusor overactivity (DO).[6] On the other hand, when the bladder cannot empty urine effectively, the associated condition is defined as detrusor underactivity (DU). Similarly, the sphincter may be either overactive or underactive. Detrusor-sphincter dyssynergia (DSD) happens in case of altered coordination between the overactive detrusor and overactive urinary sphincter, causing a dysfunctional condition, characterized by the persistence of an elevated postvoid residual (PVR) and increased detrusor pressures associated with the risk for vesico-ureteral reflux.

Urinary incontinence (UI) may be classified as urgency urinary incontinence (UUI), complaints of involuntary loss of urine associated with urgency; stress urinary incontinence (SUI), complaints of involuntary loss of urine on effort or physical exertion including sporting activities, sneezing, or coughing; and mixed urinary incontinence (MUI).

Neurogenic bladder dysfunction–related symptoms are predominantly due to the location and the extent of the neurological lesion.[7]

- Suprapontine lesions:
  - **Examples:** PD, Alzheimer's disease, stroke, TBI
  - **History:** predominantly storage symptoms
  - **Findings:** DO, insignificant PVR
- Spinal lesions between the pons and the sacral cord:
  - **Examples:** SCI, SB
  - **History:** both storage and voiding symptoms
  - **Findings:** DO, DSS, usually raised PVR
- Sacral and infrasacral lesions:
  - **Examples:** lumbar degenerative disc disease, iatrogenic pelvic nerve lesions, peripheral neuropathy (e.g., due to diabetes)
  - **History:** predominantly voiding symptoms
  - **Findings:** DU, acontractile detrusor, high PVR
- MS is a disseminated disease, so it can present different and overlapping clinical features based on the extent and localization of demyelination plaques.

Neurogenic bowel dysfunction (NBD) comprises both constipation and fecal incontinence. The latter may be due to the altered control of the anal sphincter or, mainly, to loss of liquid stool because of impacted feces in the rectum. Similar to the bladder, the distal GI tract is innervated by the SNS and PNS via the T10–L2 and S2–S4 nerve roots, respectively.

All members of the rehabilitation team take part in neurogenic bladder and bowel management through their different roles during all phases of rehabilitation.[8] However, rehabilitation does not end after in-patient hospitalization. In people with disabilities due to nervous system diseases, outpatient services are needed for longer periods to reach the highest level of functional capacity and performance, and later to sustain abilities gained from the initial rehabilitation program throughout life.[9,10]

The impact of neurogenic bladder and bowel on health-related quality of life (HRQoL) is well documented in the literature.[11,12] After SCI, persons with paraplegia prefer optimal function of bladder and bowel to ambulation, or at least both seem to be of equal importance.[13,14] With this in mind, good quality long-life management of neurogenic bladder and bowel is a high priority for the rehabilitation team.

Information and communication technology (ICT) has expanded greatly over the past decade and is now available to the majority of the world's population. Telerehabilitation services previously demanded expensive technology, special rooms, and special precautions for keeping personal information safe. At present, however, simplification has addressed many technical problems pertinent to bladder and bowel management via telerehabilitation and future improvements are a logical expectation.

In this chapter we will provide an overview of current knowledge and practice related to using telerehabilitation for bladder and bowel management along with reviewing areas that warrant further research and development.

Literature Review

METHODOLOGY

In order to determine the state of the science with regard to the use of telerehabilitation for neurogenic bladder and bowel management, the authors performed an extensive narrative research using PubMed, Scopus, and Web of Science, without finding significant original studies involving telehealth in the fields of neurogenic bladder and bowel dysfunction, but mainly expert opinions.[15] We accessed ClinicalTrials.gov on November 10, 2020, and found a recruiting study assessing the efficiency and satisfaction with telephone consultation in neuro-urology. The following search strategy took place (last update on November 15, 2020): (telerehabilitation OR telehealth OR telemedicine OR televisit OR teleconsultation) AND (bladder OR bowel OR incontinence OR continence OR urology OR gastroenterology OR coloproctology). We found 837 articles and, finally, included 23 articles (Fig. 16.1). We observed an exponential increase in the number of papers in the year 2020 (Fig. 16.2) after the COVID-19 pandemic. Most articles dealt with general interventions in urology, views, expert opinions, and guidance on telehealth. Fewer studies involved GI diseases. Most papers presented pilot studies in bladder and bowel remote management of persons with neurological diseases, presenting mainly educational/observational data on the telehealth services provided (Table 16.1).

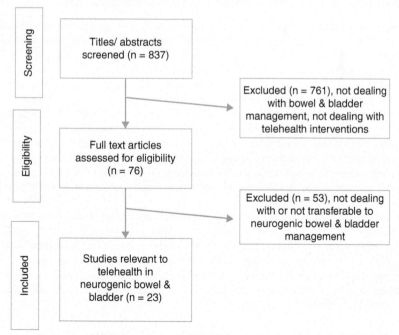

Fig. 16.1 Flow chart of our search, performed on November 15, 2020, using PubMed, Scopus, and Web of Science, and typing the following keywords: (Telerehabilitation OR telehealth OR telemedicine OR televisit OR teleconsultation) AND (bladder OR bowel OR incontinence OR continence OR urology OR gastroenterology OR coloproctology).

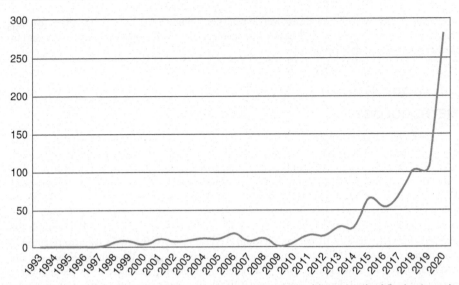

Fig. 16.2 The picture depicts the number of papers per year, obtained by typing the following terms in PubMed on November 15, 2020: (Telerehabilitation) OR (telehealth) OR (telemedicine) OR (televisit) OR (tele-consultation) AND (bladder) OR (bowel) OR (incontinence) OR (continence) OR (urology) OR (gastroenterology) OR (coloproctology). An exponential growth occurred in the year 2020, after the COVID-19 pandemic.

NONNEUROGENIC BOWEL AND BLADDER DYSFUNCTION

A recent systematic review by Novara et al. looked for urological applications of telehealth and identified 45 studies, concerning UI (n = 14), prostate cancer (n = 11), urolithiasis (n = 6), hematuria management (n = 3), urinary tract infections (UTIs; n = 5), general urology (n = 2), LUTS (n = 2), and male sexual dysfunction (n = 2).[16] The methodological quality of most studies was estimated as "good," reporting 12 studies involving randomized controlled trials (RCTs).

A vital part of telehealth interventions is represented by smartphone applications. Although most data are on nonneurogenic UI management, results can be transferable. A systematic review in urology applications, in 2015, revealed 150 applications, with one-third of them focused on calculators, diaries, and patient information, while the need for scientific approval and peer-review application validation was recognized.[17] In chronic GI disorders, another review in self-monitoring presented several applications controlling GI symptoms.[18] Comparing electronic and paper micturition charts, the same level of accuracy was documented, possibly with better adherence to electronic ones.[19]

A plethora of such interventions has been created and validated for pelvic floor muscle training, with 73 studies reported by Latorre et al.[20] Applications such as iPelvis, Kegel Trainer Pro, Tät application, and MyHealtheBladder are available, even if most of them have been not validated.[21-23] Bernard et al. highlighted the role and importance of conservative UI self-management through mobile technologies, identifying the features of data extraction, educational features, reinforcements, reminder systems, social media features, self-monitoring options, and biofeedback.[24]

NEUROGENIC BOWEL AND BLADDER DYSFUNCTION

In 2018 a narrative review of eHealth technologies for MS analyzed data from 28 eHealth solutions, finding "MS monitor" as an interactive, internet-based program for self-monitoring,

TABLE 16.1 ■ Overview of the Articles Found on Neurogenic Bladder and Bowel Telehealth Interventions.

Authors	Type	Population	Interventions	Functions	Conclusions
Jongen et al. (2016)	Utility study	Patients with multiple sclerosis (MS; n = 55)	Digital and remote communication technologies—"MS Monitor"	Interactive, internet-based program for self-monitoring, self-management, and integrated multidisciplinary care	In 46% (25/55) of the respondents, the insight into their symptoms and disabilities increased. The overall satisfaction with the program was 3.5 out of 5, and 73% (40/55) of the respondents would recommend the program to other persons with MS
Beadnall et al. (2015)	Feasibility study	Patients with MS (n = 157)	Digital and remote communication technologies—"TaDiMus"	Bladder Control Scale (BLCS); Bowel Control Scale (BWCS)	The mean time taken to complete the BLCS and BWCS was 56.6 s and 39.3 s, respectively. A total of 184 continence test sets (BLCS and BWCS) were completed; an electronic referral for formal continence review was automatically generated 128 times (68.8%) in 108 patients (68.8%), when scores ≥2 in the BLCS or BWCS were achieved
Levy et al. (2014)	Pilot study	Patients with spina bifida (n = 6)	Virtual nurse-led clinic	Support a small cohort of service users and their parents from home	Using Skype to support young people with complex needs is an effective intervention to support continence care at home
Choi et al. (2019)	Feasibility study	Patients with spina bifida (n = 5)	Mobile health application "Glowing Stars"	Integrative educational program, with health indicators for self-monitoring of voiding, defecation, skin care, taking medication, and mood status	Participants experienced an understanding of their condition, demonstrated motivation for self-management and feasibility for self-management maintenance
Sechrist et al. (2018)	Prospective observational study	Patients with spinal cord injury (n = 66)	Telemedicine (TM) visits via iPad through FaceTime	TM appointment for nonemergency needs through a liaison	26.53% (n = 26) discussed bowel and bladder, 100% of responders ranged from slightly agree to strongly agree recommending the TM program, and 88.90% (n = 40) believed the care received through TM was just as good as seeing a physician or nurse in person

Continued

TABLE 16.1 ■ Overview of the Articles Found on Neurogenic Bladder and Bowel Telehealth Interventions. —cont'd

Authors	Type	Population	Interventions	Functions	Conclusions
Yu et al. (2015)	Pilot study	Patients with spina bifida	Mobile health system called "iMHere"	To support preventive self-care for managing medications (MyMeds), neurogenic bladder (TeleCath), and bowel (BMQs), mood (Mood), and skin breakdown (SkinCare)	Telehealth usability questionnaire score was (6.52 out of 7 points, 93%). All of the participants were satisfied with the iMHere applications and would use them again in the future
Carter et al. (2019)	Proof-of-concept study	Patients with spina bifida (n = 8)	Telehealth intervention through a home urinalysis device	A system that recorded and alerted parents and urology nursing staff to signs of likely urine infection	Remote community urinalysis monitoring by parents of their child's urine was possible; the team had to manage a fluctuating telehealth workload
De Souza et al. (2017)	Pilot study	Patients with neurogenic bladder (n = 15)	Synchronous telenursing intervention by audio calls, chat, and asynchronous by email	Care delivery for neurogenic bladder patients using CIC (clean intermittent catheterization)	The potential of the telenursing intervention was demonstrated as a complement to the patients' traditional health treatment
Huri and Hamid (2020)	Expert opinion—International continence society	Neurogenic patients			Telerehabilitation is the main technology-based tool to keep neuro-urological patients out of the hospital environment. It is bridging the gap between people, physicians, and health systems, enabling everyone, especially symptomatic patients, to stay at home and communicate with physicians in virtual ways, helping to decrease the spread of the virus

self-management, and multidisciplinary care of individuals with MS.[25] Inventories to capture urological symptom data and diaries in parallel with an e-consultation were included. It was shown that through repeated use, HRQoL was increased and the quality of nursing care was improved. TaDiMuS (Tablet-based Data capture in Multiple Sclerosis), a tablet-based platform tool, which included the Bladder Control Scale and the Bowel Control Scale, proved to be an efficient, sensitive, and feasible method of screening patients for bladder and bowel dysfunction.[25]

Another population, where these interventions have been studied, is represented by SB. A nurse-led continence clinic assisted users through Skype to improve their self-care skills in a small qualitative study.[26] Glowing Stars is an Android-based application, which includes an educational module on bladder and bowel management, and an opportunity to record health indicators for self-monitoring of voiding, defecation, skin care, taking medication, and mood status.[27] In SCI, a telerehabilitation intervention using FaceTime with an iPad (Apple Inc., Cupertino, USA) was tested in 62 individuals, dealing with—amongst other concerns—bowel and bladder issues, revealing high levels of satisfaction.[28]

BENEFITS AND BARRIERS

Telehealth visits, apart from being less time-consuming, can also reduce the number of in-person visits of low acuity patients. Patients value them because of savings of time and money.[29] People are willing to participate in virtual visits (VVs) for their bladder care, specifically individuals who are more confident with internet-based communication, as well as individuals who take an active role in their own health.[30] Even if an in-person examination is required, this can still be offered following a VV.[31]

Barriers in adopting telehealth services are multifactorial. There can be aversion to change in providers and health care systems, concerns about patient privacy, and specific issues with reimbursement.[32,33] Moreover, one can ask the ethical question: "What if face-to-face visits become available or affordable only for patients with adequate resources, leaving the rest treated through telemedical consultants?"[34]

With a focus on technical adjustment, patient-related barriers include concerns about security and data protection, lack of familiarity with ICT, and difficulty with accessing a high-speed internet connection. Technological failure may significantly undermine the safety and efficacy of telehealth applications. Therefore it is important to give the patient enough time to prepare for the televisit, organize a technical service for troubleshooting, and have a backup plan in case of failure.

From a similar viewpoint, provider-related barriers include technological proficiency of doctors. As every novel health technology, it may require specific training.[35] Although telerehabilitation-related changes may appear small, they may require a significant amount of training, as they involve significant structural changes in work organization. Clinical staff may resist the adoption of telehealth for different reasons: alteration of the roles of staff members, change of the established routine clinical practice, and perceived risk of breaking down the patient-provider relationship.[29]

Telerehabilitation for Neurogenic Bladder and Bowel

INTRODUCTION

Often, compliance with therapeutic and regular follow-up care for people with a long-standing illness or health problem is unsatisfactory. Many patients face difficulties in accessing rehabilitation services, regardless of the economic situation of different countries. Various factors—such as the lack of specialized services in remote geographical areas, transportation difficulties, increased traveling risk under extreme weather conditions or natural disasters, and conditions such as the

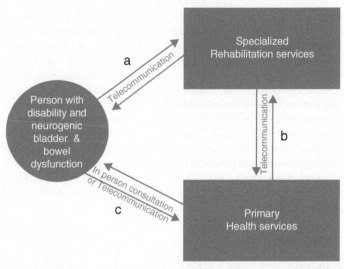

Fig. 16.3 Remote rehabilitation services for neurogenic bladder and bowel management. *(a)* Specialized health practitioner to/from patient and caregiver; *(b)* health practitioner to/from health practitioner; *(c)* nonspecialized health practitioner to/from patient and caregiver with in-person consultation or telecommunication.

COVID-19 pandemic—increase these difficulties and make access to specialized rehabilitation services almost impossible. The provision of remote health services has fortunately been simplified with the development of technology in the decade of 2010–2019, and the COVID-19 pandemic has boosted the widespread adoption of telehealth.[36]

Remote rehabilitation services concerning neurogenic bladder and bowel dysfunction may refer to:

1. Communication between specialized physicians, continence nurses, and therapists and patients at their home for reevaluation and assurance of patients' compliance and continuation of the rehabilitation program and management of neurogenic bladder and bowel (Fig. 16.3A);
2. Communication between health professionals in different geographical areas and provision of specialized knowledge to general practitioners (GPs) and other health professionals (nurses, occupational therapists, physiotherapists) in the same region as the patient and assurance of continued rehabilitation of neurogenic bladder and bowel (Fig. 16.3B);
3. The communication between GPs, nurses, and therapists and patients at their home for reevaluation and assurance of patients' compliance and continuation of the rehabilitation program and management of neurogenic bladder and bowel either in person or with telecommunication (Fig. 16.3C).

Remote health services for neurogenic bladder and bowel could reduce the cost of health care, by minimizing the number of in-person visits at specialized health care facilities, hospital readmissions, complications, and use of medication that could be avoided (e.g., use of antibiotics in misdiagnosed UTIs).[29,37]

Telerehabilitation services concerning neurogenic bladder and bowel dysfunction should only be provided by a health care team that knows and regularly cares for the specific patient. This team can also supervise and continue their therapeutic and educational program and follow-up remotely. Moreover, they can improve the patient's compliance and lessen complications with or without the collaboration of professionals of primary health services.

A web-based survey evaluated patient demographics, perceptions before use, and acceptance of VVs within an ambulatory urology setting.[30] In total, 1378 patients completed the survey.

Compared with those who were "unlikely," patients "likely" (63%) to participate in VV were younger (62 vs. 65 years), had a college education (77% vs. 65%), had previous exposure to video-conference technology (57% vs. 38%), were more comfortable discussing new symptoms (56% vs. 30%) and sensitive information (48% vs. 27%), played an active role in their health care (65% vs. 54%), traveled larger distances (>90 minutes; 69% vs. 58%), missed more work days (>1 day; 39% vs. 29%), and incurred greater expenses for their care (>$250; 52% vs. 25%).

Many studies have shown the implementation of telerehabilitation in different settings both in urology and gastroenterology.[38,39] Most studies approached telehealth adopting phone consultations and televisits, that is, digital office visits with the urologist and the patient seeing each other remotely via webcam. Another validated application involves teleconsultations, that is, electronic communication between two health care providers regarding the patient's diagnosis and/or treatment. Few studies evaluated other approaches, like telementoring, telesurgery, telerounding, or teleimaging.

TELEPHONE CONSULTATIONS

Safir et al. had 150 patients with hematuria undergoing a 20- to 25-minute long structured interview and consultation via telephone.[40] Later, these patients underwent a cystoscopy and, during this examination, they filled in a 29-question survey regarding their overall acceptance and satisfaction with the telephone consultation. The median time from consult request to appointment was 12 days, and thereafter to cystoscopy was 16 days. The patients reported high acceptance and satisfaction with the telephone consultations in terms of overall satisfaction, efficiency, convenience, friendliness, care quality, understandability, privacy, and professionalism. It was found that 98% of patients preferred phone consultation to face-to-face visits. Transportation-related issues (97%) and logistical clinic issues (65%) were identified as factors responsible for patients' preferences toward phone consultations.

TELEVISITS

Televisits provide face-to-face communication at distance better than phone calls. Video can allow evaluation of the patient's environment, physical status, and the observation of some procedures, like urinary catheterization. Most doctors perform telehealth without even realizing it, including phone calls and asynchronous messages via email or fax. These practices are usually not reimbursed, while synchronous VVs are beginning to be reimbursed by many payers. In the United States, Veterans Affairs hospitals pioneered the application of telerehabilitation with the initial attempt to deliver high-quality care in rural areas.[41] Rastogi et al. performed a cross-sectional observational study including 20,600 patients using direct-to-consumer telerehabilitation.[42] Most patients (96%) were female. Up to 84% of encounters were for UTI. In this cluster, 94% received an antibiotic, and receiving the prescription was associated with higher satisfaction with care ($P < 0.001$). The management of UTIs via telerehabilitation proved to be feasible and cost-effective, considering the lower cost of televisits compared to traditional outpatient or urgent care.

TELECONSULTATIONS

Teleconsultation has been used for decades to link tertiary-referral academic centers to smaller rural centers. This concept is particularly interesting in niche subspecialties with a dearth of centers, like neuro-urology, neuro-gastroenterology, and fetal urology. The Arkansas statewide telerehabilitation service allowed patients to combine maternal-fetal medicine and urological prenatal consultations in one visit, saving time and effort and ultimately, for most patients, providing reassurance that delivery could be accomplished locally with postnatal follow-up already arranged.[43]

OTHER TELEHEALTH APPLICATIONS

Sterbis et al. reported the first use of the robotic da Vinci Surgical System (Intuitive Surgical, Sunnyvale, USA) in urological telesurgery and the first successful telesurgical nephrectomy in an animal model.[44] They performed four right nephrectomies in porcine models using both telementoring and telesurgical approaches. Resident surgeons operated a console adjacent to the swine, while attending surgeons simultaneously operated a second console at distances of 1300 and 2400 miles from the operating room. All four procedures and both telementoring and telesurgical models were successful. Kaczmarek et al. successfully used an iPad (Apple, Cupertino, USA) for telerounding on postoperative patients,[45] while a study by Johnston et al. showed the transmission of computed tomography images of patients with renal colic to mobile devices.[46] The solutions described earlier, especially telementoring, could be an optimal way to overcome the shortage of doctors specialized in neurogenic bladder and bowel. Indeed, only few urologists are able to perform infrequent surgical procedures, like augmentation cystoplasty or creation of catheterizable cutaneous channels, so general urologists could be telementored remotely by expert ones.

Practice

Teleconsultation for neurogenic bladder and bowel rehabilitation can be performed in multiple ways. Remote long-term follow-up and management of neurogenic bladder and bowel dysfunction have been established by specialized health services using many different types of telecommunication technology either directly (Fig. 16.3A), indirectly (Fig. 16.3B), or both (Fig. 16.3A–C) with phones, mobile phones, smartphones, video calls, and emails for many years.[31] During the last decade, especially in 2020, more platforms became available for performing telerehabilitation for bladder and bowel care. In this section we will discuss the authors' historical experiences and three different approaches utilized to provide care by comprehensive neuro-urology and rehabilitation programs.

In 2010 the Spinal and Neuro-Urology Units at Careggi University Hospital, Florence, developed a telemonitoring program to ensure "closer" follow-up of patients who lived far from the hospital and had logistic barriers that prevented their attendance for in-person visits. The program was based on a web portal. Laptops and software were freely offered to the patients. The streaming platform allowed video calls and sharing of clinical documentation such as images and clinical reports among patients, physicians, GPs, and caregivers (Fig. 16.4). All data were stored in the institutional server to ensure patients' privacy and reduce the risk of data breach.

Sixteen individuals with SCI were successfully monitored with a focus on neurogenic bladder and pressure sore management. There were no adverse events and there was high patient and GP satisfaction. Still, attempts to invite nurses and physicians to participate from other public hospitals were unsuccessful, likely because their contribution would not be recognized with reimbursement.

Despite this pioneering work, this project was not sustained. With the COVID-19 outbreak in Italy, in March 2020, because of an inability to perform face-to-face visits and concerns about privacy, telephone visits started (ClinicalTrials.gov Identifier: NCT04341714).[47]

For these providers, compared to previous experience, telephone use combined with email exchanges seemed easier, faster, more intuitive, and more effective in collecting the patients' history, investigation, and diagnostic reports. In addition, the patients were very happy to communicate via phone. Subsequently, in light of the pandemic, when the clinics opened, telephone triage was performed prior to planned visits to collect relevant data and shorten the length of visits.

In September 2020 a new public online system, supported by the Italian region of Tuscany, was designed on a secure and dedicated web portal (https://televisita.sanita.toscana.it/). All specialist televisits became recognized and reimbursed by the national health system while telephone calls

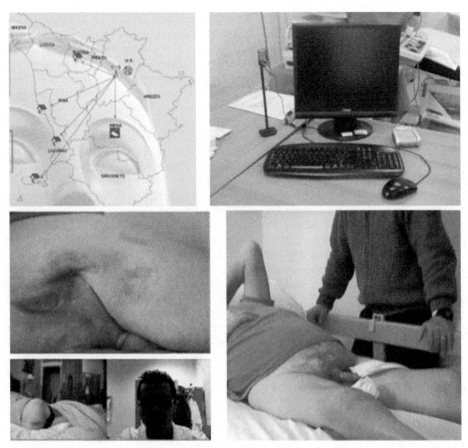

Fig. 16.4   First experience of telemonitoring by the Spinal Unit and Neuro-Urology Unit, in Florence, Italy, during 2010 to 2012.

were not reimbursed. Now patients can easily connect with smartphones, tablets, computer, or laptop, typing their social security number, while doctors have been equipped by a digital identity to create the meeting room with the patient. Likewise, another web portal for teleconsulting between nonmedical health care workers, such as nurses, physiotherapists, occupational therapists, dieticians, and patients, is now in use (https://teleconsulto.sanita.toscana.it/).

Another possibility for virtual urological care is through a store-and-forward method. The Neuro-urology Service, Unipolar Spinal Unit, Niguarda Hospital, Milan, started a phone-based consultation service at the beginning of the COVID-19 pandemic. Still, there were problems with phone lines, doctor-dependent interviews, and patients' anxiety and concerns about missing important signs and/or symptoms. In addition, one patient refused the phone consultation to avoid paying for the visit.

In response, a novel telerehabilitation service was developed based on an online questionnaire and the exchange of patients' clinical documentation. As part of development, the first issue addressed was ensuring patients' data protection. An expert legal advisor was involved to succeed with developing a safe and valid solution. Moreover, this service was offered only for follow-up visits.

The adapted workflow is depicted in. First, a phone call took place to explain the current clinic organization and assess the patients' feasibility to participate in a telerehabilitation visit.

If they accepted, patients were asked to fill in a 10-minute-long questionnaire simulating a structured interview and divided into multiple sections. To avoid operator-dependent bias, increase coherence with patients' real conditions, and limit medicolegal issues, the authors included questions from self-administered international questionnaires that were validated in Italian to assess the severity of the patient's condition. The first section collected demographic characteristics. The second section analyzed COVID-19 testing and related signs and symptoms. In the third section, the urological status was assessed, with questions on signs and symptoms of symptomatic UTIs, episodes of macrohematuria, difficulties with catheterization, and UI-related burden using validated questionnaires (see Section on "The Use of Standardized Tools for Patients' Evaluation").[48] NBD was screened with a new tool, called the Monitoring Efficacy of NBD Treatment on Response (MENTOR), in the fourth section.[49] This is a decision-making tool, delivering a final result according to a "traffic light" system (green, yellow, or red) to determine any need for treatment changes.

The online platform was delivered as a progressive web application (PWA) to limit technical problems. There was no requirement to install it, and there was automatic adaption to different systems (computers, phones, tablets). Patients were asked to send their clinical documentation from after the last check-up to doctors' institutional emails or upload them onto the developed online platform. In the absence of specific problems, the authors recommend an annual follow-up visit for all individuals with neurogenic bladder and bowel with the following examinations: bladder/bowel diary, creatinine, urinalysis, abdominal ultrasound, and urine cytology (in case of individuals with neurogenic bladder for >10 years and/or risk factors for bladder cancer like cigarette smoking).[50]

The final step was represented by medical report writing. Each patient was phoned again to discuss indications, and received the medical report based on the phone call, questionnaires, and clinical documentation provided.

Later, patients were asked to fill in a web-based survey to evaluate the offered service. The questions were based on a 10-point Likert scale and developed with the collaboration of a psychologist and a statistician.

From May 1 to June 30, 2020, 186 outpatient visits were performed. The breakdown of urgent visits, first visits, and follow-up visits was, respectively, 29 (15.6%), 25 (13.4%), and 132 (71.0%). Feasibility of the asynchronous teleurology visits was assessed by involved doctors depending on the available previous clinical documentation. In 13 (9.8%) cases, telerehabilitation was not possible. Six patients lacked appropriate ICT or were not tech-savvy, while seven individuals refused remote visits, preferring to come in person. Most patients (119, 90.2%) accepted telerehabilitation. All of them (100%) managed to complete the described telerehabilitation workflow.

The MENTOR tool allowed urologists to promptly detect patients with inappropriate bowel management (i.e., the individuals who did not obtain a green flag). Furthermore, those individuals with red flags (n = 22) were referred to the neuro-gastroenterology clinic with priority compared to the individuals with yellow flags (n = 9).

Results from the first 100 patients who answered the questionnaire and agreed to share their data for research purposes are shown in Table 16.2. The collected data showed that most patients were not worried about inappropriate management via telerehabilitation (median: 2; range: 1–10) and felt satisfied after this service (median: 10; range: 4–10). They would like the ability to continue to use this service for check-ups after the COVID-19 emergency (median: 8; range: 1–10) and suggest this approach be used for other people for check-ups (median: 9; range: 1–10).

Up to 90% of follow-up visits were accomplished via telerehabilitation. The authors believe this high proportion was due to the ease of access to the PWA and to the store-and-forward strategy. Indeed, asynchronous telerehabilitation is less difficult to implement than synchronous telerehabilitation, which requires real-time application and patients' involvement. Interestingly, when the authors started offering real-time VVs, patients preferred the store-and-forward approach for

TABLE 16.2 ■ **Results of the Evaluation Survey Filled in by the First 100 Patients Who Completed Follow-up Visits Via the Telerehabilitation service Developed by the Neuro-urology Service, Unipolar Spinal Unit, Niguarda Hospital, Milan, Italy. The Questions Were Based on a 10-Point Likert Scale.**

Item	Median (Range)
During COVID-19 pandemic, I would like to access hospital only for urgency	10 (5–10)
During COVID-19 pandemic, I support telemedicine for follow-up	10 (1–10)
During COVID-19 pandemic, I support telemedicine for first visits	7 (1–10)
The communication with doctors was easy via phone	10 (3–10)
The communication with doctors was easy via email	10 (2–10)
The upload of clinical documentation was easy	10 (2–10)
The online questionnaire was easy to fill in	10 (3–10)
The online questionnaire was long to fill in	3 (1–10)
The online questionnaire included all the aspects worthy of evaluation	9 (3–10)
The online questionnaire raised awareness about my clinical condition	7 (1–10)
I feel worried about an inappropriate management via telemedicine	2 (1–10)
I felt satisfied after the offered telemedicine service	10 (4–10)
When COVID-19 emergency is over, I would like the continuation of this telemedicine service for check-ups	8 (1–10)
When the COVID-19 emergency is over, I would like the continuation of this telemedicine service for first visits	5 (1–10)
I would recommend this approach to other people for check-ups	9 (1–10)
I would recommend this approach to other people for first visits	5 (1–10)

follow-up because it did not oblige them to stay connected at a specific time. However, store-and-forward care is no longer reimbursable, so the authors are currently offering VVs, which have also expanded care to help patients with difficulties with catheterization, who would like to talk extensively and in-depth about the diagnostic-therapeutic work-up, and to monitor skin lesions of external genitalia or stomas.

Not all rehabilitation facilities or providers have expert neuro-urologists as part of their team. Thus another model for neurogenic bladder and bowel management (Fig. 16.5) utilized in Greece is primarily based on the organization of rehabilitation health care services and the interdisciplinary method for collaborating with health professionals in different departments, hospitals, and levels of health services (B, C, D, E) on a remote communication system with the person with neurogenic bladder and bowel and/or her/his caregivers (A). This remote model assures the smooth transfer of the patient to the different components of health services and to well-informed health professionals, and facilitates interdisciplinary cooperation. Moreover, it supports the communication of specialized knowledge and, where necessary, the training of health professionals and the person with neurogenic bladder and bowel, and their caregivers and significant ones.

Flexible solutions to provide health services were incorporated in 2020, in the PRM departments of "G. Gennimatas" General Hospital and 414 Military Hospital of Special Diseases, in Athens. A care program was implemented for chronic patients with approval by the Ethical-Scientific

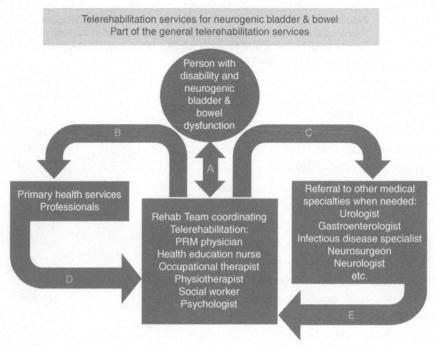

Fig. 16.5 The Greek telerehabilitation model for neurogenic bladder and bowel.

Committee, Administration, and Data Protection Offices. Consultations were first provided through phone and email, but that framework was found to be chaotic. Subsequently, a system of remote prescription of tests, medications, and other supplies (e.g., catheters for intermittent catheterizations) was developed and the potential for remote medical management was acknowledged. In this system, an electronic prescription by the physician appears on the patient's mobile phone with a barcode that is then presented to the pharmacist.

The official videoconference platform of the hospital was chosen not only to better adhere to safety and privacy issues but also to ensure formality of the meeting. A consent form is completed prior to the visit, along with bowel and bladder diaries and a questionnaire created by the members of the rehabilitation team, taking into consideration the ISCoS (International Spinal Cord Society) Lower Urinary Tract Function, Urinary Tract Infection and Bowel Function Basic Data Sets.[51–53] Variables deriving from the International Classification of Function, Disability and Health (ICF) framework (Table 16.3) were also included.[54] Twenty-seven categories were derived from the ICF core sets for neurological conditions postacute care, stroke, MS, TBI, and long-term management of SCI (https://www.icf-research-branch.org/icf-core-sets/category/8-neurologicalconditions; https://www.icf-coresets.org/en/page1.php). This questionnaire (Table 16.4) is addressed in each telerehabilitation consultation and completed by the health care professional in order to ensure a common language in remote clinical assessment between all team members.

Services focus on proper management at home, ensuring compliance with recommended care plans, medication management, and treatment of simple complications such as UTIs. If in doubt or in the presence of any red flag (i.e., failure of passage of transurethral catheter, persistent macrohematuria, unresolved or relapsing episodes of autonomic dysreflexia, acute urinary retention), or ineffective management, an in-person examination is recommended.

TABLE 16.3 ■ **Suggestions From the International Classification of Function, Disability, and Health (ICF) Categories to Be Taken Into Consideration in a Telerehabilitation Consultation for Neurogenic Bowel and Bladder Dysfunction.**

Minimum Bowel/Bladder Neurogenic Dysfunction Set

Body System/Functions	Activity and Participation	Environmental Factors
s110 Structure of brain	d230 Carrying out daily routine	e115 Products and technology for personal use in daily living
s120 Spinal cord and related structures	d410 Changing basic body position	e120 Products and technology for personal indoor and outdoor mobility and transportation
s610 Structure of urinary system	d420 Transferring oneself	e155 Design, construction, and building products and technology of buildings for private use
s810 Structure of areas of skin	d445 Hand and arm use	e310 Immediate family
b130 Energy and drive functions	d455 Moving around	
b152 Emotional functions	d465 Moving around using equipment	
b164 Higher-level cognitive functions	d520 Caring for body parts	
b525 Defecation functions	d530 Toileting	
b620 Urination functions		
b640 Sexual functions		
b710 Mobility of joint functions		
b730 Muscle power functions		
b735 Muscle tone functions		
b760 Control of voluntary movement functions		
b810 Protective functions of the skin		

Special Considerations

FIRST VISITS

It can be difficult to establish a new patient-provider relationship via telehealth. Physical examination is usually necessary during the first patient-provider visit and can detect significant findings. For instance, in case of SCI, clinical examination, assessment of lesion level, injury severity, and evaluation of sacral reflexes are necessary for understanding neurogenic bladder and bowel symptoms. In case of people with cognitive impairment (e.g., due to stroke, TBI), it may be easier for doctors to overcome patients' cognitive problems in person, while televisits may require a third person, like the caregiver and/or GP, who is well informed about the patient's history, medical conditions, and current status. The caregiver may help provide valid data about the patient's health, but is not directly involved, with associated risk of overestimation and/or underestimation of specific signs and symptoms. Therefore telehealth is feasible

TABLE 16.4 ■ **An International Classification of Function, Disability, and Health (ICF)-Based Questionnaire for Telerehabilitation Consultation for Neurogenic Bowel and Bladder Dysfunction (Under Evaluation by the Telerehabilitation Team in Athens).**

Patient Name:_____   Date Filled:_____

Medical Record Information for Telerehabilitation Session:
These fields are filled with information from patient's medical record and are guiding the health professional during the telerehabilitation session

1. Where is the neurological lesion located?	□ Supra-pontine □ Brain stem □ Supra-sacral □ Conus medullaris □ Cauda equina
2. Cause of neurological lesion	□ TSCI □ NTSCI □ MS □ Spina bifida □ Other, specify_____
3. ISNCSCI, AIS (for SCI only)	□ A □ B □ C □ D NLI:_____
4. Is there a urinary/gastrointestinal tract impairment unrelated to the neurological lesion?	□ No □ Yes, specify_____ □ Unknown
5. Are you aware of the need to empty the bowel and bladder?	□ No □ Yes □ Not applicable □ Unknown
6. How do you empty your bladder?	□ Normal voiding □ Straining □ CIC □ IC □ Urinary diversion □ Other □ Unknown
7. How do you empty your bowel?	□ Normal defecation □ Straining □ Digital stimulation □ Mini enema □ Transanal irrigation □ Colostomy □ Sacral anterior root stimulation □ Other □ Unknown
8. How long is required for defecation?	□ 0–30 min □ 30–60 min □ >1 hour □ Not applicable □ Unknown
9. Do you have any perianal problems?	□ Hemorrhoids □ Anal fissure □ Other_____ □ None
10. Have you had any surgery related to your urinary tract/bowel?	□ Indicate which and when _____

Telerehabilitation Session:
The following questions are referring to what caused the telerehabilitation session and present symptoms:

1. Telerehabilitation session scheduled due to	□ Triggered by the patient □ Triggered by rehabilitation team □ Inability to proceed with in-person visit □ Regular follow-up □ New symptoms requiring consultation □ New data affecting neurogenic bladder and bowel management
2. (i) Have you had any new symptoms of a urinary tract infection? (ii) Urinalysis—culture results: _____ _____ _____	□ No □ Fever □ New/increase incontinence □ Malaise □ Cloudy urine □ Pyuria □ Discomfort/pain over kidney/bladder or during micturition □ Autonomic dysreflexia □ Other:_____

Continued

TABLE 16.4 ■ **An International Classification of Function, Disability, and Health (ICF)-Based Questionnaire for Telerehabilitation Consultation for Neurogenic Bowel and Bladder Dysfunction (Under Evaluation by the Telerehabilitation Team in Athens).—cont'd**

3. What is the frequency you empty your bladder in a day?	_____
4. What is the frequency you empty your bowels?	☐ Daily ☐ 1–6 times/week ☐ Less than 1/week ☐ Not applicable ☐ Unknown
5. Are signs of dysreflexia (headache/perspiration/increase in blood pressure) relieved after bowel/bladder evacuation?	☐ No ☐ Yes, rarely ☐ <1/month ☐ Yes, often ☐ >1/month
6. Do you have any urinary incontinence episodes?	☐ Daily ☐ 1 or more/ week ☐ <1/week ☐ Never ☐ Not applicable
7. Do you have any fecal incontinence episodes?	☐ Daily ☐ 1or more/week ☐ <1/week ☐ Never ☐ Not applicable
8. Do you have the need to wear a diaper, pad, plug, condom catheter, ostomy bag, or other?	☐ Indicate which_____
9. Do you receive any medication related to your bladder function?	☐ Bladder relaxant ☐ Sphincter relaxant ☐ Antibiotics ☐ Other_____
10. Do you receive any medication related to your bowel function?	☐ Oral laxatives Indicate_____ ☐ Constipating agents Indicate_____
11. Has there been any change in your bowel function within the last year?	☐ Yes ☐ No ☐ Not applicable ☐ Unknown
12. Has there been any change in your bladder function within the last year?	☐ Yes ☐ No ☐ Not applicable ☐ Unknown
13. Do you have any pressure ulcers?	☐ Yes, specify where_____ ☐ No
Impact on Function	**Degree of Impairment (1–5), 8 (Not Specified), 9 (Not Relevant)**
1. Is fatigue interfering with bowel and bladder management?	
2. How is the patient feeling about dealing with bowel and bladder management?	
3. How affected is the ability of the patient to plan and coordinate bowel and bladder management?	
4. How is the pattern of defecation affected?	
5. How is the pattern of urination affected?	
6. How is sexual function affected?	
7. Is restriction in ROM impacting bowel and bladder management?	

Continued

TABLE 16.4 ▪ An International Classification of Function, Disability, and Health (ICF)-Based Questionnaire for Telerehabilitation Consultation for Neurogenic Bowel and Bladder Dysfunction (Under Evaluation by the Telerehabilitation Team in Athens).—cont'd

8. How much is impairment in muscle strength affecting bowel and bladder management?	
9. How much is muscle tone affecting bowel and bladder management?	
10. Does lack of control of voluntary movements affect bowel and bladder management?	
	Degree of Restriction in Performance (1–5), 8 (Not Specified), 9 (Not Relevant)
11. How much is carrying out a daily routine affected?	
12. How much are transfers affected?	
13. How much is moving around with/without equipment affected?	
14. How much is hand and arm use as far as bowel and bladder management affected?	
15. How much is the use of toilet affected?	
16. How much is work routine affected by bowel and bladder management?	
	Degree of Environmental Impact (–5 to +5)
17. How helpful are assistive devices and other modifications dealing with bowel and bladder management?	
18. How accessible is the toilet in terms of architectural barriers?	
19. How supportive is immediate family and/or assistants in bowel and bladder management?	

CIC, Clean intermittent catheterization; *MS,* multiple sclerosis; *NLI,* neurological level of injury; *NTSCI,* non traumatic spinal cord injury; *ROM,* range of motion; *TSCI,* traumatic spinal cord injury.

and safe in case of cognitive impairment, but doctors should be prepared to spend more time during the e-consult and make sure they have access to the patient's electronic medical record and a reliable provider or assistant who can help them examine the patient and obtain accurate information about the neurological and physical examination, appropriate imaging, and all data available to understand the patient's clinical condition. Finally, most communication is paraverbal and physicians must make eye contact and show empathy to the patient, regardless of whether they are in person or seeing a patient virtually.

LONG-TERM MANAGEMENT

Individuals with SCIs, MS, ALS, and stroke have limited functional reserve to withstand hospital infections, have mobility impairments, and usually have a solid doctor-patient relationship developed through many visits over the years.[55] Indeed, neuro-urological patients, especially those with SCI, are usually chronic and many visits may be performed with the only necessity to show clinical data, like a bladder diary, imaging studies, and laboratory tests. In this setting, telerehabilitation may be useful to save travel time. VVs may be useful to triage patients who are safe to manage at a distance from those requiring an urgent, in-person evaluation. Moreover, people with SCI may be young and thus more likely to use ICT, whereas the other individuals likely have significant physical limitations that may increase difficulty with travel. Thus the population of persons with neurological disability may represent the ideal population for tele-visits, especially for the follow-up of neurogenic bladder and bowel dysfunction, when a physical examination is not necessary.

EMERGENCIES

Emergencies are difficult to manage at distance. An urgent request for a visit should be carried out under the best conditions for both doctors and patients. The most frequent indications may entail catheter malfunction/blockade, urosepsis, and renal failure. In these cases, physical examination, interventional maneuvers (e.g., urinary catheter placement), and/or diagnostic examinations (e.g., genitourinary ultrasound in case of renal colic) are needed. Currently, phone consultations or VVs can be used for screening for which patients need to go to the emergency room or be seen in person. Nevertheless, patients with urgent concerns should be referred directly to an acute care facility.

In the future, indications for telerehabilitation may be expanded to the emergency setting through novel solutions, for example, augmented reality, virtual reality, three-dimensional (3D) printing, 5 G wireless technology, and haptic gloves to create an experience of touch to the doctor. Additionally, small home robots may be telemanipulated to perform interventional maneuvers and examination kits and applications may allow patients or caregivers to perform guided medical examinations with a remote board-certified physician (Tyto, TytoCare, Netanya, Israel). All these devices have not been applied in neurogenic bladder and bowel dysfunction yet but, in the future, they could be adapted to subspecialty-specific needs. The transition from bench to home of these novel solutions may improve patients' follow-up to daily, automated, precise, efficient, and efficacious telemonitoring, which may be associated with significantly improved outcomes.

THE USE OF STANDARDIZED TOOLS FOR PATIENT EVALUATION

The use of a checklist may be beneficial to focus the interview on the issues of primary interest in the shortest time possible.[56] The use of validated tools for evaluation presents several advantages. Scoring systems may be helpful in quantifying symptoms in an objective way, reducing the provider-dependent impact. In case of medicolegal issues, evaluating modules suggested by guidelines filled in by patients may represent proof of the patient's responses and of the disease degree. Doctors should select the appropriate tool evaluating the validation for the patient's language and paying attention to the administration modality (patient vs. health care provider).

The long and short forms of the Qualiveen and I-QOL (Incontinence Quality of Life questionnaire) for neurogenic bladder dysfunction seem optimal for telehealth.[57,58] In case of NBD, the novel MENTOR tool represents the archetype of a decision-making tool to adopt for patient evaluation. We advocate the development and use of similar decision-making tools to increase consistency, productivity, and efficiency. In this way, physicians may avoid redundancy and supersede alarming signs and symptoms. If the patients thoughtfully fill in questionnaires at home, the doctor may save time during the visit and obtain more accurate information from patients who complete the module in a safe, familiar place, and not under pressure. Similarly, the International SCI Data Sets and the International Standards for the Assessment of Autonomic Function after SCI may help clinicians to collect data in a structured and shared way.[59,60]

LEGAL AND REGULATORY ISSUES

Several authors have made recommendations to start telehealth based on expert opinion, but these suggestions should always be tailored to local health care systems and specific needs.[61,62] Indeed the activation of a telerehabilitation service requires the resolution of significant legal, privacy, and billing issues, which differ significantly across countries and hospitals.

In Europe, this process is regulated by the General Data Protection Regulation (GDPR)—Regulation UE n. 2016/679 (John, 2018). According to Article 9 of the GDPR, "… the processing of genetic data, biometric data for the purpose of uniquely identifying a natural person, data concerning health or data concerning a natural person's sex life or sexual orientation shall be prohibited." This prohibition is subject to some exceptions: in particular, Section 9, Subsect. 2, lett. (i) of the GDPR provides the following "(i) processing is necessary for reasons of public interest in the area of public health, such as protecting against serious cross-border threats to health or ensuring high standards of quality and safety of health care and of medicinal products or medical devices, on the basis of Union or Member State law which provides for suitable and specific measures to safeguard the rights and freedoms of the data subject, in particular professional secrecy." This exception perfectly fits with the situation experienced during the COVID-19 pandemic, creating the legal basis for a lawful processing of personal data of e-patients during the emergency, but some principles like minimization and security of personal data processed must be fulfilled with appropriate technical and organizational measures.

It is important to limit the circulation of sensitive data, for example, avoiding emails for file exchange, preferring an online platform where both patients and doctors can upload and download clinical documentation. We encourage the use of hospital servers instead of data remote storage (i.e., cloud services), as the improper use of patients' data may be unreported and unjustified even in case of paid services. However, complete anonymization is a chimera while offering telerehabilitation services, as it is mandatory to identify the sender of medical information, namely, the patient or the caregiver. In the Milan experience, the log-in process was based on a two-factor authentication process, that is, the patient received the form link by email and an automatically generated code by phone message, and the associated patient code was reported in an encrypted file, which was accessible to only two staff members. In addition, the minimization of identifying questions and the use of encrypted communications, like Secure Sockets Layer, to cypher the traffic between the client and the server hosting the questionnaire, can improve further security of personal data processed.

Before performance of e-consult, informed consent for telehealth should be obtained after discussion about the structure and timing of services, record keeping, scheduling, privacy, potential risks, confidentiality, and billing.

The final medical report of the televisit should be similar to the report of in-person visits specifying and describing precisely the employed telerehabilitation approaches. Moreover, considering these patients are at high risk, the authors always report contact information in case of complications to anticipate the follow-up evaluation, since we do not have long-term follow-up to evaluate the safety and efficacy of telehealth compared to standard in-person visits.

Reimbursement is an evolving topic.[31] Currently, payers may reimburse VVs, while they do not compensate phone calls and asynchronous exchange of emails or fax between patients and providers. Similarly, teleconsultations, telementoring, and telesurgery are poorly formalized.

COST-EFFECTIVENESS

The literature is not unanimous about the cost-effectiveness of telerehabilitation. Some authors have reported economic savings with telehealth compared to standard visits, besides reducing hospital infections (including COVID-19), in-hospital injuries, patients' travels, carbon dioxide production, traffic pollution, and waiting lists for emergencies or first visits, for example, Chu et al. demonstrated that patients saved an average of 277 travel miles, 290 minutes of travel time, and up to $193 per visit through urology telerehabilitation clinics.[63]

However, based upon the Milan experience, telerehabilitation was found to be a time-consuming service. Each visit took approximately 1 hour, and many steps were necessary before completing the final reports. Patient distance was outweighed by a more in-depth evaluation of clinical documentation. This consideration is significant in terms of reimbursement: telerehabilitation was not a brief visit, but a complex visit requiring appropriate reimbursement. The authors believe these long-lasting visits were due to an initial learning curve, and these visits may be successfully provided in a shorter amount of time in the future.

Recommendations and Future Research

Follow-up televisits for neurogenic bowel and bladder management represent a safe and effective solution for assessing specific treatment responses and/or reports of bladder/bowel diaries, medical imaging, and laboratory tests. Well-designed, multicenter, long-term RCTs to test the safety and efficacy of telerehabilitation applications for each disease-specific indication are recommended; in particular, cost-benefit analyses would be appropriate.

The authors believe telehealth will never completely substitute in-person visits, but it is a promising way to triage patients, differentiating cases that can be managed safely at a distance from those that require extensive in-person evaluations. Moreover, it can be an excellent way to monitor long-term patients for their compliance with prescribed management. Overall, the use of telerehabilitation for neurogenic bladder and bowel can be beneficial to shorten waiting lists for first visits and emergencies, to decrease the burden of travel on patients, to allow greater frequency of visits for patients who are managed long term, and to offer longer and high-quality face-to-face care for those in need.

Acknowledgments

Dr. Del Popolo would like to express his deep gratitude particularly to Drs. Stefania Musco and Gabriele Righi for their support and assistance. Drs. Michele Spinelli and Gianluca Sampogna thank Mr. Pierluigi Perri, Esq, for his essential contribution on medicolegal issues. Drs. Christina-Anastasia Rapidi and Antonios Kontaxakis thank Dr. Eleni Moumtzi, Dr. Prokopios Manthos, Mrs. Anna Maina, and Mr. Nikos Tsolis for their contribution in organizing telerehabilitation services.

CASE REPORT

MR was a 64-year-old man who suffered from T4 AIS B paraplegia. He developed SCI after a trauma 17 years ago. He was taking an antihypertensive drug and oxybutynin 2.5 mg t.i.d. for overactive bladder. The patient performed four clean intermittent catheterizations per day. He planned a follow-up visit 2 months after detrusor injections of botulinum toxin A (200 U), which he could not attend in person owing to restrictions due to the COVID-19 pandemic. We offered a televisit, which he accepted. The patient received the credentials to log in to our telerehabilitation platform, where he uploaded a 3-day bladder diary, a urine culture (positive for pansensitive *Escherichia coli*), a urine cytology (3/3 neg), a 7-day

Continued

CASE REPORT —cont'd

bowel diary, and a genitourinary ultrasound (irregular bladder morphology with many small diverticula, bladder-wall thickness = 4 mm, normal renal findings, fecal retention). He also filled in our question-naires. The answers excluded symptomatic UTIs, episodes of macrohematuria, and catheterization problems. However, mild urinary incontinence was assessed through Qualiveen-30. The patient filled in the MENTOR tool: the NBD score was low (8/47), but the patient referred autonomic dysreflexia due to bowel problems as a special attention symptom, so the MENTOR tool resulted "yellow." We planned a VV and explained that, before increasing the oxybutynin to 5 mg t.i.d. and/or repeating injections of botulinum toxin, we wanted to ensure he had appropriate bowel management, as UI may be solved in similar cases by effective management of neurogenic bowel. After the consultation, we sent the final medical report to the patient suggesting a visit by our gastroenterologists and a urological reevaluation after optimizing bowel management.

References

1. Malykhina AP, Wyndaele JJ, Andersson KE, et al. Do the urinary bladder and large bowel interact, in sickness or in health? ICI-RS 2011. *Neurourol Urodyn*. 2012;31(3):352–358. https://doi.org/10.1002/nau.21228.

2. Martinez L, Neshatian L, Khavari R. Neurogenic bowel dysfunction in patients with neurogenic bladder. *Curr Bladder Dysfunct Rep*. 2016;11(4):334–340. https://doi.org/10.1007/s11884-016-0390-3.

3. Emmanuel A. Neurogenic bowel dysfunction. *F1000Res*. 1928;20(8):F1000 https://doi.org/10.12688/f1000research.20529.1. Faculty Rev-1800.

4. Liao L, Madersbacher H. *Neurourology: Theory and Practice*. Netherlands: Springer; 2019. ISBN 978-94-017-7509-0.

5. D'Ancona C, Haylen B, Oelke M, et al. Standardisation Steering Committee ICS and the ICS Working Group on Terminology for Male Lower Urinary Tract & Pelvic Floor Symptoms and Dysfunction. The International Continence Society (ICS) report on the terminology for adult male lower urinary tract and pelvic floor symptoms and dysfunction. *Neurourol Urodyn*. 2019;38(2):433–477. https://doi.org/10.1002/nau.23897.

6. Wein AJ, Kavoussi LR, Partin AW, et al. *Campbell-Walsh Urology*. 11th ed.: Elsevier; 2015. ISBN: 978-9996111563.

7. Taweel WA, Seyam R. Neurogenic bladder in spinal cord injury patients. *Res Rep Urol*. 2015;7:85–99. https://doi.org/10.2147/RRU.S29644.

8. Agrawal S, Agrawal RR, Wood HM. Establishing a multidisciplinary approach to the management of neurologic disease affecting the urinary tract. *Urol Clin North Am*. 2017;44(3):377–389. https://doi.org/10.1016/j.ucl.2017.04.005. PMID: 28716319.

9. Rapidi CA, Tederko P, Moslavac S, et al. Professional Practice Committee of the UEMS-PRM Section. Evidence-based position paper on Physical and Rehabilitation Medicine (PRM) professional practice for persons with spinal cord injury. The European PRM position (UEMS PRM Section). *Eur J Phys Rehabil Med*. 2018;54(5):797–807. https://doi.org/10.23736/S1973-9087.18.05374-1.

10. Stillman MD, Hoffman JM, Barber JK, et al. Urinary tract infections and bladder management over the first year after discharge from inpatient rehabilitation. *Spinal Cord Ser Cases*. 2018;4:92. https://doi.org/10.1038/s41394-018-0125-0.

11. Emmanuel A. Managing neurogenic bowel dysfunction. *Clin Rehabil*. 2010;24(6):483–488. https://doi.org/10.1177/0269215509353253.

12. Patel DP, Elliott SP, Stoffel JT, et al. Patient reported outcomes measures in neurogenic bladder and bowel: a systematic review of the current literature. *Neurourol Urodyn*. 2016;35(1):8–14. https://doi.org/10.1002/nau.22673.

13. Anderson KD. Targeting recovery: priorities of the spinal cord-injured population. *J Neurotrauma*. 2004;21(10):1371–1383. https://doi.org/10.1089/neu.2004.21.1371.

14. Lo C, Tran Y, Anderson K, et al. Functional priorities in persons with spinal cord injury: using discrete choice experiments to determine preferences. *J Neurotrauma*. 2016;33(21):1958–1968. https://doi.org/10.1089/neu.2016.4423.

15. Huri E, Hamid R. Technology-based management of neurourology patients in the COVID-19 pandemic: is this the future? A report from the International Continence Society (ICS) institute. *Neurourol Urodyn.* 2020;39(6):1885–1888. https://doi.org/10.1002/nau.24429.

16. Novara G, Checcucci E, Crestani A, et al. Research Urology Network (RUN). Telehealth in urology: a systematic review of the literature. How much can telemedicine be useful during and after the COVID-19 pandemic? *Eur Urol.* 2020;78(6):786–811. https://doi.org/10.1016/j.eururo.2020.06.025.

17. Pereira-Azevedo N, Carrasquinho E, Cardoso de Oliveira E, et al. mHealth in urology: a review of experts' involvement in app development. *PLoS One.* 2015;10(5):e0125547. https://doi.org/10.1371/journal.pone.0125547.

18. Riaz MS, Atreja A. Personalized technologies in chronic gastrointestinal disorders: self-monitoring and remote sensor technologies. *Clin Gastroenterol Hepatol.* 2016;14(12):1697–1705. https://doi.org/10.1016/j.cgh.2016.05.009.

19. Krhut J, Gärtner M, Zvarová K, et al. Validating of a novel method for electronically recording overactive bladder symptoms in men. *Low Urin Tract Symptoms.* 2016;8(3):177–181. https://doi.org/10.1111/luts.12093.

20. Latorre GFS, de Fraga R, Seleme MR, et al. An ideal e-health system for pelvic floor muscle training adherence: systematic review. *Neurourol Urodyn.* 2019;38(1):63–80. https://doi.org/10.1002/nau.23835.

21. Grimes CL, Balk EM, Crisp CC, et al. A guide for urogynecologic patient care utilizing telemedicine during the COVID-19 pandemic: review of existing evidence. *Int Urogynecol J.* 2020;31(6):1063–1089. https://doi.org/10.1007/s00192-020-04314-4.

22. Hoffman V, Söderström L, Samuelsson E. Self-management of stress urinary incontinence via a mobile app: two-year follow-up of a randomized controlled trial. *Acta Obstet Gynecol Scand.* 2017;96(10):1180–1187. https://doi.org/10.1111/aogs.13192.

23. Goode PS, Markland AD, Echt KV, et al. A mobile telehealth program for behavioral treatment of urinary incontinence in women veterans: development and pilot evaluation of MyHealtheBladder. *Neurourol Urodyn.* 2020;39(1):432–439. https://doi.org/10.1002/nau.24226.

24. Bernard S, Boucher S, McLean L, et al. Mobile technologies for the conservative self-management of urinary incontinence: a systematic scoping review. *Int Urogynecol J.* 2020;31(6):1163–1174. https://doi.org/10.1007/s00192-019-04012-w. Epub 2019 Jul 2. PMID: 31267139.

25. Marziniak M, Brichetto G, Feys P, et al. The use of digital and remote communication technologies as a tool for multiple sclerosis management: narrative review. *JMIR Rehabil Assist Technol.* 2018;5(1):e5. https://doi.org/10.2196/rehab.7805.

26. Levy S, Henderson L, McAlpine C. Growing up with confidence: using telehealth to support continence self-care deficits amongst young people with complex needs. *Inform Prim Care.* 2014;21(3):113–117. https://doi.org/10.14236/jhi.v21i3.58.

27. Choi EK, Jung E, Ji Y, et al. A 2-step integrative education program and mHealth for self-management in Korean children with spina bifida: feasibility study. *J Pediatr Nurs.* 2019;49:e54–e62. https://doi.org/10.1016/j.pedn.2019.09.002.

28. Sechrist S, Lavoie S, Khong CM, et al. Telemedicine using an iPad in the spinal cord injury population: a utility and patient satisfaction study. *Spinal Cord Ser Cases.* 2018;4:71. https://doi.org/10.1038/s41394-018-0105-4.

29. Castaneda P, Ellimoottil C. Current use of telehealth in urology: a review. *World J Urol.* 2020;38(10):2377–2384. https://doi.org/10.1007/s00345-019-02882-9.

30. Viers BR, Pruthi S, Rivera ME, et al. Are patients willing to engage in telemedicine for their care: a survey of preuse perceptions and acceptance of remote video visits in a urological patient population. *Urology.* 2015;85(6):1233–1239. https://doi.org/10.1016/j.urology.2014.12.064.

31. Miller A, Rhee E, Gettman M, et al. The current state of telemedicine in urology. *Med Clin North Am.* 2018;102(2):387–398. https://doi.org/10.1016/j.mcna.2017.10.014.

32. Amparore D, Campi R, Checcucci E, et al. Forecasting the future of urology practice: a comprehensive review of the recommendations by International and European Associations on priority procedures during the COVID-19 pandemic. *Eur Urol Focus.* 2020;6(5):1032–1048. https://doi.org/10.1016/j.euf.2020.05.007.

33. Badalato GM, Kaag M, Lee R, et al. Role of telemedicine in urology: contemporary practice patterns and future directions. *Urology Practice.* 2020;7(2):122–126. https://doi.org/10.1097/UPJ.0000000000000094.

34. Kernebeck S, Busse TS, Böttcher MD, et al. Impact of mobile health and medical applications on clinical practice in gastroenterology. *World J Gastroenterol*. 2020;26(29):4182–4197. https://doi.org/10.3748/wjg. v26.i29.4182.

35. Ellimoottil C. Implementing telemedicine in urology: an overview of the benefits and barriers. *J Urol*. 2019;202(1):47–48. https://doi.org/10.1097/JU.0000000000000285.

36. Gadzinski AJ, Gore JL, Ellimoottil C, et al. Implementing telemedicine in response to the COVID-19 pandemic. *J Urol*. 2020;204(1):14–16. https://doi.org/10.1097/JU.0000000000001033.

37. Edison MA, Connor MJ, Miah S, et al. Understanding virtual urology clinics: a systematic review. *BJU Int*. 2020;126(5):536–546. https://doi.org/10.1111/bju.15125.

38. Ellimoottil C, Skolarus T, Gettman M, et al. Telemedicine in urology: state of the art. *Urology*. 2016;94:10–16. https://doi.org/10.1016/j.urology.2016.02.061.

39. Lee T, Kim L. Telemedicine in gastroenterology: a value-added service for patients. *Clin Gastroenterol Hepatol*. 2020;18(3):530–533. https://doi.org/10.1016/j.cgh.2019.12.005.

40. Safir IJ, Gabale S, David SA, et al. Implementation of a tele-urology program for outpatient hematuria referrals: initial results and patient satisfaction. *Urology*. 2016;97:33–39. https://doi.org/10.1016/j. urology.2016.04.066.

41. Darkins A. The growth of telehealth services in the Veterans Health Administration between 1994 and 2014: a study in the diffusion of innovation. *Telemed J E Health*. 2014;20(9):761–768. https://doi. org/10.1089/tmj.2014.0143.

42. Rastogi R, Martinez KA, Gupta N, et al. Management of urinary tract infections in direct to consumer telemedicine. *J Gen Intern Med*. 2020;35(3):643–648. https://doi.org/10.1007/s11606-019-05415-7.

43. Rabie NZ, Canon S, Patel A, et al. Prenatal diagnosis and telemedicine consultation of fetal urologic disorders. *J Telemed Telecare*. 2016;22(4):234–237. https://doi.org/10.1177/1357633X15595556.

44. Sterbis JR, Hanly EJ, Herman BC, et al. Transcontinental telesurgical nephrectomy using the da Vinci robot in a porcine model. *Urology*. 2008;71(5):971–973. https://doi.org/10.1016/j.urology.2007.11.027.

45. Kaczmarek BF, Trinh QD, Menon M, et al. Tablet telerounding. *Urology*. 2012;80(6):1383–1388. https:// doi.org/10.1016/j.urology.2012.06.060.

46. Johnston 3rd WK, Patel BN, Low RK, et al. Wireless teleradiology for renal colic and renal trauma. *J Endourol*. 2005;19(1):32–36. https://doi.org/10.1089/end.2005.19.32.

47. Chesnel C, Hentzen C, Le Breton F, et al. Efficiency and satisfaction with telephone consultation in neuro-urology: experience of the COVID-19 pandemic. *Neurourol Urodyn*. 2021;40(3):929–937. https:// www.clinicaltrials.gov/ct2/show/NCT04341714.

48. Tubaro A, Zattoni F, Prezioso D, et al.; Flow Study Group. Italian validation of the International Consultation on Incontinence Questionnaires. *BJU Int*. 2006;97(1):101–108. doi: 10.1111/j.1464-410X. 2006.05885.x.

49. Emmanuel A, Krogh K, Kirshblum S, et al. Creation and validation of a new tool for the monitoring efficacy of neurogenic bowel dysfunction treatment on response: the MENTOR tool. *Spinal Cord*. 2020;58(7):795–802. https://doi.org/10.1038/s41393-020-0424-8.

50. Sampogna G, Maltagliati M, Galfano A, et al. Experience of a tertiary referral center in managing bladder cancer in conjunction with neurogenic bladder. *Spinal Cord Ser Cases*. 2020;6(1):61. https://doi. org/10.1038/s41394-020-0302-9.

51. Biering-Sørensen F, Craggs M, Kennelly M, et al. International lower urinary tract function basic spinal cord injury data set. *Spinal Cord*. 2008;46(5):325–330. https://doi.org/10.1038/sj.sc.3102145.

52. Goetz LL, Cardenas DD, Kennelly M, et al. International spinal cord injury urinary tract infection basic data set. *Spinal Cord*. 2013;51(9):700–704. https://doi.org/10.1038/sc.2013.72.

53. Krogh K, Halvorsen A, Pettersen AL, et al. Version 2.1 of the International Spinal Cord Injury Bowel Function Basic Data Set. *Spinal Cord Ser Cases*. 2019;5:63. https://doi.org/10.1038/s41394-019-0210-z.

54. World Health Organization. *International Classification of Functioning. Disability and Health: ICF.*: *World Health Organization*; 2001. https://apps.who.int/iris/handle/10665/42407.

55. Boehm K, Ziewers S, Brandt MP, et al. Telemedicine online visits in urology during the COVID-19 pandemic—potential, risk factors, and patients' perspective. *Eur Urol*. 2020;78(1):16–20. https://doi. org/10.1016/j.eururo.2020.04.055.

56. Glavind K, Bjørk J, Lindquist AS. A retrospective study on telephone follow-up of anterior colporrhaphy by a specialized nurse. *Int Urogynecol J*. 2014;25(12):1693–1697. https://doi.org/10.1007/ s00192-014-2444-4.

57. Bonniaud V, Bryant D, Parratte B, et al. Development and validation of the short form of a urinary quality of life questionnaire: SF-Qualiveen. *J Urol*. 2008;180(6):2592–2598. https://doi.org/10.1016/j.juro.2008.08.016.
58. Schurch B, Denys P, Kozma CM, et al. Reliability and validity of the incontinence quality of life questionnaire in patients with neurogenic urinary incontinence. *Arch Phys Med Rehabil*. 2007;88(5):646–652. https://doi.org/10.1016/j.apmr.2007.02.009.
59. Biering-Sørensen F, Charlifue S, DeVivo M, et al. International spinal cord injury data sets. *Spinal Cord*. 2006;44(9):530–534. https://doi.org/10.1038/sj.sc.3101930.
60. Alexander MS, Biering-Sorensen F, Bodner D, et al. International standards to document remaining autonomic function after spinal cord injury. *Spinal Cord*. 2009;47(1):36–43. https://doi.org/10.1038/sc.2008.121.
61. Musco S, Del Popolo G, Lamartina M, et al. Neuro-urology during the COVID-19 pandemic: triage and priority of treatments. *Neurourol Urodyn*. 2020;39(7):2011–2015. https://doi.org/10.1002/nau.24460.
62. Viers BR, Lightner DJ, Rivera ME, et al. Efficiency, satisfaction, and costs for remote video visits following radical prostatectomy: a randomized controlled trial. *Eur Urol*. 2015;68(4):729–735. https://doi.org/10.1016/j.eururo.2015.04.002.
63. Chu S, Boxer R, Madison P, et al. Veterans Affairs telemedicine: bringing urologic care to remote clinics. *Urology*. 2015;86(2):255–260. https://doi.org/10.1016/j.urology.2015.04.038.

CHAPTER 17

Telerehabilitation for Treatment of Sexual Concerns

Marcalee Alexander ■ Gianluca Sampogna

Sexuality is an important part of life for persons with and without disabilities. Research has addressed the sexual concerns of persons with spinal cord injuries (SCIs),[1] multiple sclerosis,[2] stroke,[3] arthritis,[4] musculoskeletal impairments,[5] and other disabilities. Yet, the needs of persons with disabilities with regard to sexuality are commonly underaddressed.[6] This is unfortunate because, as has been shown in persons with multiple sclerosis, sexual dysfunction can have a greater negative impact on mental health related to quality of life[7] than severity of physical disability and it can be posited that this would also be the case for other disabilities.

Telerehabilitation presents an ideal opportunity for providing information about sexual health to persons with new or long-standing disabilities. Persons in acute rehabilitation are often too preoccupied with concerns such as a new stroke, traumatic brain injury (TBI), or SCI, to name a few, to focus on any information provided regarding sexuality. Additionally, older individuals may have preexisting sexual concerns that predate a new disability, such as those related to diabetes, hypertension, coronary artery disease, or neuropathy. For these individuals, the availability of sexuality treatment programs and sexual counseling can provide an opportunity to complete their reintegration into their previous lifestyle and even potentially improve their premorbid sexual function.

Review of the published literature reveals sparse information on the use of telemedicine for sexuality concerns. There is a recent Kaiser Foundation report that addresses the use of telehealth services for prescription of contraceptives for women and for treatment of sexually transmitted infections.[8] Another report addresses the use of telehealth to treat internet-based sexual addiction.[9] Moreover, a recent paper regarding the use of telemedicine for sexual medicine focused on the legal aspects of telehealth and setting up a practice with some do's and don'ts, rather than providing a review of published literature.[10] With regard to telehealth and disabilities there is a considerable amount of information available on the internet about specific sexual topics and this information has been reviewed for content;[11] however, there is little information available about how to have an actual telerehabilitation visit related to sexual concerns.

The use of electronic medical records has paved the way for the use of telerehabilitation to provide sexual counseling and remediation services. With consumers having easy access to their medication lists and their concomitant diagnoses, which they can quickly share with health care professionals, there is a new opportunity to provide access to remote, more specialized providers. Additionally, there is an opportunity for detailed aspects of the physical examination and imaging to be shared with health professionals.

In order to perform a telerehabilitation sexuality-focused visit, it is important to ensure that the basic tenets of telerehabilitation are followed. The provider needs to be in a private, well-lit space where the patient can feel comfortable that they are being properly assessed. The patient also needs to be reminded at the start of the visit that the professional will be asking them about sensitive issues; thus they need to feel comfortable with an appropriate level of privacy in their location.

It is especially important that any local laws such as HIPAA are followed and that all aspects of internet security are considered, despite any temporary clemency due to COVID-19. Additionally, it is important that any partner is allowed to attend the visit and, if necessary for physical examination, the patient should have an assistant present.

Sexual History

CHILDHOOD CONCERNS

Comprehensive assessment of sexuality after a disabling disorder starts with a review of the individual's childhood and adolescent sexual experiences. The worldwide prevalence of child abuse is 8% to 31% for girls and 3% to 17% for boys, with 9 girls and 3 boys out of 100 having experienced forced intercourse.[12] Thus it is important to be aware of this issue and assess whether the individual was raised in a healthy sexual environment or whether there were issues of abuse causing distorted sexual development. These long-standing issues are important to identify because they often lead to psychological and sexual concerns, such as anxiety, low self-esteem, and depression, which compound the impact of disability on sexuality and can also lead to medically unexplained symptoms.[13,14] Moreover, these individuals are at risk for later revictimization and high-risk sexual behavior, having multiple sex partners, teenage pregnancies, and experiencing sexual assault as adults.[13] If an individual has a history of sexual abuse, it is important to ascertain if they have access to proper counseling and treatment and that these issues are recognized in any discussions of sexuality and disability.

It is also important to assess sexual orientation and gender identity and whether there are religious or cultural issues that impact an individual's sexuality. Those individuals who are raised in a sexually restrictive religious environment may have experienced issues related to the expression of their sexual orientation or nonconforming gender identity. Moreso, they may have concerns regarding participating in sexual acts outside the context of marriage, the use of birth control, or the practice of abortion. Thus as part of a sexuality telehealth visit, it is appropriate to query the individual regarding their sexual orientation, gender identity, and whether there are any religious or cultural concerns they have regarding their sexuality.

DEMOGRAPHIC AND RELATIONSHIP ISSUES

The desire and need for sexual expression changes throughout the lifespan. It is therefore important to consider the age and relationship status of the person who is being treated. It is also important to assess the individual's premorbid level of sexual knowledge and determine whether they have an appropriate foundation of information to begin learning from. Individuals who have never achieved orgasm prior to a disability or illness need to be treated differently than individuals who are sexually experienced. Moreover, relationship status and whether individuals are married, separated, divorced, and/or living with a partner needs to be determined so that the contributions of the partner and relationship to the individual's sexual situation are identified. Nevertheless, the health professional must not fall into a practice of assuming that just because an individual is elderly that they are not sexually active or do not have an interest in sexual rehabilitation.

PREMORBID FUNCTION

Before assessing the impact of a specific disability on an individual's sexuality, it is important to determine what the individual's premorbid sexual functioning was. In the time of the electronic medical record, the health professional can often obtain a glimpse into the individual's function by assessing their medication list. Individuals with a preexisting prescription for a phosphodiesterase type 5 (PDE5) inhibitor such as sildenafil or vardenafil likely have a premorbid issue with erectile dysfunction (ED), while individuals with depression or anxiety can have sexual dysfunction either from the disorder or from treatment with a serotonin-specific reuptake inhibitor such as fluoxetine or paroxetine and are prone to loss of libido, arousal dysfunction, and orgasm dysfunction. Individuals with diabetes type 1 and 2 often have issues with neurogenic or vascular arousal dysfunction; thus it is important that an adequate premorbid history is obtained. Similarly, individuals with peripheral vascular and/or coronary artery disease often have sexual arousal dysfunction and individuals with genitourinary issues such as benign prostatic hypertrophy or postmenopausal vaginal atrophy often have concomitant issues with arousal and potentially dyspareunia. Finally, people with chronic pain can have physical issues with positioning because of the pain and because many medications that have either been previously prescribed for pain management or are in vogue now result in sexual dysfunction.

The Impact of the Individual's Disability

Once you have taken the individual's premorbid psychological and medical history into account, it is time to assess the impact of the individual's particular disability on their sexual functioning. An easy way to do this is by considering where the pathology is located on the individual's body and whether this pathology will cause a direct or indirect effect on their sexual response. People with spinal cord dysfunction probably have the most direct impact of their dysfunction on sexual response, and research has confirmed that the impact of injury on sexual response is related to the location and degree of injury in the spinal cord.[15–17] Based on this research it has been determined that the degree of preservation of the ability to perceive pinprick and light touch sensation in the T11-L2 dermatomes can help predict the retention of psychogenic genital arousal, while the maintenance of reflex responses in the S3-5 area can predict the retention of reflex genital arousal. This important information is obtained through physical examination and the International Standards to Assess Autonomic Function after SCI is a useful format to record this information.[18] With the new version of the standards, which were released in 2021, the user is prompted with a section that indicates the anticipated impact of the injury on sexual response. This facilitates comparing the anticipated impact that the injury could cause with the impact that the individual with the SCI reports, making it easier to see if there is potential for factors other than the SCI to contribute to an individual's sexual concerns.[19] For diagnoses other than SCI or SCD there can still be direct neurological effects on sexual function, such as with autonomic neuropathies associated with diabetes, surgical procedures that can negatively affect the thoracolumbar sympathetic output, or with stroke, TBI, or multiple sclerosis with damage to the central nervous system pathways involved in sexual response. However, as compared to SCI, there is substantially less research defining the impact of specific neurological injuries on human sexual arousal. Moreover, since stroke is often accompanied by comorbidities such as hypertension and diabetes that can have independent effects on sexual response, it is difficult to determine if there is any particular pattern of stroke that causes sexual dysfunction.

Orgasm is generally considered the culmination of the sexual response cycle. For persons with SCIs it has been determined that genital orgasms are improbable in persons with complete lower motor neuron SCIs affecting their sacral segments. Determination that an injury is a complete lower motor neuron injury requires the performance of an International Standards for the Neurologic Classification of SCI examination and the finding of no sensation when a gloved finger is pressed against the anal wall and no sensation at the S3-5 dermatomes. Additionally, the individual must have no bulbocavernosus reflex and no anal wink reflex, and these individuals have a patulous anus and areflexic bladder and bowel. This is not to say that these individuals may not have a nongenital orgasm; however, it is prudent to educate this group of people in particular about their options for nongenital orgasm. For people with all other levels and degrees of SCI, statistics in an untreated population have shown that approximately 50% of males and 50% of females retain the capacity for orgasm after SCI.[20] Moreover, this capacity is not based upon degree or level of injury. In light of this, it is important to inform people with SCIs that problems achieving orgasm may be multifactorial and not just related to their injury, and that it is worthwhile to work to remove potential offending agents that could contribute to orgasmic dysfunction after SCI, especially if the individual is interested in improving their orgasmic capacity.

The Need for Education and Practice

Once the potential impact of injury on a person's sexual response has been assessed, it is important to educate the patient about their sexual potential. Education about positioning helps people prepare to engage in sexual activities in advance so they can be more confident in their sexual encounters. Additionally, education about the potential for neurogenic bladder and bowel accidents and the need for assuring adequate emptying prior to sexual activity is important. Spasticity and neuropathic pain can also cause difficulty with positioning during sexual activity and the use of lubrication, satin sheets, and adequate cushioning can also be a worthwhile addition to someone's sexual repertoire.

For people with respiratory concerns, the need for oxygen during sexual activity or the use of a ventilator is an important point to discuss. Similarly, people who have sustained strokes or recent myocardial disorders need to be counseled and provided with information regarding what activities are safe for them to engage in. Individuals with arthritis may require extra lubrication and joint protection techniques during sexual activities and those with hip replacements need to maintain their operative precautions.

Generally, after basic education is provided for people with new injuries or disabilities, it is worthwhile to explain that the individual needs to go home and "practice" to see the impact of their injury or illness on their sexual function. In the case of people with SCIs, masturbation is beneficial to see what does and does not work for them from a sexual standpoint and this may be facilitated by voice-activated devices or through the use of adaptive devices if a person has decreased hand function. With a neurological injury or disorder, the change in sensation and motor function that an individual experiences must be acknowledged and explored so that the person feels comfortable with their body. More so, by masturbating, the person is able to explore their own body without the stress of pleasing a partner or worrying about how their new body works or about bladder and bowel concerns. The individual can also experience the impact of arousal and orgasm on their spasticity and pain and try out various adaptive devices and sex toys that can help stimulate their arousal and orgasm. In the case of SCI, research has shown that it takes significantly longer for women with SCIs to achieve orgasm through masturbation than able-bodied women.[15] In contrast, in men with SCIs it takes longer to achieve orgasm through masturbation but the results were not statistically significantly different than for able-bodied men.[16]

The issue of using masturbation as a means to reclaim one's sexual potential after stroke, multiple sclerosis, or with other progressive neurological issues has not been addressed. It follows, however, that eliminating the distractors of a partner and thereby decreasing stress would have a positive impact on one's ability to achieve orgasm. Decreased stress during sexual activity may also have a beneficial effect on blood pressure; however, further research is necessary to explore this potential.

The Importance of Follow-Up

Sexuality is not a static concern. After an initial visit, it is recommended that they review appropriate reading material such as Sexual Sustainability: A Guide to Having a Great Sex Life with a Spinal Cord Disorder.[21] Moreover, it is recommended that any sexual consultation performed through telerehabilitation include a follow-up session. This allows the individual to go home, explore their sexual potential, and then to come back and essentially have a confidante to discuss their findings—both positive and negative. This is an important option because the first exploration of one's sexual potential after stroke or other disability can lead to many findings and questions. Additionally, there are many other variables that affect the sexual potential of a person, regardless of the presence of a disability and these issues can surface once an individual starts to become sexually active. For instance, although people may express an interest in regaining their sexual self after an injury or illness, they may still be wrought with other medical concerns that predominate their life and the presence of a follow-up appointment with a physician or counselor can remind them of the importance of their sexuality. Additionally, the individual may realize that the problem is not the pathology, rather it is fatigue associated with their general lifestyle, and having their health professional ask them about their sexuality may remind them of its importance in their life.

Once a patient has completed the first round of sexual education, practice, and follow-up, it is worthwhile to review other issues that can be impacting a person's ability to be sexually active. Common issues can include stress and depression, which can each independently affect sexual function. The presence of a new injury or disabling illness can cause the person to feel stressed about potential health care costs, the need for assistance at home, or the potential loss of employment and the impact on the family. If an individual is a breadwinner who needs to now be taken care of by their partner, this can also be a stressor on a relationship. Depression can preexist a new disability or illness and can also occur because of a new injury. Since depression in and of itself can cause sexual dysfunction and because psychological treatment for depression is generally beyond the scope of practice of a physiatrist, this can be a red flag as to the need for referral to a psychologist for patients seen in follow-up.

Other issues that can impact the sexuality of a person with a disabling condition include the presence of children or elderly parents at home. If the person is living in a busy household without privacy this may cause an inability to explore their sexual potential and thereby diminish sexual interest, leading to decreased activity and ultimately sexual satisfaction. Loneliness can also be an issue for a person with a disability. The inability to go out into the community as frequently can be burdensome, especially if they are quarantined at home or if there are medical reasons they cannot get out. Similarly, after an injury or disabling illness occurs, the partner may be a source of sexual distress. It is not uncommon for a person with an injury or illness to continue to want to remain sexually active and emotionally and physically intimate with their partner while the partner transitions into a caregiver role and decides that they are no longer sexually interested in the person with the disability.

IATROGENIC EFFECTS

When working to improve people's sexual concerns, it is paramount to consider system-based and iatrogenic problems. A substantial variable in health care is the issue of insurance-based or hospital-based formularies that determine which medications a patient is prescribed. Unfortunately, these formularies often include medications that cause sexual side effects. Additionally, many providers are focused on their specialty or the acute problems that patients are experiencing when they are treated. This may also result in prescription of medications with sexual side effects and it is therefore important that the provider treating sexual dysfunction review and consider all of a patient's medications.

In the field of rehabilitation, antispasticity drugs, narcotics, antidepressants, antiseizure medications, and antihypertensives commonly cause sexual side effects that can compound the impact of an injury on sexual responses.

The antispasticity drug baclofen is commonly prescribed for people with spasticity. It can be used orally and intrathecally. An issue that is commonly disregarded is that both oral and intrathecal baclofen can cause sexual side effects, including difficulty with maintaining an erection and ejaculation in men and orgasmic dysfunction in women. These findings were noted in individuals with SCI, multiple sclerosis, and cerebral palsy.[22, 23] In light of this, it is important when conducting a sexuality telerehabilitation consultation to consider the issue of spasticity and what medications the patient is on for treatment. Moreover, if the patient is on baclofen it may make sense to alter the timing of the drug, decrease the dose, wean the patient from baclofen, or switch to another antispasmodic such as tizanidine, dantrium, or botulinum toxin if the patient has focal spasticity.

Over the past three decades narcotics have been used excessively for treatment of chronic pain and the impacts of opiate crisis are well known around the world. One side effect of the opiate crisis that less attention has been paid to, however, is the impact on sexual functioning and with this the impact on relationships. Issues such as loss of sex drive in both men and women,[24, 25] loss of fantasies, loss of morning erections, premature ejaculation, and ejaculation with a soft penis have been reported. The use of buprenorphine as compared to methadone or heroin has been shown to have significantly less side effects on sex drive, fantasies, and premature ejaculation.[24] Therefore it may be appropriate for individuals with low sex drive who may be on chronic opiates for pain management to be weaned to buprenorphine for concomitant management of their pain along with improvement in their sexual function.

Antidepressants are commonly used in rehabilitation and their use has particularly been touted in stroke.[26] With regard to sexuality, however, antidepressants are a double-edged sword and while depression can cause sexual dysfunction, antidepressants can do the same. Therefore when focusing on sexual rehabilitation it is important to assess the individual's use of antidepressants; if an individual is on antidepressants, determine whether the drug they are taking is likely to cause sexual side effects and if so, consider switching to a drug with less side effects such as bupropion, duloxetine, mirtazapine, or reboxetine (not available in the United States) rather than an SSRI or a tricyclic antidepressant.[27] Review of all of the potential antidepressants and their impact on sexual function is beyond the scope of this chapter; therefore the clinician is encouraged to review the impact of the specific medications the patient is on and make any clinically appropriate changes in conjunction with the individual's psychiatrist or prescribing physician.

With the opiate crisis, the use of antiseizure drugs for neuropathic pain has become more common. These drugs may also have sexual side effects. Gabapentin has been shown to cause anorgasmia in both men and women,[28, 29] although a recent randomized placebo-controlled trial showed that gabapentin was beneficial to improve sexual function in vulvodynia;[30] thus its use may be considered in patients with neuropathic pain located in the genital area. Pregabalin has also been shown to cause anorgasmia and severe delayed ejaculation and even priapism;[31, 32] however, there is also a suggestion in the literature about the enhancement of libido with pregabalin in a subject treated with it for anxiety[33] and the abuse of pregabalin for sexual purposes.[34]

Antihypertensives are also commonly used by people in rehabilitation as hypertension is a contributing factor in many disorders such as stroke, cardiac events, and amputation which can result in rehabilitation transfer. Many antihypertensives, including beta blockers such as propranolol and diuretics such as hydrochlorothiazide, can cause sexual dysfunctions. Moreover, this is a problem that can occur in men and women with hypertension.[35, 36]

It is beyond the scope of this chapter to review all of the medications that can cause sexual dysfunction. The sexual health provider is therefore encouraged to research any medications that they may be unfamiliar with when seeing a patient who is on multiple medications and complains of sexual dysfunction. It is also strongly recommended that rather than add new medications, such as PDE5 inhibitors, the prescriber considers whether current medications can be successfully adjusted in dose or in timing in order to promote successful sexual encounters or if the medications can be switched to an alternative without sexual side effects.

MORE PRACTICE AND BACK TO THE BASICS

In addition to discussing iatrogenic effects and making suggestions for changes, it is important to use balance in your discussions with patients and remind them that sexuality is not all clinical, rather it is a combination of mental or psychological and physical components. When discussing iatrogenic effects with patients, I also bring up the basics involved with good sexuality: romance, feeling good about yourself, and having a clear mind when you are sexually active. At this time I also review the issue of spectatoring (or watching yourself when you are sexually active and criticizing your technique, wondering about your partner, or why things are or are not working the way you want, so that you miss the enjoyment of the sexual encounter).

This is also a good time to bring up the issue of mindfulness and how it relates to sexual encounters. Mindfulness is the concept of being completely present in this moment, not before and not after and not in another place. Mindfulness is often practiced by stopping what you are doing, closing your eyes, and just focusing on your breathing. This could be done by feeling the breath go in and out of the nostrils or focusing on the breath going in and out of your lungs. The key component of mindfulness is to realize that our minds often wander, and it is important to bring your thoughts back to the object or focus your meditation practice. If one considers the concept of spectatoring, mindfulness is essentially the opposite, so it is not surprising that mindfulness has become a core component of sexual counseling.

One of the benefits of a telerehabilitation practice is the ability to conveniently follow-up with patients. For this reason, I recommend developing a treatment strategy with your patient at the beginning of their visits and indicate the approach you will use. I also believe it is beneficial to briefly revisit patients at intervals of around 4 weeks so that they are able to try out the impacts of medication changes. Still, it is important to do this at a frequency that makes sense to them and their lifestyle.

Second-Level Therapies

FOR WOMEN

When treating sexual dysfunction in a woman with a disability, and especially when doing so via telehealth, it is important to ensure that the woman has had an adequate gynecological and medical evaluation and that her risks of other concerns such as HPV, pregnancy, and sexually transmitted diseases are identified. There are limited options to treat female sexual dysfunction; however, the use of a clitoral vacuum suction device and the use of vibratory stimulation was shown to improve orgasmic function in women with SCI and MS.[37] Although the use of sildenafil did not reveal statistically significant benefits in women with SCIs,[38] some women with disabilities do report that its off label use is beneficial. Moreover, although its use is not approved by the US Food and Drug Administration (FDA) and further study is warranted, testosterone has been shown to have beneficial effects in improving orgasmic function for postmenopausal women.[39]

FOR MEN

Treatment of sexual dysfunctions by nonspecialists has been facilitated since the introduction of PDE5 inhibitors: sildenafil, tadalafil, vardenafil, and avanafil.[40] They are considered first-line pharmacological treatment in neurogenic ED. To date, there are no studies with high level of evidence assessing the efficacy, side effects, and patient-tailored indications across different active principles, dosages, and formulations (pill vs. oral thin film) in neurogenic ED.[41] In any case, patients should be informed about the duration of action (short- vs. long-acting drugs), possible disadvantages, and how to use the medicine (e.g., avoid food prior to taking sildenafil). Starting with lower dosages (e.g., sildenafil 50 mg or tadalafil 10 mg orally 30 or 60 minutes before sexual intercourse) and increasing progressively in case of nonresponse is prudent. Moreover, PDE5 inhibitors may be administered successfully on a daily basis (e.g., tadalafil 5 mg once daily).

In people with SCI, PDE5 inhibitors improve erectile function, retrograde ejaculation, and satisfaction. Monitoring treatment outcomes with questionnaires validated internationally, for example, the international index of erectile function (IIEF),[42] is recommended. Despite beneficial results, most neuro-urological patients require long-term therapy and have been shown to have low compliance because of side effects, principally headache, flushing, runny nose, vision changes, and stomach upset.[43] In people with high-level SCI and multiple system atrophy, PDE5 inhibitors should be used cautiously because of the risk for significant hypotension.[44] An absolute contraindication is represented by concomitant use of nitrates, which are taken on demand by spinal cord–injured individuals at risk for autonomic dysreflexia (i.e., with lesions at or above T6): the association of nitrates and PDE5 inhibitors may result into life-threatening hypotension episodes. PDE5 inhibitors are largely prescribed by virtue of tolerability and efficacy; however, the aforementioned conditions should always be considered by clinicians recommending PDE5 inhibitors.

A significant issue of these medications is with their mechanism of action. By blocking the hydrolysis of the second messenger cGMP in the cavernous tissue and favoring the accumulation of cytosolic calcium, these drugs are associated with increased arterial blood flow, provoking compression of the subtunical venous plexus, leading to penile erection.[45] They are not erection initiators, so PDE5 inhibitors require some residual nerve function and sexual stimulation to be effective. In this context, efficacy is defined as an erection, with rigidity, sufficient for satisfactory intercourse.[46]

An intermediate solution is represented by the intraurethral application of alprostadil, which is safer, but less effective.[47] Since this route of administration is not particularly invasive, especially if patients can catheterize themselves, this approach may be suggested also through televisits, controlling remotely first applications.

Mechanical devices, like vacuum erection devices (VEDs) and penile constriction rings, are associated with significant results;[48] however, these are often considered less cosmetically appealing than other means of improving erections. By using an external penile pump (either manual or battery operated), VED creates vacuum suction within the plastic cylinder placed around the penis, drawing blood into the penis to provoke erection. Simultaneously, a rubber or silicon constrictive ring tightens around the penis to maintain erection; however, it must be removed within 30 minutes to avoid very serious complications such as skin necrosis. Other significant drawbacks include pressure ulcers, petechiae, and bruising, especially in case of absent residual sensitivity at the level of external genitalia. Therefore the authors advocate the use of mechanical devices to treat neurogenic ED only in well-informed individuals, preferably (but not only) with sensitivity preserved partially.

Tertiary Care

Individuals not responding to oral drugs and/or taking medications interfering with PDE5 inhibitors may benefit from intracavernous injections of alprostadil, papaverine, or phentolamine to treat ED.[49] The authors discourage clinicians from prescribing intracavernous injections through televisits without a first training session in person. Careful dose titration and some precautions are mandatory to limit the risk for significant complications such as priapism, pain, and corpora cavernosa fibrosis. Appropriate training sessions are mandatory to teach the patient and/or the partner to perform intracavernous injections safely and effectively and to monitor for potential complications.

If the previous treatments and combinations of treatments fail, patients may ultimately desire a penile prosthesis. In one study it was reported that most (83.7%) spinal cord injured men with different types of penile prostheses reported they continued to have sexual intercourse after a mean follow-up of 7 years.[50] However, penile prostheses should be considered cautiously and only in serious ED, as they are associated with significant complications, including infection, prosthesis perforation, and mechanical failure.

Recommendations for Research

As with most other areas of telerehabilitation, there are significant needs for research to optimize the use of telerehabilitation techniques for individuals with sexual dysfunction related to disability. Optimal timing and frequency of education and training still warrants examination. For those individuals with diminished hand function or decreased mobility, the use of virtual reality for sexual satisfaction and for remote controlled masturbatory devices remains in its infancy and can be explored. Moreover, the use of sexual surrogates for persons with disabilities remains a controversial, yet unexplored topic.

CASE STUDY

BA is a 38-year-old female with T7 AIS A paraplegia and neurogenic bladder and bowel. She presents for telehealth evaluation complaining of decreased libido and anorgasmia. Her preinjury history reveals she had a positive sex life without sexual dysfunction prior to injury. She is otherwise healthy. Review of her medications reveals she has been on baclofen 20 mg four times daily for spasticity along with Lexapro 10 mg daily despite her functioning independently at a wheelchair level. During her telehealth visit she is educated about the potential effects of her medications on her sexual potential. She is gradually weaned off of the Lexapro with improvement in her libido but she remains anorgasmic. She returns for reevaluation at which point she opts to wean down on her baclofen. Her dose is gradually decreased to 20 mg daily, which she takes at bedtime. At her final visit, she reports she has regained the ability to achieve orgasm with the use of a vibrator.

References

1. Alexander MS, Marson L. The neurologic control of arousal and orgasm after with specific attention to spinal cord lesions: integrating basic and clinical sciences. *Auton Neurosci*. 2018;209:90–99. https://doi.org/10.1016/j.autneu.2017.01.005. PMID: 28222972.

2. Kessler TM, Fowler CJ, Panicker JN. Sexual dysfunction in multiple sclerosis. *Expert Rev Neurother*. 2009;9(3):341–350. https://doi.org/10.1586/14737175.9.3.341.

3. Richards A, Dean R, Burgess GH, et al. Sexuality after stroke: an exploration of current professional approaches, barriers to providing support and future directions. *Disabil Rehabil*. 2016;38(15):1471–1482. https://doi.org/10.3109/09638288.2015.1106595.

4. Newman AM. Arthritis and sexuality. *Nurs Clin North Am*. 2007;42(4):621–630. https://doi.org/10.1016/j.cnur.2007.08.006.

5. Monga T, Tan G, Ostermann HJ, et al. Sexuality and sexual adjustment of patients with chronic pain. *Disabil Rehabil*. 1998;20(9):317–329. https://doi.org/10.3109/09638289809166089.

6. Eisenberg NW, Andreski S, Mona LR. Sexuality and physical disability: a disability-affirmative approach to assessment and intervention within health care. *Curr Sex Health Rep*. 2015;7:19–29. https://doi.org/10.1007/s11930-014-0037-.

7. Schairer LC, Foley FW, Zemon V, et al. The impact of sexual dysfunction on health-related quality of life in people with multiple sclerosis. *Mult Scler*. 2014;20(5):610–616. https://doi.org/10.1177/1352458513503598.

8. Weigel G, Fredreiksen B, Ranji U, et al. Telemedicine in Sexual and Reproductive Health. Issue Brief. *Henry J. Kaiser Family Foundation*. https://www.ncsddc.org/wp-content/uploads/2020/05/KFF-Issue-Brief-Telemed-in-Sex-Repro-Health-11.2019.pdf; Accessed 25.10.20.

9. Dooley A, de la Houssaye N, Baum N. Use of telemedicine for sexual medicine patients. *Sex Med Rev*. 2020;8:507–514. https://doi.org/10.1016/j.sxmr.2020.06.001.

10. Putnam E, Maheu M. Online sexual addiction and compulsivity: integrating web resources and behavioral telehealth in treatment. *Sex Addict.* 2000;7(1-3):91–112. https://doi.org/10.1080/10720160008400209.
11. Heath B, Flicker S, Nepveux D, et al. A content analysis of youth sexual health websites: exploring their relevance and accessibility for youth with disabilities. *Health Tomorrow.* 2013;1:1–26. https://ht.journals. yorku.ca/index.php/ht/article/view/37271/33843; Accessed 25.10.20.
12. Barth J, Bermetz L, Heim E, et al. The current prevalence of child sexual abuse worldwide: a systematic review and meta-analysis. *Int J Public Health.* 2013;58:469–483. https://doi.org/10.1007/s00038-012-0426-1.
13. Lalor K, McElvaney R. Child sexual abuse, links to later sexual exploitation/high risk behavior, and prevention/treatment programs. *Trauma Violence Abuse.* 2010;11(4):159–177. https://doi.org/10.1177/1524838010378299.
14. Duncan R, Mulder R, Wilkinson S, et al. Medically unexplained symptoms and antecedent sexual abuse: an observational study of a birth cohort. *Psychosom Med.* 2019;81(7):622–628. https://doi.org/10.1097/PSY.0000000000000726.
15. Sipski ML, Alexander CJ, Rosen RC. Sexual arousal and orgasm in women: effects of spinal cord injury. *Ann Neurol.* 2001;49(1):35–44.
16. Sipski M, Alexander CJ, Gomez-Marin O. Effects of level and degree of spinal cord injury on male orgasm. *Spinal Cord.* 2006;44:798–804.
17. Sipski ML, Alexander CJ, Gomez O, et al. The effects of spinal cord injury on psychogenic sexual arousal in males. *J Urol.* 2007;177(1):247–251.
18. Alexander MS, Biering-Sorensen F, Bodner D, et al. International standards to document remaining autonomic function after spinal cord injury. *Spinal Cord.* 2009;47:36–43.
19. Wecht J, Krassioukov A, Alexander M, et al. International Standards to document Autonomic Function following SCI (ISAFSCI): second edition. *Top Spinal Cord Inj Rehabil.* 2021;27(2): https://doi.org/10.46292/sci2702-23.
20. Alexander M, Marson L. Orgasm and SCI: what do we know? *Spinal Cord.* 2018;56:538–547. https://doi.org/10.1038/s41393-017-0020-9.
21. Alexander M. Sexual sustainability: a guide to having a great sex life with a spinal cord disorder. Amazon; 2017.
22. McGehee M, Hornyak JE, Lin C, et al. Baclofen-induced sexual dysfunction. *Neurology.* 2006;67(6):1097–1098. https://doi.org/10.1212/01.wnl.0000237332.25528.ac.
23. Denys P, Mane M, Azouvi P, et al. Side effects of chronic intrathecal baclofen on erection and ejaculation in men with spinal cord lesions. *Arch Phys Med Rehab.* 1998;79(5):494–496.
24. Al-Gommer O, Sanju G, Haque S, et al. Sexual dysfunctions in male opiate users: a comparative study of heroin, methadone, and buprenorphine. *Addict Disord Their Treat.* 2007;6(3):137–143. https://doi.org/10.1097/ADT.0b013e31802b4e8c.
25. Pacheco Palha A, Esteves M. A study of the sexuality of opiate addicts. *J Sex Marital Ther.* 2002;28(5):427–437. https://doi.org/10.1080/00926230290001547.
26. Davis P, Leira EC, Jang M, et al. Effects of antidepressants on the course of disability following stroke. *Am J Geriatr.* 2011;29(12):1007–1015.
27. Schweitzer I, Maguire K, Ng C. Sexual side effects of contemporary antidepressants: review. *Aust NZ J Psychiatry.* 2009;43(9):795–808. https://doi.org/10.1080/00048670903107575.
28. Perloff MD, Thaler DE, Otis JA. Anorgasmia with gabapentin may be common in older patients. *Am J Geriatr Pharmacother.* 2011;9(3):199–203. https://doi.org/10.1016/j.amjopharm.2011.04.007.
29. Kaufman KR, Struck PJ. Gabapentin-induced sexual dysfunction. *Epilepsy & Behav.* 2011; 21(3):324–326.
30. Bachmann GA, Brown CS, Phillips NA, et al. Effect of gabapentin on sexual function in vulvodynia: a randomized, placebo-controlled trial. *Am J Obstet Gynecol.* 2019;221(1):89e1–89e8. https://doi.org/10.1016/j.ajog.2018.10.021.
31. Calabro RS, DeLuca R, Pollicino P, et al. Anorgasmia during pregabalin add-on therapy for partial seizures. *Epileptic Disord.* 2013;15:358–361.
32. Bucur M, Jeczmien P. Pregabalin and libido-case reports. *The Open Neuropsychopharmacology Journal.* 2011;4:8–9.
33. Karanc Y. Priapism associated with pregabalin. *Am J Emerg Med.* 2020;38(4):852e1–852e2.

34. Osman M, Casey P. Pregabalin abuse for enhancing sexual performance: case discussion and literature review. *Ir J Psychol Med.* 2014;31(4):281–286.

35. Viigimaa M, Vlachopoulos C, Lazaridis A, et al. Management of erectile dysfunction in hypertension: tips and tricks. *World J Cardiol.* 2014;6(9):908–915.

36. Doumas MI, Tsiodras S, Tsakiris A, Douma S, et al. Female sexual dysfunction in essential hypertension: a common problem being uncovered. *J Hypertens.* 2006;24(12):2387–2392. https://doi.org/10.1097/01.hjh.0000251898.40002.5b.

37. Alexander M, Bashir K, Marson L, et al. A randomized trial of clitoral vacuum suction versus vibratory stimulation in neurogenic female orgasmic dysfunction. *Arch Phys Med Rehabil.* 2018;99(2):299–305.

38. Alexander MS, Rosen RC, Steinberg S, et al. Sildenafil in women with sexual arousal disorder following spinal cord injury. *Spinal Cord.* 2011;49(2):273–279.

39. Achilli C, Pundir J, Ramanathan P, et al. Efficacy and safety of transdermal testosterone in postmenopausal women with hypoactive sexual desire disorder: a systematic review and meta-analysis. *Fertil Steril.* 2017;107:475–482.

40. Rees PM, Fowler CJ, Maas CP. Sexual function in men and women with neurological disorders. *Lancet.* 2007;369(9560):512–525. https://doi.org/10.1016/S0140-6736(07)60238-4.

41. Chen L, Staubli SE, Schneider MP, et al. Phosphodiesterase 5 inhibitors for the treatment of erectile dysfunction: a trade-off network meta-analysis. *Eur Urol.* 2015;68(4):674–680. https://doi.org/10.1016/j.eururo.2015.03.031.

42. Rosen RC, Riley A, Wagner G, et al. The international index of erectile function (IIEF): a multidimensional scale for assessment of erectile dysfunction. *Urology.* 1997;49(6):822–830. https://doi.org/10.1016/s0090-4295(97)00238-0.

43. Lombardi G, Macchiarella A, Cecconi F, et al. Ten years of phosphodiesterase type 5 inhibitors in spinal cord injured patients. *J Sex Med.* 2009;6(5):1248–1258. https://doi.org/10.1111/j.1743-6109.2008.01205.x.

44. Lombardi G, Nelli F, Celso M, et al. Treating erectile dysfunction and central neurological diseases with oral phosphodiesterase type 5 inhibitors. Review of the literature. *J Sex Med.* 2012;9(4):970–985. https://doi.org/10.1111/j.1743-6109.2011.02615.x.

45. Lue TF. Erectile dysfunction. *N Engl J Med.* 2000;342(24):1802–1813. https://doi.org/10.1056/NEJM200006153422407.

46. Hatzimouratidis K, Salonia A, Adaikan G, et al. Pharmacotherapy for erectile dysfunction: recommendations from the fourth International Consultation for Sexual Medicine (ICSM 2015). *J Sex Med.* 2016;13(4):465–488. https://doi.org/10.1016/j.jsxm.2016.01.016.

47. Bodner DR, Haas CA, Krueger B, et al. Intraurethral alprostadil for treatment of erectile dysfunction in patients with spinal cord injury. *Urology.* 1999;53(1):199–202. https://doi.org/10.1016/s0090-4295(98)00435-x.

48. Levine LA, Dimitriou RJ. Vacuum constriction and external erection devices in erectile dysfunction. *Urol Clin North Am.* 2001;28(2):335–341. https://doi.org/10.1016/s0094-0143(05)70142-7. ix-x.

49. Deforge D, Blackmer J, Garritty C, et al. Male erectile dysfunction following spinal cord injury: a systematic review. *Spinal Cord.* 2006;44(8):465–473. https://doi.org/10.1038/sj.sc.3101880.

50. Lombardi G, Musco S, Wyndaele JJ, et al. Treatments for erectile dysfunction in spinal cord patients: alternatives to phosphodiesterase type 5 inhibitors? A review study. *Spinal Cord.* 2015;53(12):849–854. https://doi.org/10.1038/sc.2015.116.

CHAPTER 18

Telepsychology

Ramiro Mitre

Introduction

Emma is a rehabilitation psychologist who works in a rural area and counsels 15 people per week. Whereas her colleagues could see their clients in an office in 2 days on a light schedule, Emma had to travel nearly 400 miles weekly. Her work consists of providing rehabilitation services to people with injuries or conditions that cause disability, and most of those consumers are not able to pay visits to her office. Like most rehabilitation psychologists, Emma works primarily with people who have had strokes, amputations, patients who suffer from spinal cord injury (SCI), those with traumatic brain injuries (TBIs), and she also treats co-occurring disorders like depression, anxiety, and pain.

In addition to conducting neuropsychological assessments for rehabilitation facilities and providing assistance to their patients, Emma teaches and researches at a local university and is a proud mother of two children. Naturally, she must organize her time very well to be able to fulfill all her responsibilities and this is not an easy task.

The COVID-19 pandemic forced Emma to reframe her practice and find ways to continue working. The internet quickly became indispensable and videoconferencing software that, until recently, she had no idea existed, now became her main, and most valuable, tool. Even though she was understandably reluctant at the beginning, she was able to see the advantages of this new working modality: she doubled the number of patients that she helps gain more independence and opportunities and she stopped spending long hours at the wheel—which reduced the risks fatigue causes and saved her much time. Not only does she do all of this without neglecting her work at the university, but she also spends more time with her children and in the comfort of her home.

Although Emma did not know it, what she just started is a practice that has been going on for several years and is called "telepsychology."

TELEMEDICINE AND TELEPSYCHOLOGY

Academic literature offers many terms related to telepsychology as a "new" discipline of study. The quotation marks appear for two reasons: firstly, and as we will see later, telepsychology is not really a discipline itself; and secondly, it is not so recent, temporally speaking. To understand what it is about, we must go back to another concept, one that is wider, older, and on which its procedures are based: telemedicine.

Telemedicine is a term that has many definitions. Etymologically speaking, it means "to cure at distance," and its definition varies according to the criteria applied by different authors and organizations. Essentially, it refers to the application of information and communication technologies (ICT) to improve patient outcomes and increase access to care and medical information.[1]

Although there are literally hundreds of definitions of telemedicine, the World Health Organization (WHO)[2] has adopted a rather broad concept:

The delivery of health care services, where distance is a critical factor, by all health care professionals using information and communication technologies for the exchange of valid information for diagnoses, treatment and prevention of disease and injuries, research and evaluation, and for the continuing education of health care providers, all in the interests of advancing the health of individuals and their communities (1998, p. 10).

Most definitions converge on the idea that telemedicine is a science in constant development. This is largely due to ongoing technological advances, the changing needs related to health care, and the circumstances of each society. Another element on which existing definitions agree is the purpose of telemedicine, which is to provide clinical support. The discipline intends to improve health outcomes through various types of ICT, overcoming geographical barriers, and connecting with users who are in different locations.[1]

In the field of psychology, the use of information technologies also finds many terminological variations. Several authors use synonyms such as online therapy, cybertherapy, e-therapy, telehealth, e-health, and online psychological interventions for their studies.[3,4]

From a practical point of view, "telepsychology" and "telepsychological interventions" will be used interchangeably in this chapter, denoting the American Psychological Association (APA) meaning. The APA defines telepsychology as the provision of psychological services through the use of technologies instead of, or in addition to, in-person communication, and that includes the use of telephone, email, text messaging, videoconferencing, mobile applications, and structured programs on a web page.[5]

Although there is practically no information available about rehabilitation telepsychology, dozens of studies, metaanalyses, and reviews on general telepsychology have shown very favorable results and, almost all of them, agree upon the effectiveness of telepsychological interventions.[6] For instance, Backhaus et al. performed a metaanalysis focusing on 65 articles on videoconferencing psychotherapy that found procedures to be feasible, with good user satisfaction, and similar clinical outcomes to traditional psychotherapy.[7] Varker et al. assessed the evidence for synchronous telepsychology interventions and found that video teleconferencing and telephone-delivered interventions provide an effective mode of treatment delivery.[8] Hilty et al.[9] performed a metaanalysis that suggested the efficacy of telehealth for diagnosis and assessment goals was similar to in-person treatments, and increased access to care.

This metaanalysis and most studies available—including randomized trials, reports, and less rigorous research—suggest that telepsychology is as effective as face-to-face psychotherapy, and evidence indicates positive results in process variables—such as satisfaction and rapport—outcome variables, and treatment acceptance and credibility.[10]

In the modality of telepsychology, both evidence-based psychotherapeutic treatments[11] and diagnostic and evaluation processes[9] have shown very similar results compared to in-person treatments. These findings are consistent across different populations and settings, and for numerous disorders. Proof thereof are the Practice Guidelines of the American Telemedicine Association, which state that there is no evidence of users who do not benefit from or are harmed by remote videoconferencing health care services.[12]

Telepsychological interventions can be applied to almost all cases that require psychological assistance in rehabilitation. This includes diagnoses traditionally associated with rehabilitation—such as brain damage, SCI, TBI, or amputations—and newer target populations, for example, those in intensive care units and transplant recipients.[13]

Despite the relevance and increasing use of ICT, relatively few psychologists make use of telepsychological interventions. Many, like Emma, would never have done it because they did not know what it is about, others refuse because they are afraid of it, and some mistakenly assume that it requires too much professional updating. Regardless of the reasons, there are still many barriers to overcome for millions of users to remedy time or distance limitations and access psychological services.

Telerehabilitation in Psychology

Interestingly, one of the first documented references to telemedicine was in the "psy" field. In 1959 faculty members of the Department of Psychiatry at the University of Nebraska implemented a two-way closed-circuit microwave television to share demonstrations and information with students on campus and with Norfolk State Hospital.[14]

Since then, both the uses and the technological means have changed substantially and, although telepsychology is mostly used as a way of providing services, its uses are not limited to that. The scope is very broad and comprises asynchronous media—those that include a certain time lag between transmission and reception, such as email or text messaging—and synchronous media, communications that take place in real time, commonly through videoconferencing, chat, or instant messaging.[6, 15]

Telerehabilitation, understood as a branch of telemedicine whose objective is to control rehabilitation at a distance,[16] uses many telepsychological interventions.

Telepsychology uses four general types of services:

1. Direct-to-consumer: patient-initiated synchronous two-way voice or video virtual visits;
2. Remote patient monitoring: a client at home being monitored by a clinician from a remote location using two-way video or an electronic device;
3. Store and forward: collecting clinical information and sending it electronically to another site for asynchronous evaluation;
4. Mobile health applications: mobile and wireless technologies to support the achievement of health objectives.[17]

Since technology has become so relevant in our everyday life, almost all psychologists use some technological means for their professional activity—from phone calls to arrange appointments, to bibliographic searches on the internet for research. Some psychologists use these as routine and incorporate them into their daily tasks—like Emma, who now assesses and sees all her patients through videoconferencing—and some use them only occasionally. However, information regarding the use of telepsychology for individuals with disability continues to expand, with care of individuals in some diagnostic groups having more evidence basis than others. Ownsworth et al.[18] identified and appraised 13 studies evaluating the efficacy of telerehabilitation for adults with TBI (10 randomized controlled trials and 3 pre- and postgroup studies) and found that the evidence of efficacy was somewhat mixed: telephone-based interventions showed positive effects at postintervention with reports of improvements in global functioning, posttraumatic symptoms and sleep quality, and depressive symptoms. Internet-based interventions support feasibility, but their efficacy could not be determined because of insufficient studies.

In a systematic review, Tran et al. included six studies that met the criteria to evaluate whether technology facilitates interdisciplinary teamwork for the care of people with TBI.[19] The review identified four different telehealth interventions: electronic goals systems, telerehabilitation, videoconferencing, and a point-of-care team-based information system. Both barriers and facilitators were found in the use of eHealth: on one hand, eHealth interventions seem to support interdisciplinary teams, but on the other hand, the existing literature is not enough to recognize barriers and enablers of a successful interdisciplinary telehealth model for people with TBI. Some authors like Pierce et al. state that TBI may be difficult to treat via telepsychology because of the need to coordinate care with in-person services such as medical examinations and physical therapy.[20]

Although much more research is needed, studies that focus on stroke show that teleinterventions have either better or equal effects on motor, higher cortical, and mood disorders compared with traditional face-to-face therapy and they contribute to overcoming distance barriers.[21-24] Furthermore, tools like virtual reality (VR) have demonstrated an increased motivation in users, allowing longer and more training sessions in community-dwelling stroke survivors.[25] In the field of family support, home-based teleintervention programs like that by Kim et al.[26] in South Korea have proven to be cost-effective and supportive in reducing family caregivers' burden by providing prompt, relevant information for their needs.

To date, only a few studies have focused on teleinterventions in SCI. In a review of 29 studies, Irgens et al.[27] found that the use of telehealth in people with SCI seems to be positive where treatment and follow-up are concerned, as well as having socioeconomical and environmental benefits. Research that focused on VR and SCI shows that VR may not be more effective than conventional physical therapy in improving functional performance,[28] but if VR is combined with conventional physical therapy, interventions could have a greater impact in achieving the intended effects on balance recovery after SCI.[29] Moreover, one study tested a teleintervention consisting of an hour-long counseling session each week to enhance need satisfaction, motivation, physical activity, and quality of life among adults with SCI.[30] Its findings showed that the intervention group reported greater autonomous motivation and increased their leisure time physical activity levels after 8 weeks of coaching.

As can be seen, there is little information available about telepsychology and the aforementioned conditions. However, there is even less information about the impact of telepsychology for persons with amputations. One exception is the work on phantom limb pain of Bahirat et al.[31] They have developed a mixed reality-based framework to generate a virtual phantom limb in real time to manage the pain, and it has proven to be feasible and have potential value for pain management.[32]

Although humans can be extremely resilient and can overcome many challenging circumstances, people who have suffered injuries or experienced conditions that cause disability often also experience depression, anxiety, posttraumatic stress disorder (PTSD), suicidal thoughts, social phobia, and/or substance abuse. Evidence-based psychotherapies like cognitive-behavioral therapy, family therapy, crisis management, exposure therapy, coping skills intervention, behavioral activation, and mindfulness-based interventions have shown to be successful and cost-effective.[33] Additionally, those interventions that focus on changing users' behaviors, feelings, thoughts, and relationships have been shown better than no therapy and often produce better outcomes than medications.[34]

The provision of optimal treatment for people who need psychological services is one of the biggest goals in the field. For those purposes, evidence-based practices should be adapted to the online modality. As said before, there is strong evidence that suggests that telepsychological interventions are an effective mode of treatment delivery. All the mental health conditions mentioned earlier have shown similar outcomes when teleinterventions are compared with treatments delivered in person.[35]

In addition to the intervention itself, telepsychological rehabilitation services include prevention, counseling, monitoring, evaluation, consultation, supervision, and education tasks. Evidence shows that such services can be carried out throughout the lifespan and generally in a process that involves other professionals or paraprofessionals. Because telerehabilitation is so broad, the environments in which it takes place are also broad, ranging from clinics, hospitals, and other health care settings, to schools, homes, or other community spaces.[36]

In addition to monitoring the efficacy of telepsychology on patient care, there have been some successful telehealth psychological training programs. Frank et al.[37] reviewed the literature and found that online training can improve therapist knowledge and skill in the short-term, and outcomes in use of the intervention, and satisfaction with training also showed beneficial results.

Health care providers (and especially those who work with people with disabilities) often experience higher levels of stress. Some mindfulness-based online training programs for professionals and paraprofessionals have proven to relieve stress response, increase emotional intelligence and the use of effective coping strategies, enhance resilience, and decrease anger and negative affect through a convenient, affordable, and easily accessible virtual format.[38, 39]

Whatever the services provided, telepsychology implies the use of any technological means. In 2013 the APA published its Guidelines for the Practice of Telepsychology, which emerged from the work of the Joint Task Force for the Development of Telepsychology Guidelines for Psychologists. In these guidelines, they argue that the telecommunications used in telepsychology involve the "preparation, transmission, communication, or related processing of information by electrical, electromagnetic, electromechanical, electro-optical, or electronic means" (p. 792). This includes the use of traditional and mobile telephony, videoconferencing services, email, chat, messaging, and the internet (websites, blogs, and social networks). They also point out that the information transmitted—which may be written or include images, sounds, and so on—can be synchronous or asynchronous, and that technology can:

- augment traditional in-person services (e.g., assigning reading material after the face-to-face meeting),
- be used as a service itself (such as the use of videoconferencing), and
- be combined in different ways depending on the purposes.

According to the criteria of Barnwell,[40] Brennan et al.,[36] and Rutledge,[41] Table 18.1 lists the technological tools that can be used to implement telepsychological interventions.

TABLE 18.1 ■ Commonly Used Tools in Telepsychology.

Tools	Description	Uses
Applications (apps)	A stand-alone software program designed to do a particular thing often downloaded to a mobile telephone	Psychological clinical training (simulated clinical interviews and feedback), assessment, intervention, providing instructions
Artificial intelligence	Computer systems that perform tasks that normally require human intelligence (such as visual perception, speech recognition, decision-making, etc.)	Psychological clinical training (simulated clinical interviews and feedback), assessment, and intervention
Augmented reality	The use of technology to overlay digital elements onto real experience	Delivering clinical interventions (e.g., surgical simulations and treatment for phobias and PTSD)
Bots	Programs that automatically run tasks, like gathering email addresses, posting ads, etc.	Addressing administrative issues
Captology	The study of computers as persuasive technology to influence behaviors and attitudes	Behavioral interventions
Email, text, and fax	Methods of exchanging messages between people using electronic devices	Follow-up on patient care and providing clarification of advice, creating a written record of information, providing patients with a summary of useful information (e.g., contact information for referrals, test results, and procedural information), educating patients with articles and links, extended contact with patients beyond office visits, and delivering clinical interventions
Forums and chat rooms	An online place to have conversations by posting messages (often text and images)	Delivering clinical interventions and providing a lifeline to treatment and social support

Continued

TABLE 18.1 ■ **Commonly Used Tools in Telepsychology.—Cont'd**

Tools	Description	Uses
Landline telephone	A system for transmitting voices over a distance using wire or radio by converting acoustic vibrations to electrical signals	Speaking to clients regarding administrative issues Delivering clinical interventions
Smartphone	A mobile phone with more advanced capabilities, which generally include a variety of apps and the ability to access the internet and browse the web	Speaking to clients regarding administrative issues Delivering clinical interventions
Social media	A set of internet technologies that enables social tools for collaboration, categorization, creation, and sharing	Self-publishing tools (e.g., WordPress or Twitter), aggregators and social news sites (e.g., Technorati and Digg), social networking sites (e.g., Facebook and LinkedIn), content communities (e.g., YouTube and Instagram), virtual worlds based on games or social connection (e.g., Second Life), collaborative projects that create large bodies of crowd-curated information (e.g., Wikipedia)
Tablets and iPad	Portable, flexible devices with multiple functions due to the almost limitless number of apps	Supporting rehabilitation programs and functions
The cloud	Communication network that connects a large number of computers, services, or software	Documentation storage and file transfer
User experience	The psychological impact of the user interface. It is an evaluation of how something is experienced.	Assessing the user's behavior, emotions, and attitudes about using a product, system, or service
Videoconferencing	A technology that allows users in different locations to hold face-to-face meetings without having to move to a single location together	Delivering clinical interventions
Virtual reality	A computer simulation that completely immerses a user in a simulated environment	Delivering clinical interventions (e.g., surgical simulations and treatment for phobias and PTSD)
Wearable technology	Devices that can be worn by the user that track and measure information, and allow data manipulation	Safety monitoring, health and wellness monitoring, home rehabilitation, assessment of treatment efficacy, early detection of disorders, or noncompliance
Websites	A "place" or "page" on the internet with their own address	Making and seeing upcoming appointments online, asking providers questions, getting hours and directions, accessing and downloading new patient forms

PTSD, Posttraumatic stress disorder.

Practice

To better understand the telepsychological interventions that can be implemented in rehabilitation, we will first consider the definition of Rehabilitation Psychology held by the APA:

> (…) the study and application of psychological principles on behalf of persons who have disability due to injury or illness. Rehabilitation psychologists, often within teams, assess and treat cognitive, emotional, and functional difficulties, and help people to overcome barriers to participation in life activities. Rehabilitation psychologists are involved in practice, research, and advocacy, with the broad goal of fostering independence and opportunity for people with disabilities.

As the specialty addresses behavioral and mental health challenges of people with an injury or chronic disability condition, interventions usually target their:

- mental and psychological status,
- emotional coping,
- behaviors that promote positive adaptation to disability, and
- minor adjustment issues and/or severe psychopathology.[42]

As said before, the difference between psychology and telepsychology resides in the means used and not in the ends pursued, and therefore the practical domains of the discipline are the same in both cases. Bearing those practical domains in mind, we shall next discuss the procedures used in telepsychological interventions in rehabilitation.

USE OF TELEPSYCHOLOGY FOR ASSESSMENT PURPOSES

Administration of standardized and nonstandardized tests and behavioral observations fall within the competence of rehabilitation psychologists to assess the psychological and cognitive functioning of users.

Evidence suggests that telepsychological assessments can be reliable, feasible, and accepted for many conditions, psychological, psychiatric, and neurological, and in different populations.[43–48] Not only do teleassessments provide access, convenience, and cost savings for consumers, but they also seem to be a very good resource for clarifying diagnoses, and incorporating client strengths, challenges, and preferences into treatment plans.[49]

For some time now, and especially since the COVID-19 pandemic began, many tests that required in-person interaction began to be replaced by videoconferencing, remote platforms, and other technological means.[50]

When assessing major depression, bipolar disorder, obsessive-compulsive disorder, panic disorder, substance abuse, schizophrenia, PTSD, cognitive functioning, and suicidal thinking, videoconferencing appears to be the most reliable and acceptable option; in fact, most commonly used measures for assessing those disorders have been validated in the online format and demonstrated the reliability and acceptability of videoconferencing assessment.[51]

In general, distance assessments follow the same principles as face-to-face assessments, but with some adaptations. In particular, it is suggested that psychologists adapt both their communication skills and the assessment instruments—many of which already have this new format—to telecommunication.[52]

Of course, more research and large-scale studies are still needed to ensure equivalence between remote and face-to-face evaluations, but the overall picture is very promising. In the meantime, it is recommended that before using technology in the assessment process, the clinician becomes aware of what types of tests are used, their limitations, their standardization procedures, and their quality and security.[6] At the same time, it is also recommended to consider the adaptation of all clinical interviews, behavioral records, checklists, questionnaires, and recording applications to the digital format and in a culturally sensitive manner.[53]

Cultural issues are especially important when it comes to assessment processes. Not only because of the methodological implications, such as cross-cultural equivalence or construct, method, and item bias, but also because the construct of culture itself is difficult to define and measure, and psychologists should guarantee to provide nondiscriminatory assessments.[54]

USE OF TELEPSYCHOLOGY FOR TREATMENT

Treatment in rehabilitation psychology often involves both individual and family/caregiver coping and adaptation. Individual and group interventions include counseling and psychotherapy, cognitive remediation, behavioral management, enhancing use of assistive technology, and facilitation of healthy team functioning.[55]

As the provision of telepsychological services does not differ greatly from face-to-face services, providers are advised to consider all the factors that guarantee quality services, and to commit to general competence as practitioners.[6]

Békés and Aafjes-van Doorn[56] have examined psychotherapists' attitudes toward online therapy during the COVID-19 pandemic and found that most of them acknowledged a positive attitude toward online psychotherapy, suggesting they were likely to keep using it in the future. One of the reasons for those findings might be related to the fact that synchronous interventions such as videoconference meetings have practically the same characteristics as face-to-face interaction and that asynchronous interventions offer multiple benefits.[57] Regardless of whether the interventions occur in real time or with delayed interaction, telepsychological treatments require adapting the procedures to the peculiarities of each case. These adaptations must consider adjustments in communication and in the way the working alliance is established—based on age, settings, culture, diagnoses, and so on. At the same time, providers should also adapt the techniques they use, for example, behavioral activation, live exposure, cognitive restructuring, guided imagery, and so on, for the online format.[52]

In order to achieve these goals, a few specific guidelines are provided, but broadly speaking, practitioners are encouraged to adopt best practice principles.

BEST PRACTICE PRINCIPLES IN TELEPSYCHOLOGY

Nelson et al.[51] have summarized consensus documents from several authors and associations that work in tele–mental health and they suggest adopting the following 10 principles for a telepsychology practice:

1. The basic standards of professional conduct governing psychology are not altered by the use of telehealth technologies to deliver health care, conduct research, or provide education.
2. Confidentiality of client visits, patient health records, and the integrity of information in the health care information system is essential.
3. All clients must be informed about the process, its attendant risks and benefits, and their own rights and responsibilities, and must provide adequate informed consent.
4. Telehealth services must adhere to the basic assurance of quality and professional health care in accordance with psychology's clinical standards.
5. Psychology, as a discipline, must examine how its patterns of care delivery are affected by telehealth and is responsible for developing its own processes for assuring competence in the delivery of telepsychological interventions.
6. Documentation requirements for telepsychology services must be developed that assure documentation of each client encounter with recommendations and treatment,

communication with other health care providers as appropriate, and adequate protections for client confidentiality.

7. Clinical guidelines should be based on empirical evidence and professional consensus among involved health care disciplines.

8. The integrity and therapeutic value of the relationship between clients and psychologists should be maintained and not diminished by the use of telehealth technology.

9. Psychologists do not need additional licensing to provide telepsychology services, and telehealth technologies cannot be used as a vehicle for providing services that otherwise are not legally or professionally authorized.

10. The safety of clients and practitioners must be ensured, so safe hardware and software, combined with demonstrated user competence, are essential components of safe telepsychology practice.

Special Considerations

Technology is allowing infinite possibilities in the health care field in general and in rehabilitation psychology, in particular. Although it offers many benefits, there is also another side of that coin and challenges are also present.

We shall briefly analyze some of the main benefits offered by telepsychological interventions and contrast them with their disadvantages and limitations.

BENEFITS

As discussed earlier, one of the main contributions of technology to rehabilitation practice is the removal of barriers.

If we go back to the introductory vignette, we can see how telerehabilitation becomes a cost-effective alternative for Emma. Unlike traditional rehabilitation services, telepsychology reduces the costs and difficulties related to travel.[58] But, in addition to removing geographical barriers, telepsychological interventions also make it possible to reduce problems that emerge from the socioeconomic status of users and their financial situation, contribute to reducing social isolation, help with physical limitations and mobility, and even assist in breaking down attitudinal barriers while simultaneously increasing access to specific expertise.[59] Moreover, services can be offered across the lifespan and in a continuum of care.[36]

Such benefits are not limited to clinical work but may also be present in other areas of psychological practice such as prevention, supervision, education, and research. In this way, ICT can increase the scope and quality of services and even provide services in places or settings that would otherwise be very difficult to access.

The fact that the technology makes it possible for a psychologist to be present in other cities, states, and even countries helps to overcome the maldistribution of clients and providers while reducing travel costs, difficulties that may be experienced with public transportation, and long waiting lists for treatment.[60]

On the other hand, the tools used in telepsychology do not usually require specialized equipment. Almost everyone has a phone that can be used to solve many clinical and administrative issues, and smartphones with internet access are a great tool because of all the advantages pointed out earlier. The use of software and hardware for videoconferencing offers possibilities of virtual interaction that do not require much more than a built-in webcam and adequate processing speed (which most recently built computers offer), and an average speed internet connection.[40]

Particularly in the area of telerehabilitation, videoconferencing tools have special importance because of the advantages they can bring to patients with physical disabilities by avoiding the need to travel to appointments.[61]

LIMITATIONS

Of course, new solutions also bring new challenges. Just as technology brings many benefits, it also carries risks, ethical considerations, and some drawbacks. To avoid these negative aspects, it is vital to follow best practices and specific guidelines that serve as support to reduce such risks as much as possible.

Telepsychological interventions pose challenges at different levels, such as technological, legal, deontological, and clinical; therefore psychologists must be responsible and aware of the possible risks.[53]

Even though several guidelines and standards are available, to date there is no specific protocol for telepsychological practice. That means that the implementation of the available resources varies according to the practitioner's criteria. On top of that, professional practice is also influenced by the availability of access to technology for all the intervening actors and the limitations of each type of technology.

While the great majority of technological tools are within the reach of any internet user, the alternatives are many, varied, and wide. Logically, not all of them are free of privacy risks or offer Health Insurance Portability and Accountability Act (HIPAA)-compliant service, secure digital signatures, or secure information storage, so it is recommended to pay special attention when choosing the media. It is strongly suggested that practitioners prioritize best practices and consider ethical and legal rules to avoid inappropriate use and client privacy violation, and to be aware of the security and personal data protection issues.[61]

It should be also noted that while clients value and benefit from listening to the recordings of their sessions, sometimes those recordings are done without the practitioners' knowledge, and that might pose legal issues.[62] Even if users do not record their visits to find fault with a professional, there is always the chance of a malpractice lawsuit and specialists suggest that physicians should always assume that their patients are recording their conversations.[63]

As obvious as it may sound, psychologists must have specific skills to implement technology-mediated interventions, and this is an issue that should not be neglected. These skills range from familiarity with the technological systems or devices available to fundamental knowledge and functional skills, such as policy and procedure development, and troubleshooting.[64]

Although telepsychology is having a large impact on professional practice, there are still many professionals who lack the necessary knowledge to carry out an ethical and competent practice, and there seem to be few training options available to achieve the necessary competencies.[57]

Table 18.2 synthesizes the main advantages and limitations of telepsychology.

ACCESSIBILITY AND USABILITY

Beyond the benefits and limitations posed by the practice of telepsychology, there is another issue that deserves special consideration in rehabilitation. Because of the individual characteristics of people with disabilities, practitioners should take into account the use of technology in terms of usability and accessibility.

Many of the challenges derived from ICT implementation can be overcome by adopting a "universal design" (UD) approach to technology in telerehabilitation. This would imply that all people could benefit from products and environments, without the need for adaptations or specialized design.[65] Table 18.3 illustrates the seven principles developed by North Carolina State University for technology design in order to reduce access difficulties for both users and service providers.

Recommendations

No one could deny that, although there are limitations, telepsychological interventions bring great advantages and sufficient benefits to justify the integration of ICT into the

TABLE 18.2 ■ **Advantages and Limitations of the Use of Technologies for the Provision of Psychological Services.**

Advantages	Limitations
Accessibility: technology facilitates access to groups that have challenges in attending face-to-face therapy (youngsters; people with functional disabilities; clients with reduced mobility; saturated or distant health centers; people residing in rural areas or abroad, etc.).	Unequal use: technology is not used by many people, such as the elderly.
Ease of initiation of psychotherapy: the alternative to access initial psychological help for people who have difficulties accessing a face-to-face psychological help service (e.g., people who suffer from psychological problems such as social anxiety problems, agoraphobia, depression, or suicidal ideation).	Clinical risks: there are greater challenges or inability to assist people who require care in crisis, so it is not advisable to use ICT in those cases.
Profitability and efficiency: technology reduces travel time and expenses.	Initial investment: to have the necessary technology might require a significant initial outlay.
Maintaining regularity: ICT makes it possible to maintain regular and continuous contact when continuity could not be provided in person (e.g., people who travel frequently).	Legal issues: there is a lack of knowledge and clear requirements regarding legal regulations and ethical recommendations.
Availability of information: customer information (such as medical history or test results) is easily accessible and fast for professionals and clients.	Data protection risks: client information in different media increases the risks and makes it necessary to protect personal information.
Technological features: professionals can exchange great amounts of information, and technology makes it easier to record and analyze the information collected.	Lack of professional training and need of therapeutic process adaptations to the online environment: training is barely available for psychologists who wish to perform online interventions.
There is increasing empirical support for telepsychological interventions: a growing body of research supports the use of technology in psychological interventions.	Need for more research: more empirical evidence is needed, with homogeneous and unified criteria on the type of online interventions and supports, as well as on less common psychological problems and the latest technological formats.

ICT, Information and communication technology.
Note: Recovered from Guía para la Intervención Telepsicológica. In: De la Torre Martí, M., & Pardo Cebrián, R, eds. *Colegio Oficial de Psicólogos de Madrid.* 2018:24.

therapeutic process,[53] even if there is not yet enough evidence to judge some specific issues as advantages or disadvantages.[52]

There are many resources to guide psychological practice at a distance. Most guidelines provide recommendations and orient decision-making based on ethical and legal aspects.[52] Some of them outline technological requirements, point out considerations about security and access to information, offer guidance about appropriate measures on the use of hardware and software to protect data integrity and privacy, as well as list online resources and platforms.[52]

In the not too distant future, researchers will probably develop and publish specific competencies for telepractice in psychology. In the meantime, it is suggested that in addition to considering

TABLE 18.3 ▥ Principles of Universal Design (North Carolina State University).

UD Principle 1: Equitable Use

The design is useful and marketable to people with diverse abilities.

Guidelines

- 1a. Provide the same means of use for all users: identical whenever possible; equivalent when not.

- 1b. Avoid segregating or stigmatizing any users.

- 1c. Provisions for privacy, security, and safety should be equally available to all users.

- 1d. Make the design appealing to all users.

UD Principle 2: Flexibility in Use

The design accommodates a wide range of individual preferences and abilities.

Guidelines

- 2a. Provide choice in methods of use.

- 2b. Accommodate right- or left-handed access and use.

- 2c. Facilitate the user's accuracy and precision.

- 2d. Provide adaptability to the user's pace.

UD Principle 3: Simple and Intuitive Use

Use of the design is easy to understand, regardless of the user's experience, knowledge, language skills, or current concentration level.

Guidelines

- 3a. Eliminate unnecessary complexity.

- 3b. Be consistent with user expectations and intuition.

- 3c. Accommodate a wide range of literacy and language skills.

- 3d. Arrange information consistent with its importance.

- 3e. Provide effective prompting and feedback during and after task completion.

UD Principle 4: Perceptible Information

The design communicates necessary information effectively to the user, regardless of ambient conditions or the user's sensory abilities.

Guidelines

- 4a. Use different modes (pictorial, verbal, tactile) for redundant presentation of essential information.

- 4b. Provide adequate contrast between essential information and its surroundings.

- 4c. Maximize "legibility" of essential information.

- 4d. Differentiate elements in ways that can be described (i.e., make it easy to give instructions or directions).

- 4e. Provide compatibility with a variety of techniques or devices used by people with sensory limitations.

UD Principle 5: Tolerance for Error

The design minimizes hazards and the adverse consequences of accidental or unintended actions.

Guidelines

- 5a. Arrange elements to minimize hazards and errors: most used elements, most accessible; hazardous elements eliminated, isolated, or shielded.

- 5b. Provide warnings of hazards and errors.

Continued

TABLE 18.3 ■ Principles of Universal Design (North Carolina State University).—Cont'd

• 5c. Provide fail safe features.

• 5d. Discourage unconscious action in tasks that require vigilance.

UD Principle 6: Low Physical Effort
The design can be used efficiently and comfortably and with a minimum of fatigue.

Guidelines

• 6a. Allow user to maintain a neutral body position.

• 6b. Use reasonable operating forces.

• 6c. Minimize repetitive actions.

• 6d. Minimize sustained physical effort.

UD Principle 7: Size and Space for Approach and Use
Appropriate size and space is provided for approach, reach, manipulation, and use regardless of user's body size, posture, or mobility.

Guidelines

• 7a. Provide a clear line of sight to important elements for any seated or standing user.

• 7b. Make reach to all components comfortable for any seated or standing user.

• 7c. Accommodate variations in hand and grip size.

• 7d. Provide adequate space for the use of assistive devices or personal assistance.

UD, Universal design.
© Copyright 1997 North Carolina State University, The Center for Universal Design.

the available guidelines, psychologists rely on the profession's ethics code, and the jurisdictional statutes and regulations, to adapt ethical aspects, decision-making, and professional in-person practices to telepsychology.[59]

McCord et al.[6] have identified available telepsychology guidelines, to understand similarities and differences, and organize the contents into a model of nine core practice domains influenced by practice setting and modality. Table 18.4 summarizes the core telepsychology practice domains and the tasks or considerations that operationalize each domain.

Considering that telerehabilitation is still in the first stages of development and that the speed of scientific and technological progress is increasing, two points are more than clear. On the one hand, all the information offered in this chapter is not and will not be sufficient to perform telepsychological interventions. On the other hand, and closely related, there is still a considerable way to go as far as theory and practice are concerned, and it is necessary to continue deepening scientific knowledge.

The rapid and growing advances in technology make it hard for investigators to keep up with telepsychology knowledge. A priority area of research for psychologists should be the impact of ICT on all aspects of their practice and, in the field of rehabilitation psychology, more studies are vital. Researchers should focus on the efficacy, optimal utilization, methodology, and barriers and enablers of successful teleinterventions for TBI, SCI, stroke, and other conditions that lead to disability.

Research has an intrinsic value because it leads to knowledge and we know that knowledge is power. But when it comes to helping people have better and happier lives, research becomes especially meaningful, and that is why we need to do our best: millions of people depend on us.

TABLE 18.4 ■ **Summary of Available Guidelines.**

Telepsychology Practice Domain	Tasks or Considerations
Administrative Skills	
Verification of identity and location/imposter concerns	Verify the identity of the client (or the decision-maker if the client lacks the capacity to consent to services); make it possible for the client to verify the identity and credentials of the counselor
Record keeping	Maintain notes of all contacts with clients and obtain hard or electronic copies of online communications
Billing	Outline financial arrangements, costs for types of services, reductions for outages, overage fee responsibility, etc.
Organization information	Provide clients with access to counselors' professional information, including internet presence, ownership, location, website, contact information, licensure, and regulatory bodies
Insurance/coverage	Obtain liability insurance coverage for all e-services
Assessment	
Considerations	Know evolving online assessments, limitations, and standardization procedures
Protection	Protect all online assessment data, as well as the integrity of the test instruments
Ethics and Law	
Relevant ethical codes and guidelines	Refer to and enact the ethical codes of your country and/ or profession; enact these exactly as one would in traditional in-person services. Practice according to local, state, national guidelines for your field and for telepsychology and telepsychology specialties
Remote environment	Assess for distractions, confidentiality, safety, etc.
Relevant law jurisdiction; licensure	Ensure that services are only provided within legal geographic borders; verify client's location
Mandatory reporting	Be familiar with and carry out the local laws regarding who is designated as a mandatory reporter of abuse, what duties are expected of them, and what the timelines are for reporting and to whom
Informed consent (content, age, ability to consent)	Due to unique telepsychology considerations (e.g., telephone counseling), verify a client's identity and ability to consent prior to the onset of services
Multicultural competence	Regardless of modality, be equipped to acknowledge and address multicultural considerations. Attend to any special multicultural considerations for telepsychology, especially knowing the area in which you are providing services
Psychotherapy	
Client appropriateness	Know who fits with which modality (consider research, repeated emergencies, tendency toward crises, access to resources, client's comfort, etc.); refer to in-person services when necessary; develop plan in case client's inappropriateness emerges after onset of telepsychology services
Informed consent	Inform the client of risks, benefits, and alternatives to telepsychology in language that is easily understood; inform of patient and clinician rights and responsibilities; establish patient-provider relationship; make sure client has capacity to consent

Continued

TABLE 18.4 ■ Summary of Available Guidelines.—Cont'd

Telepsychology Practice Domain	Tasks or Considerations
Professional boundaries and communication	Consider issues related to electronic communication (e.g., maintain professional language over text/email, do not forward client's texts/emails, etc.); inform client of when and how you are available and what to do in an emergency; do not interact with clients via social media and explain this policy at onset of services
Privacy and confidentiality	Regarding the use of encryption, transmission, storage, and disposal of patient health information: (a) create policies and procedures, (b) demonstrate knowledge of these issues, and (c) inform the client
Handle outages/downtime	Incorporate clinical issues into your downtime decision-making; communicate plans for downtime with clients at onset of services; make contingency plans for downtime and enact them if needed
Competency to provide the service	Effectively provide the content of the treatment at hand, regardless of the mode of communication (i.e., teleservices vs. in-person)
Termination	Know when and how to terminate services; analyze progress of treatment goals; develop follow-up plan; refer if necessary; analyze satisfaction with telepsychology services
Research and Evaluation	
Research/evaluation protocols	Consider collecting data on outcomes, satisfaction, and experiences with telepsychology for individual use (i.e., treatment planning, continuous quality improvements in service delivery) or research
Informed consent	Inform participants of the nature and purpose of the procedures/research, their ability to opt out, and their data usage only with permission
Information security of data	Keep data collected via internet surveys secure and only collect data from clients with their expressed permission
Risk Assessment	
Knowledge of local resources	Know the resources (for emergencies or in-person services when necessary), how to access them, what to do to address any lack of appropriate resources, and have a way to communicate these to the client
Emergency planning	Know what to do in an emergency or crisis and how to connect clients with local resources; have an emergency contact on file
Supervision	
Telesupervision	Be familiar with relevant literature; be competent in the technology used for telesupervision and the technology used by the supervisee for service delivery if applicable; know supervision models appropriate for telepsychology; determine if telesupervision is appropriate; give supervisee feedback and receive feedback
Technical Skills	
Counselor knowledge	Demonstrate knowledge of available evolving technology, uses of technological mediums, strengths, limitations, and effectiveness of technological mediums, and technological definitions and concepts; maintain telepsychology competence and obtain continuing education
Client communication	Translate and communicate the logistics of technology use to clients
Equipment use	Use appropriate equipment and technologies for clients' needs, including connectivity, bandwidth, software, special equipment, etc. Obtain skills relevant to troubleshooting and preventing disruptions in technology

Note: Adapted from C. McCord, P. Bernhard, M. Walsh, et al. A consolidated model for telepsychology practice. *Journal of Clinical Psychology.* 2020;76(6):5-8.

References

1. WHO Global Observatory for eHealth Series Telemedicine: Opportunities and Developments in Member States *Report on the Second Global Survey on eHealth*. Vol. 2. World Health Organization; 2009.
2. World Health Organization. *A Health Telematics Policy in Support of WHO's Health-For-All Strategy for Global Health Development: Report of the WHO Group Consultation on Health Telematics*. World Health Organization; 1998.
3. Barak A, Klein B, Proudfoot JG. Defining internet-supported therapeutic interventions. *Ann Behav Med.* 2009;38(1):4–17. https://doi.org/10.1007/s12160-009-9130-7.
4. Eysenbach G. What is e-health? *J Med Internet Res.* 2001;3(2):E20. https://doi.org/10.2196/jmir.3.2.e20.
5. American Psychological Association. Guidelines for the practice of telepsychology. *Am Psychol.* 2013;68(9):791–800. https://doi.org/10.1037/a0035001.
6. McCord C, Bernhard P, Walsh M, et al. A consolidated model for telepsychology practice. *J Clin Psychol.* 2020;76(6):1060–1082. https://doi.org/10.1002/jclp.22954.
7. Backhaus A, Agha Z, Maglione ML, et al. Videoconferencing psychotherapy: a systematic review. *Psychol Serv.* 2021;9:111–131. https://doi.org/10.1037/a0027924.
8. Varker T, Brand RM, Ward J, et al. Efficacy of synchronous telepsychology interventions for people with anxiety, depression, posttraumatic stress disorder, and adjustment disorder: a rapid evidence assessment. *Psychol Serv.* 2019;16(4):621.
9. Hilty DM, Ferrer DC, Parish MB, et al. The effectiveness of telemental health: a 2013 review. *Telemed J E Health.* 2013;19:444–454. https://doi.org/10.1089/tmj.2013.0075.
10. Waltman SH, Landry JM, Pujol LA, et al. Delivering evidence-based practices via telepsychology: illustrative case series from military treatment facilities. *Prof Psychol Res Pr.* 2019;51(3):205–213. https://doi.org/10.1037/pro0000275.
11. Gros DF, Morland LA, Greene CJ, et al. Delivery of evidence-based psychotherapy via video telehealth. *J Psychopathol Behav Assess.* 2013;35:506–521. https://doi.org/10.1007/s10862-013-9363-4.
12. American Telemedicine Association. Practice Guidelines for Video-Based Online Mental Health Services. 2013. Retrieved from http://www.americantelemed.org/docs/default-source/standards/practice-guidelines-for-video-based-online-mental-health-services.pdf?sfvrsn=6.
13. Budd MA, Hough S, Wegener ST, eds. *Practical Psychology in Medical Rehabilitation*. New York: Springer International Publishing; 2017.
14. Preston J, Brown FW, Hartley B. Using telemedicine to improve health care in distant areas. *Hosp Community Psychiatry.* 1992;43(1):25–32. https://doi.org/10.1176/ps.43.1.25.
15. Grigsby WJ. Telehealth: an assessment of growth and distribution. *J Rural Health.* 2002;18:348–358. https://doi.org/10.1111/j.1748-0361.2002.tb00896.x.
16. Zampolini M, Todeschini E, Hermens H, et al. Tele-rehabilitation: present and future. *Ann Ist Super Sanita.* 2008;44(2):125–134.
17. Mechanic OJ, Persaud Y, Kimball AB. *Telehealth systems. StatPearls.* Treasure Island (FL): StatPearls Publishing; 2020. http://europepmc.org/books/NBK459384.
18. Ownsworth T, Arnautovska U, Beadle E, et al. Efficacy of telerehabilitation for adults with traumatic brain injury: a systematic review. *J Head Trauma Rehabil.* 2018;33(4):E33–E46. https://doi.org/10.1097/HTR.0000000000000350.
19. Tran V, Lam MK, Amon KL, et al. Interdisciplinary eHealth for the care of people living with traumatic brain injury: a systematic review. *Brain Inj.* 2017;31(13-14):1701–1710.
20. Pierce BS, Perrin PB, Tyler CM, et al. The COVID-19 telepsychology revolution: a national study of pandemic-based changes in U.S. mental health care delivery. *Am Psychol.* 2020;76(1):14–25. https://doi.org/10.1037/amp0000722.
21. Sarfo FS, Ulasavets U, Opare-Sem OK, et al. Tele-rehabilitation after stroke: an updated systematic review of the literature. *J Stroke Cerebrovasc Dis.* 2018;27(9):2306–2318.
22. Al Kasab S, Adams RJ, Debenham E, et al. Medical University of South Carolina Telestroke: a telemedicine facilitated network for stroke treatment in South Carolina—a progress report. *Telemed J E Health.* 2017;23(8):674–677.
23. Chen J, Jin W, Zhang XX, et al. Telerehabilitation approaches for stroke patients: systematic review and meta-analysis of randomized controlled trials. *J Stroke Cerebrovasc Dis.* 2015;24(12):2660–2668. https://doi.org/10.1016/j.jstrokecerebrovasdis.2015.09.014.

24. Kizony R, Weiss PL, Feldman Y, et al. *Evaluation of a tele-health system for upper extremity stroke rehabilitation. 2013 International Conference on Virtual Rehabilitation (ICVR)*. New Jersey: IEEE; 2013:80–86.

25. Schröder J, van Criekinge T, Embrechts E, et al. Combining the benefits of tele-rehabilitation and virtual reality-based balance training: a systematic review on feasibility and effectiveness. *Disabil Rehabil Assist Technol*. 2019;14(1):2–11.

26. Kim SS, Kim EJ, Cheon JY, et al. The effectiveness of home-based individual tele-care intervention for stroke caregivers in South Korea. *Int Nurs Rev*. 2012;59(3):369–375.

27. Irgens I, Rekand T, Arora M, et al. Telehealth for people with spinal cord injury: a narrative review. *Spinal Cord*. 2018;56(7):643–655.

28. Miguel-Rubio D, Rubio MD, Salazar A, et al. Effectiveness of virtual reality on functional performance after spinal cord injury: a systematic review and meta-analysis of randomized controlled trials. *J Clin Med*. 2020;9(7):2065.

29. Miguel-Rubio AD, Rubio MD, Salazar A, et al. Is virtual reality effective for balance recovery in patients with spinal cord injury? A systematic review and meta-analysis. *J Clin Med*. 2020;9(9):2861.

30. Chemtob K, Rocchi M, Arbour-Nicitopoulos K, et al. Using tele-health to enhance motivation, leisure time physical activity, and quality of life in adults with spinal cord injury: a self-determination theory-based pilot randomized control trial. *Psychol Sport Exerc*. 2019;43:243–252.

31. Bahirat, K., Annaswamy, T., Prabhakaran, B. Mr. MAPP: Mixed Reality for MAnaging Phantom Pain. In *Proceedings of the 25th ACM International Conference on Multimedia* 2017:1558-1566.

32. Annaswamy M, Bahirat K, Raval G, et al. Clinical feasibility and preliminary outcomes of a novel mixed reality based system to manage phantom pain for patients with lower limb amputation: a pilot study. medRxiv. Published online January 1, 2020:2020.08.29.20133009. doi:10.1101/2020.08.29.20133009.

33. Cook SC, Schwartz AC, Kaslow NJ. Evidence-based psychotherapy: advantages and challenges. *Neurotherapeutics*. 2017;14(3):537–545.

34. David D, Lynn SJ, Montgomery GH. An introduction to the science and practice of evidence-based psychotherapy. In: David D, Lynn SJ, Montgomery GH, eds. *Evidence-Based Psychotherapy: The State of the Science and Practice*. Wiley-Blackwell; 2018:1–10.

35. Chen CK, Nehrig N, Wash L, et al. When distance brings us closer: leveraging tele-psychotherapy to build deeper connection. *Couns Psychol Q*. 2020:1–14.

36. Brennan D, Tindall L, Theodoros D, et al. A blueprint for telerehabilitation guidelines. *Int J Telerehabilitation*. 2010;2(2):31–34. https://doi.org/10.5195/ijt.2010.6063.

37. Frank HE, Becker-Haimes EM, Kendall PC. Therapist training in evidence-based interventions for mental health: a systematic review of training. *Clin Psychol*. 2020;27(3):e12330.

38. Jung YH, Ha TM, Oh CY, et al. The effects of an online mind-body training program on stress, coping strategies, emotional intelligence, resilience and psychological state. *PloS One*. 2016;11(8):e0159841.

39. Lee D, Lee WJ, Choi SH, et al. Long-term beneficial effects of an online mind-body training program on stress and psychological outcomes in female healthcare providers: a non-randomized controlled study. *Medicine*. 2020;99(32):e21027.

40. Barnwell SS. A telepsychology primer. *J Health Serv Psychol*. 2019;45(2):48–56. https://doi.org/10.1007/bf03544680.

41. Rutledge P. *Media Psychology: What You Need to Know and How to Use It. Practical Psychology in Medical Rehabilitation*. New York: Springer International Publishing; 2017:513–532. https://doi.org/10.1007/978-3-319-34034-0_56.

42. Cox DR, Hess DW, Hibbard MR, et al. Specialty practice in rehabilitation psychology. *Prof Psychol Res Pr*. 2010;41(1):82–88. https://doi.org/10.1037/a0016411.

43. Brearly TW, Shura RD, Martindale SL, et al. Neuropsychological test administration by videoconference: a systematic review and meta-analysis. *Neuropsychol Rev*. 2017;27(2):174–186.

44. Galusha-Glasscock JM, Horton DK, Weiner MF, et al. Video teleconference administration of the repeatable battery for the assessment of neuropsychological status. *Arch Clin Neuropsychol*. 2016;31(1):8–11.

45. Grady B, Myers K, Nelson EL, et al. Evidence-based practice for telemental health. *Telemed J E Health*. 2011;17(2):131–148.

46. Jong M. Managing suicides via videoconferencing in a remote northern community in Canada. *Int J Circumpolar Health*. 2004;63(4):422–428.

47. Miller ET, Neal DJ, Roberts LJ, et al. Test-retest reliability of alcohol measures: is there a difference between Internet-based assessment and traditional methods? *Psychol Addict Behav*. 2002;16(1):56–63.

48. Wadsworth HE, Dhima K, Womack KB, et al. Validity of teleneuropsychological assessment in older patients with cognitive disorders. *Arch Clin Neuropsychol.* 2018;33(8):1040–1045. https://doi.org/10.1093/arclin/acx140.

49. Harrell KM, Wilkins SS, Connor MG, et al. Telemedicine and the evaluation of cognitive impairment: the additive value of neuropsychological assessment. *J Am Med Dir Assoc.* 2014;15(8):600–606. https://doi.org/10.1016/j.jamda.2014.04.015.

50. American Psychological Association. Guidance on psychological tele-assessment during the COVID-19 crisis. 2020. http://www.apaservices.org/practice/reimbursement/health-codes/testing/tele-assessment-covid-19.

51. Nelson EL, Bui TN, Velasquez SE. Telepsychology: research and practice overview. *Child Adolesc Psychiatr Clin N Am.* 2011;20(1):67–79. https://doi.org/10.1016/j.chc.2010.08.005.

52. Martí MD, Cebrián RP. Guía para la Intervención Telepsicológica. Colegio oficial de la Psicología de Madrid. 2017:7-36. https://www.copmadrid.org/web/img_db/publicaciones/guia-para-la-intervencion-telepsicologica-5c1b5a8602018.pdf.

53. Ramos Torio, R., Alemán Déniz, J. M., Ferrer Román, C., et al. Guía para la práctica de la Telepsicología. *Consejo General de la Psicología España.* 2017:7-36. https://doi.org/10.23923/cop.telepsicologia.2017

54. Rossier J, Duarte ME. Testing and assessment in an international context: cross- and multi-cultural issues. In: Athanasou J, Perera H, eds. *International Handbook of Career Guidance.* Cham: Springer; 2019. https://doi.org/10.1007/978-3-030-25153-6_28.

55. American Psychological Association. Rehabilitation Psychology. 2015. https://www.apa.org/ed/graduate/specialize/rehabilitation.

56. Békés V, Aafjes-van Doorn K. Psychotherapists' attitudes toward online therapy during the COVID-19 pandemic. *J Psychother Integr.* 2020;30(2):238–247. https://doi.org/10.1037/int0000214.

57. Cooper SE, Campbell LF, Smucker Barnwell S. Telepsychology: a primer for counseling psychologists. *Couns Psychol.* 2019;47(8):1074–1114. https://doi.org/10.1177/0011000019895276.

58. Marzano G, Ochoa-Siguencia L, Pellegrino A. Towards a new wave of telerehabilitation applications. *Perspective.* 2017;1(1):1–9.

59. Martin JN, Millán F, Campbell LF. Telepsychology practice: primer and first steps. *Pract Innov.* 2020;5(2):114–127. https://doi.org/10.1037/pri0000111.

60. Nelson E-L, Bui T. Rural telepsychology services for children and adolescents. *J Clin Psychol.* 2010;66(4):490–501. https://doi.org/10.1002/jclp.20682.

61. Rutledge CM, Kott K, Schweickert PA, et al. Telehealth and eHealth in nurse practitioner training: current perspectives. *Adv Med Educ Pract.* 2017;8:399.

62. Mercer, E. Recording Doctor Visits Is Just Another Step Toward Patients Taking Ownership over Their Own Care. 2020. https://opmed.doximity.com/articles/recording-doctor-visits-is-just-another-step-toward-patients-taking-ownership-over-their-own-care?_csrf_attempted=yes.

63. Woods, J. A. Audio-Video Recording of Patient Visits. 2020. https://home.svmic.com/resources/newsletters/145/audio-video-recording-of-patient-visits.

64. McCord CE, Saenz JJ, Armstrong TW, et al. Training the next generation of counseling psychologists in the practice of telepsychology. *Couns Psychol Q.* 2015;28(3):324–344.

65. Connell, B. R., Jones, M., Mace, R., et al. Steinfeld, Molly Story, & Gregg Vanderheiden–The Center for Universal Design (1997): The Principles of Universal Design, Version 2.0. Raleigh, NC: North Carolina State University.

CHAPTER 19

Telephysical Therapy

Mohit Arora ■ Camila Quel De Oliveira

Introduction

Physical therapy, also known as physiotherapy, is a health care profession that uses evidence-based kinesiology, exercise prescription, health education, mobilization, electrical and physical agents to treat acute or chronic pain, movement and physical impairments resulting from injury, trauma, or illness typically of musculoskeletal, cardiovascular, respiratory, neurological, and endocrinological origins. Physical therapy is concerned with human function and movement and maximizing physical potential to identify and promote health-related quality of life and movement potential.[1]

Physical therapy is used to improve a patient's physical functions through physical examination, diagnosis, prognosis, patient education, physical intervention, rehabilitation, disease prevention, and health promotion. Physical therapy is practiced by physical therapists (or physiotherapists). Physical therapists can help people at any stage of life when movement and function are threatened by aging, injury, diseases, disorders, conditions, or environmental factors.[2] Maximizing movement is an important benefit of physical therapy as pain-free movement is crucial to quality of life, ability to earn a living, and independence. Personalized care is emphasized through treatment plans for each person's individual needs, challenges, and goals regardless of whether the individual is dealing with a chronic condition or recovering from injury, or wants to prevent future injury and chronic disease. Physical therapists provide customized care in hospitals, private practices, outpatient clinics, homes, schools, sports and fitness facilities, work settings, and nursing homes. They promote recovery by empowering people to be active participants in their care by working collaboratively with other health care professionals.

Physical therapists are also key members of the health care team in other important areas. Physical therapy is an important part of international efforts to avoid overuse of opioids. In some situations, dosed appropriately, prescription opioids are an appropriate part of medical treatment. However, the Centers for Disease Control and Prevention urges health care providers to reduce the use of opioids in favor of safe alternatives like physical therapy for most long-term pain. Opioid risks include depression and mood disorders, overdose, and addiction, plus withdrawal symptoms when stopping use. Physical therapy can also help people avoid and/or delay surgery. For some conditions, including meniscal tears and knee osteoarthritis, rotator cuff tears, spinal stenosis, and degenerative disc disease, treatment by a physical therapist is as effective as surgery. Moreover, in conjunction with medical management or nonoperative orthopedic care provided by a physical medicine and rehabilitation physician, orthopedist, or even primary care specialist, many patients can avoid the need for surgery altogether.

Telerehabilitation and Telerehabilitation in Physical Therapy

Telerehabilitation has been defined as "the delivery of rehabilitation services via information and communication technologies" and encompasses services that include assessment, prevention, treatment, education, and counseling.[3] Telerehabilitation in physical therapy (TelePT) is a sub-component of telerehabilitation, defined as delivering physical therapy services to patients at a distance using information and communication technologies (ICTs).[4]

In the late 1990s telePT was used for one-on-one physical therapy[5,6] and for monitoring the progress of people with stroke during rehabilitation.[7] Over the last decade, telePT has been widely used for consultations, assessment, and treatment in a range of conditions. It has also been used to deliver education-based interventions and promote physical fitness and well-being.[8] On the one hand, technology may contribute to sedentary behavior (e.g., playing computer games or working in front of a computer for prolonged periods in a seated position) across different age groups and socioeconomic levels. On the other hand, using technology, such as smartphone applications and wearable devices, can provide innovative solutions to increase physical activity and reduce sedentary behavior.[9]

Currently, more than 6.8 billion people use mobile phones worldwide. An analysis conducted in 2013 revealed that over 40,000 health and fitness applications are currently available to the public, and over half of smartphone users report having downloaded such applications.[10] More specifically, in physical therapy, Machado et al. conducted a systematic review of mobile applications targeted at people with low back pain. They included 61 apps in their analyses out of over 700 available apps in iTunes and Google Play between 2015 and 2017.[11]

People of all ages with a variety of symptoms and medical conditions may be candidates for telePT, for example, people with balance disorders, people seeking pre- and postoperative care, management of chronic pain, amputation care, people with neurological conditions (like stroke, spinal cord injury [SCI], traumatic brain injury [TBI]) receiving home-based rehabilitation, and so on (Table 19.1). TelePT has been proven valuable in improving postoperative outcomes and functional recovery in surgical patients, where patients considered telePT as a positive experience and suitable for those with long traveling distances or mobility issues, flexible exercise hours, and the ability to integrate exercises into daily life directly.[12-14] Also, telePT has been valuable

TABLE 19.1 ▪ Some of the Potential Uses of TelePT.

Technology	Population	Potential Use
mHealth	Chronic disease management in elderly	Reminding people to undergo scheduled exercise[95]
mHealth	Various disabilities	Allow patients to record and share their health measures and send them electronically to physicians and/or specialists[96]
Online technology/ mHealth	Various disabilities in aging population	• Allow for greater access to health care provisions • Availability of care • Supports self-management • Prevention in routine care. This will reduce unnecessary admissions and helps to reduce health care costs in an aging population[97]
mHealth	Various acute and chronic conditions	Function as self-assessment, screening and testing tools and symptom checkers, goal setters, and treatment/exercise logs and prescribers
Interactive websites	Musculoskeletal conditions in all age groups	Tailored and progressive home exercise programs (HEPs) and monitoring compliance[98]

in overcoming the discontinuities that may arise in communication between the hospital and another health care provider and primary care facilities for treating complex surgical cases in the community.[15]

There is also growing evidence showing positive effects of telePT on clinical outcomes in patients with certain types of cancer,[16, 17] neurological disorders,[18–20] sports injuries,[21] cardiac disease and rehabilitation,[22, 23] musculoskeletal disorders,[6] chronic pain,[24] chronic obstructive pulmonary disease (COPD),[25] and pelvic floor disorders.[26] TelePT has been delivered in various formats: smartphone applications, web-based use of activity trackers (pedometers), videoconference, and text messages to monitor conditions, deliver exercise, and educational strategies.

ROLE OF TELEPT IN INITIAL CONSULTATION AND ASSESSMENT

Some of the common assessment items of a conventional physical therapy session are easily collected via telePT. Therefore an initial telePT consultation can include subjective assessment, observational analysis of function, posture and gait, quality of movement, observation of active range of motion, pain tolerance, and irritability. In an initial consultation, if telePT is being delivered in addition to face-to-face sessions, the therapist should identify the need for investigation before attending face-to-face appointments. Education is another important component of treatment in chronic pain and disease management, exercise interventions, review, and program updates. TelePT can successfully deliver interventions targeting education.

Some assessment components such as manual tests for strength and mobility, neurological examination of reflexes and sensation, motor control assessments, and special tests for diagnostic purposes can be challenging to conduct via telePT. Therapists can seek alternative ways of obtaining these data by questioning the patient, acquiring it from their physician, and considering the need for a complimentary face-to-face appointment. There are challenges in delivering interventions that involve manual guidance or specialized equipment such as joint manipulation or body-weight support treadmill training. In those cases, the therapist should seek alternative interventions. Although carers may assist in delivering some simple interventions such as supporting a limb during an active-assisted exercise, it is the therapist's responsibility to ensure the patient's safety during the session.

The use of telePT has been proven effective for an initial consultation in musculoskeletal conditions,[27, 28] neurological conditions,[29–31] and delivering rehabilitation consultations using a low-bandwidth internet-based telePT for remote areas.[32] TelePT has been now widely used in assessing range of motion[33, 34] and muscle strength[33] and in diagnosing conditions like low back pain,[35] shoulder disorders,[36] knee conditions,[37] and other nonarticular lower-limb conditions.[38]

ROLE OF TELEPT IN ADVOCATING EDUCATION AND TREATMENT

The role of the physical therapist in the management of chronic conditions has changed in the past decades. Self-management interventions, including education and strategies to increase physical activity, have superior results to hands-on physical therapy interventions.[39] Self-management is the individual's ability to manage the symptoms, treatment, physical and psychosocial consequences, and lifestyle changes inherent in living with a chronic condition. Patient education, empowerment, and monitoring are key components for the success of self-management strategies.[40]

Self-management strategies consisting of educational modules delivered via email or websites have been successful in increasing physical activity participation in people with acquired brain injuries,[41] reducing pain and disability in chronic low back pain,[39] and improving quality of life for people with COPD.[42] To increase adherence and motivation, online educational modules can be supplemented with weekly phone calls or videoconferencing for monitoring, which can significantly reduce face-to-face time with therapists and, in turn, reduce costs related to long-standing disease management.

TelePT has been widely used for delivering education and treatment for various disorders, such as stroke, SCI, brain injury, cardiovascular disease, and amputation. A meta-analysis of 12 studies involving stroke survivors suggested that telerehabilitation can be a suitable alternative to usual rehabilitation care, especially in remote or underserved areas. The outcomes included in this meta-analysis were activities of daily living, balance scale, and motor functions.[43] Another review in adults with TBI found that structured telephone interventions were effective for improving some outcomes (but not physical function outcomes) following TBI. The review included 10 randomized controlled trials looking at the feasibility and/or effectiveness of telephone-based and internet-based interventions.[44] TelePT has also been widely used in people with spinal cord disease.[30, 31, 45] A systematic review of telerehabilitation and mobile health (mHealth) interventions suggested the potential to improve health-related outcomes in people with SCI in home and community settings.[46] This review included nine studies delivering a telerehabilitation intervention via phone or video call facility (such as Skype, Scopia, Tandberg conferencing equipment, and CareCall system). Also, some of these studies used adjunct technologies to deliver the intervention and capture real-time outcomes, such as the eTDS bundle, ReJoyce workstation, a powered toothbrush, adapted flosser, and/or oral irrigator.[46] In the last few years, telerehabilitation has been gaining popularity for prevention, such as cardiovascular diseases. A meta-analysis, including 13 studies, suggested insufficient evidence in reducing overall cardiovascular risk.[47]

Another area where telerehabilitation has been widely used is people with lower-limb amputation, ulcer, and weight management.[48] Telerehabilitation can promote better/faster healing of wounds and better adherence to self-care regimens, both of which may reduce health care costs for individuals with long-distance travel time.[49]

ROLE OF TELEPT IN PROMOTING PHYSICAL ACTIVITIES

Physical inactivity has been identified as a global epidemic by the World Health Organization (WHO). It is the fourth leading risk factor for global mortality,[50] contributing to approximately 3.2 million deaths annually worldwide. The Americas region has the highest prevalence of inactivity, followed by the Eastern Mediterranean region.[51] The cost related to physical inactivity on health care systems is overwhelming. In the United Kingdom, the annual cost is $11.2 billion;[52] in Canada, the cost is approximately $6.8 billion per year.[53] The United States spends more than 75% of the $2 trillion annual health care budget on physical inactivity–related hospitalizations.[54] To combat this growing epidemic globally, the WHO and many countries like Canada, the UK, and the United States have developed Physical Activity Guidelines.[55–57]

Technologies for self-tracking have become increasingly popular within the general population. At the same time, health care professionals embrace the opportunities they perceive through using what has been dubbed "mHealth" to promote the public's health.[58] This electronic monitoring of human health behavior is fast becoming an area of increasing research focusing on "sensor fusion" using single systems or devices.[59]

Many studies have provided evidence on the effectiveness of fitness technology to engage people in various types of exercise programs. A systematic review suggested positive results such as weight loss and changes in health risk behavior in individuals with inactive lifestyle in studies that used mixed technology-based physical activity interventions (web-based technology, mobile phones, and accelerometers).[60] Some of the commonly used devices that measure and track physical activity are as follows.

Pedometers

They count and monitor the number of steps taken while walking, jogging, and running. They can also provide distance covered and caloric expenditure. Studies have shown that some pedometers provide a valid and reliable measure of step counts during walking,[61, 62] and pedometer-based walking increases physical activity.[63] Bravata and colleagues studied efficacy of pedometers and reported that setting a step goal for a day on a pedometer was a key predictor for increasing physical activity by 27% over the baseline value. Programs such as pedometer-based walking were also associated with significant decreases in body mass index (BMI), body weight, and systolic blood pressure.[64, 65]

Accelerometers

They record body acceleration from minute to minute, providing detailed information about the frequency, duration, intensity, and movement patterns. They are more expensive than pedometers and used more widely in research.

Heart Rate Monitors

They are used primarily to assess exercise intensity for individuals with cardiac conditions and highly trained competitive athletes. These devices can also estimate exercise energy expenditure. The use of heart rate monitor data in conjunction with an accelerometer can improve energy expenditure by 20% during physical activity.[66] Some devices monitor heart rate and body motion at the same time to provide valid and reliable physical activity measures.[67-69]

Interactive Video Games

They promote physical activities, improve aerobic capacity, and promote fitness level, for example, Dance-Dance Revolution, Wii Sports, and Sony Play Station. *Exergaming* is the term given to interactive digital games in which the player actively moves. Bailey and McInnis evaluated the enjoyment and 10-minute energy demand of six different exergaming systems and treadmill walking for children of normal and above-normal BMIs. The associated metabolic equivalent (MET) levels were in the moderate- to vigorous-intensity ranges.[70]

Fitness Smart Trackers

Fitness trackers can monitor daily steps, heart rate, physical and sports activities, and sleep, such as smartwatches and wrist bands.

Smartphone Applications

They allow users to track physical activities such as jogging/biking routes, workout data, and comprehensive workout history.[10] Some smartphone applications provide professional virtual reality coaching to promote physical activity.

Many organizations and institutions are now utilizing interactive games to promote physical activity in children, adolescents, and older adults. Warburton and colleagues reported that an interactive video cycling game significantly increased heart rate and energy expenditure as compared to traditional cycling at constant, submaximal workloads.[71] Interactive games are not exclusively for children and also hold promise for promoting functional independence, improving balance, preventing falls, reducing premature disability, and maintaining health by increasing adults' and seniors' physical activity levels.[72] The elderly population who completed a 3-month video dancing intervention (30 minutes per session, twice weekly) showed improved balance confidence, mental health, and time walking along a narrow path.[73]

Fitness technology often utilizes behavior change techniques, such as goal setting, feedback, rewards, and social factors to increase the individual's adherence to physical activity.[10] Providing feedback such as reminders, text messages, and real-time alerts is essential for tracking goals and increasing activity levels. Some fitness trackers' features are to vibrate, ping, or display a congratulatory message when a goal has been achieved. Users can easily share their progress with their friends on social media as a great motivational tool.[10] Technology-based fitness tools provide a less costly alternative to one-on-one therapy, are simple to use, and provide meaningful outputs to users. Studies have found that fitness trackers, such as wrist-worn devices, have acceptable reliability and validity comparable to research-standard devices in the laboratory.[10]

Many reviews looking at the effectiveness of different digital interventions for different conditions have been published in the last decade. A review published in 2017 involving 27 studies suggested that digital interventions that include health education, goal setting, self-monitoring, and parent involvement can significantly improve adolescents' dietary and physical activity behaviors. This review also found that the studies delivering interventions using websites as a platform are more effective than interventions delivered using digital platforms such as apps, text messages, and social media.[74] Another review suggested positive effects of ICTs in physical activity interventions for children and adolescents, especially when used with other delivery approaches, such as the face-to-face method.[75] An overview of reviews published in 2011 identified 12 recommendations for practice associated with increased effectiveness in dietary and physical activity interventions.[76]

PERFORMANCE OF TELEPHYSICAL THERAPY

TelePT aims to overcome barriers and provide equitable access to physical therapy. TelePT also can help overcome barriers to face-to-face consultations, such as clinic scheduling and logistics, difficulties with transportation because of distance or financial issues, adverse weather, disasters, pandemics, and secondary conditions. There are various ways of administering telePT. The first two described here are traditional methods, but the latter two have evolved with advancing technology.

Synchronous

Health information is delivered in real time. This can be done through interactive video with the client and health professional present at the same time, such as through videoconferencing. It can be used for an initial consultation and for diagnosing and treating clients.[77] This requires high bandwidth, constant connectivity, and investment in related hardware.

Asynchronous or Store and Forward

Health information is collected at the client site and then transferred for assessment to a physical therapist located at another site. An example of this is a person tracking their own activity or steps on a particular day, and then this information is sent to the physical therapist to monitor. Another example is using newer technology such as virtual reality or "wearables" to store and forward data back to the therapist. This is generally used for assessing or monitoring progress with an exercise routine. This is less dependent on constant connectivity but more complicated to administer. There is a time delay between when a message is sent from one party and received by the second party.[77]

Mobile Health or mHealth

This is a special form of digital health, including mobile phone applications available directly to consumers. They are inexpensive and have built-in software functionality for accessing health information in a timely way.[78] mHealth is seen as a potential means for worldwide change because of its high reach and low-cost solutions.[79] Smartphone applications represent a new and emerging way to deliver telePT that promotes active participation from both the physical therapist and the client throughout the course of treatment.

Hybrid Model

This is usually a combination of synchronous and asynchronous telePT.

TelePT in Clinical Practice

The rapid evolution of technology has allowed physical therapy to deliver health care in a new, remote fashion. For example, videoconferencing allows for the provision of consultations, diagnostic assessments, and delivery of treatment interventions and provides verbal and visual interaction between the therapist and the client. In clinical practice, the use of telePT has been proven effective for initial consultation purposes, disease management, and advocating different types of therapy, for example, groups versus one-on-one, strengthening versus conditioning, and maintenance versus ongoing active therapy. The following telePT model of care can be applied to disorders or conditions that physical therapy treats. There are specific challenges that come with technology when managing a disorder or condition using telePT. These challenges are manageable and are usually outweighed by the benefits that come with telePT, also explained earlier in this chapter. The following figure depicts an overarching theoretical model on how telePT can be used and implemented in many different ways, targeting a different population with different disorders (Fig. 19.1).

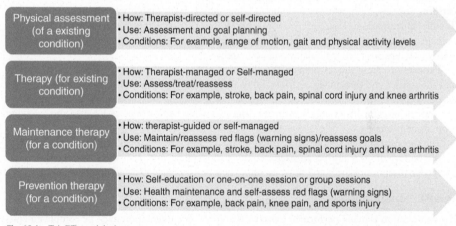

Physical assessment (of a existing condition)
- How: Therapist-directed or self-directed
- Use: Assessment and goal planning
- Conditions: For example, range of motion, gait and physical activity levels

Therapy (for existing condition)
- How: Therapist-managed or Self-managed
- Use: Assess/treat/reassess
- Conditions: For example, stroke, back pain, spinal cord injury and knee arthritis

Maintenance therapy (for a condition)
- How: therapist-guided or self-managed
- Use: Maintain/reassess red flags (warning signs)/reassess goals
- Conditions: For example, stroke, back pain, spinal cord injury and knee arthritis

Prevention therapy (for a condition)
- How: Self-education or one-on-one session or group sessions
- Use: Health maintenance and self-assess red flags (warning signs)
- Conditions: For example, back pain, knee pain, and sports injury

Fig. 19.1 TelePT model of care.

Some of the important criteria for implementing telePT in clinical practice are as follows.

ELIGIBILITY FOR TELEPHYSICAL THERAPY

Before considering telePT, it is important to assess the patient suitability and potential risks of delivering physical therapy interventions remotely. Previous to an initial consultation, it is important to verify.

Home Setting

This includes the patient's accommodation type (house, unit, assisted living), physical environment (decluttered, adequate light and space), and who they live with.

Need for Assistance

Consider the need for a family member or carer to assist during sessions, especially for people with mental and neurological disorders, or who are elderly or frail.

Patient Complexity and Characteristics

Patients who demonstrate risky behaviors, such as disinhibition, poor insight, poor judgment, poor impulse control, or a significant cognitive impairment (Mini-Mental State Examination <21), or who present suicidal ideation will require a risk mitigation plan.

Technology Available

Confirm electricity is available for the connection, if internet coverage is available, and if there is a landline or mobile phone number to contact the patient in the case of problems with the internet connection (in the case of videoconference).

PREPARATION FOR TELEPT SESSIONS

Before delivering telePT interventions via teleconference, the therapist must consider the environment where the therapist is as it determines the type of exercises that they can demonstrate to the patient. A larger room and a plinth are good options to demonstrate exercises in lying, sitting, or standing positions. Furthermore, it is important to prepare the exercises that the patient will perform, and any equipment needed and to know their current mobility levels before the session. The therapist should be aware of relevant comorbidities that may impact therapy, such as low back pain, poor vision, or hearing and consider the patient's level of risk-taking, cognitive level, and ability to follow instructions quickly and accurately.

Patients or carers should prepare their therapy environment, declutter, remove trip hazards, and allow space and camera visuals for walking and turning. Equipment or room markings may be needed as part of the preparation for mobility/standing training and collecting outcome measures. The patient or carer may roughly estimate distances using large strides as 1 meter and knowing room dimensions.

The therapist should educate the patient on the importance of providing continuous feedback on discomfort or pain during an exercise. The patient must not push their limb/body beyond acceptable discomfort levels and must monitor their performance to avoid potential injuries.

TelePT Consultation

If a consultation is being performed between therapists, documentation must be completed contemporaneously by therapists at both ends of the telePT consultation. It is advisable to document within the client notes, including time and date of consultation, consent for any intervention delivered, attendees (everyone present in a visit should be recorded), detailed assessment and clinical notes, outcomes discussed, recommended actions, and responsibility for action specifically designated to an individual. Documentation should also include a statement such as "consultation conducted via synchronous clinical video telehealth." Some other implementation considerations are therapist checklist, room requirements, patient information, documentation, confidentiality, and evaluation.

BENEFITS AND CHALLENGES OF TELEPT

In general, telePT reduces the costs and enhances accessibility for both health care providers and patients compared with traditional inpatient or person-to-person rehabilitation. TelePT can increase accessibility and help overcome geographical barriers, allowing a person to stay more closely connected with a physical therapist after an initial in-person visit. TelePT can also help people living in remote areas where physical therapy is not accessible. Because of the elimination of geographical barriers, telePT saves traveling time, money, and the negative environmental impact of travel when compared with in-person visits. Moreover, the lack of a physical waiting room makes waiting for an appointment more functional. Finally, telePT may aid in the early assessment of a health problem or secondary health condition, and it is believed that people who take part in telePT are more likely to comply and adhere to their exercise program.

TelePT also has other advantages related to safety and preparedness. A physical therapist can provide safe and effective telePT customized to a person's specific needs and goals for their own living environment rather than in the artificial environment of a clinic, gym, or hospital. In the elderly population, telePT is also more convenient and an optimal way to address falling concerns in conjunction with family member and caregiver involvement. In a world where face-to-face access to physical therapy services is vulnerable (during an emergency situation like the COVID-19 pandemic) as well as where the gap between the supply of and demand for physical therapy services is widening, telePT allows physical therapists to continue to provide services at a distance.[80, 81]

Despite good quality research in telePT, there are challenges and barriers to its use in organizational, personal, and technical arenas in both developing and developed countries. Some common organizational challenges are lack of national telePT policies and clinical guidelines,[82, 83] lack of eHealth resources[82] or access to exercise equipment for patients,[84] lack of government support for sustainability,[83] lack of training for stakeholders,[85] and need for ICT infrastructure.[83, 85, 86] Some common personal challenges include cost; personal feelings about the effectiveness of telePT; privacy and confidentiality;[87, 88] service acceptance, adherence, and satisfaction;[82, 87, 89] knowledge and skills required to use and access the technology;[90] lack of personal contact (face-to-face meeting) and empathy;[91, 92] and unwillingness to give up a paper culture.[89] Technical challenges include slow internet or limited network coverage,[85, 87, 90] availability and knowledge of installation of complex software,[85] relying on computers (hardware failure or limitations) or smart phones,[85] and associated costs.[84]

Special Considerations in TelePT

Most costs involved with telePT involve setting up the telePT services. When specific new applications are used, they are an investment in the longer term. While these applications provide an exciting new outlet for physical therapy to proceed toward the future, a thorough assessment of how they can be adapted to suit health care's current needs is important as is an assessment of sustainability of the business model.

The technology that is being used must be accessible and allowed in the country with no restrictions. Easy navigation of the technology with a limited need for training is important for both the physical therapist and the client. Avoidance of software installation and complex processes is beneficial as is the ability to adapt to the clients' needs and disabilities. Integration with other software and technologies using application programming interface (API) and syncing information in real time is also important. Accessibility of technology also means, however, that it must be accessible within your country/organization/state and that both the client and professional have access to use the technology. Some commonly used platforms for video communication are Zoom, FaceTime, Skype, WhatsApp, and Microsoft Teams.

While a business model needs to consider a few different options to cater to persons from different age groups and with different types of disability, the physical therapist must be aware of the platform's and software's quality and data protection.[93] Each country has its own Data Protection Act to protect the client's information and rights. Some key data protection principles are that data should be used fairly and lawfully; used in a way that is adequate, relevant, and accurate; kept only for the necessary time period; and protected and handled with confidentiality at all times according to local ethical regulations. Additionally, the technology used needs to conform to required levels of security as mandated by state or country laws and provision of the safe and secure passage of data over internet through end-to-end encryption.

The physical therapist performing telePT needs to have a prior understanding of what the end-user's needs and expectations are. For example, what is the purpose of the telePT session? Is it consultation, delivering an intervention or both? Involvement of family or caregiver during the telePT is crucial and, where possible, involving families and carers as partners in treatment and care planning brings valuable knowledge and insights about the consumer and resources to assist in their recovery.

In addition to factors such as goal setting, self-efficacy, and motivation, other factors can affect a patient's ability to respond positively to a home exercise program. While demographics such as age and gender have been shown to have little effect on these rates,[94] other factors may affect compliance with telePT, such as levels of physical activity at baseline, mental health issues, the quality of the patient's social support system, perceived barriers to exercise, health literacy, time commitment, and cost of treatment.

One final consideration when performing telePT is the need for disclaimers and legal acknowledgments. A disclaimer is a statement denying responsibility intended to prevent civil liability arising for particular acts or omissions in the real world. On the other hand, disclaimers also serve as a warning to users. Disclaimers give clients realistic expectations for a therapy outcome or service that is being delivered. However, this is often not enough to guarantee legal protection.

Recommendations for Future Actions and Research

As the value of telerehabilitation is increasingly acknowledged, efforts should be directed to address the challenges for developing telePT in individual countries for future routine care and for emergency preparedness. This will involve advocating for a national telerehabilitation plan and policies. Moreover, physical therapy experts around the world should come together to develop clinical guidelines for telePT.

There are many areas where research into telerehabilitation and telePT is necessary. Studies need to determine the effect of specific protocols for telerehabilitation and telePT on key outcome measures for patients. Long-term effects, costs, benefits, and associated risks should be assessed. More knowledge of the treatment burden for people with different disabilities could help guide decisions about minimally worthwhile treatment effects.

Studies need to include outcomes to track the impact of telePT and telecare on working practices, productivity, and resource use and to target physical therapy programs administered via these applications to identify any rehabilitation or home exercise program advances. Studies also need to determine smartphone applications' effectiveness to improve health behaviors as compared with in-person rehabilitation.

Nevertheless, current and future studies must minimize bias through such activities as randomly allocating participants to groups, use concealed allocations, and blind assessors. Studies must report between-group differences for all outcomes and ensure they have a sufficient sample size to detect clinically important differences. Finally, studies must follow reporting guidelines.

CASE STUDY #1   AP, 42 YEAR-OLD MALE, COMPUTER ENGINEER

AP has been experiencing low back pain for the last 3 months. After his first visit to a GP, he has been advised to see a physical therapist for his treatment. He does not have the capacity to visit a physical therapist because he has limited time, lives in a remote area, and is in acute pain. He contacted a physical therapy service in a nearby region and asked for telePT services. The following schedule was advocated as a part of his treatment based on the model of care depicted earlier:

- *Timepoint 0 Administrative Consultation*: Done via a telephone call by the receptionist. This call was regarding AP's preference about the mode of telePT technology, platform familiarity and accessibility, and any health data that he would like to share with the therapist before the initial consultation.
- *Timepoint 1 TelePT Initial Consultation:* Done via Zoom.
  - *Assessment*—A therapist-guided approach was used where the therapist started an interactive discussion by asking a few questions related to AP's signs and symptoms, characteristics of pain, pain intensity, as well as his physical activity level (using data from his smartwatch that he shared with the therapist prior). The physical assessment included assessments such as an active straight leg raise test in supine and spine active range of motion in standing.
  - *Goal planning*—During this consultation, short-term goals were set, including education about posture and building upon some general physical conditioning activities (daily walks after work). The physical therapist also provided AP with some home exercise pamphlets via email.
- *Timepoint 2 TelePT Follow-Up Visit*: Done via Zoom
  - *Reassessment*: A therapist-guided approach was used where the therapist started an interactive discussion on AP's current signs and symptoms, characteristics of pain, his compliance with advised exercises
  - *Goal planning*: During this e-visit, AP was given a progressive self-guided home exercise program using an interactive website and educated about his long-term goals.
- *Timepoint X Maintenance TelePT*: Done using an interactive website. When he does his exercises each day, he was directed to fill an online form about his daily signs and symptoms, and a plan was then customized according to his situation.
  - *Maintain*: AP has been doing all the prescribed exercise and has been 80% compliant (statistics from interactive website).
  - *Goals*: AP has been progressing well, and his pain is 60% less than his baseline pain score (statistics from the interactive website).

CASE STUDY #2   KD, 36 YEAR-OLD FEMALE, EXECUTIVE ASSISTANT

KD has been experiencing knee pain for the last 2 months. After her first visit to a doctor, she has been advised to see a physical therapist for her treatment. She lives in a remote area, is in a lot of pain, and cannot travel. She contacted a physical therapy service about telePT. The following schedule was used as a part of her treatment:

- *Timepoint 0 Administrative Consultation*: Done via a telephone call by the receptionist. This call was regarding KD's preference about the mode of telePT technology, platform familiarity and accessibility, and any health data that she would like to share with the therapist before the initial consultation.
- *Timepoint 1 TelePT Initial Consultation*: Done via telephone call (KD has minimal access to high-speed internet).
  - *Assessment*—A therapist-directed approach was used. The therapist received and reviewed some of KD's assessment sent via email before her appointment. The therapist started the conversation with an interactive discussion by asking a few in-depth questions about KD's condition. The therapist also discussed KD's knee range of motion, pain characteristics, and activities that ease and exaggerate her pain.
  - *Goal planning*—During this consultation, short-term goals were also set, including education about posture, self-management of pain, and building upon some general physical conditioning activities. She was given home exercise pamphlets via email.
- *Timepoint 2 TelePT Follow-Up Visit:* Done via telephone.
  - *Reassessment*: A therapist-guided approach was used where the therapist started an interactive discussion about KD's current signs and symptoms, characteristics of pain, and her compliance with advised exercises. During each follow-up visit, she was also asked to rate the intensity of her pain and compliance with the exercise prescribed.
  - *Goal planning*: During this visit, she was also provided with a progressive self-guided home exercise program (via email) and educated about her long-term goals.

References

1. World Confederation for Physical Therapy (WCPT). Policy statement: description of physical therapy. http://www.wcpt.org/policy/ps-descriptionPT#appendix_1; Accessed 15.12.20.
2. World Health Organization. Classification of health workforce statistics. WHO, Geneva. www.who.int/hrh/statistics/workforce_statistics; Accessed 05.12.20.
3. Brennan D, Tindall L, Theodoros D, et al. A blueprint for telerehabilitation guidelines. *Int J Telerehabil.* 2010;2(2):31–34.
4. Laver KE, Schoene D, Crotty M, et al. Telerehabilitation services for stroke. *Cochrane Database Syst Rev.* 2013;2013(12):CD010255.
5. Gal N, Andrei D, Nemeş DI, et al. A Kinect based intelligent e-rehabilitation system in physical therapy. *Stud Health Technol Inform.* 2015;210:489–493.
6. Mani S, Sharma S, Omar B, et al. Validity and reliability of Internet-based physiotherapy assessment for musculoskeletal disorders: a systematic review. *J Telemed Telecare.* 2017;23(3):379–391.
7. Jagos H, David V, Haller M, et al. A framework for (tele-) monitoring of the rehabilitation progress in stroke patients: eHealth 2015 Special Issue. *Appl Clin Inform.* 2015;6(4):757–768.
8. Peretti A, Amenta F, Tayebati SK, et al. Telerehabilitation: review of the state-of-the-art and areas of application. *JMIR Rehabil Assist Technol.* 2017;4(2):e7.
9. Heyward V, Gibson A. *Excerpt from Advanced Fitness Assessment and Exercise Prescription.* 7th ed. http://www.humankinetics.com/excerpts/excerpts/technology-can-boost-physical-activity-promotion-nbsp; Accessed 05.12.20
10. Sullivan AN, Lachman ME. Behavior change with fitness technology in sedentary adults: a review of the evidence for increasing physical activity. *Front Public Health.* 2016;4:289.
11. Machado GC, Pinheiro MB, Lee H, et al. Smartphone apps for the self-management of low back pain: a systematic review. *Best Pract Res Clin Rheumatol.* 2016;30(6):1098–1109.
12. Beaver K, Tysver-Robinson D, Campbell M, et al. Comparing hospital and telephone follow-up after treatment for breast cancer: randomised equivalence trial. *BMJ.* 2009;338:a3147.
13. van Egmond MA, van der Schaaf M, Vredeveld T, et al. Effectiveness of physiotherapy with telerehabilitation in surgical patients: a systematic review and meta-analysis. *Physiotherapy.* 2018;104(3):277–298.
14. Latham NK, Harris BA, Bean JF, et al. Effect of a home-based exercise program on functional recovery following rehabilitation after hip fracture: a randomized clinical trial. *JAMA.* 2014;311(7):700–708.
15. Forster AJ, Murff HJ, Peterson JF, et al. The incidence and severity of adverse events affecting patients after discharge from the hospital. *Ann Intern Med.* 2003;138(3):161–167.
16. Head BA, Studts JL, Bumpous JM, et al. Development of a telehealth intervention for head and neck cancer patients. *Telemed J E Health.* 2009;15(1):44–52.
17. van Egmond MA, Engelbert RHH, Klinkenbijl JHG, et al. Physiotherapy with telerehabilitation in patients with complicated postoperative recovery after esophageal cancer surgery: feasibility study. *J Med Internet Res.* 2020;22(6):e16056.
18. Burdea GC, Cioi D, Kale A, et al. Robotics and gaming to improve ankle strength, motor control, and function in children with cerebral palsy--a case study series. *IEEE Trans Neural Syst Rehabil Eng.* 2013;21(2):165–173.
19. Carey JR, Durfee WK, Bhatt E, et al. Comparison of finger tracking versus simple movement training via telerehabilitation to alter hand function and cortical reorganization after stroke. *Neurorehabil Neural Repair.* 2007;21(3):216–232.
20. Huijgen BC, Vollenbroek-Hutten MM, Zampolini M, et al. Feasibility of a home-based telerehabilitation system compared to usual care: arm/hand function in patients with stroke, traumatic brain injury and multiple sclerosis. *J Telemed Telecare.* 2008;14(5):249–256.
21. Russell TG, Blumke R, Richardson B, et al. Telerehabilitation mediated physiotherapy assessment of ankle disorders. *Physiother Res Int.* 2010;15(3):167–175.
22. Fletcher GF, Chiaramida AJ, LeMay MR, et al. Telephonically-monitored home exercise early after coronary artery bypass surgery. *Chest.* 1984;86(2):198–202.
23. Smart N, Haluska B, Jeffriess L, et al. Predictors of a sustained response to exercise training in patients with chronic heart failure: a telemonitoring study. *Am Heart J.* 2005;150(6):1240–1247.
24. Krein SL, Kadri R, Hughes M, et al. Pedometer-based internet-mediated intervention for adults with chronic low back pain: randomized controlled trial. *J Med Internet Res.* 2013;15(8):e181.

25. Tsai LL, McNamara RJ, Moddel C, et al. Home-based telerehabilitation via real-time videoconferencing improves endurance exercise capacity in patients with COPD: the randomized controlled TeleR study. *Respirology*. 2017;22(4):699–707.

26. Sjöström M, Umefjord G, Stenlund H, et al. Internet-based treatment of stress urinary incontinence: 1- and 2-year results of a randomized controlled trial with a focus on pelvic floor muscle training. *BJU Int*. 2015;116(6):955–964.

27. Aarnio P, Lamminen H, Lepistö J, et al. A prospective study of teleconferencing for orthopaedic consultations. *J Telemed Telecare*. 1999;5(1):62–66.

28. Ohinmaa A, Vuolio S, Haukipuro K, et al. A cost-minimization analysis of orthopaedic consultations using videoconferencing in comparison with conventional consulting. *J Telemed Telecare*. 2002;8(5):283–289.

29. Savard L, Borstad A, Tkachuck J, et al. Telerehabilitation consultations for clients with neurologic diagnoses: cases from rural Minnesota and American Samoa. *NeuroRehabilitation*. 2003;18(2):93–102.

30. Arora M, Harvey LA, Glinsky JV, et al. Telephone-based management of pressure ulcers in people with spinal cord injury in low- and middle-income countries: a randomised controlled trial. *Spinal Cord*. 2017;55(2):141–147.

31. Irgens I, Rekand T, Arora M, et al. Telehealth for people with spinal cord injury: a narrative review. *Spinal Cord*. 2018;56(7):643–655.

32. Lemaire ED, Boudrias Y. Greene G. Low-bandwidth, Internet-based videoconferencing for physical rehabilitation consultations. *J Telemed Telecare*. 2001;7(2):82–89.

33. Laskowski ER, Johnson SE, Shelerud RA, et al. The telemedicine musculoskeletal examination. *Mayo Clin Proc*. 2020;95(8):1715–1731.

34. Dent PA Jr., Wilke B, Terkonda S, et al. Validation of teleconference-based goniometry for measuring elbow joint range of motion. *Cureus*. 2020;12(2):e6925.

35. Truter P, Russell T, Fary R. The validity of physical therapy assessment of low back pain via telerehabilitation in a clinical setting. *Telemedicine and e-Health*. 2013;20(2):161–167.

36. Steele L, Lade H, McKenzie S, et al. Assessment and diagnosis of musculoskeletal shoulder disorders over the Internet. *Int J Telemed Appl*. 2012;2012:945745.

37. Richardson BR, Truter P, Blumke R, et al. Physiotherapy assessment and diagnosis of musculoskeletal disorders of the knee via telerehabilitation. *J Telemed Telecare*. 2017;23(1):88–95.

38. Russell T, Truter P, Blumke R, et al. The diagnostic accuracy of telerehabilitation for nonarticular lower-limb musculoskeletal disorders. *Telemed J E Health*. 2010;16(5):585–594.

39. Du S, Hu L, Dong J, et al. Self-management program for chronic low back pain: a systematic review and meta-analysis. *Patient Educ Couns*. 2017;100(1):37–49.

40. Barlow J, Wright C, Sheasby J, et al. Self-management approaches for people with chronic conditions: a review. *Patient Educ Couns*. 2002;48(2):177–187.

41. Jones TM, Dear BF, Hush JM, et al. myMoves program: feasibility and acceptability study of a remotely delivered self-management program for increasing physical activity among adults with acquired brain injury living in the community. *Phys Ther*. 2016;96(12):1982–1993.

42. Cannon D, Buys N, Sriram KB, et al. The effects of chronic obstructive pulmonary disease self-management interventions on improvement of quality of life in COPD patients: a meta-analysis. *Respir Med*. 2016;121:81–90.

43. Tchero H, Tabue Teguo M, Lannuzel A, et al. Telerehabilitation for stroke survivors: systematic review and meta-analysis. *J Med Internet Res*. 2018;20(10):e10867.

44. Ownsworth T, Arnautovska U, Beadle E, et al. Efficacy of telerehabilitation for adults with traumatic brain injury: a systematic review. *J Head Trauma Rehabil*. 2018;33(4):e33–e46.

45. Arora M, Harvey LA, Lavrencic L, et al. A telephone-based version of the spinal cord injury–secondary conditions scale: a reliability and validity study. *Spinal Cord*. 2016;54(5):402–405.

46. Wellbeloved-Stone CA, Weppner JL, Valdez RS. A systematic review of telerehabilitation and mHealth interventions for spinal cord injury. *Curr Phys Med Rehabil*. 2016;4(4):295–311.

47. Merriel SW, Andrews V, Salisbury C. Telehealth interventions for primary prevention of cardiovascular disease: a systematic review and meta-analysis. *Prev Med*. 2014;64:88–95.

48. Barnason S, Zimmerman L, Schulz P, et al. Weight management telehealth intervention for overweight and obese rural cardiac rehabilitation participants: a randomised trial. *J Clin Nurs*. 2019;28(9-10):1808–1818.

49. Rintala DH, Krouskop TA, Wright JV, et al. Telerehabilitation for veterans with a lower-limb amputation or ulcer: technical acceptability of data. *J Rehabil Res Dev.* 2004;41(3B):481–490.

50. Pate RR, Pratt M, Blair SN, et al. Physical activity and public health. A recommendation from the Centers for Disease Control and Prevention and the American College of Sports Medicine. *JAMA.* 1995;273(5):402–407.

51. World Health Organisation. Health topics: physical activity. 2014. http://www.who.int/topics/physical_activity/en/; Accessed 05.12.20.

52. NHS Health Scotland. Costing the burden of ill health related to physical inactivity for Scotland. 2012. http://www.healthscotland.com/uploads/documents/20437-D1physicalinactivityscotland12final.pdf; Accessed 06.12.20.

53. Janssen I. Health care costs of physical inactivity in Canadian adults. *Appl Physiol Nutr Metab.* 2012;37(4):803–806.

54. Li J. Improving chronic disease self-management through social networks. *Popul Health Manag.* 2013;16(5):285–287.

55. Department of Health and Social Care. UK Physical Activity Guidelines. 2019. https://assets.publishing.service.gov.uk/government/uploads/system/uploads/attachment_data/file/832868/uk-chief-medical-officers-physical-activity-guidelines.pdf; Accessed 15.12.20.

56. Piercy KL, Troiano RP, Ballard RM, et al. The physical activity guidelines for Americans. *JAMA.* 2018;320(19):2020–2028.

57. Tremblay MS, Warburton DE, Janssen I, et al. New Canadian physical activity guidelines. *Appl Physiol Nutr Metab.* 2011;36(1):36–46. 7-58.

58. Lupton D. Quantifying the body: monitoring and measuring health in the age of mHealth technologies. *Critical Public Health.* 2013;23(4):393–403.

59. Lowe SA, ÓLaighin G. Monitoring human health behaviour in one's living environment: a technological review. *Med Eng Phys.* 2014;36(2):147–168.

60. Hassett L, van den Berg M, Lindley RI, et al. Effect of affordable technology on physical activity levels and mobility outcomes in rehabilitation: a protocol for the Activity and MObility UsiNg Technology (AMOUNT) rehabilitation trial. *BMJ Open.* 2016;6(6):e012074.

61. Holbrook EA, Barreira TV, Kang M. Validity and reliability of Omron pedometers for prescribed and self-paced walking. *Med Sci Sports Exerc.* 2009;41(3):670–674.

62. Hasson RE, Haller J, Pober DM, et al. Validity of the Omron HJ-112 pedometer during treadmill walking. *Med Sci Sports Exerc.* 2009;41(4):805–809.

63. Williams DM, Matthews CE, Rutt C, et al. Interventions to increase walking behavior. *Med Sci Sports Exerc.* 2008;40(suppl 7):S567–S573.

64. Bravata DM, Smith-Spangler C, Sundaram V, et al. Using pedometers to increase physical activity and improve health: a systematic review. *JAMA.* 2007;298(19):2296–2304.

65. Richardson CR, Newton TL, Abraham JJ, et al. A meta-analysis of pedometer-based walking interventions and weight loss. *Ann Fam Med.* 2008;6(1):69–77.

66. Strath SJ, Brage S, Ekelund ULF. Integration of physiological and accelerometer data to improve physical activity assessment. *Med Sci Sports Exerc.* 2005;37(suppl 11):S563–S571.

67. Barreira TV, Kang M, Caputo JL, et al. Validation of the Actiheart monitor for the measurement of physical activity. *Int J Exerc Sci.* 2009;2(1):60–71.

68. Crouter SE, Churilla JR, Bassett Jr. DR. Accuracy of the Actiheart for the assessment of energy expenditure in adults. *Eur J Clin Nutr.* 2008;62(6):704–711.

69. Zakeri I, Adolph AL, Puyau MR, et al. Application of cross-sectional time series modeling for the prediction of energy expenditure from heart rate and accelerometry. *J Appl Physiol (1985).* 2008;104(6):1665–1673.

70. Bailey BW, McInnis K. Energy cost of exergaming: a comparison of the energy cost of 6 forms of exergaming. *Arch Pediatr Adolesc Med.* 2011;165(7):597–602.

71. Warburton DE, Charlesworth S, Ivey A, et al. A systematic review of the evidence for Canada's physical activity guidelines for adults. *Int J Behav Nutr Phys Act.* 2010;7:39.

72. Hamm J, Money AG, Atwal A, et al. Fall prevention intervention technologies: a conceptual framework and survey of the state of the art. *J Biomed Inform.* 2016;59:319–345.

73. Studenski S, Perera S, Patel K, et al. Gait speed and survival in older adults. *JAMA.* 2011;305(1):50–58.

74. Rose T, Barker M, Maria Jacob C, et al. A systematic review of digital interventions for improving the diet and physical activity behaviors of adolescents. *J Adolesc Health.* 2017;61(6):669–677.

75. Lau PWC, Lau EY, Wong DP, et al. A systematic review of information and communication technology-based interventions for promoting physical activity behavior change in children and adolescents. *J Med Internet Res.* 2011;13(3):e48.
76. Greaves CJ, Sheppard KE, Abraham C, et al. Systematic review of reviews of intervention components associated with increased effectiveness in dietary and physical activity interventions. *BMC Public Health.* 2011;11(1):119.
77. Marcoux RM, Vogenberg FR. Telehealth: applications from a legal and regulatory perspective. *P T.* 2016;41(9):567–570.
78. Gogia S, Hartvigsen G. Rationale, history, and basics of telehealth. In: Fundamentals of Telemedicine and Telehealth. Chapter 2. Academic Press; 2020.
79. Dicianno BE, Parmanto B, Fairman AD, et al. Perspectives on the evolution of mobile (mHealth) technologies and application to rehabilitation. *Phys Ther.* 2015;95(3):397–405.
80. Boldrini P, Bernetti A, Fiore P. Impact of COVID-19 outbreak on rehabilitation services and physical and rehabilitation medicine physicians' activities in Italy. An official document of the Italian PRM Society (SIMFER). *Eur J Phys Rehabil Med.* 2020;56(3):316–318.
81. O'Connell CM, Eriks-Hoogland I, Middleton JW. Now, more than ever, our community is needed: spinal cord injury care during a global pandemic. *Spinal Cord Ser Cases.* 2020;6(1):18.
82. Ho K, Al-Shorjabji N, Brown E, et al. Applying the resilient health system framework for universal health coverage. *Stud Health Technol Inform.* 2016;231:54–62.
83. Marcelo A, Ganesh J, Mohan J, et al. Governance and management of national telehealth programs in Asia. *Stud Health Technol Inform.* 2015;209:95–101.
84. Leochico CFD, Espiritu AI, Ignacio SD, et al. Challenges to the emergence of telerehabilitation in a developing country: a systematic review. *Front Neurol.* 2020;11:1007.
85. Marcelo A, Adejumo A, Luna D. Health informatics for development: a three-pronged strategy of partnerships, standards, and mobile health. Contribution of the IMIA Working Group on health informatics for development. *Yearb Med Inform.* 2011;6:96–101.
86. Nguyen QT, Naguib RN, Abd Ghani MK, et al. An analysis of the healthcare informatics and systems in Southeast Asia: a current perspective from seven countries. *Int J Electron Healthc.* 2008; 4(2):184–207.
87. Macrohon BC, Cristobal FL. The effect on patient and health provider satisfaction regarding health care delivery using the teleconsultation program of the Ateneo de Zamboanga University-School of Medicine (ADZU-SOM) in rural Western Mindanao. *Acta Med Philipp.* 2013;47(4):18–22.
88. Sahu M, Grover A, Joshi A. Role of mobile phone technology in health education in Asian and African countries: a systematic review. *Int J Electron Healthc.* 2014;7(4):269–286.
89. Mandirola Brieux HF, Benitez S, Otero C, et al. Cultural problems associated with the implementation of eHealth. *Stud Health Technol Inform.* 2017;245:1213.
90. Leochico CFD, Valera MJS. Follow-up consultations through telerehabilitation for wheelchair recipients with paraplegia in a developing country: a case report. *Spinal Cord Ser Cases.* 2020;6(1):58.
91. Ramos RM, Cheng PGF, Jonas SM. Validation of an mHealth app for depression screening and monitoring (psychologist in a pocket): correlational study and concurrence analysis. *JMIR Mhealth Uhealth.* 2019;7(9):e12051.
92. Hernandez JPT. Network diffusion and technology acceptance of a nurse chatbot for chronic disease self-management support: a theoretical perspective. *J Med Invest.* 2019;66(1.2):24–30.
93. Karen Finnin. Data security in digital practice. 2019. https://www.karenfinnin.com/data-security-in-digital-practice/.
94. DiMatteo MR. Variations in patients' adherence to medical recommendations: a quantitative review of 50 years of research. *Med Care.* 2004;42(3):200–209.
95. West D. How mobile devices are transforming healthcare. *Issues in Technology Innovation.* 2012;18:1–10.
96. NHS Choices. Health tools: interactive tools, smartphone apps and podcasts. http://www.nhs.uk/tools/pages/toolslibrary.aspx?Tag=&Page=1; Accessed 02.12.20.
97. Scottish Centre for Telehealth & Telecare. Supporting improvement, integration and innovation - Business Plan 2012-2015. http://sctt.org.uk/programmes/; Accessed 25.11.20.
98. Dean SG, Smith JA, Payne S, et al. Managing time: an interpretative phenomenological analysis of patients' and physiotherapists' perceptions of adherence to therapeutic exercise for low back pain. *Disabil Rehabil.* 2005;27(11):625–636.

CHAPTER 20

Teleoccupational Therapy

Carl Froilan D. Leochico ▪ Nishu Tyagi

Introduction

Eleanor Roosevelt once said, "The purpose of life, after all, is to live it, to taste experience to the utmost, to reach out eagerly and without fear for newer and richer experience." Living life to the fullest is what occupational therapy practitioners (OTPs) aim for their clients to achieve, as advocated by the American Occupational Therapy Association.[1] The practice of occupational therapy (OT) is directed toward enabling clients with or without disability to participate in functional tasks that are of significant meaning to them and intrinsically related to their "health, self-esteem, social competence, happiness, and satisfaction with life."[2]

Traditionally, an OT client receives in-person individualized initial evaluation, shared goal setting (with family and OTP), customized interventions, and regular reevaluations to ensure that the desired outcomes are being met.[1] In line with evidence-based practice, the OTP provides a holistic approach to patient care by also evaluating and modifying the client's environment, whether at home, school, workplace, or leisure.

Unfortunately, barriers to accessing in-person OT services exist in various health care settings around the world. Some of these barriers are related to urbanization of health care services, shortage of OTPs, lack of nearby OT facilities, transportation issues, time conflicts, social stigma, socioeconomic and language challenges, geographical limitations, travel and weather restrictions, functional mobility impairments, and immunocompromised clients.[3-8] Recently, social distancing and health risks related to the COVID-19 pandemic have also become an additional significant barrier to rehabilitation access worldwide.[9] With the increasing evidence that the aforementioned barriers can be addressed by telerehabilitation, various OT stakeholders (i.e., OTPs, clients, carers, families, remote health care providers, OT students, society) have been given the opportunity to virtually reach out to each other and achieve common goals.[10, 11]

Telerehabilitation in Occupational Therapy

Telerehabilitation in OT may be referred to by various other terms such as telehealth, telemedicine, teletherapy, teleoccupational therapy, telecare, telepractice, and digital or virtual care, among others. Telerehabilitation refers to the use of any form of information and communications technology (ICT) to "deliver clinical services at a distance by linking clinician to client, caregiver, or any person(s) involved in client care" (e.g., remote therapist or local health care provider) for "evaluation, intervention, monitoring, supervision, and consultation," consistent with the full scope of OT practice (e.g., health promotion, habilitation, rehabilitation, etc.).[12, 13] In 2014 the World Federation of Occupational Therapists (WFOT) recognized telerehabilitation as a viable method to deliver client-centered OT services when accessing in-person care is "not possible, practical or optimal," and/or when telerehabilitation is "mutually acceptable to the client and provider."[13] For instance telerehabilitation may be appropriate to (1) bridge the gap between specialists and clients; (2) enable access to rehabilitation especially in geographically isolated and disadvantaged areas; (3) reduce travel or waiting times; (4) minimize direct and indirect expenses; (5) personalize care; (6) promote clients' active engagement in their natural environment; and/or (7) protect people from COVID-19.[3,9]

Similar to other rehabilitation disciplines adopting telerehabilitation as a service delivery model, OT that is conducted from a distance should observe all applicable jurisdictional, institutional, and professional regulations and policies.[13] Ideally, OTPs should be trained and culturally competent to deliver services remotely to clients with the same standards of care as traditional or in-person encounters within the natural limitations of telerehabilitation.[11, 13] Telerehabilitation should not be viewed as a new OT intervention, but rather a new way of delivering usual care.[14]

Current Evidence

OT services may be delivered via telerehabilitation to clients across all ages and in any phase of the care spectrum.[15] Telerehabilitation has been widely used for various conditions or purposes, such as "wheelchair prescription, neurological assessment, adaptive equipment, prescription and home modification, ergonomic assessment, school-based practice, early intervention services, health and wellness programming, and rehabilitation for individuals who have experienced stroke, breast cancer, traumatic brain injury, polytrauma, Parkinson's disease, and other neurological and orthopedic impairments."[14]

By using ICT that ranges from simple low-cost telephone interviews to advanced internet-enabled gamified virtual rehabilitation with robot telepresence, telerehabilitation can be performed by OTPs according to the "individuals, groups, or cultures they serve, contextualized to the occupations and interests of clients."[13, 16, 17] With a client-centered approach, the choice of appropriate technology is determined by each client's needs, resources, digital capacity, and preferences, and is guided by the OTP to ensure that real-world trade-offs are recognized and balanced (i.e., benefits outweigh the risks inherent to telerehabilitation).[18] In clinical practice, the chosen technology is usually the simplest and least expensive that can meet the client's OT goals. For instance, in resource-limited countries with an unstable internet connection (if any), the following store and forward techniques may be used: text messaging; sending private messages on social media; emailing short video clips of a client performing common activities of daily living (ADLs); sending ancillary or imaging results; and forwarding links to exercise videos or useful online health-related resources.[6, 8]

For a structured presentation of the growing body of evidence supporting the use of telerehabilitation as an OT service delivery model, two conceptual frameworks are presented as follows:

1. *Person-Environment-Occupation-Performance (PEOP) Model*
   The PEOP model emphasizes the client's functional performance within his/her natural, often least restrictive, environment.[19] Using this model, telerehabilitation can facilitate skills development, environmental modification, and/or healthy behavior adoption or reinforcement.[20]

2. *Coaching Model (CM)*
   Following the principles of early intervention (EI), the CM used in telerehabilitation is founded on the active and huge role of the clients and their primary carers, who are empowered and guided by the remote OTP to develop, implement, and sustain therapeutic interventions.[21, 22]

In addition, research on telerehabilitation-delivered OT services can also be presented according to its primary focus or objective, such as teleevaluation (e.g., conducting remote assessments, establishing reliability of remote assessments), teleintervention (e.g., employing preventative, habilitative, or rehabilitative strategies), teleconsultation (e.g., providing health-related advices),

TABLE 20.1 ■ **Examples of General and Specific Practice Areas in Occupational Therapy (OT) That Can Benefit From Telerehabilitation.**

General Practice Areas[a]	Specific Areas or Conditions
Academic education	Teaching OT students on interprofessional education[26]
Children and youth	Children with special needs[27] Early intervention services[28] Students with visual and fine motor deficits affecting handwriting skills[11,18]
Developmental disabilities	Autism spectrum disorder[11,18] Cerebral palsy[11,18]
Health and wellness	Obesity[29] Physical inactivity (deconditioning)[30]
Home and community health	Chronic diseases, such as diabetes mellitus, heart failure, hypertension[31] Home safety[32]
Mental health	Depression[18] Posttraumatic stress disorder[33]
Productive aging	Aging in place[34] Community-dwelling older adults[18]
Rehabilitation and disability	Acquired brain injuries[11] Adults with mobility impairments needing wheelchair or seating devices[18] Breast cancer[11] Dementia[35] Patients awaiting discharge from inpatient medical and orthopedic wards[11] Spinal cord injury[11] Stroke[11,18] Traumatic brain injury[11,18]
Work and industry	Analysis of workspaces[25] Injury prevention[25]

[a]Adapted from the special interest sections of the American Occupational Therapy Association (American Occupational Therapy Association [n.d.];[36] Cason [2012][25]).

and/or telemonitoring (e.g., obtaining health-related information and following through of clients with chronic conditions).[23,24] Essentially all practice areas within the scope of OT can potentially utilize telerehabilitation for at least some components of care.[23,25] Table 20.1 presents a shortlist of these practice areas based primarily on recent systematic reviews.

Teleevaluation and teleconsultation present both opportunities and limitations. Physical examination, functional assessment, and other OT-specific measures may be challenging to administer accurately and safely at a distance. In order to acquire these particular competencies, clinicians in general can attend formal and/or informal education and training opportunities on practical and creative techniques to circumvent the absence of hands-on evaluations.[37] A significant amount of knowledge can also be gained from the growing body of literature that describes teleevaluation for various conditions or services (see Table 20.2). The reliability and validity of common assessment tools administered via telerehabilitation have been established in previous studies, but further research is warranted for other useful tools and conditions as well.[23] It is crucial that clients are properly and adequately evaluated during the teleconsultation before appropriate OT assessment, diagnosis, and plan-of-care can be formulated.

In 2019 Hung and Fong published a systematic review of the current evidence on telerehabilitation in OT practice, wherein they analyzed 15 articles with the following study designs

TABLE 20.2 ■ **Examples of Teleevaluation Services and Tools Applicable to Occupational Therapy (OT) in the Literature.**[a]

Teleevaluation Services	References
Adaptive equipment prescription and home modification	Sanford et al. (2009)
Cognitive screening	Abdolahi et al. (2014); Stillerova et al. (2016)
Ergonomic assessment	Baker & Jacobs (2012)
Home assessment	Hoffman & Russell (2008); Nix & Comans (2017)[38]
Lymphedema assessment	Galiano-Castillo et al. (2013)
Neurological examination	Boes et al. (2020)
Orthopedic (hand) assessment	Worboys et al. (2017)
Pain assessment of orthopedic or neurological conditions	Wahezi et al. (2020)
Special tests for orthopedic or neurological examination	Verduzco-Gutierrez et al. (2020)
Wheelchair prescription	Schein et al. (2010); Schein et al. (2011)
Reliable Teleevaluation Tools	**References**
Canadian Occupational Performance Measure	Dreyer et al. (2001)
Ergonomic Assessment Tool for Arthritis	Backman et al. (2008)
European Stroke Scale	Palsbo et al. (2007)
Functional Independence Measure	Hoffmann et al. (2008)
Functional Reach Test	Palsbo et al. (2007)
Jamar Dynamometer	Hoffmann et al. (2008)
Kohlman Evaluation of Living Skills	Dreyer et al. (2001)
Mini-Mental State Examination	Ciemins et al. (2009); McEachern et al. (2014)
Montreal Cognitive Assessment	Abdolahi et al. (2014); Stillerova et al. (2016)
Nine-Hole Peg Test	Hoffmann et al. (2008)
Preston Pinch Gauge	Hoffmann et al. (2008)
Timed Up and Go Test	Hwang et al. (2016)
Unified Parkinson's Disease Rating Scale	Hoffmann et al. (2008)

[a]Largely based on the telehealth position paper of the American Occupational Therapy Association (American Occupational Therapy Association [AOTA][23]).

and corresponding levels of evidence: three randomized controlled trials (RCTs) (level II), eight quasiexperimental studies (level III), one single-group postintervention trial (class III), and three single-case studies (class IV).[11] Their search was limited to articles published from 2008 to 2017. The patients included in the reviewed articles were aged 2 to 70 years and had different medical conditions (Table 20.1). All accessed telerehabilitation services at home, except for one program where services were accessed in a community center. The majority of patients were accompanied by a significant other (i.e., parent or carer) for technical support and in-person assistance in assessment, treatment, or monitoring. Telerehabilitation was conducted using different hardware (e.g., telephone, smartphone, personal computer, iPad, digital camera, external web camera, robot, sensor glove) and software (e.g., videoconferencing platforms, customized mobile applications, web-based applications, instant messaging system, videogames, screen avatar) in either synchronous, asynchronous, or hybrid (mixed) formats.

An example of a telerehabilitation study in which the PEOP model is applicable with focus on teleintervention is one RCT that recruited 99 adult patients with subacute stroke assigned to either treatment group (i.e., hand robot-assisted device coupled with home exercise program) or control group (i.e., traditional home exercise program only). All patients exercised for 3 hours for 5 days a week for 8 consecutive weeks. Pretest-posttest comparisons showed statistically significant changes in most domains on the Stroke Impact Scale and the Center for Epidemiologic Studies Depression Scale for both groups.[39] In a similar earlier report, a 54-year-old patient with right medullary pyramidal infarct that completed 38 hours of robotic-assisted training plus 47 hours of home exercises demonstrated clinically important improvements on the Action Research Arm Test, Functional Ability Scale, Fugl-Meyer Assessment, and a portion of the Wolf Motor Function Test.[40] Telerehabilitation in these studies might have applied the PEOP model of care to facilitate motor and functional recovery.

In another RCT, the CM was applied with focus on telemonitoring. Twenty-four children with spastic hemiplegic cerebral palsy and mild-to-moderate functional impairment were recruited. The children's primary carers received in-person training in performing standardized assessments and function-based treatments at home. Those assigned to the treatment group received closer supervision or guidance by a remote OTP through hybrid telemonitoring using a web-based camera software. Equal improvement in satisfaction with occupational performance was observed in both groups, but greater improvements in dexterity and functional performance were seen in the treatment group.[41] In another study, collaborative OT sessions with parents of children with autism spectrum disorder (ASD) were conducted initially in-clinic, followed by online sessions for 6 weeks. The CM seemed to have been employed through use of family schedules, sensory diets, and archived webcam sessions. Results showed improved carryover of home interventions by "providing opportunities for parents to ask questions, review sensory techniques, and understand the therapist's clinical reasoning."[42] Ensuring active family participation in patient care through remote consistent coaching is indeed vital in telerehabilitation.

Consistent with the PEOP model, each person's home or environment (e.g., for work, study, or leisure) is as unique as the performance needs of the individual. With proper modifications, the surroundings of a person with disability can provide support for daily activities, instead of magnifying the functional loss arising from injury or illness.[43] Typically, OTPs perform a predischarge environmental assessment for inpatients to ensure person-environment fit and safe transition to home.[38,44] Telerehabilitation may be performed in lieu of in-person environmental assessment and intervention for various reasons, including, but not limited to, the following:

- Factors on the side of the OTP: lack of manpower, time constraints, heavy workload including administrative tasks, travel costs, distance, nonpayment by insurance carriers, compensation, health risk (e.g., COVID-19); and
- Factors on the side of the client: willingness, privacy, time constraints, health risk (e.g., COVID-19).[38]

The rehabilitation medicine physician and/or OTP can virtually examine the client's actual living setup or workplace ergonomics and analyze ADL performance within a natural environment. Through telerehabilitation, preferably using synchronous means (e.g., video call) over asynchronous means (e.g., taking photos and identification of potential hazards), environmental assessments can be conducted to identify existing architectural barriers that may be overlooked by the client or family.[38] Using a mobile-based application capable of measuring actual distances and inserting pieces of durable medical equipment into a virtually created floor plan may also be helpful and practical.[44] Depending on the assessment, appropriate home or environmental interventions can be instituted in the form of architectural modifications (e.g., durable medical equipment, ramp to front door, grab bar, improved lighting, removal of clutter, motion sensor light switch, fall-preventive measures), adaptive equipment (e.g., long-handled reacher), personal assistance (e.g., family or caregiver education), durable medical equipment (e.g., bedside commode), identification of things misused (e.g., use of towel bar to help get off the toilet), mobility equipment (e.g., walker, wheelchair), prosthetics (e.g., hearing aid, magnifying glass), and even technological adaptations and solutions (e.g., adjusting the phone settings for users with visual impairment, using voiceover screen reader).[43,44] Currently, however, it is difficult to make comparisons across studies and determine which forms of environmental intervention, either delivered face-to-face or through telerehabilitation, are most appropriate for a given client or case because of variations in methodologies in the literature.[45] Future research on best practices in home modification, especially when delivered through telerehabilitation, is recommended.

Nonetheless, a subjective individualized approach should take precedence over a mere objective checklist in recommending environmental modifications, which ultimately depend on the client's and family's needs, goals, and resources.[46] For instance frail elderly patients with prior fall episodes at home would most likely prefer to continue "aging in place" despite environmental barriers that can result in further disability, but this does not mean they are not amenable to home modifications or advice.[45] Proper and practical patient education can help them understand that home modifications and assistive technologies can delay dependence in functional activities, enhance carer self-efficacy, decrease mortality, and minimize costs for assistance and health care.[45,47–50] A longitudinal study has shown that home modifications can reduce long-term difficulty with ADLs (i.e., up to 6 months), and each month of waiting for a home modification to be instituted can worsen functional dependence.[51] Hence, a timely environmental intervention should be implemented as soon as a problem is identified.

Appropriate environmental interventions are proven effective in preventing falls, according to the results of a systematic review and metaanalysis consistent with Cochrane findings.[46,52] Three-fourths or 75% of the following criteria should be met for an environmental intervention to be considered high quality or intensity:

1. A comprehensive evaluation process of hazard identification and priority setting taking into account both personal risk and environmental audit;
2. The use of an assessment tool validated for the broad range of potential fall hazards;
3. Inclusion of formal or observational evaluation of the functional capacity (physical capacity, behavior, functional vision, habits) of the person within the context of their environment; and
4. Provision of adequate follow-up by the health professional and support for adaptations and modifications.[46]

Lastly, when performing an environmental assessment and intervention, the rehabilitation medicine physician and/or OTP must keep in mind the following four dimensions of the home:

1. Physical dimension: referring to home structure (e.g., width of doorframes, height of steps, height of toilet), materials and finishes, services and facilities, space, ambient conditions, and location;
2. Temporal dimension: referring to current and future family health and setup (e.g., aging family members, growth of children, resale value of the house);
3. Occupational dimension: referring to modifications for self-care and domestic activities; and
4. Societal dimension: referring to economic and political conditions affecting resources and control of people over their homes, such as "government policies, national standards, individual service restrictions, guidelines, and costs."[38,53]

The unprecedented interruption of in-person access to OT services during the COVID-19 pandemic put new and old clients at a disadvantage, with the vast majority of OTPs and students in a potential dilemma.[18,54] The usual barriers to telerehabilitation may also apply to OT in various health care settings worldwide (e.g., lack of acceptance, resources, digital capacity). Of special note, however, the lack of telerehabilitation education, training, and experience among a number of current OTPs and their students may be a huge concern especially among non- or slow adopters of the technology. Appropriate relevant awareness campaigns and educational opportunities for stakeholders should, therefore, be provided or enhanced.

Interprofessional Education Through Telerehabilitation

Students now are the future drivers and users of telerehabilitation in OT. In order to prepare them for the continued modernization of health care delivery in many parts of the world, restructuring of the current academic curriculum may be necessary.[55] Integrating telerehabilitation and interprofessional education (IPE) in teaching-learning activities can help students recognize the value of alternative service delivery models in the midst of workforce shortage, unequal distribution of resources, COVID-19, and other challenges to in-person health care access.[56] A team-based approach to patient care consists of interacting with and learning with and from all the members of the rehabilitation team, which consists of, but are not limited to, the physiatrist, physiotherapist, speech-language pathologist, psychologist, prosthetist-orthotist, dietician, social worker, and rehabilitation nurse, among others.

The core values of IPE (e.g., values, ethics, responsibilities, collaboration, teamwork, mutual respect amid professional practice differences) may be incorporated in various course materials and contents. For instance, in one setting, the College of Nursing collaborated with the Department of Rehabilitation Sciences in the College of Allied Health in the same university to provide opportunities for students to work harmoniously together despite the physical distance via videoconferencing.[26] Creating a structured learning online environment such as role-playing or simulations prior to an actual telerehabilitation session with a real client under the remote supervision of a teacher-clinician can help develop "webside" manners, teleevaluation, teleconsultation, teleintervention, and telemonitoring competencies, among others.[26,57] Theoretical knowledge and virtual clinical experiences can also help orient trainees on the complexities of health care, barriers to telerehabilitation, reimbursement policies, medicolegal implications, jurisdiction, and other practical issues they may face in practice.

Recommendations for Future Research

Despite the development of cutting-edge technologies, there remains to be a huge gap in evidence-based telerehabilitation practice in OT. It is difficult to generalize the results of existing relevant studies in the midst of absent universal or standard patient eligibility criteria for different pathologies, limited sample size, and varying telerehabilitation protocols, technologies, and outcomes measures. Studies on the long-term effects, cost-effectiveness, client and provider characteristics that best suit telerehabilitation, medicolegal risk management, effective strategies to ensure data privacy and security, and reliability of remote (clinician-administered) and in-person (carer-administered) OT assessments are recommended.[11,18]

Summary

There is a growing trend of telerehabilitation adoption worldwide during a health crisis that caught stakeholders unprepared for the sudden interruption of health care access. Through telerehabilitation, OT practitioners and clients can remain connected and achieve meaningful rehabilitation goals together. Various technologies can be leveraged within the context of the objectives, resources, and competencies on both sides. Educational opportunities to equip current and future stakeholders are necessary to utilize telerehabilitation effectively, safely, and wisely.

CASE STUDIES

CASE 1: SPINAL CORD INJURY

MB is a 36-year-old male from India with L2 American Spinal Injury Association (ASIA) Impairment Scale (AIS) grade B paraplegia due to fall with fracture. With 0/5 muscle strength on bilateral lower extremities, he was rendered bedridden and dependent in ADLs. He completed 4 weeks of inpatient spinal cord injury (SCI) rehabilitation, wherein he developed his skills in bed mobility, transfers, and wheelchair use. Due to the COVID-19 pandemic he was prematurely discharged home and offered to undergo telerehabilitation. He lives round 159 km away from the hospital.

MB and his carers were oriented on the telerehabilitation process, benefits, limitations, and risk management. Due to fluctuating internet in his home, he opted to use hybrid telerehabilitation (e.g., text messaging, phone call, sending of audio-video recordings of in-home exercise sessions to the occupational therapy practitioner [OTP] in-charge through WhatsApp and/or email). He underwent 8 weeks of telerehabilitation, consisting of physiotherapy, occupational therapy, and home modifications, with regular follow-ups with a physiatrist. Through several recordings over time, improvements in his functional skills were observed (e.g., turning, rolling, supine-to-sit; activities of daily living including lower garment dressing, commode transfers; bed-to-wheelchair transfers and performing wheelies). The OTP evaluated the videos every week and made one follow-up call per week to give further advice and encouragement and to address queries.

At the end of 8 weeks, MB completed the SCI Measure through a phone interview and was remotely assessed live through WhatsApp videoconferencing with the telerehabilitation team. He also shared images of low-cost bathroom modifications he did at home and videos of his functional training sessions showing independent transfer to and from his two-wheeler scooter. Infographic and other resource materials (e.g., relevant YouTube videos) on proper bedsore care and hygiene were sent to the client and carer. After 8 weeks of telerehabilitation, MB became confident, motivated, and functionally independent in most ADLs.

This example used both PEOP and coaching models. Teleevaluation, teleintervention, and telemonitoring were conducted through synchronous and/or asynchronous means, whichever applicable.

CASE 2: LOW BACK PAIN

VS is a 40-year-old male call-center agent and exercise enthusiast who is complaining of low back pain. After being evaluated and medically managed by a physiatrist through teleconsultation as suffering from paralumbar strain, he was referred to an OTP for a back school program through telerehabilitation.

The OTP conducted initial evaluation through live videoconferencing using a secure platform. He reported low back pain, graded 5/10 on the numeric rating scale, which started approximately 2 months prior. The pain was aggravated by long hours of sitting at work and his weekend warrior workout routine. Because of the pain, he found it difficult to carry his 3-year-old child, sit and drive in heavy traffic, and go back to the gym. With the help of his wife, a nonclinician who provided in-person assist in certain parts of the physical examination under remote guidance of the OTP, straight leg raise (SLR) test was performed and found to be positive on the left side. Crossed SLR test was negative. The client had forward-head and slouched sitting posture and was hyperlordotic in resting standing position. Muscle strength of the bilateral lower limbs seemed unremarkable on functional strength testing (e.g., high marches, partial squats, tip-toes on one leg, stair-climbing). On ergonomic assessment, the chair he used for working at home was too high and the arm rests too far apart for his relatively short slim stature. He would slouch to reach forward to his desktop computer.

Since the schedules of the client and OTP did not allow them to meet synchronously on a regular basis, they decided to use instant messaging and exchange of video or image files to show demonstration and return-demonstration of neck, shoulder, back and core stabilization exercises, postural awareness techniques, and makeshift ergonomic adjustments (e.g., placement of pillows between him and the armrests, foot rest, aligning the desktop computer screen at or slightly below eye level). Proper back mechanics were also reinforced through infographic materials sent by the OTP. After about 2 weeks, they had a live video consultation and the client reported fewer occurrences of pain.

This example primarily employed the Person-Environment-Occupation-Performance (PEOP) model. It also shows the potential role of an in-person assistant, who can either be a nonclinician or clinician, that can help relay health-related information to the remote OTP during teleevaluation. Clinical reasoning can guide the OTP to select and apply appropriate ICT for teleinterventions aligned with the client's occupation, resources, schedule, goals, context, and environment.

CASE 3: CEREBRAL PALSY

RT is a 5-year-old only child of a single mom. She has spastic hemiplegia due to cerebral palsy. She complained of difficulty using her right upper limb for school-related tasks in preparation for enrollment

Continued

in a special education class. While her mother goes to work, she is brought to her 55-year-old aunt who lives next door, where her hobbies include playing computer games and watching YouTube videos. She regularly attended in-person occupational therapy sessions before the pandemic.

At the start of the city lockdown, telerehabilitation was offered to the client and family. However, the aunt admitted having difficulty in operating a laptop and required remote basic technical training conducted by the OTP with in-person assistance from the client's mother. She learned how to turn on and off the laptop, connect to the internet, log in on a secure videoconferencing platform using the mother's personal email account, and adjust the web camera and speaker volume. When troubleshooting was necessary, she easily reached the OTP via phone.

The child had telerehabilitation 1 hour every other day; the OTP shared her screen on the chosen videoconferencing platform to show the slide presentation she prepared for each session. Each presentation followed a storyline that entailed active participation in upper limb exercises and bimanual activities. Activity worksheets emailed by the OTP were printed by the mother before each session. Available school and household items were also prepared by the mother, as instructed by the OTP based on the learning activities for the day. To improve strength, the following items were used: binder clips, clothespins, hair ties, masking tape (e.g., to form shapes and letters), Play-Doh, and rubber bands. To improve fine motor skills, the following items were used: beads, coins, Lego, playing cards, puzzle board, spinning tops, and stickers. To improve school-related task performance, the following items were used: art papers, crayons, glue, paint set, pencil, ruler, and white board with marker and eraser. The level of difficulty of activities was varied and adjusted based on RT's tolerance and rate of progress. Homework was also given to ensure carryover of functional gains. The OTP and mother agreed on reward cards (e.g., additional 15-minute screen time for game or video, favorite ice cream, stay up 1 hour past bedtime) that were given to RT as positive reinforcement every time she accumulated a certain number of points from the individual activities.

Scheduled video-based teleconsultations were conducted with the mother, aunt, and OTP to obtain feedback and adjust the pacing of the telerehabilitation sessions accordingly. The mother said, "Being a single parent has always been difficult, especially pre-pandemic when I had to allot time to bring and fetch RT to/from the rehabilitation center regularly. Now with telerehabilitation, a lot of time and effort have been saved. Telerehabilitation also made it easier to reach out to the OTP to discuss RT's progress and adjust our goals and expectations. Aunt and I are also learning a lot from the activities which we can reinforce on RT during our free time."

This example used the coaching model, highlighting the role of the client's carers to set up and facilitate the telerehabilitation. Teleintervention was conducted through synchronous means and was reinforced through a home exercise program.

CASE 4: STROKE

AB is a 45-year-old right-handed female with hypertension who suffered a right-sided ischemic stroke. She used to attend regular in-person rehabilitation sessions within the city until her family moved to the country. She is ambulatory with modified independence in some ADLs (score of 2 on the Modified Rankin Scale). She is an officer of the stroke support group of the hospital she used to go to for rehabilitation. She remains in touch with the support group and rehabilitation staff through social media. She wants to maintain her improvements from rehabilitation, but there is no nearby rehabilitation facility in their new place.

The client enrolled in the telerehabilitation program at the same hospital she used to go to in-person. She was able to participate in a group teletherapy with other community-dwelling members of the stroke support group who had had similar functional capacities and needs. All of them consented through electronic means to participate in group activities consisting of a wellness program for reconditioning and recreational activities for bimanual and task-specific training facilitated remotely by an OTP. The participants met synchronously once a week for 2 hours per session through a common secure platform and complied with asynchronous home exercises monitored by their assigned OTP buddies through a social media platform's private group chat. Safety risks were managed by ensuring a reliable family member was always on standby and co-located with each participant.

This example primarily used the coaching model and emphasized the potential role of telerehabilitation to connect to patients in rural areas without easy access to in-person or community-based rehabilitation. By leveraging low-cost and locally available technologies, clients could maintain their motor and functional improvements, as well as their social skills and emotional and mental well-being.

Acknowledgment

The authors would like to acknowledge Ms. Ruby Aikat of the Amity Institute of Occupational Therapy at the Amity University, Noida, India for her contribution to the literature search on telerehabilitation applications in occupational therapy.

References

1. American Occupational Therapy Association. (n.d.-a). About Occupational Therapy. https://www.aota.org/about-occupational-therapy.aspx; Accessed February 20, 2021.
2. Clark FA, Parham D, Carlson ME, et al. Occupational science: academic innovation in the service of occupational therapy's future. *Am J Occup Ther*. 1991;45(4):300–310. https://doi.org/10.5014/ajot.45.4.300.
3. Corey T. Perspectives of occupational therapy practitioners on benefits and barriers on providing occupational therapy services via telehealth. *Student Capstone Projects*. 2019. Retrieved from https://soar.usa.edu/capstones/12.
4. Gardner K, Bundy A, Dew A. Perspectives of rural carers on benefits and barriers of receiving occupational therapy via information and communication technologies. *Aust Occup Ther J*. 2016;63(2):117–122. https://doi.org/10.1111/1440-1630.12256.
5. Hoffmann T, Cantoni N. Occupational therapy services for adult neurological clients in Queensland and therapists' use of telehealth to provide services. *Aust Occup Ther J*. 2008; 55(4):239–248. https://doi.org/10.1111/j.1440-1630.2007.00693.x.
6. Leochico CFD, Valera MJS. Follow-up consultations through telerehabilitation for wheelchair recipients with paraplegia in a developing country: a case report. *Spinal Cord Ser Cases*. 2020;6(1):58. https://doi.org/10.1038/s41394-020-0310-9.
7. Nobakht Z, Rassafiani M, Hosseini SA, et al. Telehealth in occupational therapy: a scoping review. *Int J Ther Rehabil*. 2017;24(12):534–538. https://doi.org/10.12968/ijtr.2017.24.12.534.
8. Tyagi N, Amar Goel S, Alexander M. Improving quality of life after spinal cord injury in India with telehealth. *Spinal Cord Ser Cases*. 2019;5(1):70. https://doi.org/10.1038/s41394-019-0212-x.
9. Pan American Health Organization & World Health Organization. Rehabilitation considerations during the COVID-19 outbreak. 2020. https://iris.paho.org/handle/10665.2/52035.
10. Cason J. Telehealth and occupational therapy: integral to the triple aim of health care reform. *Am J Occup Ther*. 2015;69(2):1–8. https://doi.org/10.5014/ajot.2015.692003.
11. Hung KN, Fong K. N. K. G. Effects of telerehabilitation in occupational therapy practice: a systematic review. *Hong Kong J Occup Ther*. 2019;32(1):3–21. https://doi.org/10.1177/1569186119849119.
12. Occupational Therapy Australia. Telehealth Guidelines 2020. 2020. https://otaus.com.au/publicassets/553c6eae-ad6c-ea11-9404-005056be13b5/OTA.
13. World Federation of Occupational Therapists. World Federation of Occupational Therapists' position statement on telehealth. *Int J Telerehabilitation*. 2014;6(1):37–40. https://doi.org/10.5195/IJT.2014.6153.
14. Cason J. Telehealth: a rapidly developing service delivery model for occupational therapy. *Int J Telerehabilitation*. 2014;6(1):29–36. https://doi.org/10.5195/ijt.2014.6148.
15. Brennan D, Tindall L, Theodoros D, et al. A blueprint for telerehabilitation guidelines. *International Journal of Telerehabilitation*. 2010;2(2):31–34. https://doi.org/10.5195/IJT.2010.6063.
16. Hegel MT, Lyons KD, Hull JG, et al. Feasibility study of a randomized controlled trial of a telephone-delivered problem-solving-occupational therapy intervention to reduce participation restrictions in rural breast cancer survivors undergoing chemotherapy. *Psychooncology*. 2011;20(10):1092–1101. https://doi.org/10.1002/pon.1830.
17. Reifenberg G, Gabrosek G, Tanner K, et al. Feasibility of pediatric game-based neurorehabilitation using telehealth technologies: a case report. *Am J Occup Ther*. 2017;71(3). https://doi.org/10.5014/ajot.2017.024976. 7103190040p1.
18. Sarsak HI. Telerehabilitation services: a successful paradigm for occupational therapy clinical services? *Int Phys Med Rehabil J*. 2020;5(2):93–98. https://doi.org/10.15406/ipmrj.2020.05.00237.
19. Smith D, Hudson S. Using the person–environment–occupational performance conceptual model as an analyzing framework for health literacy. *J Commun Healthc*. 2012;5(1):11–13. https://doi.org/10.1179/1753807611Y.0000000021.
20. Cason J. An introduction to telehealth as a service delivery model within occupational therapy. *OT Practice*. 2012;17(7):CE1–CE8.

21. Kessler D, Graham F. The use of coaching in occupational therapy: an integrative review. *Aust Occup Ther J.* 2015;62(3):160–176. https://doi.org/10.1111/1440-1630.12175.

22. Little LM, Pope E, Wallisch A, et al. Occupation-based coaching by means of telehealth for families of young children with autism spectrum disorder. *Am J Occup Ther.* 2018;72(2). https://doi.org/10.5014/ajot.2018.024786. 7202205020p1.

23. American Occupational Therapy Association (AOTA). Telehealth in occupational therapy. *Am J Occup Ther.* 2018;72(Suppl 2). https://doi.org/10.5014/ajot.2018.72S219. 7212410059p1.

24. Jacobs K, Cason J, McCullough A. The process for the formulation of the International Telehealth Position Statement for occupational therapy. *Int J Telerehabilitation.* 2015;7(1):21–32. https://doi.org/10.5195/IJT.2015.6163.

25. Cason J. Telehealth opportunities in occupational therapy through the Affordable Care Act. *Am J Occup Ther.* 2012;66(2):131–136. https://doi.org/10.5014/ajot.2012.662001.

26. Ciro C, Randall K, Robinson C, et al. Telehealth and interprofessional education. *OT Practice.* 2015;20(7):7–10.

27. Gallagher TE. Augmentation of special-needs services and information to students and teachers "ASSIST"—a telehealth innovation providing school-based medical interventions. *Hawaii Med J.* 2004;63(10):300–309. http://www.ncbi.nlm.nih.gov/pubmed/15570717.

28. Cason J. Telerehabilitation: an adjunct service delivery model for early intervention services. *Int J Telerehabilitation.* 2011;3(1):19–30. https://doi.org/10.5195/IJT.2011.6071.

29. Neubeck L, Redfern J, Fernandez R, et al. Telehealth interventions for the secondary prevention of coronary heart disease: a systematic review. *Eur J Cardiovasc Prev Rehabil.* 2009;16(3):281–289. https://doi.org/10.1097/HJR.0b013e32832a4e7a.

30. Harada ND, Dhanani S, Elrod M, et al. Feasibility study of home telerehabilitation for physically inactive veterans. *J Rehabil Res Dev.* 2010;47(5):465. https://doi.org/10.1682/JRRD.2009.09.0149.

31. Darkins A, Ryan P, Kobb R, et al. Care coordination/home telehealth: the systematic implementation of health informatics, home telehealth, and disease management to support the care of veteran patients with chronic conditions. *Telemed J E Health.* 2008;14(10):1118–1126. https://doi.org/10.1089/tmj.2008.0021.

32. Breeden LE. Occupational therapy home safety intervention via telehealth. *Int J Telerehabilitation.* 2016;8(1):29–40. https://doi.org/10.5195/IJT.2016.6183.

33. Germain V, Marchand A, Bouchard S, et al. Effectiveness of cognitive behavioural therapy administered by videoconference for posttraumatic stress disorder. *Cogn Behav Ther.* 2009;38(1):42–53. https://doi.org/10.1080/16506070802473494.

34. Mann WC, ed. *Smart Technology for Aging, Disability, and Independence.* Hoboken, NJ: John Wiley & Sons; 2005. https://doi.org/10.1002/0471743941.

35. Hori M, Kubota M, Ando K, et al. The effect of videophone communication (with skype and webcam) for elderly patients with dementia and their caregivers. *Gan To Kagaku Ryoho.* 2009;36(Suppl 1):36–38. http://www.ncbi.nlm.nih.gov/pubmed/20443395.

36. American Occupational Therapy Association. (n.d.-b). Special Interest Sections. 2021. https://www.aota.org/Practice/Manage/SIS.aspx.

37. Leochico C, Espiritu A, Ignacio S, et al. Challenges to the emergence of telerehabilitation in a developing country: a systematic review. *Front Neurol.* 2020;11:1007. https://doi.org/10.3389/fneur.2020.01007.

38. Nix J, Comans T. Home Quick – occupational therapy home visits using mHealth, to facilitate discharge from acute admission back to the community. *Int J Telerehabilitation.* 2017;9(1):47–54. https://doi.org/10.5195/IJT.2017.6218.

39. Linder SM, Rosenfeldt AB, Bay RC, et al. Improving quality of life and depression after stroke through telerehabilitation. *Am J Occup Ther.* 2015;69(2). https://doi.org/10.5014/ajot.2015.014498.69022900 20p1.

40. Linder SM, Reiss A, Buchanan S, et al. Incorporating robotic-assisted telerehabilitation in a home program to improve arm function following stroke. *J Neurol Phys Ther.* 2013;37(3):125–132. https://doi.org/10.1097/NPT.0b013e31829fa808.

41. Ferre CL, Brandão M, Surana B, et al. Caregiver-directed home-based intensive bimanual training in young children with unilateral spastic cerebral palsy: a randomized trial. *Dev Med Child Neurol.* 2017;59(5):497–504. https://doi.org/10.1111/dmcn.13330.

42. Gibbs V, Toth-Cohen S. Family-centered occupational therapy and telerehabilitation for children with autism spectrum disorders. *Occup Ther Health Care.* 2011;25(4):298–314. https://doi.org/10.3109/07380577.2011.606460.

43. Stark S. Creating disability in the home: the role of environmental barriers in the United States. *Disabil Soc.* 2001;16(1):37–49. https://doi.org/10.1080/713662037.

44. Tsai C-Y, Miller AS, Huang V, et al. The feasibility and usability of a mobile application for performing home evaluations. *Spinal Cord Ser Cases.* 2019;5(1):76. https://doi.org/10.1038/s41394-019-0219-3.

45. Stark S, Landsbaum A, Palmer JL, et al. Client-centred home modifications improve daily activity performance of older adults. *Can J Occup Ther.* 2009;76(Suppl 1):235–245. https://doi.org/10.1177/0008417 40907600s09.

46. Clemson L, Mackenzie L, Ballinger C, et al. Environmental interventions to prevent falls in community-dwelling older people. *J Aging Health.* 2008;20(8):954–971. https://doi.org/10.1177/0898264 308324672.

47. Gitlin LN, Corcoran M. Expanding caregiver ability to use environmental solutions for problems of bathing and incontinence in the elderly with dementia. *Technol Disabil.* 1993;2(1):12–22. https://doi.org/10.3233/TAD-1993-2104.

48. Gitlin LN, Corcoran M, Winter L, et al. A randomized, controlled trial of a home environmental intervention. *Gerontologist.* 2001;41(1):4–14. https://doi.org/10.1093/geront/41.1.4.

49. Gitlin LN, Hauck WW, Winter L, et al. Effect of an in-home occupational and physical therapy intervention on reducing mortality in functionally vulnerable older people: preliminary findings. *J Am Geriatr Soc.* 2006;54(6):950–955. https://doi.org/10.1111/j.1532-5415.2006.00733.x.

50. Mann WC, Ottenbacher KJ, Fraas L, et al. Effectiveness of assistive technology and environmental interventions in maintaining independence and reducing home care costs for the frail elderly. A randomized controlled trial. *Arch Fam Med.* 1999;8(3):210–217.

51. Petersson I, Kottorp A, Bergström J, et al. Longitudinal changes in everyday life after home modifications for people aging with disabilities. *Scand J Occup Ther.* 2009;16(2):78–87. https://doi.org/10.1080/11038120802409747.

52. Gillespie LD, Robertson MC, Gillespie WJ, et al. Interventions for preventing falls in older people living in the community. *Cochrane Database Syst Rev.* 2012;2012(9):CD007146. https://doi.org/10.1002/14651858.CD007146.pub3.

53. Aplin T, de Jonge D, Gustafsson L. Understanding the dimensions of home that impact on home modification decision making. *Aust Occup Ther J.* 2013;60(2):101–109. https://doi.org/10.1111/1440-1630.12022.

54. Hoel V, Zweck Cvon, Ledgerd R, World Federation of Occupational Therapists The impact of Covid-19 for occupational therapy: findings and recommendations of a global survey. *World Fed Occup Ther Bull.* 2021. https://doi.org/10.1080/14473828.2020.1855044.

55. Burrage, M. M. Telehealth and Rehabilitation: Extending Occupational Therapy Services to Rural Mississippi. [Thesis]. University of Southern Mississippi; 2019.

56. Leochico CFD. Adoption of telerehabilitation in a developing country before and during the COVID-19 pandemic. *Ann Phys Rehabil Med.* 2020;63(6):563–564. https://doi.org/10.1016/j.rehab.2020.06.001.

57. Leochico CF, Mojica JA. Telerehabilitation as a teaching-learning tool for medical interns. *PARM Proceedings.* 2017;9(1):39–43.

CHAPTER 21

Telerehabilitation for Hand and Upper Extremity Conditions

Lisa Kozden ▦ Tiffany Pritchett ▦ Nishu Tyagi ▦ Carl Froilan D. Leochico

Introduction

Rehabilitation of the hand and upper extremity requires a clinician to be knowledgeable as well as creative due to the complex, intricate, and functional design of this most valuable human tool. Having an in-depth understanding of the anatomical, physiological, neurological, and psychosocial functions of the upper limb is crucial for the clinician when evaluating a client, setting goals, and developing a treatment program. When using telerehabilitation to conduct this same process, the clinician must rely on both past experience and intuitive guidance to provide valuable service to clients in need of individualized care.

The unique nature of upper extremity rehabilitation embraces the strengths of both occupational and physical therapy professions.[1] The philosophical tenets of physical therapy include evaluation and treatment of the musculoskeletal and neurological systems using clinical measurements, physical agent modalities, manual therapy techniques, and therapeutic exercises. Occupational therapy tenets include evaluation and treatment of these same systems, while focusing more often on functional assessments, behavioral and environmental modifications, orthotic fabrication, and psychosocial approaches. Through the use of meaningful activities, occupational therapists are able to promote subconscious functional movements of the upper extremity embedded in occupation.[2] Occupational therapists commonly utilize both biomechanical and occupation-centered interventions in upper extremity rehabilitation. Therefore they must continue using evidence-based yet practical approaches to reflect the unique benefits of the two treatment principles.[1]

On a worldwide basis, upper extremity conditions are both prevalent and costly, particularly in the areas of work-related musculoskeletal disorders (WMSDs) and neurological conditions such as cerebral vascular accidents (CVAs).[3-7] In developing countries, muscular pain in the neck and upper limbs accounts for up to 42% of work-related injuries, impacting not only employees' health, quality of life, and occupational performance but also the overall public health system of the countries in which they reside.[6] Although the prevalence of CVAs resulting in upper extremity dysfunction has decreased in developed countries over the last 40 years, developing countries have experienced just the opposite scenario.[7] The increased prevalence of CVA in developing countries places undue stress on already fragile systems that are unable to meet the growing demand by people in need of health care and social services.[7]

According to the US Department of Labor Statistics in 2018, there were 286,810 upper extremity injuries, which accounted for almost 32% of all nonfatal occupational injuries and illnesses resulting in days away from work.[8] From January to December of 2009, over 92,000 patients were diagnosed with an upper extremity injury, resulting in approximately 3,468,996 people with upper extremity injuries visiting emergency departments in the United States.[9] The incidence of upper extremity injuries is 1130 cases per 100,000 people per year, implying that an individual has a 1-in-88 chance of incurring an upper extremity injury needing emergency medical care in any given year.[9] According to the Centers for Disease Control and Prevention (CDC), upper extremity disorders most frequently occur among people who engage in work requiring frequent repetitive and resistive tasks.[10] These conditions affect the nerves, tendons, and muscles of the neck, shoulder, elbow, wrist, and hand, for which organizations pay more than USD 2.1 billion in direct and indirect workers' compensation costs.[10] These medical costs have created a negative impact on the financial status of the American health care system.

Telerehabilitation and Neurological Conditions

The COVID-19 pandemic has catalyzed the unprecedented shift to alternative delivery methods of hand rehabilitation in various health care settings throughout the world in order to prevent or address the devastating functional consequences of hand conditions left untreated. Telerehabilitation is a viable option that existed even pre-pandemic, albeit not as popular then as now. Nonetheless, it is found to be feasible, logical, and practical specifically for hand rehabilitation for several reasons: (1) potential ability to maximize neuroplasticity or neuromuscular recovery; (2) adaptation in the client's home or work environment; and (3) promotion of client's active engagement in the rehabilitation process.[11]

Upper extremity telerehabilitation, particularly for neurological conditions including strokes and spinal cord injuries, may involve technological home or workplace-based solutions which can increase the number of repetitions and duration of training required to promote neuroplasticity. A potential for spontaneous recovery and neuroplastic adaptation may be achieved using an intensive telerehabilitation program in which the client can engage for a longer period in the home environment, as compared with the same intensity of in-clinic rehabilitation program. The client typically performs this in-clinic program for fewer hours with no reassurance of functional carryover at home or in the workplace. The usual frequency of in-clinic stroke rehabilitation sessions may provide substantially less activities to maximize neuroplasticity, for which 300 repetitions of task-specific upper extremity activity are recommended.[12, 13] Aside from frequency, continuous progression of exercise intensity is needed to improve motor skill that can likewise be facilitated remotely by a trained clinician. In addition, functional gains may be more sustained and contextualized through telerehabilitation as the client actively performs exercises using actual household items relevant to day-to-day living. It is important for the clinician to evaluate the client's natural environment and provide appropriate recommendations for adaptation or modification. As long as the client consents, telerehabilitation may provide clinicians with the opportunity to observe and analyze the client's environmental context with higher accuracy as compared with in-clinic evaluations, wherein verbal reports from the client or caregiver may not be as accurate and informative.

In order to increase the amount of rehabilitation received by the clients and minimize costs, involvement of reliable co-located family members or caregivers during and after the telerehabilitation sessions may seem logical.[14] In a randomized, noninferiority clinical trial that compared stroke home-based telerehabilitation with in-clinic therapy, there was noted improvement in motor status and patient knowledge about stroke with either approach.[14] A meta-analysis showed moderate, albeit limited, evidence that stroke telerehabilitation of varied approaches (i.e., videogame-driven, virtual reality) is comparable with in-clinic rehabilitation in terms of functional improvement and motor gain.[15] Nonetheless, a Cochrane review argued that telerehabilitation is still emerging and understandably more studies are required for more definitive conclusions.[16]

Although telerehabilitation has the potential to promote and sustain functional improvements, it should be emphasized that no "one telerehabilitation program fits all." For instance, impairments in tone and sensation of the hand, attention, cognition, and consciousness are some factors that may limit manipulation of household or makeshift items used for telerehabilitation.

The effectiveness of various telerehabilitation approaches depends on the type and severity of the disease, along with accompanying impairments and comorbid conditions.[17] Hence, a creative and individualized telerehabilitation program must be carefully prepared. Clients with lifelong conditions, such as degenerative joint disease and neurological diseases such as stroke, polyneuropathies, and spinal cord injuries, for whom long-term in-clinic rehabilitation may be costly, monotonous, and burdensome, may be transitioned to pure telerehabilitation or hybrid telerehabilitation (i.e., mixed in-clinic and home-based virtual rehabilitation).

Telerehabilitation and Musculoskeletal Conditions

Acute and postsurgical conditions initially require a hands-on approach to treatment, which can later be transitioned to telerehabilitation to ensure proper and sustained supervision by a clinician. Generally, in-clinic approach is advised for initial comprehensive evaluation of acute and postsurgical hand conditions and for instituting appropriate meticulous interventions, such as wound care, edema management, and orthotic fabrication. Following this initial phase of treatment, which may involve as few as two or three in-clinic visits, telerehabilitation sessions may then follow for further promotion of healing and function incorporating client/caregiver education and home exercise programs. The decision to transition to telerehabilitation should be based on the sound clinical judgment of the clinician and informed consent and cooperation of the client. The clinician must consider the various biopsychosocial factors affecting the client's participation with telerehabilitation, such as cognitive, visual or hearing impairments, lack of caregiver support, loss of fine motor skills, incoordination, and technical resources and capacity.

Chronic and nonsurgical conditions, such as tendinopathies, fractures with immobilization protocols, and cumulative trauma disorders, may be treated with either a pure or hybrid telerehabilitation approach. During evaluation, clinicians must gather adequate subjective and objective information to establish an effective and practical home exercise program with the client. After establishing rapport with the client, the clinician can develop an occupational profile and encourage the client to incorporate objects and activities from the natural environment. In this way, the clinician can observe the client's occupational performance and make recommendations as needed. For instance, if a client with lateral epicondylosis reports pain and difficulty with specific tasks, the clinician can educate the client regarding behavior modification as it impacts occupations of self-care, work, or leisure.

Because telerehabilitation is different from an in-clinic therapy experience, establishment of rapport between clinician and client is imperative. This rapport will be the foundation upon which the clinician may initiate client education, promote understanding and acceptance of "skilled education" and the advantages of remotely supervised home-based interventions, and assure clients that their needs and goals will be met through the therapeutic process in spite of the distance. In reality, the process does not occur in a sequenced, step-by-step fashion. Rather, it is fluid and dynamic, allowing clinicians and clients to exchange ideas on what will work best, while maintaining their focus on preidentified clinical outcomes. As with in-clinic sessions, reassessments are needed to continually reflect on the current treatment plan and make appropriate adjustments as needed.

Once a plan of care is established, the clinician can assist the client in identifying actual household items as well as accessible make-shift exercise equipment that can be used during the telerehabilitation sessions. For instance, if dumbbells or exercise bands are unavailable for upper limb strengthening exercises, a client can use a handheld plastic stapler (weighing approximately half a pound), canned vegetables (1 pound), unopened bottle of water (450 mL), or empty wine bottle (750 mL; 1 pound), half gallon of milk (4–5 pounds), or full gallon of milk (8 pounds).[18] Utilizing table-tops, kitchen counters, and doorways at home in performing self-assisted range of motion or active-assisted range of motion (aided by a reliable caregiver) can allow the client to engage in home exercise programs without purchasing additional equipment. Transitioning to active range of motion exercises in functional reaching patterns, shoulder flexion and external rotation, and elbow, wrist, and finger extension can be incorporated in everyday home activities. Tools needed for basic and instrumental activities of daily living (ADL) during telerehabilitation sessions can help improve impairments and improve specific skills. For instance, utilizing buttons, zippers, and fasteners can improve mobility and fine motor coordination, while allowing the client to regain independence and self-confidence in the area of dressing.

Therapeutic exercises can be an integral part of a telerehabilitation intervention when improving hand function. However, addressing impairments through exercise may be challenging without manual guidance from the clinician or use of specific equipment, such as resistance bands and putty, which are typically available during in-clinic rehabilitation. Clinicians are encouraged to utilize their clinical judgment and reasoning to overcome this challenge. For instance a toolkit of therapeutic items may be carefully curated together with the client or family to help address certain deficits in performance skills and achieve rehabilitation goals. If the client lives within a reasonable distance from the rehabilitation center, a family member or caregiver may be asked to pick up therapeutic tool kits from the clinician for use during their telerehabilitation appointments. The clinician may also choose to mail or deliver the toolkits to the client as another option.

Special Considerations

Clinicians treating clients with upper extremity conditions have traditionally utilized patient-rated outcome (PRO) assessments to promote a client-centered and occupation-centered treatment approach. PRO assessments typically address client engagement in occupation and elicit important subjective information relevant to function.[19] Such data may be required to evaluate client function and justify the need for therapeutic services. Commonly used PRO assessments include the Disabilities of the Arm, Shoulder, and Hand (DASH) Inventory, Quick DASH (QDASH) Scale, and Patient-Rated Wrist Evaluation (PRWE).[19-21] In a scoping review of outcome measures for stroke telerehabilitation, the most commonly used tools include the Fugl-Meyer Assessment of Stroke Recovery (FMA) and the Box and Block Test (BBT).[22] These psychometrically sound assessments address function and provide clinicians a systematic method to adequately evaluate occupational performance within a telerehabilitation delivery system.

Telerehabilitation in this area of practice does limit clinicians' ability to offer hands-on treatment techniques, such as orthotic fabrication, manual therapy, wound/scar management, and certain modalities for addressing pain and edema. Clinicians must ensure that communication and education of the clients and caregivers are clear, concise, and easily understood to ensure positive outcomes and avoid misconceptions or unmet expectations.

There is undoubtedly significant potential in the area of telerehabilitation in addressing upper extremity dysfunction, although many challenges remain within this upcoming field of practice. Fear of technology and operability by health care providers as well as clients may decrease willingness to utilize this mode of care.[23] Learning new technology skills may be a source of apprehension particularly among clients, who may be significantly limited physically as well as cognitively. Inflexibility in transitioning from the "hands-on" in-clinic approach to a virtual medium of service delivery and concerns regarding effectiveness and ability to achieve rehabilitation goals have potential negative impact on the emergence of telerehabilitation, including hand telerehabilitation. A paradigm shift facilitated by clinicians' open-mindedness and practical clinical reasoning, along with clients' empowerment and active participation in the treatment process, may help pave the way to greater adoption of telerehabilitation for various conditions.[24]

State licensure issues, which include professional portability, have the potential to limit telerehabilitation services. Within the United States, clinicians must be licensed within the state they are practicing as well as within the state the client is receiving the care.[25] Clinicians must abide by state laws and regulations related to telehealth as well as state occupational therapy licensing board regulations and policies. Inconsistent laws, regulations, and policies among states (and even within states) necessitate the need to continually check state statutes and occupational therapy practice regulations and policies to ensure compliance when delivering services via telehealth.[26] Licensure laws in conjunction with lack of reimbursement and payment systems currently impede a greater platform for delivery of telerehabilitation services. In addition, the need for research supporting telerehabilitation as a service delivery model and development of outcome measures specifically for the use of evaluating and measuring progress through telerehabilitation are imperative for its continued use in various health care settings.

Special considerations must be contemplated when assessing which clients will successfully participate in telerehabilitation. Clients who are used to receiving skilled in-clinic therapy have the potential to demonstrate significant physical and cognitive deficits, which can impact their ability to independently participate in telerehabilitation. Clients with diagnoses affecting upper extremity function, such as stroke and traumatic brain injury, may also present with visual, visuoperceptual, and cognitive deficits (i.e., impulsivity, decreased comprehension, inability to follow verbal/visual directions, distractibility). These individuals may be at a disadvantage and will require clinicians' clinical judgment to evaluate the need for adaptive technology, equipment, or adaptive therapeutic materials in order to allow for increased accessibility to this population.[26] Clinicians may recommend in-clinic sessions or a hybrid approach in addition to significant support by caregivers or personal care assistants during virtual appointments.

Technology continues to improve, grow, and expand as new sensory-based rehabilitation, virtual environments, and video image-based telerehabilitation are being introduced. Nevertheless, availability of technology to individuals across socioeconomic levels and practice settings (including remote and rural areas) and limitations related to internet accessibility impact the availability of telerehabilitation as well as fluidity of video sessions with "freezing," lagging, or dropped/interrupted sessions. These technology-related limitations in conjunction with predetermined length of sessions (e.g., 45 minutes) can significantly impact the success and quality of care. Thus for each telerehabilitation session, there should be a backup plan for failings in technology, which may include phone call follow-ups to minimize the impact on the therapeutic sessions. The type of telerehabilitation delivered will also determine the type of technology equipment required to participate in the sessions. For example, a client who is being treated for a distal radius fracture may need to be seated throughout the session while completing range of motion exercises and would require the use of a desktop or laptop computer. Alternatively, a client who is in phase 3 of a recovery of rotator cuff repair, initiating active range of motion at the shoulder through functional reaching and moving around their home environment, may require the use of mobile device such as a smartphone, tablet, or laptop. These devices also allow the individual to easily move around the environment and provide multiple visual points of movement and function.

Telerehabilitation limits physical examination and hands-on techniques typically utilized by health care professionals. These techniques include manual manipulation, custom splinting, and use of kinesiotaping and other modalities in clinic or hospital settings. Furthermore, at this time it limits the use of typical outcome measures of upper limb function including dynamometers, goniometers, nine-hole peg tests, and the Jebsen test among others. More research on outcome measures for evaluating hand and upper extremity conditions through telerehabilitation is, therefore, recommended.

Areas for Future Research

Unquestionably, the COVID-19 pandemic caused a massive shift in delivering hand and upper extremity rehabilitation services and opened avenues for future research. Clinicians must now shift their client-centered approach from using a hands-on technique in the clinic to incorporating a hands-off approach in the virtual and natural environment of the client. Fortunately, this shift offers clinicians, educators, and researchers more opportunities to examine and explore the benefits of treating clients using both traditional and telerehabilitation approaches in a hybrid model of practice. For instance, researchers have identified the following areas for future studies: communication with clients, education, and self-management; functional outcomes and therapists' adherence to treatment guidelines; clients' perceptions of and satisfaction levels with services provided; efficacy of telerehabilitation in various phases of the healing process (acute vs. chronic); and the socioeconomic implications of this hybrid approach on clinicians, clients, and reimbursement systems on a global basis.[27, 28] Since the onset of the COVID-19 pandemic, researchers also found the most at-risk populations to be older adults with chronic health conditions. During long periods of quarantine, they often experience a decrease in overall strength and endurance, which may further complicate the symptoms of their upper extremity conditions.[29] The overall lesson is that health care providers must remain flexible, thinking outside of traditional means of treatment and ready to use alternative, skilled, and client-centered clinical approaches that optimize client outcomes and prevent further decline in function, most especially in the area of upper extremity care. This client-centered and holistic approach to care is central to the philosophy of occupational therapy; therefore integration of telerehabilitation services should be a natural transition into practice for occupational therapists.

CASE STUDY

GUILLAIN-BARRÉ SYNDROME

Stephanie is a 65-year-old female who presented with progressive distal paresthesia, numbness of fingers and toes, diffuse weakness, and subjective dysphagia. She was admitted to the neurointensive care unit and intubated for respiratory support. She was further treated with intravenous immunoglobulin (IVIG) for 5 days, and underwent a tracheostomy and PEG placement. She was weaned from the ventilator and transferred to acute inpatient rehabilitation, with the diagnosis of Guillain-Barré syndrome. She completed 8 weeks of acute inpatient rehabilitation, where she progressed to a regular diet and thin liquids and PEG tube was removed. She was discharged home and referred to outpatient occupational therapy for evaluation. Stephanie was discharged home at the start of the COVID-19 crisis and therefore her initial occupational evaluation was completed via high-end videoconferencing (telerehabilitation). During the 45-minute session, Stephanie and her husband were present, and her occupational history, profile, and performance skills and patterns were assessed by the occupational therapist in the setting of her home environment. Stephanie participated in occupations and demonstrated active range of motion in her bilateral upper extremities. This allowed the OT to observe limited range of motion, strength, and compensatory movements in her dominant right upper extremity, primarily in her shoulder. Through observation, Stephanie's right scapula was protracted and elevated with mild upward rotation and moderate scapular winging. A home exercise program was initiated during the initial evaluation with education and hands-on training provided by her husband to Stephanie on passive range of motion techniques through the virtual video session. Follow-up sessions were completed through continued telehealth sessions with emphasis on increasing active range of motion in her right glenohumeral joint to promote increased functional reaching required for bathing (washing hair), upper body dressing and home management tasks (reaching into cabinets) through the use of MedBridge for continued progression of her home exercise program. MedBridge is an online educational platform for patient education and generates customized home exercise programs for clients by their therapists through the use of pictures and video demonstration. Stephanie plateaued with her active range of motion in her upper extremity, unable to achieve greater than 110 degrees of shoulder flexion without shoulder elevation and lateral trunk flexion. The occupational therapist requested an in-clinic appointment to address scapular mobility, wherein the therapist completed scapular glides and distraction due to increased tightness and muscle shortening in her periscapular muscles. After completion of the remaining plan of care, Stephanie was able to achieve full range of motion throughout her dominant upper extremity with equal strength to her contralateral upper extremity.

CHRONIC WRIST PAIN

Kelly is a 46-year-old female who was referred to occupational therapy for chronic pain in her left non-dominant wrist. She reported having pain along the ulnar aspect of her wrist which began approximately 3 months prior and has worsened over time. She reports 8/10 pain with any weight-bearing into her wrist, especially during workouts. She is unable to perform planking or spinning, and is also unable to grip and rotate objects such as lifting pots and pans when cooking for her family.

Upon inspection of her left wrist (as compared to her right), her therapist noted increased edema at the area of the ulnar styloid. When asked to grasp and rotate her water bottle into full supination and pronation, Kelly reported increase in pain. Her therapist then asked to observe the positioning of her scapulae and upper body posture from behind and from the side. Her therapist also observed her active reaching overhead bilaterally and unilaterally. Kelly presented with a protracted, depressed, and downwardly rotated with mild winging of L scapula at rest, which inhibited full active abduction as compared to the contralateral side. She also noted that Kelly stands with a forward head position and kyphotic posturing of the shoulders (with L humeral head sitting in more anterior position than the R). The therapist explained how this proximal positioning of the L shoulder girdle can contribute increased stress to the distal joints of the extremity in weight-bearing positions, such as planking and spinning. Increased edema and resistive gripping of objects at end range supination/pronation can increase pressure on the ligaments at the ulnar wrist, causing pain.

After evaluation, Kelly's therapist recommended the use of supportive gloves with gel padded inserts to decrease wrist extension in weight-bearing positions as well as applying kinesiotape to ulnar wrist to decrease edema and increase support during weight-bearing exercises. The therapist also recommended a proximal strengthening program for upper body posturing. At a 2-week follow-up, the client reported making modifications to workouts, wearing the gloves and applying the tape. Client reported 0/10 pain at rest and 1–2/10 with full weight-bearing using tape and gloves during workouts.

DISTAL RADIUS FRACTURE WITH COMPLEX REGIONAL PAIN SYNDROME

Jane is a 60-year-old female who works as a bank teller. She tripped over a bag of money as she entered the bank vault and fell onto her right dominant outstretched hand and arm, incurring a displaced articular fracture of the distal radius. After undergoing an open reduction internal fixation surgery to repair the fracture, Jane was referred to a certified hand therapist at 3 weeks post-op and was instructed to wear a wrist immobilization orthosis. Because of the delay in being referred to therapy, her wrist and hand became very edematous, painful, and stiff. Jane was evaluated in the clinic for her initial evaluation and the therapist recommended that she begin a home program including removal of the orthosis, active range of motion of the upper extremity in all planes, edema/pain management, and use of hand for everyday activities whenever possible.

As a result of the prolonged immobilization period, Jane began to present with symptoms consistent with complex regional pain syndrome (CRPS), including constant burning pain at rest and with activity, fluctuating edema, stiffness of wrist/hand, and skin color changes. Jane received in-clinic hand therapy services by an occupational therapist for a few weeks before the COVID-19 pandemic began. During the quarantine period, Jane began telerehabilitation visits twice a week to monitor the progress of her home program.

During the virtual visits, the therapist recommended additional pain management and behavior modification techniques as the therapist was able to observe Jane within her home environment. These visits were also crucial to monitor and advance her home exercise program as needed. For instance, the therapist was able to instruct Jane's spouse on how to apply kinesiotape to her hand and upper extremity to provide pain relief to the hypersensitive superficial nerves that were limiting Jane's function throughout the day (See video 21.1). The therapist was also able to monitor and assess Jane's ability to cope with the isolation and intense pain she was feeling on a day-to-day basis. As Jane reported her functional challenges to the therapist, she was able to work together with her therapist to adjust and modify her program to provide maximum benefit during the 2-month quarantine period. These virtual visits provided not only benefits to Jane's physical health, but to her psychosocial health as well. Because of telerehabilitation, the occupational hand therapist was able to fulfill her role as a clinician dedicated to promoting the holistic health and occupational performance of her client.

CASE STUDY

STROKE

Pam is a 60-year-old, female, left-handed, housewife, with unremarkable past medical history. One day prior to admission, she woke up feeling dizzy. Her family noticed her to have slurring and difficulty in standing up. She was brought to the nearest hospital, which was 2 hours away from their house without traffic. Upon arrival in the emergency room, her blood pressure was noted to be 190/100 mmHg. She was alert and not in cardiopulmonary distress. She could follow commands and was oriented to three spheres. She was noted to have dysarthria and dysmetria with failed finger-to-nose test on the left. All her limbs had good strength and sensation. Computed tomography (CT) scan showed left cerebellar bleed of about 3 cm. She was admitted and medically managed as cerebrovascular disease. Rehabilitation began as soon as day 1 post-stroke and consisted of physical therapy for her balance and occupational therapy for her incoordination. After 7 days, she was medically cleared to go home. Before discharge, she was reassessed to be moderately assisted with most ADL, especially bimanual activities. She was advised to continue rehabilitation at home. However, her family claimed that they could not bring her regularly to the hospital for rehabilitation since the husband has daytime work and two children had to go to school. Only her 16-year-old niece who lives next door could assist her from time to time at home. Hence, telerehabilitation was arranged.

The physiatrist, occupational therapist, and speech-language pathologist who attended to the patient in the hospital were put in charge of her telerehabilitation program to ensure rapport, familiarity with the case, and continuity of care. During the first telerehabilitation session 5 days from hospital discharge, the patient was reassessed to have the following rehabilitation problems: difficulty writing with her left hand, incoordination, and dysarthria. The rehabilitation team agreed to achieve the following telerehabilitation short-term goals: (1) improved coordination and ease in performing ADL and (2) improved articulation.

The telerehabilitation program consisted of both synchronous and asynchronous techniques. Tele–occupational therapy and tele–speech therapy sessions were done three times a week for 1 month before medical follow-up through videoconferencing. Through screen-sharing function of the videoconferencing platform, the therapist was able to show freely available videos on YouTube that demonstrate basic techniques in handwriting. Each step was explained carefully and demonstrated to train the affected left hand. Part-practice and whole-practice of specific ADLs were also trained through real-time telerehabilitation. Speech training consisted of remote live supervision of oral motor, reading, and breathing exercises, as well as store and forward techniques such as sending of electronic brochures containing home program and exercise diary.

References

1. MacDermid JC. OT and PT are equally foundational to hand therapy. *J Hand Ther.* 2019;32(4):409–410. https://doi.org/10.1016/j.jht.2019.10.002.
2. Weinstock-Zlotnick G, Mehta SP. A systematic review of the benefits of occupation-based intervention for patients with upper extremity musculoskeletal disorders. *J Hand Ther.* 2019;32(2):141–152. https://doi.org/10.1016/j.jht.2018.04.001.
3. Piedrahita H. Costs of work-related musculoskeletal disorders (MSDs) in developing countries: Colombia case. *Int J Occup Saf Ergon.* 2006;12(4):379–386. https://doi.org/10.1080/10803548.2006.11076696.
4. Van Eerd D, Munhall C, Irvin E, et al. Effectiveness of workplace interventions in the prevention of upper extremity musculoskeletal disorders and symptoms: an update of the evidence. *Occup Environ Med.* 2016;73(1):62–70. https://doi.org/10.1136/oemed-2015-102992.
5. Shankar S, Kumar RN, Mohankumar P, et al. Prevalence of work-related musculoskeletal injuries among South Indian hand screen-printing workers. *Work.* 2017;58(2):163–172. https://doi.org/10.3233/WOR-172612.
6. Nguyen TH, Hoang DL, Hoang TG, et al. Prevalence and characteristics of multisite musculoskeletal symptoms among district hospital nurses in Haiphong, Vietnam. *Biomed Res Int.* 2020;2020:3254605. https://doi.org/10.1155/2020/3254605.
7. Hughes CML, Padilla A, Hintze A, et al. Developing an mHealth app for post-stroke upper limb rehabilitation: feedback from US and Ethiopian rehabilitation clinicians. *Health Informatics J.* 2019;26(2):1104–1117. https://doi.org/10.1177/1460458219868356.
8. U.S. Department of Labor Statistics. Injuries, Illnesses and Fatalities. 2018. https://www.bls.gov/iif/oshwc/osh/case/cd_r19_2018.htm; Accessed September 2, 2020.

9. Ootes D, Lambers KT, Ring DC. The epidemiology of upper extremity injuries presenting to the emergency department in the United States. *HAND.* 2012;7(1):18–22. https://doi.org/10.1007/s11552-011-9383-z.

10. Centers for Disease Control and Prevention. (n.d.). The National Institute for Occupational Safety and Health (NIOSH). 2020. https://www.cdc.gov/niosh/docs/96-115/diseas.html#Musculoskeletal Disorders of the Upper Extremities.

11. Fluet GG, Patel J, Qiu Q, et al. Motor skill changes and neurophysiologic adaptation to recovery-oriented virtual rehabilitation of hand function in a person with subacute stroke: a case study. *Disabil Rehabil.* 2017;39(15):1524–1531. https://doi.org/10.1080/09638288.2016.1226421.

12. Birkenmeier RL, Prager EM, Lang CE. Translating animal doses of task-specific training to people with chronic stroke in 1-hour therapy sessions: a proof-of-concept study. *Neurorehabil Neural Repair.* 2010;24(7):620–635. https://doi.org/10.1177/1545968310361957.

13. Lang CE, MacDonald JR, Gnip C. Counting repetitions: an observational study of outpatient therapy for people with hemiparesis post-stroke. *J Neurol Phys Ther.* 2007;31(1):3–10. https://doi.org/10.1097/01.NPT.0000260568.31746.34.

14. Stinear CM, Lang CE, Zeiler S, et al. Advances and challenges in stroke rehabilitation. *Lancet Neurol.* 2020;19(4):348–360. https://doi.org/10.1016/S1474-4422(19)30415-6.

15. Chen J, Jin W, Zhang X-X, et al. Telerehabilitation approaches for stroke patients: systematic review and meta-analysis of randomized controlled trials. *J Stroke Cerebrovasc Dis.* 2015;24(12):2660–2668. https://doi.org/10.1016/j.jstrokecerebrovasdis.2015.09.014.

16. Laver KE, Adey-Wakeling Z, Crotty M, et al. Telerehabilitation services for stroke. *Cochrane Database Syst Rev.* 2020;1(1):CD010255. https://doi.org/10.1002/14651858.CD010255.pub3.

17. Staszuk A, Wiatrak B, Tadeusiewicz R, et al. Telerehabilitation approach for patients with hand impairment. *Acta Bioeng Biomech.* 2016;18(4):55–62. . http://www.ncbi.nlm.nih.gov/pubmed/28133379.

18. Tanaka MJ, Oh LS, Martin SD, et al. Telemedicine in the era of COVID-19. *J Bone Jt Surg Am.* 2020;102(12):e57. https://doi.org/10.2106/JBJS.20.00609.

19. Valdes K, MacDermid J, Algar L, et al. Hand therapist use of patient report outcome (PRO) in practice: a survey study. *J Hand Ther.* 2014;27(4):299–308. https://doi.org/10.1016/j.jht.2014.07.001.

20. Hudak PL, Amadio PC, Bombardier C, et al. Development of an upper extremity outcome measure: the DASH (disabilities of the arm, shoulder, and head). *Am J Ind Med.* 1996;29(6):602–608. https://doi.org/10.1002/(SICI)1097-0274(199606)29:6<602::AID-AJIM4>3.0.CO;2-L.

21. MacDermid JC. Development of a scale for patient rating of wrist pain and disability. *J Hand Ther.* 1996;9(2):178–183. https://doi.org/10.1016/S0894-1130(96)80076-7.

22. Veras M, Kairy D, Rogante M, et al. Scoping review of outcome measures used in telerehabilitation and virtual reality for post-stroke rehabilitation. *J Telemed Telecare.* 2017;23(6):567–587. https://doi.org/10.1177/1357633X16656235.

23. Leochico C, Espiritu A, Ignacio S, et al. Challenges to the emergence of telerehabilitation in a developing country: a systematic review. *Front Neurol.* 2020;11:1007. https://doi.org/10.3389/fneur.2020.01007.

24. Theodoros D, Russell T. Telerehabilitation: current perspectives. *Stud Health Technol Inform.* 2008;131:191–209. http://www.ncbi.nlm.nih.gov/pubmed/18431862.

25. American Occupational Therapy Association Telerehabilitation position paper. *Am J Occup Ther.* 2005;59(6):656–660. https://doi.org/10.5014/ajot.59.6.656.

26. Jacobs, K., McCormack, G. (Eds.). Occupational Therapy Manager (6th ed). 2019. Bethesda, MD: AOTA Press. https://doi.org/10.7139/2017.978-1-56900-592-7

27. Pugliese M, Wolff A. The value of communication, education, and self-management in providing guideline-based care: lessons learned from musculoskeletal telerehabilitation during the COVID-19 crisis. *HSS J.* 2020;16(Suppl 1):1–4. https://doi.org/10.1007/s11420-020-09784-2.

28. Turolla A, Rossettini G, Viceconti A, et al. Musculoskeletal physical therapy during the COVID-19 pandemic: is telerehabilitation the answer? *Phys Ther.* 2020;100(8):1260–1264. https://doi.org/10.1093/ptj/pzaa093.

29. Vieira ER, Richard L, da Silva RA. Perspectives on research and health practice in physical and occupational therapy in geriatrics during and post COVID-19. *Phys Occup Ther Geriatr.* 2020;38(3):199–202. https://doi.org/10.1080/02703181.2020.1786906.

CHAPTER 22

Telerehabilitation for Exercise in Neurological Disability

Ashraf S. Gorgey ▓ Jacob A. Goldsmith ▓ Melodie Anderson
▓ Teodoro Castillo

Disability is an umbrella term describing a state of decreased functioning associated with disease, disorder, injury, or other health conditions. Disability may be experienced as an impairment, activity limitation, or participation restriction, and refers to the negative aspects of an individual's health condition and environmental and personal factors.[1,2] Disabilities are diverse and heterogeneous, encompassing congenital conditions present at birth (e.g., cerebral palsy), developmental conditions (e.g., autism, attention deficit hyperactivity disorder [ADHD]), traumatic injuries (e.g., traumatic brain injury [TBI], spinal cord injury [SCI]), and chronic conditions (e.g., diabetes). Disabilities may be progressive (e.g., muscular dystrophy), static (e.g., limb loss), or intermittent (e.g., some forms of multiple sclerosis [MS]). Individuals with disabilities are vulnerable to deficiencies in health care services, and may experience greater vulnerability to secondary and comorbid conditions.[3,4]

Advancement in medical care has increased the life expectancy of the general population and persons with disabilities. This increase in life expectancy for persons with disabilities is associated with secondary chronic conditions, which are currently responsible for 60% of the global disease burden, and 80% in developing countries.[5] According to the World Health Organization report on disability in 2011, one billion people globally experience disability; that is, every alternate household has a person with disability.[6] As of 2017 half of the persons with disabilities cannot afford health care and are 50% more likely to suffer catastrophic health expenditure. These individuals have the same general health care needs as others but are twice as likely to experience inadequacy in health providers' skills and facilities, three times more likely to be denied health care, and four times more likely to be mistreated in the health care system.[7]

The economic burden of disability and associated medical comorbidities has continued to rise at an alarming rate. Individuals with disability are more likely to suffer from obesity, muscle atrophy, osteoporosis, accelerated atherogenesis, type 2 diabetes mellitus, and other complications that increase the risk of stroke, coronary heart disease, and cardiometabolic disorders.[8-14] Reduction in the level of physical activity and associated sedentary lifestyle are primary factors that lead to the development of secondary complications.[15,16]

Physical Activity in Individuals With Disability

For several decades, the scientific community has realized the impact of neurological disorders on the well-being of society, families, and individuals. Neurological disorders are diseases of the central and peripheral nervous systems. These disorders include Alzheimer's disease and other dementias, epilepsy, stroke, MS, Parkinson's disease (PD), and traumatic disorders due to trauma to the head or spinal cord (TBI and SCI, respectively).[2] These medical conditions can result in a low quality of life, social isolation, and psychosomatic impairment.[17–19] Individuals with neurological disability require frequent, specialized, and interdisciplinary health care addressing mobility, autonomic function,[20,21] as well as other potential secondary complications.[4,22,23]

Many neurological disorders have common symptoms of reduced motor function, increased fatigue, and reduced physical activity levels.[24,25] The physical activity levels of individuals with disability are only 40% of the general population.[26] The American College of Sports Medicine and the American Heart Association recommend healthy adults engage in 150 minutes of moderate-intensity exercise per week to maintain cardiorespiratory fitness.[27] Guidelines for individuals with disability have highlighted the importance of improving physical activity levels.[28] For instance, in 2017, the updated guidelines recommended that persons with SCI engage in routine physical activity for at least 20 to 30 minutes two to three times per week, to attenuate cardiovascular comorbidities.[15,29] A prominent symptom of neurological disorders is progressive neuromuscular weakness.[30] Therefore the recommendations have highlighted the significance of engaging in strength training programs to enhance musculoskeletal integrity. With respect to SCIs, approximately 50% of individuals with SCI engage in no leisure-time physical activity (LTPA) such as sports, wheeling, or walking for pleasure or exercise.[31] Indeed, increased physical activity levels and exercise have been shown to have positive effects on disease outcomes in various neurological disorders.[24,32]

Several reports have indicated significant barriers to improving physical activity levels and exercise adherence in persons with disabilities.[33] These barriers include costs of exercise facilities, limited access to facilities, lack of adequate transportation, and lack of motivation.[34–39] For example, a lack of background knowledge on dealing with persons with SCI, and failure to provide appropriate exercise routines based on the individual's neurological level and spared muscle function act as barriers to exercise.[34] This highlights the importance of improving exercise individualization and physical activity adherence among persons with disability. Telerehabilitation (TR) programs to increase physical activity and exercise have been successfully used in many neurological disorders, including stroke, TBI, dementia, PD, SCI, and MS.

Telerehabilitation for Individuals With Disabilities

The World Health Organization defines rehabilitation as a set of interventions needed when a person is experiencing limitations in everyday functioning due to aging or health condition, including chronic diseases or disorders, injuries, or traumas. Rehabilitation requires one-on-one interaction between clinicians and patients. This interaction works toward a number of beneficial outcomes including solving existing medical, social, and psychological consequences via routine physical and diagnostic evaluations, as well as the use of different laboratory and imaging procedures. Rehabilitation is a patient-centered health intervention for individuals with complex needs that may be delivered through specialized rehabilitation programs or integrated into the health care programs and services, such as primary and mental health care.

Telehealth communication has emerged as a promising avenue to improve rehabilitation, and long-term physical activity and exercise compliance. Home TR aims to improve clinical outcomes and access to care while reducing complications, hospitalizations, and clinic or emergency room visits. Overall, TR offers "healing from a distance" by delivering health services remotely through information and communication technologies. TR goes beyond telemedicine, offering clinical and nonclinical services, including providing patients and caregivers with education through distance learning, training, and administrative meetings and presentations.

TR is a relatively new subdiscipline of telemedicine and eHealth where communication and information technology can have a positive impact on health and well-being.[40] This improved care coordination between specialty providers, clients, caregivers, and local clinical providers avoids unguided rehabilitation services offered by paramedical and rehabilitation personnel at remote locations without a physiatrist's diagnosis and prescription. Most importantly, TR has the potential to exceed traditional care and management strategies for the lifelong care of people with disability.

Advances in videoconferencing software allow for safe and continuous monitoring of at-home exercise regimens.[41] The rapid evolution of TR technologies has led to wearable devices connected to web-based apps on mobile devices that record and store physiological data (e.g., heart rate, blood pressure, glucose levels). Although a relatively new avenue of research, many studies have reported increased physical activity levels, cardiorespiratory fitness, and high exercise adherence levels in individuals using TR programs. Inexpensive home-based telecommunication programs may represent an effective rehabilitation option for clinicians to overcome adherence and commitment issues while improving health following disability. Moreover, these programs may reduce the health costs associated with lengthy rehabilitation for people with disabilities while allowing facilities to connect with patients more effectively by providing services via internet and video technologies.

Applications of Telerehabilitation in Conjunction With Endurance Exercise Training

SPINAL CORD INJURY

Various forms of home-based aerobic exercise programs have been utilized, including cycle ergometry,[42] functional electrical stimulation lower-extremity cycling (FES-LEC),[43] lower-extremity training,[44] and walking[45] (Table 22.1). A recent study with four participants (chronic SCI, various levels of injury) examined the feasibility of a remotely delivered exercise program. Participants engaged in a web-based home exercise program consisting of 30 to 45 minutes of aerobic exercise using an arm ergometer at moderate intensity (~60% of heart rate reserve) three times per week for 8 weeks. This study had 100% adherence, and the majority of participants demonstrated improved levels of physical activity, aerobic capacity, and life satisfaction.[46] Another study examined a home-based physical activity intervention on health-related quality of life in inactive individuals with chronic SCI (<T4). Participants randomly assigned to the intervention group completed four 45-minute moderate intensity (60%–65% of peak oxygen uptake) arm ergometry exercise sessions per week for 6 weeks. Exercise self-efficacy and the physical and psychological quality of life domains were improved.[42]

Several case studies have also demonstrated FES-LEC telephone-based exercise interventions to be feasible and effective long-term exercise strategies (e.g., 56 months) to improve adherence, body composition, and muscle hypertrophy among the SCI population.[47–49]

OTHER NEUROLOGICAL DISORDERS

Additional neurological disorders have benefited from TR, specifically for exercise purposes. A case report of a 67-year-old woman with PD demonstrated that 4 months (16 sessions with four 1-hour sessions/week) of a home exercise program targeting motor symptoms of PD elicited improvements in gait, endurance, balance confidence, and quality of life. The participant's satisfaction with the program was also high.[50] A randomized controlled trial (RCT) examined the efficacy of a lower-extremity intensive function training (LIFT) compared to an attention control group receiving upper-extremity bimanual training in children with cerebral palsy. Twenty-four children with unilateral spastic cerebral palsy were randomized to receive 90 hours of LIFT or an equivalent dose of attention control (2 hours/day, 5 days/week) for 9 weeks. LIFT showed greater improvement for the 1-minute walk test and overall walking ability compared to an intensity and time-equated control condition.[44]

TABLE 22.1 ■ **Studies Examining Home-Based Endurance Exercise Training.**

Endurance Exercise Studies

Author, Year	Design	Disability	TSI	Sample Size	Injury Level	Platform	Exercise	Duration	Outcomes
Latimer et al. (2006)	RCT	SCI	19.34 ± 19.79 years	26	Multiple levels	Telephone	Physical activity	8 wks	Activity level Motivation Confidence
Arbour-Nicitopoulos et al. (2009)	RCT	SCI	18.01 ± 14.16 (INT) 11.75 ± 9.82 (CON) years	44	Multiple levels	In-home Telephone	Resistance bands	10 wks	LTPA Self-efficacy
Dolbow et al. (2012)	Case series	SCI	12 ± 13.26 years	17	C4-T11	Telephone	FES-LEC	16 wks	Adherence
Dolbow et al. (2012)	Case study	SCI	18 months	1	C5	Telephone	FES-LEC	9 wks	Body composition Seat pressure QOL
Dolbow et al. (2012)	Case study	SCI	33 years	1	C4	Telephone	FES-LEC	24 wks	Body composition EE QOL
Arbour-Nicitopoulos et al. (2014)	Prospective	SCI	14.5 ± 12.7 years	65	Multiple levels	Telephone	LTPA	6 months	LTPA
Lai et al. (2016)	Case series	SCI	25.8 ± 4.3 years	4	T1-T2, T10-T11, C4-C5, T2-T3	Web-based	Arm ergometer	8 wks	Adherence Aerobic capacity Life satisfaction
Dolbow et al. (2017)	Case study	Tetraplegia	33 years	1	C4	Telephone	FES-LEC	56 months	Body composition BMD

Continued

TABLE 22.1 ■ **Studies Examining Home-Based Endurance Exercise Training.—Cont'd**

Endurance Exercise Studies

Author, Year	Design	Disability	TSI	Sample Size	Injury Level	Platform	Exercise	Duration	Outcomes
Coulter et al. (2017)	RCT	SCI	13 ± 11.6 (INT) 15.7 ± 9.7 (CON) years	24	C3/4-L3	Web-based	Aerobic, strength, stretching, balance	8 wks	Compliance 6MPT 6MWT
Nightingale et al. (2018)	RCT	SCI	>1 year	19	<T4	In-home	Arm ergometer	6 wks	QOL Self-efficacy
Braga et al. (2018)	Feasibility study	ALS	7.6 ± 4.12 months	10	NA	In-home telemonitoring	Walking	6 months	Compliance Function
Chatto et al. (2018)	Case report	PD	2 years	1	NA	In-home	Motor learning	4 months	Gait Endurance Balance Confidence Quality of life
Surana et al. (2019)	RCT	Cerebral palsy	NA	24	NA	In-home	Lower-extremity functional training	9 wks	Gait capacity and performance
Paul et al. (2019)	RCT feasibility study	MS	NA	90	NA	Web-based	Strength, aerobic, balance	6 months	Adherence Walking Balance Resource use
Plow et al. (2019)	RCT	MS	12.7 ± 8.6 years	208	NA	Telephone	Walking program	12 wks	Fatigue Physical activity Quality of life Step count

ALS, Amyotrophic lateral sclerosis; CON, control; EE, energy expenditure; FES-LEC, functional electrical stimulation lower-extremity cycling; INT, intervention; LTPA, leisure-time physical activity; MS, multiple sclerosis; PD, Parkinson's disease; Pop, population; RCT, randomized controlled trial; SCI, spinal cord injury; TSI, time since injury or onset; Wks, weeks; 6MWT, six-minute walk test; 6MPT, six-minute push test.

A recent single-blinded RCT examined the effects of a telephone-delivered intervention on fatigue, physical activity levels, and quality of life in adults with MS. Participants (n = 208) were randomized to one of three groups: a contact-control intervention, physical activity only group, and a physical activity plus fatigue self-management intervention. Over the 12-week training period, the fatigue self-management group significantly improved self-reported fatigue and physical activity levels compared to the contact-control intervention. There were no significant differences between the fatigue self-management group and the physical activity only group. The physical activity only group had significant improvements compared to the control group on moderate-to-vigorous exercise and step count, while there were no significant differences in quality of life between groups.[45] A recent study examining telemonitoring of a home-based exercise program in individuals with amyotrophic lateral sclerosis (ALS) showed improvements in function and high compliance.[51] Benefits of TR have also been reported in dementia[52] and MS.[53, 54]

Home-based telecommunication exercise programs may represent an effective and inexpensive option to improve the health of individuals with disability while overcoming common adherence and commitment issues. Indeed, home-based exercise programs effectively improve exercise endurance and physical activity in individuals with disabilities.[55, 56] However, few RCTs have investigated the effect of endurance exercise in persons with disabilities. The present data suggest TR programs are safe, feasible, and effective at increasing physical activity levels while improving cardiorespiratory health, body composition, and quality of life.

Applications of Telerehabilitation in Conjunction With Resistance Exercise Training

SPINAL CORD INJURY

Skeletal muscle atrophy is associated with disuse and resultant reductions in physical activity levels, mechanical loading of bone, and subsequent decline of bone mineral density (BMD).[57] Specifically, in SCI, maintaining lean mass below the injury level is associated with improvements in body composition, metabolic health, and mitochondrial density and activity.[58, 59] Therefore the preservation of skeletal muscle size and function is necessary for proper metabolism and has clinical implications. Adherence to a long-term exercise program is vital to achieve and maintain increases in muscle size and function. Longitudinal changes in exercise studies indicate that fat and lean mass are favorably altered in response to exercise, but these alterations regress to that of preintervention levels following 2.5 years of exercise cessation.[60] Home-based TR exercise programs may offer a strategy for improving adherence to long-term resistance training programs to attenuate the health risks and secondary complications.[41] Various forms of home-based resistance exercise programs have been utilized, including neuromuscular electrical stimulation resistance training (NMES-RT)[41, 61] and upper body resistance band exercises[62–64] (Table 22.2). A recent pilot study found favorable changes in muscle hypertrophy and intramuscular fat following 8 weeks of twice-weekly NMES-RT. Another study evaluating electrical stimulation training over 2 years found favorable changes in torque, fatigue, and BMD.

Individuals with paraplegia can develop shoulder problems over time, including chronic pain.[62] This may interfere with activities of daily living and quality of life. Van Straaten investigated the effectiveness of 12 weeks of a high-dose home exercise TR program for manual wheelchair users with SCI on shoulder pain and function. Sixteen participants engaged in rotator cuff and scapular stabilization exercises (three sets of 30 repetitions) three times weekly for 12 weeks under the supervision of a physical therapist via videoconferencing. Shoulder pain and function improved following the intervention.[64] Another study examined the effect of 8 weeks of a scapula-focused

TABLE 22.2 ■ Studies Examining Home-Based Resistance Exercise Training.

Resistance Exercise Studies

Author, Year	Design	Disability	TSI	Sample Size	Injury Level	Platform	Exercise	Duration	Outcomes
Mahoney et al. (2005)	Before-after trial	SCI	13.4 ± 6.5 years	5	C5-C10	Telephone	NMES	12 wks	Hypertrophy Glucose Insulin
Sabatier et al. (2006)	Longitudinal	SCI	13.4 ± 6.5 years	5	C5-T10	Telephone	NMES	18 wks	Muscle fatigue Compliance Arterial diameter
Nawoczenski et al. (2006)	Clinical trial	SCI Spina bifida	17.0 ± 13.3 (INT) 9.2 ± 5.8 (CON) years	41	Multiple levels	In-home Telephone	Resistance bands	8 wks	Shoulder pain and function
Shields and Dudley-Javoroski (2006)	Case series	SCI	6 wks	7	C5-T10	In-home	NMES	2 years	Compliance Torque Fatigue BMD
Dudley-Javoroski and Shields (2008)	Case report	SCI	7 wks	1	T4	In-home	NMES	4.6 years	Torque Fatigue BMD
Kern et al. (2010)	Longitudinal prospective	SCI	9 months to 9 years	25	T12-L5 conus/cauda equina	In-home	FES	2 years	Hypertrophy Force output
Kemp et al. (2011)	RCT	Paraplegia	>5 years	80	Multiple levels	In-home	Resistance bands	12 wks	Strength QOL Pain
Mulroy et al. (2011)	RCT	Paraplegia	17.9 ± 9.2 (INT) 22.3 ± 11.8 (CON) years	80	Multiple levels	In-home	Resistance bands	12 wks	Shoulder pain QOL

Continued

TABLE 22.2 ■ Studies Examining Home-Based Resistance Exercise Training. —Cont'd

Resistance Exercise Studies

Author, Year	Design	Disability	TSI	Sample Size	Injury Level	Platform	Exercise	Duration	Outcomes
Sasso and Buckus (2013)	Case study	SCI	28 years	1	T12	In-home	Resistance band circuit	12 wks	Strength Pain $VO_{2\ Peak}$ Cholesterol
Van Staaten et al. (2014)	Repeated measures	SCI 1 post-polio	16 (3.7–41.8) years[a]	16	C6-T8 and below	Videoconference	Resistance bands	12 wks	Shoulder pain and function
Chumbler et al. (2015)	RCT	Stroke	<24 months	52	NA	In-home	Strength and balance exercises	3 months	Satisfaction with care Fall-related self-efficacy
Gorgey et al. (2017)	Case series	SCI	>1 year	5	C5-T11	Web-based	NMES	8 wks	Body composition Hypertrophy Compliance
Dodakian et al. (2017)	Repeated measures	Stroke	24 (21–36) wks	12	NA	Videoconference	Arm motor therapy games	28 days	Compliance Arm motor status Depression
Vloothuis et al. (2019)	RCT	Stroke	36 (28–57) (INT) 37 (26–55) (CON) days	66	NA	In-home caregiver-mediated	Individualized exercises	8 wks	Mobility Length of stay Strength
Cramer et al. (2019)	RCT	Stroke	132 ± 65 (INT) 129 ± 59 (CON) days	124	NA	In-home	Arm motor therapy	6–8 wks	Motor function

[a]Years in a wheelchair.

BMD, Bone mineral density; CON, control; INT, intervention; NMES, neuromuscular electrical stimulation; Pop, population; QOL, quality of life; RCT, randomized controlled trial; SCI, spinal cord injury; TSI, time since injury or onset; Wks, weeks.

exercise intervention on pain and functional disability in individuals with SCI and shoulder impingement syndrome. Forty-one manual wheelchair users (with SCI and spina bifida) with (n = 21) and without shoulder impingement symptoms (n = 20) participated in this clinical trial. The intervention group received home-based exercise instruction consisting of stretching and strengthening exercises and demonstrated significant improvement in shoulder pain, function, and satisfaction.[65]

OTHER NEUROLOGICAL DISORDERS

Supervised rehabilitation can improve functional recovery after stroke, but only a minority of individuals still undergo supervised rehabilitation 1 month after discharge,[66] which may be due to limited access, cost, or compliance.[67] In a recent RCT, home-based TR was compared to a dose and intensity-matched therapy delivered in a traditional in-clinic setting for stroke patients. Substantial gains were seen in arm motor function regardless of in-home or in-clinic setting, suggesting that TR has the potential to substantially improve access to rehabilitation therapy on a large scale.[68] Another RCT examining the effects of 8 weeks of caregiver-mediated exercise e-Health program versus usual care in stroke patients also reported no significant between-group differences in mobility or length of stay.[69] Twelve stroke patients (3–24 months poststroke) with arm motor deficits participated in 28 days of in-home TR. Sessions consisted of 1 hour of individualized exercises, games, stroke education, and an optional hour of free play. Arm motor status improved, and compliance was excellent (97.9%).[67]

A multisite single-blinded RCT examined the effects of a multifaceted stroke TR intervention on fall-related self-efficacy and satisfaction with care. Fifty-two veterans (<24 months poststroke) were randomized to either an intervention or usual care group. The 3-month intervention consisted of exercise and adaptive strategies. The intervention improved satisfaction with care, however no improvements were seen in fall-related self-efficacy.[70] Other reports have indicated that poststroke patients receiving rehabilitation treatments in a familiar environment experienced less mortality and dependence than those undergoing conventional care, and they obtained earlier reintegration and better quality of life.[71-74] Moreover a few RCTs in poststroke patients demonstrated that motor rehabilitation treatments delivered via TR resulted in similar outcomes as standard rehabilitation care.[75-77]

Exercise can positively affect health outcomes and attenuate secondary complications associated with various disorders. As previously stated, the benefits of exercise are lost following a period of disuse, highlighting the need for continuous, possibly lifelong exercise in individuals with disabilities. The current data suggest TR programs are safe, feasible, and effective at increasing physical activity levels while improving muscular strength, body composition, and quality of life. TR may be particularly relevant to individuals with denervated muscles that require rehabilitation over a long duration. However, few RCTs have investigated the effect of home-based resistance exercise in populations with disabilities.

Technological Advances and Future Directions

Many recent technological advances, including powered exoskeletons, virtual reality (VR), brain-computer interface (BCI), motorized orthoses, and other assistive devices, have enabled improved health outcomes and walking ability in individuals with disabilities. Powered exoskeletons are wearable robotic units (motorized orthoses) controlled by computer boards that power a system of motors, pneumatics levers, or hydraulics to restore locomotion.[78-80] Exoskeletons offer independence in standing and walking with minimal metabolic cost while facilitating improvements in quality of life.[78, 79, 81, 82] BCI establishes a direct link between neural signals generated in the brain and external devices in an attempt to restore communication and movement.[83, 84] It has been successfully used to elicit motor improvements poststroke[85] and improve quality of life in ALS.[86] VR is a technology that describes a computer-generated scenario in which the users can interact, and also facilitates biofeedback and multimodal sensory stimuli, which can be interactively used.[87,88] In-home VR training has also produced positive outcomes after stroke,[89] cerebral palsy,[90] and PD.[91] Several home-based advanced techniques are efficacious in improving health and well-being (Table 22.3).

SPINAL CORD INJURY

A crossover design study with 13 participants compared two in-home telesupervised 6-week exercise treatments (1 hour per day, 5 days per week). Conventional therapy consisted of strength training, computer games played with a trackball, and electrical stimulation. In contrast, the Rehabilitation Joystick for Computerized Exercise (ReJoyce) therapy consisted of FES exercise therapy using the ReJoyce to perform exercises associated with activities of daily living. Participants were randomized to receive either conventional treatment or ReJoyce therapy first separated by a 1-month washout period. The action research arm test and the ReJoyce automated hand function test both improved in the ReJoyce group compared to the conventional group.[92]

In another study, 12 individuals with chronic incomplete SCI used an unsupervised home-based, mobile version of lower-limb VR training for 4 weeks (16–20 sessions of 30–45 minutes each) on lower-limb muscle strength, balance, and functional mobility. Sessions consisted of motivating training scenarios and combined action observation and execution. Significant improvements were seen in lower-limb muscle strength, balance, and functional mobility. The improvements in functional mobility were still observed at 2 to 3 months posttreatment.[87]

OTHER NEUROLOGICAL DISORDERS

A recent RCT examined the effect of aerobic exercise on motor function in PD. Participants were randomly assigned to either an at-home aerobic exercise group (n = 65) or a stretching active control group (n = 65). Both interventions were home-based, and both groups received a motivational app and remote supervision. Sessions consisted of 30 to 45 minutes of training three times per week for 6 weeks. The aerobic exercise group showed improvements in motor scores compared to the stretching active control group.[91] In another RCT, 76 PD patients were randomly assigned to a remotely supervised home-based VR balance training (n = 38) versus in-clinic sensory integration balance training (SIBT; n = 38). Participants engaged in 21 sessions of 50 minutes each, 3 days per week, for 7 weeks. Home-based VR training consisted of graded "exergames" using the Nintendo Wii Fit System, while SIBT included exercises to improve postural stability. Participants improved on the Berg Balance Scale, Dynamic Gait Index, but there were no differences in fall frequency. The total cost of rehabilitation using TeleWii was lower than that of SIBT.[93] Other studies have also demonstrated the benefits of home-based Nintendo Wii training in PD.[94, 95]

Another RCT evaluated 12 weeks of in-home physical therapy using a VR gaming system to improve balance in individuals with TBI. Sixty-three individuals (n = 32, home-based control; n = 31, VR) at least 1-year post-TBI demonstrated improvements in balance regardless of group.[89, 90, 96] In another study, 30 individuals with stroke underwent 20, 45-minute training sessions three times weekly in the clinic or in the home. Both groups demonstrated improvements in the reacquisition of locomotor skills associated with balance, and the in-home group incurred lower costs.[89] In a 3-month proof-of-concept pilot study, three adolescents with hemiplegic cerebral palsy engaged in at-home VR video game-based TR exercises of the plegic hand (30 minutes/day, 5 days/week) using a sensor glove and videogame console. Hand function

TABLE 22.3 ■ **Studies Examining Home-Based Exercise Training Utilizing Technological Advances.**

Technological Advances Exercise Studies

Author, Year	Design	Disability	TSI	Sample Size	Injury Level	Platform	Exercise	Duration	Outcomes
Golomb et al. (2010)	Proof-of-concept pilot study	Cerebral palsy	NA	3	NA	Web-based VR	Hand exercises	3 months	Finger range of motion Bone health Handgrip function
Kowalczewski et al. (2011)	Crossover RCT	SCI	3.6 ± 2.1	13	C5-C7 ASI A	Web-based	FES arm	6 wks	Hand function
Ortiz-Gutiérrez et al. (2013)	Preliminary	MS	NA	47	NA	In-home	Xbox KinectVR	10 wks	Balance Postural control
Rupp et al. (2015)	Prospective Proof-of-concept	iSCI	5.8 ± 5.4	25	AIS n = 7-C; n = 18-D	In-home Robotic locomotor training	Motorized orthosis	8 wks	Functional mobility
Lloréns et al. (2015)	RCT	Stroke	>6 months	30	NA	In-home	VR	8 wks	Balance
Linder et al. (2015)	Multisite RCT	Stroke	<6 months	99	NA	In-home	Robot-assisted upper-extremity exercises	8 wks	Quality of life Depression Stroke impact scale
Villiger et al. (2017)	Before-after trial	iSCI	8.0 ± 4.5	12	C4-L3	In-home	VR	4 wks	Mobility Strength Balance
Gandolfi et al. (2017)	RCT	PD	NA	76	NA	In-home	VR	7 wks	Balance Dynamic gait Fall frequency

Continued

TABLE 22.3 ■ **Studies Examining Home-Based Exercise Training Utilizing Technological Advances.** —Cont'd

Technological Advances Exercise Studies

Author, Year	Design	Disability	TSI	Sample Size	Injury Level	Platform	Exercise	Duration	Outcomes
Tefertiller et al. (2019)	RCT	TBI	>1 year	95	NA	In-home	VR	12 wks	Balance
Van der Kolk et al. (2019)	RCT	PD	41 (16–87) (INT) 38 (19–81) (CON) months	130	NA	In-home	Cycle ergometer	6 months	Motor function
Isernia et al. (2020)	Pilot study	PD	NA	31	NA	In-home	VR	4 months	Functional mobility Quality of life Balance

AIS, American Spinal Injury Association Impairment scale; *FES*, functional electrical stimulation; *iSCI*, incomplete spinal cord injury; *MS*, multiple sclerosis; *PD*, Parkinson's disease; *Pop*, population; *RCT*, randomized controlled trial; *TSI*, time since injury; *Wks*, weeks; *VR*, virtual reality.

improved in all three participants.[90] A multisite RCT examined the effects of home-based robot-assisted rehabilitation coupled with a home exercise program versus a home exercise program alone on depression and quality of life poststroke. Ninety-nine people (<6 months after stroke) were randomized into either group for 8 weeks. Both interventions improved measures of depression and quality of life.[97]

A recent pilot multicenter study examined the efficiency and efficacy of a VR TR program in 31 PD outpatients. All participants performed in-clinic training (12 45-minute sessions, three sessions/week) for 1 month and were then assigned to an in-home intervention or a usual care control group. The in-home intervention consisted of 60 45-minute sessions, five sessions/week for 3 months. Following the in-clinic program, improvements were seen in functional mobility, balance, upper-limb mobility, global cognitive function, memory, and quality of life. After the in-home intervention, there was an additional enhancement for upper-limb mobility, whereas the control group showed worsening in balance and functional mobility 7 months postintervention.[98]

A preliminary study examined a 10-week VR TR program on postural control in MS patients. Forty-seven MS patients were assigned to either a control group (physiotherapy twice/week, 40 minutes/session) or an intervention group (four sessions/week, 20 minutes/session, 40 sessions total). The VR intervention consisted of videoconference TR using the Xbox 360 and Kinect console. Improvements in general balance and postural control were seen in both groups.[99]

Although the data are limited, the current data regarding the effect of these technologies on continued rehabilitation in patients with disabilities are promising. Although significant differences may not be seen between traditional usual care compared to TR programs, TR programs may represent an important alternative to standard in-clinic rehabilitation treatments. Future studies evaluating the combination of these technologies with home-based TR programs would be of great value.

Telerehabilitation Compared to Traditional Face-to-Face Usual Care

Although TR cannot replace interventions that require conventional face-to-face therapy, technological advances and information communication technology have made TR a more robust, accessible, usable, adaptable, convenient, and/or economical alternative. Due to the increasing life expectancy of people with disabilities, TR is a vital modality that can improve care coordination between the specialists at the centers, the local providers, and the patients and their respective caregivers.

One of the major challenges is whether TR can be an effective alternative to face-to-face rehabilitation therapy. TR will not replace a face-to-face assessment and evaluation if the clinician needs to perform a "hands-on" physical evaluation. Moreover, different situations may necessitate intense hands-on therapy, specialty equipment, exercise machines, and modalities for acute diseases and disorders, thus requiring a clinic setting. However, for chronic disease, TR is a viable option as the intensity of therapy is likely low and can be offered over a longer duration in the comfort of the patient's own home. Overall, TR improves accessibility, reduces cost, increases geographic accessibility, and extends limited resources, thus justifying its applicability and use. It allows multiple specialists, local and remote, to offer patient-centered care to a highly variable population with chronic disability. TR also facilitates rehabilitation in the client's environment, workplace, and community that helps in self-management of chronic conditions. The World Health Organization promotes attention to individuals' ability to function effectively in their environment.[100, 101] Indeed, there is growing evidence that supports the benefits of delivering TR in the client's environment because it provides a real-time assessment and can identify issues that can be addressed during the visit or set up a plan of care with the providers in the community. Hoenig et al. found that in-home TR programs can be delivered to adults with mobility impairments.[102] TR also allows caregiver participation, which does not happen in a face-to-face clinic setting if the caregivers are not present. Clinicians should be aware that patients rely on caregivers for their care at home and in the community and should be considered part of the team. Caregiver participation in assessment and treatment plans can have a significant role in the overall well-being of the person with a disability at home and in the community. There is strong evidence that behavioral therapy and vocational rehabilitation interventions are more effective if deployed in the natural environment rather than in a clinical setting.[103–106]

Individuals with disabilities have an increased likelihood of contracting infectious diseases, partly due to reduced immune function and partly to the high level of contact with wheelchairs and assistive devices (tires transfer virus to hands). Home-based TR offers a solution to this and limits exposure. TR approaches are likely to reduce infection, promote wellness, and encourage uninterrupted physical activity programs. However, TR programs require access to high-speed internet, computers, and knowledge of and familiarization with techniques to ensure proper exercise form and safety. Remote TR programs also lack the controlled environment of traditional face-to-face usual care, which may make exercise setup and performance difficult for individuals without a caregiver. Traditional face-to-face health care provides the benefit of genuine social interaction, more accurate determination of exercise form and intensity, and monitoring of physiological responses to exercise (blood pressure, heart rate, etc.).

Rehabilitation clinicians need to educate health care providers as well as patients, caregivers, and their families about the benefits of TR. There is a need to acknowledge biases with regard to face-to-face therapy, encourage the use of TR, and develop and offer new evidence-based innovations focused on providing patient-centered care with their local medical and rehabilitation providers in their homes and community. With the advancement of technology, the rehabilitation team can provide accessible, cost-effective, and timely specialty care to persons with disability in the comfort of their home or community.

Summary and Conclusions

The advent of telehealth technologies has allowed for several potential home-based exercise and rehabilitation interventions to be delivered and monitored remotely. TR programs provide increased access to health care, improved outcomes, and reduced travel time and costs, specifically for those living in rural areas. Moreover, these programs can provide lifelong care for individuals with a chronic disability with the goal of overall mental-medical wellness and optimizing functional mobility. TR videoconferencing programs provide freedom to perform exercise in one's personal space while facilitating long-term rehabilitation and beneficial, sustained lifestyle changes. Various forms of TR have been effectively utilized to improve exercise adherence and enhance health outcomes in individuals with disabilities. Both endurance and resistance strength training can be used to improve cardiorespiratory fitness, body composition, muscle size and function, and quality of life. These studies have demonstrated TR formats to be feasible, safe, and effective in enhancing health measures in persons with disabilities. Overall, few RCTs have evaluated home-based TR programs' effectiveness, specifically with regard to resistance training. Therefore there is a need for RCTs assessing the efficacy of home-based TR exercise programs. Future studies should investigate new technologies in a home-based TR format such as robotic orthoses, including exoskeletons, VR, and BCI.

STUDIES

In a study by Dolbow et al., 17 veterans with SCI (C4-T11) completed 16 weeks (two 8-week periods) of three times weekly home-based FES-LEC. Cycling duration increased over 16 weeks, three times weekly, with a goal of between 40 and 60 minutes of continuous active FES cycling. Exercise adherence was 71.7% and 62.9% for periods 1 and 2, respectively.[43]

In another study, 26 participants were randomized to an intervention group or control group. Participants formed implementation intentions, and both groups were asked to engage in 30 minutes of moderate-to-heavy intensity physical activity three times per week for 8 weeks. Participants in the intervention group engaged in more physical activity and experienced sustained motivation and greater confidence to schedule activity than the control condition.[55] A single-blinded RCT of 44 individuals with SCI evaluated a 10-week TR program on LTPA. Participants reported significantly greater LTPA, scheduling, self-efficacy at 5 and 10 weeks.[107] Another study evaluated the effectiveness of an individualized telephone-counseling program in 65 individuals with SCI over 6 months. Fifty-three of 65 participants participated in an effectiveness evaluation. This study demonstrated a trend for more clients engaging in moderate-to-heavy intensity LTPA at 6 months (52%) versus baseline (35%).[108] An RCT that included 24 individuals with SCI (C3/4-L3) the 6-minute push test or the 6-minute walk test. Four participants achieved 100% compliance (>twice per week), five achieved a 50% to 100% compliance rate (one to two times per week).[109]

References

1. Leonardi M, et al. The definition of disability: what is in a name? *Lancet*. 2006;368(9543):1219–1221.
2. World Health Organization. *Neurological disorders: public health challenges*. World Health Organization; 2006.
3. Turk MA. *Secondary conditions and disability. Workshop on Disability in America*. Washington, DC: National Academies Press; 2006.
4. Kinne S, Patrick DL, Doyle DL. Prevalence of secondary conditions among people with disabilities. *Am J Public Health*. 2004;94(3):443–445.
5. Pruitt S. *Innovative care for chronic conditions: building blocks for action: global report*. World Health Organization; 2002.
6. World Health Organization. Better health for people with disabilities: infographic. 2016. https://www.euro.who.int/en/health-topics/Life-stages/disability-and-rehabilitation/multimedia/infographic-better-health-for-people-with-disabilities.
7. World Health Organization. World Bank (2011). World report on disability. Geneva. World Health Organization. 2013. 15.
8. DeVivo MJ. Causes and costs of spinal cord injury in the United States. *Spinal Cord*. 1997;35(12):809–813.
9. Gorgey AS, et al. Effects of spinal cord injury on body composition and metabolic profile—Part I. *J Spinal Cord Med*. 2014;37(6):693–702.
10. Phillips WT, et al. Effect of spinal cord injury on the heart and cardiovascular fitness. *Curr Probl Cardiol*. 1998;23(11):641–716.
11. Kocina P. Body composition of spinal cord injured adults. *Sports Med*. 1997;23(1):48–60.
12. Mickens MN, et al. Leisure-time physical activity, anthropometrics, and body composition as predictors of quality of life domains after spinal cord injury: an exploratory cross-sectional study. *Neural Regen Res*. 2021:17. Accepted February 26, 2021.
13. Lollar DJ. Public health and disability: emerging opportunities. *Public Health Rep*. 2002;117(2):131.
14. Wilber N, et al. Disability as a public health issue: findings and reflections from the Massachusetts survey of secondary conditions. *Milbank Q*. 2002;80(2):393–421.
15. Ginis KAM, et al. Evidence-based scientific exercise guidelines for adults with spinal cord injury: an update and a new guideline. *Spinal Cord*. 2018;56(4):308–321.
16. Van der Ploeg HP, et al. Physical activity for people with a disability. *Sports Med*. 2004;34(10):639–649.
17. DeVivo MJ. Epidemiology of traumatic spinal cord injury: trends and future implications. *Spinal Cord*. 2012;50(5):365–372.
18. Gerhart KA, et al. Long-term spinal cord injury: functional changes over time. *Arch Phys Med Rehabil*. 1993;74(10):1030–1034.

19. Kennedy P, Lude P, Taylor N. Quality of life, social participation, appraisals and coping post spinal cord injury: a review of four community samples. *Spinal Cord*. 2006;44(2):95–105.

20. Curtin CM, et al. Who are the women and men in Veterans Health Administration's current spinal cord injury population? *J Rehabil Res Dev*. 2012;49(3):351–360.

21. Dryden D, et al. Utilization of health services following spinal cord injury: a 6-year follow-up study. *Spinal Cord*. 2004;42(9):513–525.

22. Post M, Van C. Leeuwen. Psychosocial issues in spinal cord injury: a review. Spinal Cord. 2012; 50(5):382–389.

23. Cobb J, et al. An exploratory analysis of the potential association between SCI secondary health conditions and daily activities. *Top Spinal Cord Inj Rehabil*. 2014;20(4):277–288.

24. Pedersen BK, Saltin B. Exercise as medicine–evidence for prescribing exercise as therapy in 26 different chronic diseases. *Scand J Med Sci Sports*. 2015;25:1–72.

25. Ellis T, Motl RW. Physical activity behavior change in persons with neurologic disorders: overview and examples from Parkinson disease and multiple sclerosis. *J Neurol Phys Ther*. 2013;37(2):85–90.

26. Buchholz AC, McGillivray CF, Pencharz PB. Physical activity levels are low in free-living adults with chronic paraplegia. *Obes Res*. 2003;11(4):563–570.

27. Pescatello LS, Riebe D, Thompson PD. *ACSM's Guidelines for Exercise Testing and Prescription*. Lippincott Williams & Wilkins; 2014.

28. Haskell WL, et al. Physical activity and public health: updated recommendation for adults from the American College of Sports Medicine and the American Heart Association. *Circulation*. 2007;116(9):1081.

29. Evans N, et al. Exercise recommendations and considerations for persons with spinal cord injury. *Arch Phys Med Rehabil*. 2015;96(9):1749–1750.

30. Lexell J. Muscle structure and function in chronic neurological disorders: the potential of exercise to improve activities of daily living. *Exerc Sport Sci Rev*. 2000;28(2):80–84.

31. Ginis KAM, et al. Leisure time physical activity in a population-based sample of people with spinal cord injury part I: demographic and injury-related correlates. *Arch Phys Med Rehabil*. 2010;91(5):722–728.

32. Halabchi F, et al. Exercise prescription for patients with multiple sclerosis, potential benefits and practical recommendations. *BMC Neurol*. 2017;17(1):185.

33. Rimmer JH, et al. Physical activity participation among persons with disabilities: barriers and facilitators. *Am J Prevent Med*. 2004;26(5):419–425.

34. Gorgey AS. Exercise awareness and barriers after spinal cord injury. *World J Orthop*. 2014;5(3):158.

35. Beatty PW, et al. Access to health care services among people with chronic or disabling conditions: patterns and predictors. *Arch Phys Med Rehabil*. 2003;84(10):1417–1425.

36. Stillman MD, et al. Health care utilization and barriers experienced by individuals with spinal cord injury. *Arch Phys Med Rehabil*. 2014;95(6):1114–1126.

37. Knox K, et al. Access to traumatic spinal cord injury care in Saskatchewan, Canada: a qualitative study on community healthcare provider perspectives. *Can J Disabil Stud*. 2014;3(3):83–103.

38. LaVela SL, et al. Geographical proximity and health care utilization in veterans with SCI&D in the USA. *Soc Sci Med*. 2004;59(11):2387–2399.

39. Goodridge D, et al. Access to health and support services: perspectives of people living with a long-term traumatic spinal cord injury in rural and urban areas. *Disability and Rehabilitation*. 2015;37(16):1401–1410.

40. Parmanto B, Saptono A. Telerehabilitation: state-of-the-art from an informatics perspective. *Int J Telerehabil*. 2009;1(1):73.

41. Gorgey AS, et al. A feasibility pilot using telehealth videoconference monitoring of home-based NMES resistance training in persons with spinal cord injury. *Spinal Cord Ser Cases*. 2017;3(1):1–8.

42. Nightingale TE, et al. Home-based exercise enhances health-related quality of life in persons with spinal cord injury: a randomized controlled trial. *Arch Phys Med Rehabil*. 2018;99(10):1998–2006. e1.

43. Dolbow DR, et al. Exercise adherence during home-based functional electrical stimulation cycling by individuals with spinal cord injury. *Am J Phys Med Rehabil*. 2012;91(11):922–930.

44. Surana BK, et al. Effectiveness of lower-extremity functional training (LIFT) in young children with unilateral spastic cerebral palsy: a randomized controlled trial. *Neurorehabil Neural Repair*. 2019;33(10):862–872.

45. Plow M, et al. Randomized controlled trial of a telephone-delivered physical activity and fatigue self-management interventions in adults with multiple sclerosis. *Arch Phys Med Rehabil*. 2019;100(11):2006–2014.

46. Lai B, et al. Teleexercise for persons with spinal cord injury: a mixed-methods feasibility case series. *JMIR Rehabil Assist Technol.* 2016;3(2):e8.

47. Dolbow DR, et al. Report of practicability of a 6-month home-based functional electrical stimulation cycling program in an individual with tetraplegia. *J Spinal Cord Med.* 2012;35(3):182–186.

48. Dolbow D, et al. Feasibility of home-based functional electrical stimulation cycling: case report. *Spinal Cord.* 2012;50(2):170–171.

49. Dolbow DR, et al. Effects of a fifty-six month electrical stimulation cycling program after tetraplegia: case report. *J Spinal Cord Med.* 2017;40(4):485–488.

50. Chatto CA, et al. Use of a telehealth system to enhance a home exercise program for a person with Parkinson disease: a case report. *J Neurol Phys Ther.* 2018;42(1):22–29.

51. Braga ACM, et al. The role of moderate aerobic exercise as determined by cardiopulmonary exercise testing in ALS. *Neurol Res Int.* 2018;2018:8218697.

52. Dal Bello-Haas VP, et al. Lessons learned: feasibility and acceptability of a telehealth-delivered exercise intervention for rural-dwelling individuals with dementia and their caregivers. *Rural Remote Health.* 2014;14(3):2715.

53. Paul L, et al. Web-based physiotherapy for people affected by multiple sclerosis: a single blind, randomized controlled feasibility study. *Clin Rehabil.* 2019;33(3):473–484.

54. Amatya B, et al. Effectiveness of telerehabilitation interventions in persons with multiple sclerosis: a systematic review. *Mult Scler Relat Disord.* 2015;4(4):358–369.

55. Latimer AE, Ginis KAM, Arbour KP. The efficacy of an implementation intention intervention for promoting physical activity among individuals with spinal cord injury: a randomized controlled trial. *Rehabil Psych.* 2006;51(4):273.

56. Keyser RE, et al. Improved upper-body endurance following a 12-week home exercise program for manual wheelchair users. *J Rehabil Res Dev.* 2003;40(6):501.

57. Giangregorio L, McCartney N. Bone loss and muscle atrophy in spinal cord injury: epidemiology, fracture prediction, and rehabilitation strategies. *J Spinal Cord Med.* 2006; 29(5):489–500.

58. Gorgey AS, Gater DR. Insulin growth factors may explain relationship between spasticity and skeletal muscle size in men with spinal cord injury. *J Rehabil Res Dev.* 2012;49(3):373–380.

59. O'Brien LC, et al. Skeletal muscle mitochondrial mass is linked to lipid and metabolic profile in individuals with spinal cord injury. *Eur J Appl Physiol.* 2017;117(11):2137–2147.

60. Gorgey AS, et al. Longitudinal changes in body composition and metabolic profile between exercise clinical trials in men with chronic spinal cord injury. *J Spinal Cord Med.* 2016;39(6):699–712.

61. Sabatier M, et al. Electrically stimulated resistance training in SCI individuals increases muscle fatigue resistance but not femoral artery size or blood flow. *Spinal Cord.* 2006;44(4):227–233.

62. Kemp BJ, et al. Effects of reduction in shoulder pain on quality of life and community activities among people living long-term with SCI paraplegia: a randomized control trial. *J Spinal Cord Med.* 2011;34(3):278–284.

63. Sasso E, Backus D. Home-based circuit resistance training to overcome barriers to exercise for people with spinal cord injury: a case study. *J Neurol Phys Ther.* 2013;37(2):65–71.

64. Van Straaten MG, et al. Effectiveness of home exercise on pain, function, and strength of manual wheelchair users with spinal cord injury: a high-dose shoulder program with telerehabilitation. *Arch Phys Med Rehabil.* 2014;95(10):1810–1817.

65. Nawoczenski DA, et al. Clinical trial of exercise for shoulder pain in chronic spinal injury. *Phys Ther.* 2006;86(12):1604–1618.

66. Koh GC-H, et al. Effect of duration, participation rate, and supervision during community rehabilitation on functional outcomes in the first poststroke year in Singapore. *Arch Phys Med Rehabil.* 2012;93(2):279–286.

67. Dodakian L, et al. A home-based telerehabilitation program for patients with stroke. *Neurorehabil Neural Repair.* 2017;31(10–11):923–933.

68. Cramer S, Dodakian L, Le V. National Institutes of Health StrokeNet Telerehab Investigators: efficacy of home-based telerehabilitation vs in-clinic therapy for adults after stroke: a randomized clinical trial. *JAMA Neurol.* 2019;76:1079–1087.

69. Vloothuis JD, et al. Caregiver-mediated exercises with e-health support for early supported discharge after stroke (CARE4STROKE): a randomized controlled trial. *PloS One.* 2019;14(4):e0214241.

70. Chumbler NR, et al. A randomized controlled trial on stroke telerehabilitation: the effects on falls self-efficacy and satisfaction with care. *J Telemed Telecare*. 2015;21(3):139–143.

71. Jelcic N, et al. Feasibility and efficacy of cognitive telerehabilitation in early Alzheimer's disease: a pilot study. *Clin Interv Aging*. 1605;2014:9.

72. Fearon P, Langhorne P. Early Supported Discharge Trialists. Services for reducing duration of hospital care for acute stroke patients. *Cochrane Database Syst Rev*. 2012;2012(9):CD000443.

73. Mas MÀ, Inzitari M. A critical review of Early Supported Discharge for stroke patients: from evidence to implementation into practice. *Int J Stroke*. 2015;10(1):7–12.

74. Langhorne P, Widen-Holmqvist L. Early supported discharge after stroke. *J Rehabil Med*. 2007;39(2):103–108.

75. Finkelstein, J., J. Wood E. Cha. Impact of physical telerehabilitation on functional outcomes in seniors with mobility limitations. In: 2012 Annual International Conference of the IEEE Engineering in Medicine and Biology Society. San Diego, California, USA; 2012:3.

76. Cikajlo I, et al. Telerehabilitation using virtual reality task can improve balance in patients with stroke. *Disabil Rehabil*. 2012;34(1):13–18.

77. Piron L, et al. Exercises for paretic upper limb after stroke: a combined virtual-reality and telemedicine approach. *J Rehabil Med*. 2009;41(12):1016–1020.

78. Gorgey AS, Sumrell R, Goetz LL. Exoskeletal assisted rehabilitation after spinal cord injury. In: Webster J, Murphy D, eds. *Atlas of Orthoses and Assistive Devices*. Elsevier; 2019:440–447.

79. Miller LE, Zimmermann AK, Herbert WG. Clinical effectiveness and safety of powered exoskeleton-assisted walking in patients with spinal cord injury: systematic review with meta-analysis. *Med Devices (Auckl)*. 2016;9:455.

80. Gorgey AS. Robotic exoskeletons: the current pros and cons. *World J Orthop*. 2018;9(9):112.

81. Gorgey AS, et al. Effects of Testosterone and Evoked Resistance Exercise after Spinal Cord Injury (TEREX-SCI): study protocol for a randomised controlled trial. *BMJ Open*. 2017;7(4):e014125.

82. Gorgey AS, Holman ME. The future of SCI rehabilitation: understanding the impact of exoskeletons on gait mechanics. *J Spinal Cord Med*. 2018;41(5):544–546.

83. Collinger JL, et al. Functional priorities, assistive technology, and brain-computer interfaces after spinal cord injury. *J Rehabil Res Dev*. 2013;50(2):145.

84. Schwartz AB, et al. Brain-controlled interfaces: movement restoration with neural prosthetics. *Neuron*. 2006;52(1):205–220.

85. Johnson N, et al. Combined rTMS and virtual reality brain–computer interface training for motor recovery after stroke. *J Neural Eng*. 2018;15(1):016009.

86. Kübler A, et al. Patients with ALS can use sensorimotor rhythms to operate a brain-computer interface. *Neurology*. 2005;64(10):1775–1777.

87. Villiger M, et al. Home-based virtual reality-augmented training improves lower limb muscle strength, balance, and functional mobility following chronic incomplete spinal cord injury. *Front Neurol*. 2017;8:635.

88. Luque-Moreno C, et al. A decade of progress using virtual reality for poststroke lower extremity rehabilitation: systematic review of the intervention methods. *Res Int*. 2015;2015:342529.

89. Lloréns R, et al. Effectiveness, usability, and cost-benefit of a virtual reality-based telerehabilitation program for balance recovery after stroke: a randomized controlled trial. *Arch Phys Med Rehabil*. 2015;96(3):418–425.

90. Golomb MR, et al. In-home virtual reality videogame telerehabilitation in adolescents with hemiplegic cerebral palsy. *Arch Phys Med Rehabil*. 2010;91(1):1–8.

91. van der Kolk NM, et al. Effectiveness of home-based and remotely supervised aerobic exercise in Parkinson's disease: a double-blind, randomised controlled trial. *Lancet Neurol*. 2019;18(11):998–1008.

92. Kowalczewski J, et al. In-home tele-rehabilitation improves tetraplegic hand function. *Neurorehabil Neural Repair*. 2011;25(5):412–422.

93. Gandolfi M, et al. Virtual reality telerehabilitation for postural instability in Parkinson's disease: a multi-center, single-blind, randomized, controlled trial. *Biomed Res Int*. 2017;2017:7962826.

94. Esculier J-F, et al. Home-based balance training programme using Wii Fit with balance board for Parkinson's disease: a pilot study. *J Rehabil Med*. 2012;44(2):144–150.

95. Zalecki T, et al. Visual feedback training using WII Fit improves balance in Parkinson's disease. *Folia Med Cracov*. 2013;53(1):65–78.

96. Tefertiller C, et al. Results from a randomized controlled trial to address balance deficits after traumatic brain injury. *Arch Phys Med Rehabil.* 2019;100(8):1409–1416.
97. Linder SM, et al. Improving quality of life and depression after stroke through telerehabilitation. *Am J Occup Ther.* 2015;69(2). 6902290020p1-6902290020p10.
98. Isernia S, et al. Effects of an innovative telerehabilitation intervention for people with Parkinson's disease on quality of life, motor, and non-motor abilities. *Front Neurol.* 2020;11:846.
99. Ortiz-Gutiérrez R, et al. A telerehabilitation program improves postural control in multiple sclerosis patients: a Spanish preliminary study. *Int J Environ Res Public Health.* 2013;10(11):5697–5710.
100. Kuipers P, et al. Using ICF-Environment factors to enhance the continuum of outpatient ABI rehabilitation: an exploratory study. *Disabil Rehabil.* 2009;31(2):144–151.
101. Weinstein RS, et al. Integrating telemedicine and telehealth: putting it all together. *Stud Health Technol Inform.* 2008;131:23–38.
102. Hoenig H, et al. Development of a teletechnology protocol for in-home rehabilitation. *J Rehabil Res Dev.* 2006;43(2):287.
103. De Beurs E, et al. Treatment of panic disorder with agoraphobia: comparison of fluvoxamine, placebo, and psychological panic management combined with exposure and of exposure in vivo alone. *Am J Psychiatry.* 1995;152(5):683–691.
104. Mersch PPA. The treatment of social phobia: the differential effectiveness of exposure in vivo and an integration of exposure in vivo, rational emotive therapy and social skills training. *Behav Res Ther.* 1995;33(3):259–269.
105. Öst L-G, Thulin U, Ramnerö J. Cognitive behavior therapy vs exposure in vivo in the treatment of panic disorder with agoraphobia. *Behav Res Ther.* 2004;42(10):1105–1127.
106. Vlaeyen JW, et al. The treatment of fear of movement/(re) injury in chronic low back pain: further evidence on the effectiveness of exposure in vivo. *Clin J Pain.* 2002;18(4):251–261.
107. Arbour-Nicitopoulos KP, Ginis KA. Latimer AE. Planning, leisure-time physical activity, and coping self-efficacy in persons with spinal cord injury: a randomized controlled trial. *Arch Phys Med Rehabil.* 2009;90(12):2003–2011.
108. Arbour-Nicitopoulos KP, et al. Get in motion: an evaluation of the reach and effectiveness of a physical activity telephone counseling service for Canadians living with spinal cord injury. *PM&R.* 2014;6(12):1088–1096.
109. Coulter EH, et al. The effectiveness and satisfaction of web-based physiotherapy in people with spinal cord injury: a pilot randomised controlled trial. *Spinal Cord.* 2017;55(4):383–389.

CHAPTER 23

Telerehabilitation in Speech-Language Pathology

Kerry J. Davis ▪ Dana Pagliuco

Introduction

According to the National Institute on Deafness and other Communication Disorders,[1] 7.7% of US children aged 3 to 17 had a disorder related to voice, speech, language, and swallowing within the past year. In adults, approximately 4% of the US population have experienced a voice issue during the last 12 months, with additional speech disorders including stuttering and acquired language disorders related to stroke or traumatic brain injury.[1] Speech and language therapy is a critical intervention to promote language development and minimize potential gaps in skill development, including communication, social-emotional, cognition, and self-advocacy.[2] Additionally, speech-language pathologists (SLPs) support those who may have difficulty chewing and swallowing, a disorder known as dysphagia, in their ability to manage food safely during mealtimes.[3]

Telerehabilitation is one potential venue for providing speech and language therapy. Since 2006, the national accrediting board for SLPs, the American Speech Hearing and Language Association (ASHA), has supported remote service delivery as a viable option for those clients who could not access qualified providers. Telerehabilitation has provided a valuable service to children in remote areas where specialists are not readily available.[4]

As the COVID-19 pandemic spread across the world in 2020, many medical institutions were forced to close and in-person therapy was no longer available. Many health care providers, including SLPs, suddenly had to rethink how to provide effective therapy and looked to telerehabilitation as a possible option. Most of this chapter will discuss the benefits and considerations specifically related to speech and language therapy in children in the United States, including those with developmental speech and language disorders and neurologically based disabilities. However, many of the interventions and considerations apply to pediatric and adult populations around the world.

Telerehabilitation in Speech and Language Therapy

The ability of clients to access teletherapy depends upon four main components: insurance and state regulations, accessibility to an appropriate learning environment, technology access, and client profile.[3] Public and private insurers have specific policies regarding payment to providers and out-of-pocket costs to the family. During the COVID-19 crisis many insurers across the United States temporarily expanded coverage allowing more access to therapy than had been previously possible.[2] However, many licensing restrictions remained in place. Licensure rules differ across states for speech-language pathology. In telerehabilitation for speech and language therapy, the onus lies upon the practicing clinician to abide by both the individual state regulations and those established by ASHA. This includes understanding the rules governing where the therapy takes place, and where the client is receiving services. For example, a therapist in Massachusetts providing therapy to a client in New Hampshire may be subject to the licensure and business regulations in both Massachusetts and New Hampshire.

Another consideration is technology use and access. According to the Pew Research Center an average of 58% of US school-aged children have internet at home to complete school work. This number is similar for adults aged 50 to 64 where 59% of this age group consistently have access to broadband services.[5] Further, the National Center for Education Statistics[6] conducted a survey indicating that 17% of children aged 3 to 18 do not have reliable access to a laptop or desktop computer. According to both sources, disproportionate access persists across socioeconomic class and race. This results in possible gaps in telerehabilitation across groups of clients who need prescribed speech and language therapy services.

Accessibility also includes navigating the physical computer or tablet and HIPAA-compliant telerehabilitation software platforms, to protect patient privacy. For younger children or individuals with severe disabilities, accessibility is reliant upon caregivers for technology setup, logging into the session, and navigating the use of the tablet, desktop, or laptop computer. Further considerations should be given to client and caregiver independence using a touchscreen, trackpad, or external mouse, as these features are often required for more interactive therapy activities.

Finally, the client's profile should be carefully assessed for eligibility in telerehabilitation. ASHA notes that therapists should consider physical characteristics such as hearing and visual impairments, attention and behavioral issues, cultural considerations (including needing an interpreter), and caregiver support for access and troubleshooting. While none of these factors automatically disqualify a client from assessment or receiving teletherapy services, therapists should consider whether telerehabilitation is a viable and appropriate means of support. In many such cases, assessments and service delivery models may be adjusted to develop the most appropriate plan of care.

Service Delivery Models

Traditional speech therapy intervention includes physical face-to-face interactions. The client comes to the speech therapy room or the SLP provides intervention at the client's home. Caregivers report positive experiences using telerehabilitation at home.[7, 8] Telerehabilitation therapy can be effective as a primary means of synchronous (real-time) online therapy, or in combination with other options as highlighted later.

HYBRID THERAPY

Hybrid intervention may include a combination of in-person therapy, synchronous, and asynchronous online sessions.[3] For example, the therapist may initially need to see a client in person to provide hands-on cueing for oral motor positioning to determine what may work for intervention during specific articulation or oral motor feeding tasks. Once this has been determined, the client can be followed using the same approach within an online venue. Additionally, the client may upload videos of their progress in between sessions to a secure online platform for the therapist to assess progress. In this way the client benefits from real-time feedback and the therapist can track progress over time.

CONSULTATIVE

This model provides a broader, more inclusive approach to intervention. In a caregiver survey conducted by Tenforde et al.,[7] families perceived consultation across providers to be helpful in establishing consistency of care between home, school, and outpatient therapy. Like in-person visits, a consultative approach may include the therapist implementing a virtual treatment session, while additional providers (i.e., other medical professionals, caregivers, or support staff) observe the session through a shared screen feature. If there are multiple team members present during the therapy session, it may be helpful to turn off the audio and video portion of other providers to minimize distracting the client. As part of the consultative model, the clinician can use a portion of the session to allow for comments and team feedback. This can be helpful in providing concrete strategies for intervention.

MULTIDISCIPLINARY MODEL

A multidisciplinary model of intervention may be helpful when the client could benefit from the expertise of more than one professional at one time. For example, a child with feeding and swallowing issues may be best evaluated by both an SLP and an occupational therapist to address both oral motor and swallowing safety, but also fine motor, positioning, and self-feeding skills. This allows both disciplines to assess the client while minimizing the demands upon the client and family. Like the consultative model of intervention, this model allows the client to benefit from the perspectives of different disciplines simultaneously to provide a more comprehensive view of the client's current skills and treatment needs.

GROUP THERAPY

Group therapy may be a viable option for some telehealth participants. Walker et al.[9] found that telerehabilitation provided in a group format may reduce a sense of social isolation amongst participants diagnosed with aphasia. Research on the efficacy of telerehabilitation and group speech-language therapy continues to be an emerging area of need. Therapists choosing this option must continue to consider client privacy needs within a group setting.

ASYNCHRONOUS OPTION

An asynchronous, or a "store and forward" option may be helpful for the clinician when evaluating how a specific intervention is working or being implemented. In this case, the client records a short video clip of a given activity and uploads the video to a secure portal for the clinician to review ahead of the live session. This allows the clinician to view how a goal is being addressed within a specific setting or with specific caregivers. Conversely, asynchronous exercises or home programs may be created by the clinician and sent to the client or client's family in order to provide a model that can be reviewed as necessary. This option may be helpful when providing services within a consultative model.

Use in Assessment

In order to establish measurable therapy goals, the clinician must first perform a speech, language, or swallowing evaluation. A cursory intake of skills through a previsit form may help the clinician best prepare for assessment. This intake form may include the client's medical history and current speech, language, and/or dysphagia needs. A wide variety of online standardized assessments are available through major testing publishing companies. Commonly used articulation, vocabulary, and language tests can be administered by the clinician sharing the screen to allow the examinee to view pictures from each standardized test. The examinee can respond verbally, or by using the mouse or touchscreen. In some cases, external devices such as document cameras can serve as another way the examinee can view the test items or materials. For checklist or parent survey assessment tools, the item can be scanned and emailed, or sent by a hyperlink for the parent to complete and return. If this proves too cumbersome, the clinician can review the items with the parent during the virtual session.

For less standardized measures or skills best captured through observation, clinicians can coordinate with caregivers to set up an environment conducive to gathering information. This may include appropriate seating and positioning (seated at a table or highchair) and having toys from home available to observe play skills. For a feeding or swallowing assessment, therapists may observe the client's oral motor skills and interactions with food, including related items (cups, bottles, utensils, etc.). Therapists may experience issues when trying to assess some aspects related to swallowing or voice, so this may present as a challenge while supporting a client remotely.[10] Caregiver interview is also a critical component of informal assessment procedures. As with all telerehabilitation visits, the client and family member should be set up in a relatively quiet, distraction-free environment. To ensure privacy compliance, all sessions should be completed in a private setting, not in a public place.

Use in Special Populations

While research remains scant specific to diagnosis, telerehabilitation has been notably successful in children with developmental delays and neurological disorders such as autism.[11] Some positive findings have emerged in the research related to treatment of voice, aphasia, and traumatic brain injury, though the amount of research specific to such diagnosis remains limited to primarily case studies with small populations.[10] Specific to speech disorders some positive results have been found in children with a diagnosis of stuttering[12] and childhood apraxia of speech (CAS).[13] In children receiving school-based intervention, results of treatment appear to be equally as effective in treating children with speech sound disorders in person compared to an online venue.[14] As with face-to-face sessions, crafting an online session with children who have significant attention issues or those who are minimally verbal may require additional clinical accommodations. For children with significant attention issues, accommodations may include a combination of visual supports and movement breaks.

Finally, for those clients who do not attend well to a screen, or seem too young to benefit, a short period of intervention may be appropriate in the form of parent coaching and education. This may include setting up items ahead of time, and then the therapist coaching how to use specific toys or items to facilitate language and play skills. The therapist serves as a guide to support the client's needs by direct caregiver instruction.[15, 16]

Use in Practice

Like a traditional therapy session, client engagement is imperative for desired outcomes within a virtual treatment session. For a clinician whose experience lies primarily in traditional therapy delivery, the transition to teletherapy can pose challenges in lesson planning and execution. Fortunately, through the assistance of features built into telerehabilitation platforms and both subscription-based and free online resources, clinicians have the tools to effectively target a variety of speech, language, and feeding/swallowing goal areas.

Leveraging Functions and Features of Online Platforms

SCREEN SHARE

Many HIPAA-compliant telehealth platforms have built-in features to create an interactive session. The most important interactive feature is the "screen share" tool, which allows both the clinician and the client to simultaneously view what is on the clinician's computer screen.

The clinician is given the option to share their entire screen, or share only a specific application, so that other browsers and applications on a clinician's computer may remain private. This is often recommended in order to remain HIPAA compliant. When sharing the entire screen, a client may be accidentally exposed to private health information found on a medical documentation system, clinician therapy schedule, or an email application. However, the entire screen share feature may be useful when a lesson requires the clinician to toggle between two applications. In this case, care should be taken to minimize or close all browsers intended to remain out of view of the client.

One screen share option includes an interactive whiteboard feature. An intended blank slate—therapists can utilize this feature as they see fit. Common options include written or visual schedules, Venn diagrams, and to replicate language programs like the Expanding Expressions Tool[17] by Sara L. Smith or the Story Grammar Marker[18] by MindWing Concepts. Other sharing options to facilitate interaction include sharing computer audio and sharing mouse control. Sharing computer audio allows both the client and clinician to hear audio playing on the clinician's computer. Sharing mouse or trackpad control allows the client to interact with the clinician's shared screen. This feature is necessary for student participation in standardized assessments, but it also increases engagement with the variety of online treatment materials that require turn taking and direct selections. Control settings can be manipulated quickly for those clients who may be unable, or unwilling, to relinquish control of the mouse or trackpad.

While in screen share mode, clinicians will have access to a toolbar for text and annotation. Options include line drawing, highlighting, free text, shapes, stamps, and a laser pointer feature.[3] These tools give clinicians the ability to quickly provide scaffolding for individual learner needs. The stamp feature can be utilized to represent a token reinforcement schedule like a star chart for earning a preferred object or desired activity. This toolbar can also be utilized by the client when accessing the mouse-share feature, which can be helpful for marking choices during receptive language testing and treatment. The client may place a stamp or hover the laser pointer over their answer selection. This helps to reduce expressive language demands like labeling the stimulus number. This may also help reduce the reliance upon a caregiver to report the child's answer.

VIEW, BACKGROUND, AND SPECIAL FEATURES

Telerehabilitation platforms provide numerous options regarding how the clinician and client can view each other and themselves. Typically, when in screen share mode, the video image of each participant is reduced in size in order to focus the view on the clinician's screen. This should be considered during the treatment of certain diagnoses where visual models of the clinician are necessary. For example, when treating clients with speech sound disorders, there is evidence to support providing visual models of the sound in conjunction with specific gesture cues.[19] Therapists may need to remove screen share mode in these instances. The client's ability to see themselves may serve as a source of visual feedback, which can improve direct imitation of an articulatory target. However, there are options to hide the view of the client for individuals who may be distracted by their own image.

The virtual waiting room feature allows clients to be admitted into the teletherapy session at the clinician's discretion. This feature helps support patient privacy laws and ensures that individuals cannot enter the platform during another client's session. Clients can be easily moved into and out of the virtual waiting room, which is particularly useful during multidisciplinary evaluations or co-treatment sessions. This gives providers the opportunity to discuss evaluation results and develop a service delivery plan before presenting this information directly to the client.

Some videoconferencing and telerehabilitation platforms offer the option to record sessions for later review. This feature is used most often for asynchronous service delivery models but may also be a useful tool for multidisciplinary collaboration and caregiver education. Clinicians may record portions of a session to demonstrate the use of a specific technique to another provider or to elaborate on treatment plan recommendations for a parent. Therapists should exercise caution when using the screen recording feature to ensure they are remaining HIPAA compliant and within accordance of state law regarding audio and video recordings. Clinicians must receive the appropriate consent to distribute any recorded video or audio containing private health information.

The last built-in feature to discuss includes the use of green screen and preset backgrounds. A user has the option to create virtually any background from a digital photograph or internet image. This feature may be utilized for the purposes of increasing professionalism when having to provide teletherapy from home, or as a creative measure to improve engagement with specific clients. Therapy sessions can suddenly be transported to a playground, outer space, or to a specific ecosystem to reinforce a curriculum-based vocabulary unit.

Using External Accessories and Tools

Until now, we have only described features provided directly by the telerehabilitation platform. While these features help provide accessibility to a variety of computer-based resources for therapy, there are several other avenues clinicians can use to adapt their traditional therapy materials for virtual use.

A lightweight, portable, documentation camera that is inserted into the universal serial bus (USB) port of a computer provides an additional camera source that is projected on the computer monitor during screen sharing. Documentation cameras, or "DocCams," can be utilized to project therapy materials a clinician physically has on hand. This can include worksheets, flashcards, handmade materials, crafts, board games, or toys. A documentation camera is particularly helpful during interventions targeting dysphagia and feeding disorders. The DocCam can easily visualize cooking demonstrations and food play while the desktop or laptop remains in a stable position. The DocCam can be used to demonstrate therapeutic techniques to caregivers that are not easily visualized with a traditional webcam. Examples include thickening liquids according to a specific dysphagia diet or demonstrating physical prompts on a mannequin for breastfeeding, bottle feeding, cup drinking, or spoon feeding.

Many computer platforms provide compatibility with mobile technology devices allowing for a screen share option. The screen share feature allows clinicians to use interactive applications on their mobile device, eliminating the need for a direct internet connection. Using this screen share option, clinicians can display a technology-based augmentative alternative communication (AAC) system in order to provide a visual model to the client or caregiver for a navigational sequence. This can help the clinician teach caregivers how to make changes to a specific button or feature on the AAC system, or model technology use in real time.

For clients working on voice therapy and vocal intensity, additional accessories may be needed. In a pilot study of older patients participating in voice therapy, Quinn et al. noted the benefits of accessories to help with feedback and audio clarity.[20] The authors included the use of an external microphone such as a headset or monitoring systems such as a sound pressure level meter to provide feedback to both the clinician and client. Clinicians must continually explore external accessories and web-based resources to maximize treatment outcomes.

Web-Based Resources

While teletherapy has existed since the early 2000s, this service delivery was brought into the spotlight during the COVID-19 global pandemic beginning in 2020. During this time, clinicians and educators across the world were faced with a sudden shift to virtual services. Several companies that had previously catered to providing analog therapy materials adapted, while new companies catering to digital resources flourished. As teletherapy continues to gain traction as an effective alternative to in-person services, the market for assessment and treatment resources will continue to grow and improve. In the interest of remaining relevant through the expansion of teletherapy resources, the following section will not focus on listing specific websites or online subscriptions. Instead, this text will aim to provide the reader with the necessary skill set for selecting appropriate materials for a variety of speech, language, and swallowing goals.

When planning for a teletherapy session, a clinician must first decide on the purpose of the material itself. For play breaks and reinforcement, the internet can provide an endless number of free videos and websites customizable to a client's interest while addressing goals. Similarly, websites offering virtual dice, spinners, or adapted versions of classic games like Connect 4 and Chutes and Ladders may be an engaging complement to drill-based treatment like articulation or syntax targets. In many instances, utilizing a "DocCam" or screen sharing PDF files may be enough for a successful session.

FIVES Model for Choosing Resources

For other clients, it is necessary to find an interactive resource that contains the speech or language targets built into the activity. Evaluating materials using the "FIVES Criteria" developed by Sean Sweeney MS, MEd, CCC-SLP can help guide clinical decision-making when purchasing online products and subscriptions. The FIVES Criteria (which stands for *F*airly priced, *I*nteractive, *V*isual, *E*ducationally relevant, and *S*pecific) was created as a model to help professionals decide what electronic and mobile app resources were adaptable for use in intervention.[21]

FAIRLY PRICED

Determining whether a web-based material is fairly priced is most dependent upon its ability to be utilized across a variety of sessions and a variety of clients.[22] A monthly subscription-based service that provides materials for a variety of ages and a variety of speech and language targets may be worthwhile for a clinician with a varied but primarily virtual caseload. This same service is likely not a great value for a clinician who has only a few teletherapy clients, or who is providing teletherapy services in a primarily consultative or parent coaching model. Currently, there are many online resources that are free or provided at low cost to clinicians, making teletherapy resources just as accessible as traditional therapy resources.

INTERACTIVE AND VISUAL

When adapting the FIVES model to teletherapy, the interactive and visual components are of greatest importance. A survey of SLPs following the COVID-19 pandemic revealed that a majority of SLPs reported increased workload and decreased confidence in their ability to provide quality intervention when compared with an in-person service delivery.[23] In addition to a multitude of logistical obstacles, creating interactive treatment sessions was a concern for many clinicians. Therapists should consider the time and resources spent on web-based versus physical materials used with a documentation camera. In many cases, web-based materials may be more accessible and less time-consuming for treatment planning and preparation. For example, online streaming services and e-books can replace physical picture books. Applications that simulate situations like doll house play, a tea party, or a hair salon provide the opportunity to target vocabulary and concept development, comprehension for question forms and directions, and pragmatic elements of language during pretend-play schemas.

EDUCATIONALLY RELEVANT AND SPECIFIC

Finding materials that are educationally relevant and specific to therapy objectives can be particularly important for school-based clinicians, who must focus on how the child's disability impacts their educational performance.[24] Collaboration with school and medically based SLPs can help clinicians target therapy goals while simultaneously accessing curriculum content. Currently, several online marketplace sites exist as a means for educators and therapists to create, buy, and sell digital resources with therapy objectives or curriculum units in mind.

Considerations Across the Lifespan

Many of the strategies mentioned in this chapter may also be applicable to an older population who present with disorders such as Parkinson's disease, amyotrophic lateral sclerosis, and cerebral vascular accidents (CVAs). For those requiring voice intervention, research supports efficacy of treatment in patients with Parkinson's disease.[10,25,26] The role of the SLP in supporting clients with ALS may including supporting use of AAC devices and monitoring the progression of the disease and understanding how this may affect communication and swallowing intervention. Further telerehabilitation may be used to support patients as a means of social connection in those with cognitive-communicative disorders or aphasia as a result of CVA.

Therapists should consider physical limitations that may accompany these disorders and affect access. This may include assessing mouse, trackpad, or touchscreen features, and understanding the patient's comfort using technology. As in pediatric patients, caregiver support may be indicated for setting up and managing the telerehabilitation session.

Outcomes and Recommendations for Future Research

In summary, telerehabilitation has some evidence for use in a wide range of speech and language disorders including aphasia, articulation disorders, autism, dysarthria, dysphagia, fluency disorders, language and cognitive disorders, and voice disorders.[19] Many of these speech and language disorders result as a sequela of larger developmental or neurological conditions (e.g., traumatic brain injury, CVA, progressive neurological diseases, autism, and genetic syndromes). Therefore use of telerehabilitation may prove effective across the lifespan.

The efficacy of telerehabilitation across settings and specific populations requires further research. Schools are currently the most common setting in which telerehabilitation services are delivered, and there is a strong body of evidence to support this as a service delivery model.[27–31] Research supports that school-aged children receiving speech telerehabilitation were at least equivalent in effectiveness and efficiency as traditional onsite speech therapy as assessed using functional communication measures established by ASHA.[32] Similarly, telerehabilitation for adolescents and adults appears to be promising, though research in this area remains emerging.[10]

Further research is needed comparing service delivery models for specific diagnoses, particularly those that have evidence for hands-on techniques that are not feasible for the therapist to provide through a virtual platform. For example, further research is needed for motor speech disorders such as apraxia and dysarthria. Some research exists for the efficacy of telerehabilitation and the use of the Lee Silverman Program for Voice Disorders.[10, 26] However, research is needed for other evidence-based methods for motor planning disorders, for example, tactile facilitation methods such as the Dynamic Temporal and Tactile Cueing and Prompts for Restructuring Oral Muscular Phonetic Targets treatment programs for CAS.[33] Knowing this, studies comparing outcome measures for clients with apraxia who receive in-person or teletherapy are needed in order to further define the scope of teletherapy for the inclusion or exclusion of certain populations. Additionally, further research may be indicated to determine the efficacy of these techniques when provided by caregivers with clinician oversight.

Finally, research should also aim to analyze outcome measures across the previously mentioned telerehabilitation service delivery models of consultative, hybrid, group, multidisciplinary, and asynchronous. The evidence of these models remains relatively nascent for use in pediatric therapy[12] and adults.[10] This will help clinicians create evidence-based treatment plans and potentially increase stakeholder support and acceptance of tele-therapy as a consistent treatment option. Currently in the United States, many private and public insurance policies do not provide consistent reimbursement for teletherapy services, making these services less accessible across socioeconomic populations. Further research that supports the efficacy for teletherapy will be crucial for obtaining reimbursement from a variety of payer sources, allowing for greater accessibility of speech and language therapy to the broader population.

CASE STUDY 1

ES is a 6-year-old with a history of intracranial hemorrhage, right-sided weakness, and a severe phono-logical disorder complicated by oral motor weakness and dysarthria. She was evaluated in person, with one follow-up in-person visit. During the first follow-up visit, the clinician spent time determining how to cue ES for proper placement of her articulators. The therapist spent time with the mother demonstrating how to support ES at home. The remaining weekly sessions were provided online using the same kinds of cueing with the client's mother providing support. The patient's mother occasionally uploaded videos of the client working on his goals so that the speech-language pathologist could provide feedback as needed. This method of service delivery allowed ES to benefit from a combination of synchronous and asynchronous methods of intervention.

CASE STUDY 2

AB is a 3-year-old with autism receiving therapy at a preschool and applied behavioral analysis at home. She is currently being seen for language therapy. She has a short attention span, and team members are looking for ideas to help participation. During the session, AB earns stars for participation which then earns her a break. She is interested in looking at the clinician's box of small dolls during "break time." AB also has her own doll which she shares with the clinician during his break. Providers then discuss how this strategy may help motivate AB to participate longer in therapy sessions both online and in person.

CASE STUDY 3

AR (a 7-year-old child) is being treated for language deficits incurred by a traumatic brain injury. The client also has a premorbid diagnosis of attention deficit hyperactivity disorder and auditory process-ing deficits. The clinician presents a written checklist of activities to help keep the client on task. The clinician builds in movement breaks into the schedule to help with attention. One break includes the client using the trampoline in the nearby space, another includes dance videos from the online website *GoNoodle*, which includes short songs and body movements. In addition to completing the more direct activities, AR can work on his goals of following directions through movement which helps with sustain-ing attention.

CASE STUDY 4

Telerehabilitation can also support those children who require technology to communicate, also known as augmentative alternative communication.

A 15-year-old male with severe dysarthria uses a speech-generating device to communicate. The therapist is teaching the client how to build sentences by selecting a series of buttons on a touchscreen that mirror the client's speech-generative device. While the therapist is not able to physically guide the client to locate the items on her device, the highlight feature allows the SLP to model expectations using screen share.

References

1. National Institute on Deafness and Other Communication Disorders. Quick statistics about voice, speech, language. 2016. https://www.nidcd.nih.gov/health/statistics/quick-statistics-voice-speech-language.
2. American Speech Hearing Language Association. Payment and coverage considerations for telepractice services during Coronavirus/COVID-19. 2020. https://www.asha.org/practice/reimbursement/payment-and-coverage-considerations-for-telepractice-services-during-coronavirus.
3. American Speech Hearing Language Association. Telepractice. 2020. https://www.asha.org/Practice-Portal/Professional-Issues/Telepractice/#collapse_1.
4. Fairweather GC, Lincoln MA, Ramsden R. Speech-language pathology teletherapy in rural and remote educational settings: decreasing service inequities. *Int J Speech Lang Pathol*. 2016;18(6):592–602. https://doi.org/10.3109/17549507.2016.1143973.
5. Pew Research Center. Internet broadband fact sheet. 2020. https://www.pewresearch.org/internet/fact-sheet/internet-broadband/.
6. National Center for Education Statistics. Digest of Education Statistics. National Center for Education Statistics. 2018. https://nces.ed.gov/programs/digest/d18/tables/dt18_702.40.asp.
7. Tenforde AS, Borgstrom H, Polich G, et al. Outpatient physical, occupational, and speech therapy synchronous telemedicine: a survey study of patient satisfaction with virtual visits during the COVID-19 pandemic. *Am J Phys Med Rehabil*. 2020;99:977–981.
8. Wales D, Skinner L, Hayman M. The efficacy of telehealth-delivered speech and language intervention for primary school-age children: a systematic review. *Int J Telerehabil*. 2017;9(1):55–70.
9. Walker JP, Price K, Watson J. Promoting social connections in a synchronous telepractice, aphasia communication group. *Perspectives of the ASHA Special Interest Groups*. 2018;3(18):32–42.
10. Weinder K, Lowman J. Telepractice for adult speech-language pathology services: a systematic review. *Perspectives of the ASHA Special Interest Groups*. 2020;5:326–338.
11. Boisvert M, Lang R, Andrianopoulos Telepractice in the assessment and treatment of individuals with autism spectrum disorders: a systematic review. *Dev Neurorehabil*. 2010;13(6):423–432.
12. Ryer JE, Poll GH. The effectiveness of hybrid telepractice and in-person fluency treatment for a school-aged child: a case study. *Perspectives of the ASHA Special Interest Groups*. 2020;5(4):1085–1097.
13. Thomas DC, McCabe P, Ballard KJ, et al. Telehealth delivery of Rapid Syllable Transitions (ReST) treatment for childhood apraxia of speech. *Int J Lang Commun Disord*. 2016;51(6):654–671.
14. Sanchez D, Reiner JF, Sadlon R, et al. Systematic review of school telehealth evaluations. *J Sch Nurs*. 2019;35(1):61–76.
15. Roberts M, Curtis P, Sone B, et al. Association of parent training with child language development. A systematic review and meta-analysis. *JAMA Pediatr*. 2019;173(7):671–680.
16. Snodgrass M, Chung M, Biller M. Telepractice in speech-language therapy: the use of online technologies for parent training and coaching. *Commun Disord Q*. 2016;38(4):242–254.
17. Expanding Expression Tool. https://www.expandingexpression.com/.
18. Story Grammar Marker. https://mindwingconcepts.com/.
19. American Speech-Language-Hearing Association. Speech sound disorders: articulation and phonology (practice portal). 2020. www.asha.org/Practice-Portal/Clinical-Topics/Articulation-and-Phonology/.
20. Quinn R, Park S, Theodoros D, et al. Delivering group speech maintenance therapy via telerehabilitation to people with Parkinson's disease: a pilot study. *Int J Speech Lang Pathol*. 2018;21(4):385–394.
21. Davis K, Sweeney S. Reading, writing and AAC: mobile technology strategies for literacy and language development. *Perspect Augment Altern Commun*. 2015;24:19–25.
22. Sweeney, S. The FIVES Criteria: for evaluating and integrating simple technology resources in speech and language interventions. 2010. http://www.scribd.com/doc44503715/Fives-Booklet.
23. Sylvan L, Goldstein E, Crandall M. Capturing a moment in time: a survey of school-based speech-language pathologists' experiences in the immediate aftermath of the COVID-19 public health emergency. *Perspectives of the ASHA Special Interest Groups*. 2020;5(6):1735–1749.
24. American Speech-Language-Hearing Association. Documentation in schools (practice portal). 2016. www.asha.org/Practice-Portal/Professional-Issues/Documentation-in-Schools/.
25. Rangarathnam B, McCullough G, Pickett H, et al. Telepractice versus in-person delivery of voice therapy for primary muscle tension dysphonia. *Am J Speech Lang Pathol*. 2015;23(3):386–399.

26. Theodoros D, Ramig L. Telepractice supported delivery of LSVT LOUD. *Perspect Neurophysiol Neurogenic Speech Lang Disord.* 2011;21(3):107–119.

27. Gabel R, Grogan-Johnson S, Alvares R, et al. A field study of telepractice for school intervention using the ASHA NOMS K-12 database. *Commun Disord Q.* 2013;35:44–53.

28. Grogan-Johnson S, Alvares R, Rowan L, et al. A pilot study comparing the effectiveness of speech language therapy provided by telemedicine with conventional on-site therapy. *J Telemed Telecare.* 2010;16:134–139.

29. Grogan-Johnson S, Gabel R, Taylor J, et al. A pilot exploration of speech sound disorder intervention delivered by telehealth to school-aged children. *Int J Telerehabil.* 2011;3:31–42.

30. Lewis C, Packman A, Onslow M, et al. A phase II trial of telehealth delivery of the Lidcombe program of early stuttering intervention. *Am J Speech Lang Pathol.* 2008;17:139–149.

31. McCullough A. Viability and effectiveness of teletherapy for pre-school children with special needs. *Int J Lang Commun Disord.* 2001;36:321–326.

32. Short L, Rea T, Houston B, et al. Positive outcomes for speech telepractice as evidence for reimbursement policy change. *Perspectives of the ASHA Special Interest Groups.* 2016;1(18):3–11.

33. McAllister A, Broden M, Gonzalez Lindh M, et al. Oral sensory-motor intervention for children and adolescents (3-18 years) with developmental or early acquired speech disorders: a review of the literature 2000-2017. *Ann Otolaryngol Rhinol.* 2018;5(5):1221.

34. American Speech Hearing Language Association. Scope of practice in speech language pathology. 2016. https://www.asha.org/policy/sp2016-00343/.

35. Strand EA. Dynamic temporal and tactile cueing: a treatment strategy for childhood apraxia of speech. *Am J Speech Lang Pathol.* 2020;29(1):30–48.

CHAPTER 24

Pediatric Telerehabilitation

Joshua Alexander

Introduction

The American Board of Physical Medicine and Rehabilitation (ABPMR) describes pediatric rehabilitation medicine (PRM) as "the subspecialty that uses an interdisciplinary approach to address the prevention, diagnosis, treatment, and management of congenital and childhood-onset physical impairments including related or secondary medical, physical, functional, psychosocial, cognitive, and vocational limitations or conditions, with an understanding of the life course of disability."[1]

The ultimate goals of a pediatric rehabilitation program are to help pediatric patients reach adulthood as happy, healthy, and independent as possible. This is usually achieved by simultaneously enhancing their health, helping them avoid secondary complications of their condition, and maximizing their function either through regaining skills after injury or functional loss (rehabilitation) or by learning new skills in the context of a previously present disability (habilitation).

HISTORY OF PEDIATRIC REHABILITATION

Applying the principles of rehabilitation medicine to the care of children became critical in the mid-20th century when the polio epidemic reached its peak. Early PRM physicians such as Dr. George Deaver (who pioneered the concept of activities of daily living and was one of the founding members of the American Academy for Cerebral Palsy) and Dr. Jesse Wright (inventor of the rocking bed used for respiratory support) combined a multidisciplinary approach to care with the rehabilitation technologies of the day to help children stricken with the disease regain their independence in self-care skills and mobility.[2,3]

In the 1970s, physiatrists who were interested in pediatric rehabilitation joined together to offer educational programs on pediatric topics and host networking opportunities at national meetings of the American Academy of Physical Medicine and Rehabilitation (AAPMR). In 1983 this group became the AAPMR's Pediatric Special Interest Group. Two decades later, in 2003, the ABPMR began offering subspecialty certification in PRM "in order to enhance the quality of care available to individuals with pediatric rehabilitation needs and their families."[4]

CURRENT DISTRIBUTION OF PRM PHYSICIANS

While there are over 10,000 board-certified physiatrists in the United States today,[5] less than 3% of them are PRM physicians. As can be seen in Table 24.1, there is also a significantly unequal distribution of these subspecialists across the country with four states having more than 20 PRM physicians each while thirteen states have none at all. Even in states with practicing PRM physicians, children with disabilities living in rural areas often have to travel long distances to gain access to their care.[6,7]

TABLE 24.1 ■ **Geographic Distribution of 293 Board-Certified Pediatric Rehabilitation Medicine Physicians in the United States.**

293 Pediatric Physiatrists

Alabama	5	Alaska	0	Arizona	3
Arkansas	1	California	23	Colorado	12
Connecticut	1	Delaware	5	DC	6
Florida	10	Georgia	3	Hawaii	1
Idaho	2	Illinois	14	Indiana	4
Iowa	1	Kansas	0	Kentucky	2
Louisiana	3	Maine	0	Maryland	9
Mass.	6	Michigan	11	Minnesota	19
Mississippi	0	Missouri	10	Montana	0
Nebraska	0	Nevada	0	New Hampshire	0
New Jersey	12	New Mexico	0	New York	22
NC	8	North Dakota	0	Ohio	29
Oklahoma	0	Oregon	3	Pennsylvania	15
Rhode Island	0	SC	1	South Dakota	2
Tennessee	1	Texas	22	Utah	5
Vermont	1	Virginia	4	Washington	9
West Virginia	1	Wisconsin	6	Wyoming	0
Puerto Rico	2				

American Board of Physical Medicine and Rehabilitation. https://www.abpmr.org/PhysicianSearch/Search; Accessed 31.01.21.

There are far fewer physicians practicing PRM outside the United States. Table 24.2 lists the number of Physical Medicine and Rehabilitation providers from throughout the world who are members of the American Academy for Cerebral Palsy and Developmental Medicine, an international organization "dedicated to providing multidisciplinary scientific education and promoting excellence in research and services for the benefit of people with and at risk for cerebral palsy and other childhood-onset disabilities" (https://www.aacpdm.org/about; Accessed 31.01.21).

Telerehabilitation offers a means to overcome this disparity in the geographic distribution of PRM specialists and improve access to care for children with disabilities and their families regardless of where they live throughout the world.

PEDIATRIC CONDITIONS THAT MOST BENEFIT FROM TELEREHABILITATION

Although procedures most often performed by PRM physicians (like botulinum toxin injections and baclofen pump refills) cannot be offered directly through telerehabilitation, the majority of patients with conditions commonly seen in a pediatric rehabilitation practice can be served well, saving them and their families significant amounts of time, travel, and cost. Table 24.3 provides a list of common conditions seen in PRM that can benefit from telerehabilitation interventions.

TABLE 24.2 ▪ **Numbers of AACPDM Members in Each Country Who Practice Physical Medicine and Rehabilitation.**

307 Member Listings

Argentina	1	Armenia	1	Australia	6
Brazil	1	Canada	12	Costa Rica	1
Ghana	1	Israel	2	Italy	1
Japan	2	Korea	9	Luxembourg	1
Mexico	7	Netherlands	9	Philippines	1
People's Republic of China	3	Poland	3		
Qatar	1	Spain	1	Taiwan	2
Thailand	1	Turkey	2	United States	239

AACPDM, American Academy of Cerebral Palsy & Developmental Medicine. American Academy of Cerebral Palsy & Developmental Medicine. Accessed 31.01.21.

TABLE 24.3 ▪ **Common Conditions in Pediatric Telerehabilitation.**

Anoxic brain injury	Limb deficiencies
Cerebral palsy	Neuromuscular diseases
Cognitive assessments	Spasticity management
Concussion	Spina bifida
Counseling	Spinal cord injury
Feeding difficulties	Stroke
Gait abnormality	Traumatic brain injury

Pediatric Telerehabilitation

HISTORY

In the mid- to late-1990s, advances in two-way videoconferencing technologies helped lead to the establishment of the first telerehabilitation programs for children with special needs in the United States.

In 1994 the Specialized Interdisciplinary Consultation Telemedicine Project, one of the five clinical projects that were part of a larger National Library of Medicine grant, provided real time, multidisciplinary team-to-team consultation services for children with special health and behavioral needs in rural Iowa communities, particularly in their school environments. This clinical research program placed an emphasis on evaluating the efficacy of the telerehabilitation medium for coordinated, team-to-team–based care for children with disabilities. While some parents (10%–12%) reported technical problems during the telerehabilitation sessions, usually with poor audio and camera movement, the vast majority of parents felt the quality of care provided was good to excellent and reported they were satisfied or very satisfied with the care their child received via telerehabilitation.[8]

In 1995 the Children's Medical Services of the State of Georgia contracted with the Department of Pediatrics of the Medical College of Georgia (MCG) and the MCG Telemedicine Center to develop telemedicine programs to provide subspecialty care for children with special health care needs. Most of these telemedicine consultations (35%) involved pediatric allergy/immunology. Other subspecialties included pulmonology (29%), neurology (19%), and genetics (16%). Overall, families were satisfied with the services they received and the authors concluded that telemedicine was "an acceptable means of delivering specific pediatric subspecialty consultation services to children with special health care needs, living in rural areas distant to tertiary centers."[9]

In 1996 and 1997, two remote telemedicine clinics were established at nursing schools and linked to an interdisciplinary team at the University of Texas Medical Branch to improve access for children with special health care needs living in Texas. These clinics were evaluated to determine if the tertiary interdisciplinary team could effectively assess and plan interventions for children with special health care needs and to assess patient and caregiver satisfaction with this intervention. The interdisciplinary team and the patients and their families were highly satisfied with this arrangement.[10]

TelAbility was the first pediatric telerehabilitation program created by, and provided through, a PM&R department. Founded in 1998, this community-oriented, interdisciplinary program used multiple internet-based telecommunications technologies (including real-time video clinics, multipoint virtual interdisciplinary educational programs, searchable online expertise directories, chat rooms, listservs, and more) to improve the lives of young children with disabilities. The goal of this program was to use telerehabilitation to provide comprehensive, coordinated, family-centered care to children with disabilities across the state of North Carolina and to offer education, training, and peer support for people who cared for them. Instead of using the hub-and-spoke model popular at the time, TelAbility used a lattice-like network of early intervention centers, specialized day care centers, and private pediatric therapy offices to build a virtual community of caring that shared knowledge, resources, and access points.[11]

Throughout the first two decades of the 21st century, growth of pediatric telerehabilitation programs was slowed by restricted payment for services, liability and licensure issues, concerns over HIPAA compliance, and other constraints. Many of these limitations were subsequently removed by the Coronavirus Aid, Relief, and Economic Security Act of 2020, leading to accelerated adoption in the use of virtual medical and therapy services for children with disabilities and their families. While it is not yet known if these new policies will outlast the state of emergency related to the COVID-19 pandemic, more and more people have been given the opportunity to provide or receive telerehabilitation care and have discovered its many benefits.

PERFORMANCE OF TELEREHABILITATION USING DIFFERENT TECHNIQUES IN THIS SPECIALTY

Like other forms of telerehabilitation, pediatric telerehabilitation can be offered through multiple delivery mechanisms, including asynchronous/store and forward, real-time virtual visits, and remote monitoring.

In asynchronous/store and forward telerehabilitation, photos, videos, and other recordings are captured, stored, and sent to providers who then review them and provide interpretation and/or feedback at a later time. Examples include a photo of a pressure ulcer or ill-fitting brace or a video of a child's gait pattern or movement disorder. This approach can be more effective than an in-person examination in some cases because it allows for the capture and sharing of an action or movement that might not be present during a clinic visit. It also eliminates the chance that an examination may be limited by a pediatric patient's diminished ability to cooperate due to a change in their daily routine (having to travel to a doctor's office), an unfamiliar environment (the examination room in a doctor's office or medical center), and/or the presence of a stranger (the examiner).[12]

Virtual visits offer the opportunity for two-way interactions between the provider and the patient/patient's family. This allows for real-time feedback between the two sites that can optimize the examination, offer virtual mentorship, facilitate education, and provide an enhanced understanding of the patient's natural environment. Because it eliminates the need to travel to a distant location, virtual visits often enable other providers or family members to attend the visit, improving communication, care coordination, and compliance with recommendations.

While not yet as commonly utilized, remote patient monitoring (RPM) uses digital technologies to collect health-related data from individuals in one location and electronically transmit that information securely to health care providers in a different location for their assessment and recommendations.[13] This can enable providers to monitor a patient's health and functional status to anticipate and prevent secondary complications of their condition and optimize their independence. RPM is already being used to facilitate follow-up of neonatal intensive care unit (NICU) graduates, monitor cardiac function in pediatric patients with congenital heart disease, and follow patients with seizure disorders.[14, 15]

Wearable technologies that seamlessly download data into a parent's smartphone or physician's secure electronic medical record will soon enable providers to keep track of their patient's activity levels (heart rate, step counts), range of motion (through goniometric measuring devices embedded in clothing or through real-time video movement analysis at home or in the community), participation in the community (through GPS-tracking devices), and more.

Practice

USE OF PEDIATRIC TELEREHABILITATION FOR INITIAL CONSULTATION PURPOSES

These delivery systems can be used in a myriad of ways to provide comprehensive consultations, problem-focused services, therapy services, education, mentorship, and support.

Comprehensive Consultations

Telerehabilitation allows experts in PRM to provide direct comprehensive consultations to their patients in their homes, schools, early intervention centers, pediatric long-term care facilities, and other locales (the author has personal experience in providing teleconsultations to patients on the beach, in the parking lot of a fast food restaurant, and even in the middle of a corn field!). While these locations may be more convenient for the family, each presents a unique challenge to gather sufficient information through parent and patient interview and virtual examination through observation of the video.

Tips for providing direct consultations include positioning the patient and camera to optimize the video and audio input (still often limited by the family's internet speeds at home or on the road) and utilizing a second person (or a robotic mount with remote pan-tilt capability) to hold the camera/phone while the first facilitates the examination (imagine trying to perform a range of motion assessment with one hand while holding a phone in the other—doable, but suboptimal). Instructing the parent to flip the camera on the phone from mirror to distant image can improve the quality of a gait evaluation (which should be repeated to include front, back, and side views of the patient walking). The use of peripheral devices (e.g., thermometer, otoscope, stethoscope) attached to the parent's phone can enhance the cardiac, pulmonary, and ear, nose, and throat examination in a cooperative child.

When providing pediatric telerehabilitation consultations at a facility, other members of the child's care team can be invited to attend and contribute to an interdisciplinary discussion of the patient's needs. Local care providers (including nurses, therapists, child service coordinators, and others) can provide valuable information and help facilitate the examination.

There is also a place for pediatric telerehabilitation consultations in the medical inpatient and outpatient settings. Inpatient consultations to an NICU where a child with spina bifida was just born or to a pediatric intensive care unit to help treat a patient with a traumatic brain injury or spinal cord injury are just a few examples. In the outpatient setting, pediatric telerehabilitation consults directed to pediatricians can help augment the care the child receives in their medical home.

Problem-Focused Services

Potential applications for the use of pediatric telerehabilitation are limited only by the availability of appropriate technology, sufficient connectivity, and the imagination of the practitioner. Here are just a few of the many problem-focused services that can be provided (and sometimes enhanced) through pediatric telerehabilitation.

Brace Checks

With appropriate lighting and camera angles, both asynchronous and real-time interactive video-conferencing can enable a clinician to evaluate the size and fit of an ankle foot orthosis (AFO) or other types of brace and determine if a new one is indicated.

Pressure Ulcers

In similar fashion, pressure ulcer size can be evaluated and monitored through store and forward photo capture or through real-time facilitated examination. As technology continues to improve, real-time and/or remote monitoring of skin pressure mapping at brace or wheelchair cushion interfaces may reduce the incidence of pressure ulcer development.

Movement Disorders

Parents of children with disability sometimes report concerns about their child's new or chronic, but intermittent, movement disorder that is not present during an in-person clinic visit. Telerehabilitation technologies (real-time videoconferencing, asynchronous sharing of video recordings) enable the parent or local provider to capture a concerning movement pattern and share it with the clinician who can then make a diagnosis or suggest further evaluations such as EEG monitoring for a possible seizure disorder.

Gait Evaluations

In certain cases (a reluctant child, a specific terrain, etc.) telerehabilitation can enable a clinician to view a patient's gait more fully than during an in-person visit. Asking the child to give a tour of their house, walk to their room, or walk up and down the stairs at home can offer more information about the child's function in their natural environment than merely having them walk back and forth down a clinic hallway. Future technology may even allow for more objective kinematic and kinetic evaluations as telerehabilitation moves gait laboratories out of the confines of academic research centers and into the community.

Spasticity Management

While botulinum toxins cannot be virtually administered (yet), there is still a role for pediatric telerehabilitation in spasticity management. Instead of asking patients to return to the office to follow up on the effects of a toxin injection, one should consider scheduling a telerehabilitation visit facilitated by the patient's local therapist who can share their experience treating the child, provide a proxy assessment of tone using the Modified Ashworth Scale, and enable a visual assessment of the child's range of motion and movement patterns.

Care Coordination

Telerehabilitation can support and enhance the interdisciplinary nature of pediatric rehabilitation through multisite videoconferencing that facilitates communication and care coordination among PRM physicians, primary care providers, other subspecialists, school personnel, local therapists, child service coordinators, family members, social workers, psychologists, nutritionists, and others.

USE OF PEDIATRIC TELEREHABILITATION FOR DIFFERENT TYPES OF THERAPY

Like telemedical services, pediatric therapy services can be provided (and sometimes enhanced) through the use of telerehabilitation.

Pediatric occupational therapists, physical therapists, and speech-language pathologists have been providing telerehabilitation therapies for children with disabilities for over a decade in rehabilitation centers, schools, and private practice settings.

Here are several commonly used pediatric telepractice interventions:

Virtual Therapy Services

Prior to 2020, virtual therapy services performed in the school setting were often provided to overcome a paucity of school therapists, especially in more rural areas. Private speech-language pathologists were contracted to offer services as part of the child's individualized education plan where they provided visual and auditory information via videoconferencing and computer-based programs to help with cognitive, oral motor, and assistive technology training. Post-COVID-19, school systems, early intervention centers, and private pediatric therapy practices have embraced the use of teletherapy services to continue to serve their patients and their families. In-person and hands-on therapy has shifted to virtual observation, coaching, and home exercise program instruction for the child's caregivers. A recent systematic review of teletherapy practices found that using a coaching approach during sessions and scheduling regular virtual therapy visits (as opposed to having the family contact the provider on an as-needed basis) were more frequently associated with improved outcomes.[16]

Home Evaluations

Before discharge from a pediatric acute inpatient rehabilitation program, family members can provide inpatient therapists with a tour of the child's home/discharge destination so that therapists can identify potential physical barriers, arrange for necessary equipment and/or modifications, and work together to ensure that proper family training has been performed to optimally support the child's return home. In the outpatient setting, therapists can use these virtual home tours to order appropriate equipment like lifts that work well in the patient's bedroom and bath/shower chairs that fit well in the child's bathroom.

Feeding Therapy

Pediatric feeding therapy sessions, often provided by pediatric speech therapists and occupational therapists, can be extended into the home through an arrangement where therapists can mentor and coach parents as they watch and listen to them feed their child. Positioning, equipment, and behavioral modifications can be made in real time as the therapist evaluates a feeding session and provides feedback to the parent to optimize feeding safety and efficacy.

Mobility Assessments

Whether the patient ambulates or uses a wheelchair for community mobility, new wearable technologies and other remote monitoring devices will allow providers to follow their patient's activity levels, gait parameters, and mobility in the community. Goniometers, accelerometers, and

GPS-tracking devices will be linked to a phone-based app and then downloaded to a cloud database, enabling the recording of movement in the child's various natural environments (home, school, community) at various times of the day, with no direct observation required.

Behavioral Mentoring/Coaching for Parents

Pediatric psychologists and behavior therapists can use real-time videoconferencing to evaluate episodes and offer training and support to parents as they work to decrease behavior challenges that can arise around bedtime routines, potty training, and mealtimes. They can also use telerehabilitation technologies to coach parents and other caregivers to help reduce self-abusive behaviors, as well as aggressive behaviors toward others.

Nutritional Assessment and Coaching

Telerehabilitation technologies also enable pediatric dieticians to provide patient and family-centered nutritional counseling and coaching. During a home visit, the dietician can even peer into the family's pantry and refrigerator to get a better idea of the foods the family keeps at home. This approach can supplement and often confirm the self-reports of patients and their families, leading to a more useful assessment of the child's and family's home diets.

USE OF PEDIATRIC TELEREHABILITATION FOR EDUCATION, MENTORSHIP, AND SUPPORT PROGRAMS

Telerehabilitation technologies provide a convenient way for pediatric rehabilitation physicians and therapists to access education, mentorship, and support in their chosen fields. In the current environment of limited travel due to the COVID-19 pandemic, webinars, listservs, and virtual conferences and meetings have become the de facto means to connect, share information, and collaborate with other providers within and between institutions, disciplines, and countries.

Parents also benefit from online resources and programs. Sources for web-based education, mentorship, and support for parents include national and international organizations that provide information about their child's condition, information on related resources, online support groups, virtual mindfulness sessions, and community listservs.

Finally, pre-teen and teenaged patients can use web and smartphone apps to learn more about their condition, participate in virtual support groups, and get online counseling as they navigate their way through childhood and transition to life as an adult.

Special Considerations in Pediatric Telerehabilitation

As the popular pediatric saying goes, "Children are not just small adults." In a similar fashion, pediatric telerehabilitation differs from other types of telerehabilitation in many ways, including the age of users, their comfort with technology, end-user locations, time savings, informed consent, and more.

There are currently two major generations of parents of children with disabilities—Generation Xers who are somewhat facile with technology use, and Millennials who grew up as digital natives and who have easily adopted new technologies and information-sharing platforms. While some older adult patients may struggle with telerehabilitation technology, most parents of children with disabilities are familiar with web-based videoconferencing, phone apps, and digital life. This makes it easier to enroll users in pediatric telerehabilitation programs, as long as they have sufficient interest in participating, and sufficient bandwidth at home. Once a visit has begun, younger parents and their children are usually comfortable with virtual interactions and are more tolerant of, and better able to correct, occasional technological problems that may occur during a session.

Potential originating sites for pediatric telerehabilitation visits mirror the common locations where children with disabilities go each day to receive care and education. Pediatric therapists who are required to provide early intervention services in the child's natural environment[17] can use telerehabilitation to provide visits in the child's home and day care center. Other effective sites for telerehabilitation service provision include early intervention centers and schools where school personnel can facilitate a medical examination, and therapists, social workers, audiologists, and others can work virtually with special education teachers to provide related services mandated under the Individuals with Disabilities Education Act.[18]

Health care locations that are useful originating sites for telerehabilitation services include primary care offices, pediatric specialty clinics, rural health care centers, and pediatric nursing and long-term care facilities. Other common sites include patients' homes (where proxy examinations can sometimes be facilitated by home health care providers), and wheelchair clinics or prosthetic/orthotic practices where the virtual provider can offer their expertise as part of a multidisciplinary fitting team. Other, less common (and less ideal) telerehabilitation examination locations provided by the author have included inside family cars (some parked, others driving down the highway!), and a farmer's field, where the examiner could assess the effectiveness of a child's AFO as the patient walked on uneven terrain, stepping over and between rows of tobacco plants.

When calculating time savings related to pediatric telerehabilitation services, there are numerous beneficiaries of a virtual visit. The provider saves travel time (especially important for early intervention professionals who sometimes travel great distances only to discover that the child/family are not available for a home visit), the parent(s) save both travel time and time missed from work, and the school-aged child avoids missing classes.[19, 20] As mentioned previously, asynchronous store and forward telerehabilitation can help capture a finding that might otherwise be unavailable in a child who is unwilling to cooperate during an in-person examination.

Since children are not allowed to give true informed consent until they are age 18, it is imperative that (when informed consent is required) the provider obtain parental or guardian consent prior to commencing a pediatric telerehabilitation visit. In cases where the parent or guardian may not be able to attend the visit (school-based services is one example), a form that provides consent for a certain time period can be completed and kept on file.

Finally, compared with their adult counterparts, pediatric patients often have shorter attention spans and demand more play and reward during therapy sessions. In addition to encouragement from the therapist or caregiver, pediatric telerehabilitation has the potential to maintain patient engagement through virtual gamification of range of motion, strengthening, balance, and coordination exercises.[21]

As technology continues to improve, we will likely see a host of new virtual therapy programs that will encourage pediatric patient participation through the use of rewards from points scored, levels achieved, and opportunities for virtual socialization with others during exercise.

Recommendations for the Further Advancement of Pediatric Telerehabilitation

Despite its 25-year history, pediatric telerehabilitation is still in its infancy. Perhaps, in light of the recent acceleration in use due to COVID-19, it has reached toddlerhood, starting to more boldly explore its potential as it continues to gain strength. In either case, its further development is contingent upon many factors.

1. Further research should be performed to demonstrate the relative efficacy of medical and therapeutic assessments and interventions delivered in this new virtual world. Safety, efficacy, access to and quality of care, effects on health care costs, and provider and patient/family satisfaction must all be evaluated.

2. Payment for virtual services should be on par with in-person delivery and should cover visits wherever the child is located (hospital, home, school, etc.). Positive and negative effects of telerehabilitation services should be studied under both fee-for-service and value-based care structures.

3. Interstate licensure opportunities should be offered throughout the United States to enable provision of telerehabilitation services across the country.

4. Residency and graduate student training programs should include telerehabilitation training and education to prepare graduates for future virtual interdisciplinary collaborations.

5. Product innovations, such as technology-enhanced clothing, haptic transmission, and virtual therapy programs, must become cheaper and more available to users from all geographic and financial groups. Programs like fitness communities for pediatric patients with disabilities, and international communities of caring, should be implemented to encourage multisite collaborative provision of care and support.

In the end, interested parties should invest their time and energy to continue to develop, promote, and support pediatric telerehabilitation programs that will move children with disabilities and their families closer to a world of health and information equity, optimization of function, and equal opportunity for a well-lived life.

CASE STUDY

A 2.5-year-old male with spastic diplegic cerebral palsy, feeding difficulties, and developmental delay lives in a rural area that is over 150 miles away from the medical center where he receives most of his specialty medical care. He receives weekly occupational, physical, and speech therapy services through his local early intervention team. He visits his pediatric rehabilitation medicine physician every 3 months, but his mother (who is his primary caregiver at home) cannot take the entire day off to make the trip because she will miss too much work, so his aunt takes him and shares what she learns. His therapists send quarterly reports to the physiatrist but do not have any further communication with her.

An opportunity arises for the family and therapists to try out an internet-based videoconference pediatric telerehabilitation visit at their local early intervention center a few blocks away. The child, his mother, his aunt, and his therapists enter the room that is outfitted with toys, a floor mat, and some chairs. The pediatric rehabilitation medicine physician and a pediatric nutritionist connect in from the hospital. Together, they participate in a 45-minute virtual visit, where the physiatrist performs a history, getting direct input from the mother, the aunt, and the therapists, and then, with the help of the early intervention team, is able to perform a facilitated neuromusculoskeletal examination and gait evaluation.

The physiatrist, nutritionist, and therapists provide their insight and discuss their impressions and recommendations, which are shared in real time with the patient's family. Decisions are made and agreed upon by the entire care team at both sites and recorded in the patient's electronic medical record. More than half a day in travel time, effort, and cost is saved, multiple voices are able to attend, provide input, discussion and care coordination, and everyone leaves the visit with a better sense of next steps in this child's care. All participants appreciated the opportunity to work together as a team on behalf of the child and family and all look forward to their next pediatric telerehabilitation visit.

References

1. American Board of Physical Medicine and Rehabilitation. Pediatric rehabilitation medicine. https://www.abpmr.org/Subspecialties/PRM; Accessed 30.09.21.

2. Flanagan SR, Diller L. Dr. George Deaver: the grandfather of rehabilitation medicine. PM&R. 2013;5:355–359. https://doi.org/10.1016/j.pmrj.2013.03.031.

3. Alexander M, Turk MA, Ayyangar R. Dr. Jessie Wright: breaking new ground in pediatric physical medicine and rehabilitation. PM&R. 2013;5:739–746. https://doi.org/10.1016/j.pmrj.2013.07.006.

4. American Board of Physical Medicine and Rehabilitation. Pediatric rehabilitation medicine. https://www.abpmr.org/Subspecialties/PRM; Accessed 27.09.20.

5. Association of Academic Physiatrists. Growing Need for Physiatrists. http://www.physiatry.org/page/WhatIsPhysiatry; Accessed 30.09.21.

6. Skinner AC, Slifkin RT. Rural/urban differences in barriers to and burden of care for children with special health care needs. *J Rural Health.* 2007;23(2):150–157. https://doi.org/10.1111/j.1748-0361.2007.00082.x. PMID: 17397371.

7. Marcin JP, Ellis J, Mawis R, et al. Using telemedicine to provide pediatric subspecialty care to children with special health care needs in an underserved rural community. *Pediatrics.* 2004;113(1 Pt 1):1–6. https://doi.org/10.1542/peds.113.1.1. PMID: 14702439.

8. Harper DC. Telemedicine for children with disabilities. *Child Health Care.* 2006;35(1):11–27.

9. Karp WB, Grigsby RK, McSwiggan-Hardin M, et al. Use of telemedicine for children with special health care needs. *Pediatrics.* 2000;105(4 Pt 1):843–847. https://doi.org/10.1542/peds.105.4.843.

10. Robinson SS, Seale DE, Tiernan KM, et al. Use of telemedicine to follow special needs children. *Telemed J E Health.* 2003;9(1):57–61.

11. Gregory P, Alexander J, Satinsky J. Clinical telerehabilitation: applications for physiatrists. *PM R.* 2011;3(7):647–656. https://doi.org/10.1016/j.pmrj.2011.02.024.

12. Langkamp DL, McManus MD, Blakemore SD. Telemedicine for children with developmental disabilities: a more effective clinical process than office-based care. *Telemed J E Health.* 2015;21(2):110–114.

13. https://www.cchpca.org/what-is-telehealth/?category=remote-patient-monitoring..

14. Satou GM, Rheuban K, Alverson D, et al. American Heart Association Congenital Cardiac Disease Committee of the Council on Cardiovascular Disease in the Young and Council on Quality Care and Outcomes Research. Telemedicine in pediatric cardiology: a scientific statement from the American Heart Association. *Circulation.* 2017;135(11):e648–e678. https://doi.org/10.1161/CIR.0000000000000478. Epub 2017 Feb 13. PMID: 28193604.

15. Lavin B, Dormond C, Scantlebury MH, et al. Bridging the healthcare gap: building the case for epilepsy virtual clinics in the current healthcare environment. *Epilepsy Behav.* 2020;111:107262 https://doi.org/10.1016/j.yebeh.2020.107262. Epub ahead of print. PMID: 32645620; PMCID: PMC7336918.

16. Camden C, Pratte G, Fallon F, et al. Diversity of practices in telerehabilitation for children with disabilities and effective intervention characteristics: results from a systematic review. *Disabil Rehabil.* 2020;42(24):3424–3436. DOI: 10.1080/09638288.2019.1595750.

17. Adams RC, Tapia C. Early intervention, IDEA Part C Services, and the medical home: collaboration for best practice and best outcomes. *Pediatrics.* 2013;132:e1073–e1088.

18. IDEA Section 300.34 Related Services. https://sites.ed.gov/idea/regs/b/a/300.34; Accessed 30.09.21.

19. Burke BL JR, Hall RW. Section on Telehealth Care. Telemedicine: pediatric applications. *Pediatrics.* 2015;136(1):e293–e308. https://doi.org/10.1542/peds.2015-1517. PMID: 26122813; PMCID: PMC5754191.

20. Dullet NW, Geraghty EM, Kaufman T, et al. Impact of a university-based outpatient telemedicine program on time savings, travel costs, and environmental pollutants. *Value Health.* 2017;20(4):542–546. https://doi.org/10.1016/j.jval.2017.01.014. Epub 2017 Mar 6. PMID: 28407995.

21. Burdea GC, Jain A, Rabin B, et al. Long-term hand tele-rehabilitation on the PlayStation 3: benefits and challenges. *Conf Proc IEEE Eng Med Biol Soc.* 2011;2011:1835–1838. https://doi.org/10.1109/IEMBS.2011.6090522. PMID: 22254686.

CHAPTER 25

Surgical Rehabilitation Across Countries: A Model for Planning in Telerehabilitation

Jan Fridén ▨ Ines Bersch ▨ Fabrizio Fiumedinisi ▨ Silvia Schibli ▨ Sabrina Koch-Borner

Introduction

Telerehabilitation, supported by the worldwide use of smartphones, broadband internet, and computers, is a useful method in the intricate setup of the holistic treatment and rehabilitation of individuals with spinal cord injuries, traumatic brain injuries, strokes, and other causes of motor function impairment. Telerehabilitation provides additional diagnostic and therapeutic support to a wide range of patient populations with motor dysfunctions: from previous simple telephone calls for follow-up of patients in remote areas after discharge from the hospital to video-assisted examinations and therapies reaching other continents.

Telerehabilitation concepts are not new. In 1993 Delaplain and coworkers upgraded the rehabilitation process and established the use of videoconferencing for physiotherapy consultations and rehabilitation instructions from the Tripler Army Medical Center in Hawaii (Oahu) halfway across the Pacific Ocean to the Kwajalein Atoll (army base).[1] Telerehabilitation studies addressing postcardiac surgery rehabilitation are relatively abundant,[2] while studies in the field of surgical rehabilitation of patients with major motor dysfunctions are sparse. There are studies in hand surgery that show equivalent results as in physical follow-ups, a high degree of patient satisfaction, and no increased frequency of complications.[3,4] However, the patient selection in those studies consisted of more standardized procedures that usually required only postoperative training instructions or immobilization. Moreover, none of the studies included rare diseases or telerehabilitation across national borders.[5] Our structured international telerehabilitation approach integrated in our regular upper-limb reconstructive surgery service is new. The location of the Swiss Paraplegic Centre in the middle of Europe, and the fact that most of our team members are fluent in speaking and writing in English, French, German, and Italian, both facilitate communication.

Our outreach services, Nottwil Tetrahand and the International FES Centre at the Swiss Paraplegic Centre, have evolved rapidly over the last few years, in a large part due to the use of telerehabilitation and the increased demand for international services. Nottwil Tetrahand has tried to assure that treatment quality of telerehabilitation is safe, effective, patient-centered, timely, efficient, and equitable.[6] We believe that the traditional medical setting needs to be adapted to the new technological possibilities as much as possible.

A medical examination and the planning and execution of a rehabilitation program demand for a physical contact with hands-on practice at a certain time. This means that a physical examination

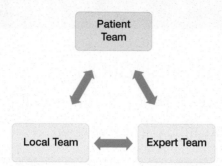

Fig. 25.1   A three-part relationship allowing patient to easily reach local and remote experts and vice versa. This structure provides a safety net for the patient. For details see Table 25.2.

by a physician and/or therapist is vital before a defined rehabilitation protocol can be initiated. Furthermore, a thorough patient evaluation is essential for the best possible rehabilitation outcomes and therefore requires high-quality input from the local health care team. In addition, and with our focus on surgical rehabilitation, a number of physical prerequisites need to be fulfilled before any preparatory measures for surgery are taken (see later).

The combination of telerehabilitation patient guidance and local health care professionals can guarantee continuous rehabilitation support and communication in all directions (Fig. 25.1). This is particularly important in surgical services to avoid/detect a potentially unfavorable evolution of a postoperative state, allowing for early countermeasures to commence. Furthermore, with the aid of the local health care professionals, follow-up checks including physical examination, as well as evaluations, are performed more efficiently and with more focus on medical details.

Accessibility and Data Security

We provide patient care with the belief that accessibility to our specialized services is important. Our homepage informs patients and colleagues about our services and how to connect with us. A shared email inbox is checked frequently to ensure patients and external colleagues a quick response to simple questions. For more complicated/technical questions or a specific patient request for a telerehabilitation session, planning is necessary. Patient data sent to us by a referring physician or other health professional need patient's approval. Data are then stored in personalized, limited-access special folders in a separate archive according to the Swiss Paraplegic Centre security regulations as described in the internal document "medical data storage."

Cross-border health care provides all European Union (EU)/European Economic Area (EEA) citizens with the opportunity to receive treatment in other EU/EEA countries.[5] Switzerland is not part of the EU but has a bilateral agreement with the EU and the European Free Trade Association countries, which enables patients to receive treatment in Switzerland paid for by their insurance. This means that an EU citizen can request medical treatment abroad according to the social insurance rules. All treatments abroad must, however, be approved in advance by the national health insurance in the patient's home country. Upon approval, a so-called S2 form is sent abroad for processing. National health services or health insurers generally grant authorization for treatment of rare diseases that are not available in home country or that are of documented better quality abroad. This applies provided that the treatment in question is also delivered for patients living in the country referred to. For non-European citizens, a deposit of the entire cost of care is required before the patient can undergo surgery and subsequent postoperative rehabilitation. In addition, two postoperative telerehabilitation consultations are charged (2 × 250 CHF = 500 CHF [≈560 USD]).

Our telerehabilitation platform is MS Teams. After giving consent to participate, we invite patients to join the platform and inform the patient that no recording whatsoever takes place; however, question and answer notes are taken and added to the patient's chart.

Telerehabilitation in Upper-Extremity Surgery

Our telerehabilitation program involves the remote assessments of preselected patients suitable for surgical reconstruction of arm and hand function. Additionally, it includes follow-ups at fixed times after reconstructive surgery, as well as per request communications with patients and therapists during the course of postsurgery rehabilitation. It does not, however, provide rehabilitation services through telecommunication technology directly to patients at home without the physical presence of a therapist.

Rehabilitative, reconstructive surgery for persons with disabilities includes several challenges. It is obvious that teaching, for example, contracture prevention in a patient with spinal cord injury or traumatic brain injury requires close contact with the patient. Also, it is evident that surgical reconstruction of the upper extremity in these or other patient groups necessitates both thorough expert physical examination and additional tests (electromyography [EMG], magnetic resonance imaging [MRI], joint range of motion, motor point mapping, spasticity, and pain analyses). However, initial contact via telerehabilitation can successfully address key issues about feasibility before intervention (Table 25.1). For the upper extremities, examinations and tests are almost

TABLE 25.1 ■ Telemedicine Q&A Level 1 Used for Primary Assessment of Suitability for Surgery.

Topic #[a]	Questions	Answers	Considerations	Decision
1	Medical, physical, mental, social factors satisfactory?	Yes/No	Timing, motivation, rehabilitation status OK?	Yes: full preop assessment. Motor point mapping needed (nerve transfer)? No: surgery contraindicated
2	Patient's goal?	COPM[b]	Goals realistic?	Yes: full preop assessment No: surgery contraindicated
3	Spasticity? Where?	Yes/No	Affecting decision-making?	Yes: continue conservative treatment No: no contraindication to surgery
4	Pain? Yes/No, Where?	Yes/No	Affecting decision-making? Further treatment?	Yes: continue conservative treatment No: no contraindication to surgery
5	Comorbidities?	Yes/No	Affecting decision-making?	Yes: continue conservative treatment No: no contraindication to surgery
6	Medication? What?	Yes/No	Affecting decision-making?	Yes: continue conservative treatment No: no contraindication to surgery

[a]Note: Topics 1 and 2 require "YES" under "Considerations" to qualify for next step in preparation for surgery. If "NO" surgery is contraindicated.
[b]Canadian Occupational Performance Measure.[7]

exclusively undertaken with the patient sitting in an electric or manual wheelchair. This facilitates targeted physical revaluation of upper-extremity functions and allows for primary assessment of whether surgical reconstruction is a treatment option. Telerehabilitation is also a patient-oriented, cost-efficient tool to improve and assure posthospital discharge rehabilitation on site after the return to home/local rehabilitation. Our telerehabilitation postsurgery starts with multiple weeks of inpatient care including therapy—three to four times daily for motor relearning and training of transferred or reinnervating muscle functions. Subsequently, at the time of discharge, detailed written instructions with didactic illustrations about what, how, and when to train new and previous motor functions together with general instructions about training of trunk stability, shoulder mobility, and other key functions to optimize arm and hand functions are provided. The gradual transition of muscle functions into patient performance and ability in daily life is also clearly outlined in these instructions. At our follow-up telerehabilitation contacts, all these functions and abilities are tested in a patient-specific manner, depending on the surgeries performed.

International Telerehabilitation Services

By working with and through other rehabilitation centers outside Switzerland, we have gradually built mutual understanding and trust to offer patients telerehabilitation consultations across several national borders. Typically, the cooperative rehabilitation unit or our unit requests a date and time for consultation. To obtain a time-efficient consultation and to meet the patient's expectations, we have structured the consultations into three levels depending on the expected complexity of the case to be presented (Table 25.2). The consultations include follow-ups at 6 and 12 months postsurgery, as well as new patients. One to two follow-ups (15 minutes each) and one new patient for primary assessment (30 minutes) usually can be performed in a 1-hour clinic. Often, a complication-free patient can be followed up at Level 2 or 3 (Table 25.2). The follow-up patients report their perceived outcomes including scoring how well they have reached their prioritized goals (performance and satisfaction) according to the Canadian Occupational Performance Measures (COPM).[7] Patients' scores are then compared with the corresponding scores for the identical activities reported preoperatively. Since this is our primary outcome measurement, it is crucial for both the referring rehabilitation provider and our own unit to verify that the patient has reached or has clearly improved their skills so they can reach their preoperatively defined goals.

For primary telerehabilitation assessments, background patient information (e.g., medical history, level of lesion, upper-extremity muscle, and sensory status) has already been emailed to our coordinator. Typically, planning and reconstruction strategies for patients with confounding factors such as comorbidities, pressure sores, severe pain, and spasticity are also discussed separately prior to the video visit.

TABLE 25.2 ■ Telerehabilitation Three-Level Settings in Nottwil Reconstructive Upper-Extremity Surgery Unit.

Level of Consultation	At Patient's End	At Expert Team's End
Level 1	Patient[a] + rehabilitation team	Physician + therapist[b] and assistant
Level 2	Patient + physician or therapist	Physician + therapist
Level 3	Patient + personal assistant or relative	Physician + therapist or assistant

[a]Patient > 18 years of age and has agreed to participate in telerehabilitation consultation.
[b]Therapist specialized in surgical rehabilitation after CNS lesions.

ELECTRICAL STIMULATION IN DIAGNOSTICS AND TREATMENT

Electrical stimulation is an integral part of the diagnostics and treatment before and after rehabilitative surgery of the upper extremities. It can effectively be applied for improvement of body structure and function or activity and participation in people with neurological diseases.[8–12] In parallel with the increased attention and application of nerve transfers to restore lost functions in tetraplegia, electrical stimulation plays a growing role to confirm excitability of donor nerves as well as differentiate between fully or partially denervated and innervated target muscles suitable for neurotization. Recently, Bersch and coworkers presented several studies addressing the functional integrity of selected, topographically defined stimulation points (motor point mapping) in the upper extremity.[13,14] This is now included in our standard protocol for patient assessment prior to determining whether to perform nerve transfer surgery.

A person with a neurological disease who decides to use either functional electrical stimulation (FES) or neuromuscular electrical stimulation (NMES) often needs to commit to long-term use. The mode of action in NMES is stimulation of an efferent nerve that finally leads to a contraction of a muscle or muscle group. The contractions elicited in this way do not necessarily bring a function that can be used in everyday life. The latter is the aim of FES. For the supervising therapist, this implies supporting a patient over the entire treatment period, coaching the stimulation setup including the stimulation that is embedded in exercises or daily activities, changing parameters or stimulation duty cycles, and answering questions that arise in the practical management of the technical equipment. When implementing electrical stimulation for the upper extremities one should be aware of both the advantages and obstacles that might occur.

Application of FES or NMES goes beyond an inpatient rehabilitation or takes place in a domestic setting from the beginning. Furthermore, the stimulation treatment can be continued in outpatient therapies supported by physio- or occupational therapists without special expertise in applying FES or NMES. Once the individually programmed device has been instructed either to the patient or the caregiver physically, the follow-up can be conducted online. Depending on the stimulation focus and target, the instruction requires equipment and sufficient comprehension in the execution by the end user. For example, in case of reconstructive Tetrahand surgery preconditioning of a donor or recipient muscle, NMES is applied for strengthening[8] or direct muscle stimulation for maintenance of muscle properties.[9] Hereby, the execution of stimulation involves one or two muscles, which means that one or two pairs of electrodes must be placed. In muscle strengthening, the stimulation is usually combined with an explicit exercise. For this purpose, an online follow-up provides all the necessary requirements and can be done with a mobile phone, tablet, or laptop. Online support can also be provided if functional tasks are supported by electrical stimulation (FES) during outpatient therapy, performed by physiotherapists or occupational therapists. This might take place as co-treatments. It is feasible and straightforward to modify stimulation parameters, electrode placements, and exercises in this context.

Online follow-ups require well-structured preparation of the stimulation schedule, the preprogrammed device, the combined exercises if indicated, and the necessary communication tools (mobile phone, tablet, and laptop). Most stimulation devices are not user-friendly for people with impaired motor control of the arm and hand. Therefore understanding the settings and the physical handling of the device and the electrodes is often shared between the person affected and a caregiver. However, adaptations in stimulation programs and troubleshooting in case of stimulator failures need to be secured. The latter must be solved smoothly and should not occur frequently. Otherwise, experience has shown that this is a cause for abandoning the stimulation. Open-mindedness, flexibility, and perseverance are needed from all parts in device settings and adjustments of the treatment. Explanations and instructions from the therapist must be precise. The technical equipment on the patient's side must be satisfactory so that high-quality visual and acoustic transmission can be obtained.

It is important to eliminate barriers from the very beginning or to reduce them to a minimum. The communication channel and online platform to be considered must be defined. The patient defines his or her options and the therapist follows them. If the patient has no technical affinity, it is recommended in advance to involve people from the patient's environment who are willing to be present during the online consultations. Technical ignorance, antipathy toward virtual forms of communication, and fear of doing something wrong or appearing ignorant must be taken seriously and should be reduced with professional assistance. Unfortunately, there are also limitations in setting up telerehabilitation for electrical stimulation consultations and support. The patient must have internet access and a device that allows video transmission. Generally, tetraplegic persons need a supporting person to help with the stimulation and the online consultation. On the side of the consultant and her/his employer, the usage of multiple online channels should be allowed with the necessary security regarding data protection. Additionally, insurance companies must also accept this form of consultation as a professional service as the therapists will charge for it at an identical level to hands-on treatment.

Future Recommendations

We have found that our telerehabilitation services have resulted in increased collaboration with other professionals and an increase in visits to our unit for hands-on participation in the various steps of pre-, peri-, and postoperative treatment. We believe this collaboration promotes state-of-the-art care and improves interprofessional exchange of information. In addition, case discussions across local and national borders with and without patients can improve the treatment of patients with spinal cord injury (Fig. 25.2).

As of February 1, 2021, we have organized 53 Level 1 telerehabilitation conferences across borders: 15 countries, 5 continents (Table 25.3). In addition, we have completed 90 international

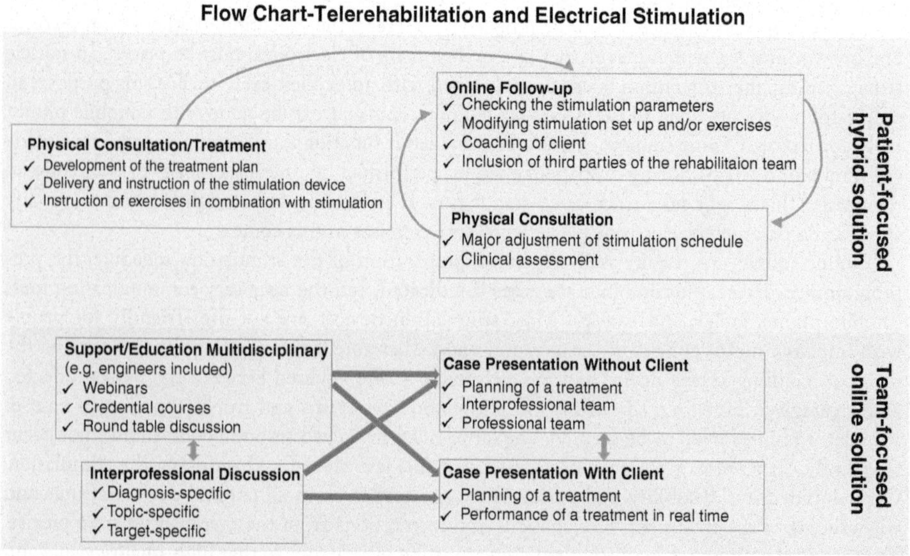

Flow Chart-Telerehabilitation and Electrical Stimulation

Physical Consultation/Treatment
✓ Development of the treatment plan
✓ Delivery and instruction of the stimulation device
✓ Instruction of exercises in combination with stimulation

Online Follow-up
✓ Checking the stimulation parameters
✓ Modifying stimulation set up and/or exercises
✓ Coaching of client
✓ Inclusion of third parties of the rehabilitaion team

Physical Consultation
✓ Major adjustment of stimulation schedule
✓ Clinical assessment

Patient-focused hybrid solution

Support/Education Multidisciplinary
(e.g. engineers included)
✓ Webinars
✓ Credential courses
✓ Round table discussion

Case Presentation Without Client
✓ Planning of a treatment
✓ Interprofessional team
✓ Professional team

Interprofessional Discussion
✓ Diagnosis-specific
✓ Topic-specific
✓ Target-specific

Case Presentation With Client
✓ Planning of a treatment
✓ Performance of a treatment in real time

Team-focused online solution

Fig. 25.2 Potential applications of telerehabilitation in the context of electrical stimulation (*blue*: patient-focused, *green*: professionals-focused).

TABLE 25.3 ▪ **Nottwil Reconstructive Upper-Extremity Surgery Telerehabilitation Consultations.**

Country	Consultation	Physician's Advice	Therapist's Advice
USA	5	2	3
Colombia	4		3
Brazil	3	5	2
South Africa	2	3	
Greece	3	2	
Cyprus	2	8	15
Portugal	2	1	
France	1	3	4
Slovenia	2		1
Great Britain	3	5	2
Netherlands	15		
Germany	5	8	16
Poland	2	2	
Luxembourg	2	2	2
Turkey	2	1	

Level 2 to 3 telerehabilitation sessions. Based on the vast interest and positive patient feedback, we believe that this service will grow.

LIMITATIONS

Telerehabilitation for rehabilitative surgery is an important diagnostic and follow-up tool, as it allows for initial assessment as well as control and continuity of postsurgery training after discharge. There are, however, obvious barriers in telerehabilitation, and it can be particularly difficult for those in the rehabilitation field. Many of us work closely with our patients, and we know too well how challenging it is to teach specific motor relearning exercises for someone with a spinal cord injury or monitor a patient's progression from a traumatic brain injury. Rigorous preparation and the multilevel, multiprofessional three-part relationship is thus necessary to (Figs. 25.1 and 25.2) provide a safety net for the patient.

We have faced a separate but incredibly important challenge with splinting before and after surgery. All splints made in-house, whether in an inpatient or outpatient setting, are custom-made and molded individually to obtain the exact position required, depending on the treatment goals. At our telerehabilitation consultations, control of the splint fitting cannot be 100% accurate. We have also observed multiple times that prefabricated, standard splints are suboptimal in terms of hand position. Typically, our splints should be configured with the wrist in intrinsic plus position, pronated forearm, wrist in 30° of extension, finger metacarpo-phalangeal (MCP) joints in 80° of flexion, proximal inter-phalangeal (PIP) in full extension, and thumb slightly abducted (Fig. 25.3). If not, the splint must be adjusted. This can be organized via all levels of consultations (Levels 1–3).

RESEARCH

Introducing and expanding an auxiliary health care service as described earlier necessitates a careful analysis of factors affecting the final treatment outcomes. A logical primary subject

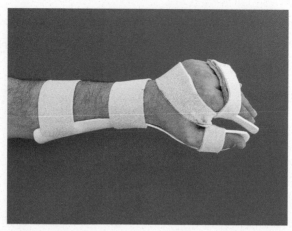

Fig. 25.3 Safe intrinsic plus splint position after grip reconstruction—wrist and PIP joints extended, MCP joints flexed.

for research is to question the patients, their relatives, caregivers, therapists, and physicians about their experiences. This approach would of course include tips about how to improve the telerehabilitation service. Additionally, it is pertinent for us to document the type and amount of training performed at home versus locally and if the outcomes and complication rates are different. Since our primary outcome measurement tool is the COPM, which itself is suitable for a telerehabilitation setting, this comparison should be straightforward to perform. Also, we wonder if questions can be addressed and answered with the same accuracy in telerehabilitation as in standard consultations. Traditional communication tools and social interactions may be impaired or misinterpreted, for example, gestures, facial expressions, eye contact, expressions of empathy, or fear.

FUTURE PERSPECTIVES AND RECOMMENDATIONS

The hybrid system of consultations with the physical presence of patient and experts combined with various settings of online consultations for assessments, postop controls, and treatment, for example, electrical stimulation, improves the care, monitoring, and general support of patients participating in surgical rehabilitation. Well-prepared telerehabilitaton sessions are cost-efficient, but most importantly, they add value to the patients. However, it is imperative that the health system recognizes, promotes, and expands the added value of telerehabilitation, especially for people with neurological dysfunctions, for example, individuals with tetraplegia or stroke who are limited in mobility. Despite its limitations and the challenges in practicing across borders, we believe that this method of rehabilitation has a great potential to facilitate patient's access to expert assessments, treatment in selected cases, and control of rehabilitation progress. Hence, it should be regarded as equal to physical consultations and reimbursement should be comparable. Finally, although collected data are not for sale, the legal framework for the collection and processing of personal information, General Data Protection Regulation (GDPR), needs to be understood and adhered to in the particular telerehabilitation setting in which one practices.

CASE STUDY 1

A 28-year-old woman fell from a climbing wall at age 5 years and sustained a proximal ulna fracture including subluxation of the radial head (Monteggia fracture). Initially, a primary closed reduction attempt was done, followed by a second one due to remaining dislocation. Five days later, compartment syndrome was diagnosed, and her palmar forearm was decompressed. An additional four operations did not improve function or position. At age of 7 years, all treatment and rehabilitation efforts were discontinued, and she had to adapt to functional loss and deformity. The patient emailed our Tetrahand service 18 years later with the question of whether her function could be improved. She had a severe right wrist flexion contracture, inability to use the fingers properly, thumb-in-palm deformity, and an overall underdeveloped arm length and atrophic musculature. After checking her medical documentation, we invited her to the Swiss Paraplegic Centre for consultation and assessment of her Volkmann's contracture.

Her right arm was smaller than the left arm but with full sensation in her hand. Her wrist was in a 40° flexed resting position with slightly flexed fingers and a scar along the entire palmar forearm with massive adhesions to the flexor tendons. Active wrist extension was visible, as well as finger and wrist flexion, but the flexor tendons were severely adhered to the skin and subcutaneous tissue, thus restraining any active wrist motion. The extensor carpi ulnaris tendon was subluxated palmarly, which by activation caused an even more pronounced wrist flexion. All wrist and finger extensor muscles demonstrated fully innervated lower motor neuron function as evidenced by electrical stimulation.[14] At this time point we offered her a surgical procedure to correct her flexion deformity followed by intensive postoperative therapy.

One year later she informed us that she wanted to undergo the surgical intervention and the postop rehabilitation as outlined. Once again, we invited to come to the facility for a face-to-face consultation to check if her function remained the same. At this point, we also did our standard presurgery assessments as well as documented her prioritized goals according to the COPM.

Her primary goals were to have a more normal appearance of her hand, to be able to hold, for example, a cucumber while cutting with the left hand, and to tap her laptop keyboard more skillfully (Fig. 25.4A). After this consultation, all necessary preoperative assessments were performed via email or video.

The surgery took place on January 28, 2020. The intervention included extensive adhesiolysis of the flexor tendons and muscle bellies, neurolysis of the median nerve along the entire forearm, lengthening of all wrist and superficial finger flexor tendons, and transposition of the subluxated extensor carpi ulnaris tendon to the extensor carpi radialis brevis.

On the first day after surgery, passive mobility of the wrist ranged from full flexion to 20° of extension. Active extension reached 0°. She had to wear a thermoplastic splint around-the-clock except for her therapy sessions. After 4 weeks of intensive therapy, her wrist showed a passive mobility up to 40° slightly in radial deviation and active extension to 10°. Active ulnar deviation as well as active finger extension remained difficult because of the long-term non-use.

Due to COVID-19, she had to proceed with the training by herself once back in her country of residence. To maintain control of her progress and to provide guidance, we agreed on video calls. Four and half months after surgery she reported how much more frequently and skillfully she was able to use her hand in daily activities. At our telerehabilitation consultation, we were able to verify that the resting position of the wrist was still in 10° flexion, but she had passive mobility to 50° extension. Actively she was able to extend her wrist to neutral position and slightly beyond. She had still 2- to 3-cm distance between fingertips and palm. We instructed her to proceed with her defined exercises. Four months later, she was incredibly happy, as her primary goal of a more normal looking hand was reached and visible to everyone; however, she could still not make a fist, because of remaining tightness of the intrinsic hand muscles. In our video call, we instructed her in detail how to treat the stiffness.

Currently, 1 year after surgery she has continued to make progress. She has already reached some of her other goals (Fig. 25.4B) and her COPM scores have changed substantially, for both performance and satisfaction (Fig. 25.5). According to the patient, her telerehabilitation follow-ups were instrumental for her recovery.

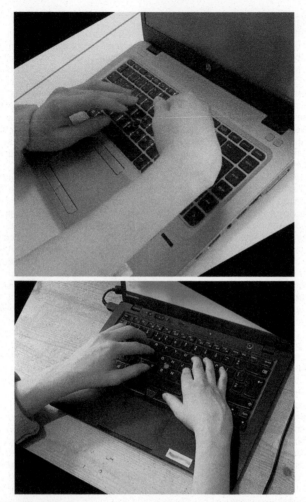

Fig. 25.4   Preoperative (A) and postoperative (B) images of patient tapping keyboard. For details see Case Study 1.

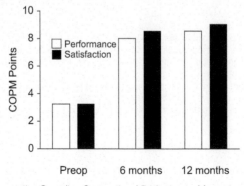

Fig. 25.5   Pre- and postoperative Canadian Occupational Performance Measures scores for patient in Case Study 1.

CASE STUDY 2

A 29-year-old man has a tetraplegia C6 AIS B after a water sport accident. After primary stabilization in the country where he sustained his accident, he decided to do his primary rehabilitation at the Swiss Paraplegic Center. In our Tetrahand expert group, all tetraplegic patients are assessed and informed about conservative and surgical interventions to improve their arm/hand function.

This patient continued to have intact shoulder muscle control, active elbow flexion, wrist extension, and wrist flexion. However, triceps function as well as finger and thumb extension and flexion were missing (Fig. 25.6A). Since he was less than 1 year post-SCI, we performed targeted motor point mappings for potential nerve transfers.[13,14] These mappings demonstrated intact lower motor neurons for key muscle functions. All other parameters were also satisfactory and thus we planned surgical intervention.

In July 2020 the patient underwent double, bilateral nerve transfers of the supinator motor branches to the posterior interosseous nerve (S-PIN) and the brachialis motor branches to the anterior interosseous nerve (B-AIN) to improve grip function and hand opening. Postoperatively, he was treated as an inpatient for 2 weeks. The first days after surgery he used an electric wheelchair to unload the nerve transfers. We instructed the patient to perform finger and thumb extension, 10 repetitions, three to five times per day as an assistant blocked the supination movement to mimic the original movement governed by the donor nerve. The assisting person extended the fingers and thumb and the patient imagined these movements. The same type of training was applied for flexion of the fingers and thumb. As soon as a distinct movement of the new function was visible, the external resistance of the original movement direction was reduced. These guided exercises were performed during the rehabilitation phase and thereafter the patient performed them independently at home according to a written protocol. During his inpatient stay, the patient was instructed to repeat the regenerating movements every day for the next 6 months.

In January 2021 we saw the patient for his 6-month postsurgical telerehabilitation Level 2 consultation to determine any visible improvements. The patient was pleased with the improvements he had achieved. He has a more open hand and reported that he was able to flex the fingertips when his wrist is stabilized. To be able to examine the functions in a more precise way, we instructed his wife to stabilize the wrist in different positions and instructed him to do different movements. A clear extension of the fingers (Fig. 25.6B) as well as ulnar deviation of the wrist were visible. The deep finger flexors were active with the wrist in an extended position. With help of the assistant, and under our guidance, all these tests could be readily undertaken and documented via telerehabilitation. We informed the patient that we had confirmed the first signs of reinnervation 6 months after surgery. We advised and instructed him to proceed with the active motor training and to keep all the joints supple by passive mobilization exercises performed by himself or by a caregiver. We will follow up the patient in 6 months for his annual follow-up and together with the patient plan further reconstructions.

These cases demonstrate how telerehabilitation consultations allow for clinical controls before and after surgery and for adjustments of rehabilitation protocols when necessary. As can be seen, telerehabilitation assists us to actively invite our patients to connect with us for questions, advice, and guidance when needed.

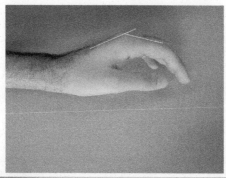

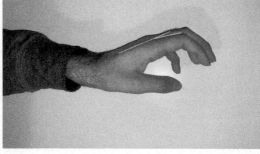

Fig. 25.6 Preoperative (A) and 6-month postoperative (B) pictures of patients who underwent bilateral nerve transfers for restoration of finger and thumb flexors and extensors. Both images depict posture of the hand when patient is asked to extend his fingers. Note the increased extension in the MCP joints in (B) compared with (A). For details see Case Study 2.

References

1. Delaplain CB, Lindborg CE, Norton SA, et al. Tripler pioneers telemedicine across the Pacific. *Hawaii Med J.* 1993;52:338–339.
2. Scalvini S, Zanelli E, Comini L, et al. Home-based exercise rehabilitation with telemedicine following cardiac surgery. *J Telemed Telecare.* 2009;15(6):297–301.
3. Grandizio LC, Foster BK, Klena JC. Telemedicine in hand and upper-extremity surgery. *J Hand Surg Am.* 2020;45(3):239–242.
4. Grandizio LC, Mettler AW, Caselli ME, et al. Telemedicine after upper extremity surgery: a prospective study of program implementation. *J Hand Surg Am.* 2020;45(9):795–801.
5. European Commission Patient's right to accessing healthcare in any EU*/EEA* country. Directive 2011/24/EU on patients' rights in cross-border healthcare. *Manual for patients.* 2019:1–34.
6. Schwamm LE. Telehealth: seven strategies to successfully implement disruptive technology and transform health care. *Health Affairs.* 2014;33:200–206.
7. Law M, Baptiste S, McColl M, et al. The Canadian occupational performance measure: an outcome measure for occupational therapy. *Can J Occup Ther.* 1990;57(2):82–87.
8. Kapadia N, Moineau B, Popovic MR. Functional electrical stimulation therapy for retraining reaching and grasping after spinal cord injury and stroke. *Front Neurosci.* 2020;14:718.
9. Sharif H, Gammage K, Chun S, et al. Effects of FES-ambulation training on locomotor function and health-related quality of life in individuals with spinal cord injury. *Top Spinal Cord Inj Rehabil.* 2014;20(1):58–69.
10. Popovic MR, Kapadia N, Zivanovic V, et al. Functional electrical stimulation therapy of voluntary grasping versus only conventional rehabilitation for patients with subacute incomplete tetraplegia: a randomized clinical trial. *Neurorehabil Neural Repair.* 2011;25(5):433–442.

11. Bersch I, Fridén J. Role of functional electrical stimulation in tetraplegia hand surgery. *Arch Phys Med Rehabil.* 2016;97(suppl 6):S154–S159.
12. Bersch I, Fridén J. Upper and lower motor neuron lesions in tetraplegia: implications for surgical nerve transfer to restore hand function. *J Appl Physiol.* 2020;129(5):1214–1219.
13. Bersch I, Koch-Borner S, Fridén J. Electrical stimulation-a mapping system for hand dysfunction in tetraplegia. *Spinal Cord.* 2018;56(5):516–522.
14. Bersch I, Koch-Borner S, Fridén J. Motor point topography of fundamental grip actuators in tetraplegia: implications in nerve transfer surgery. *J Neurotrauma.* 2020;37(3):441–447.

CHAPTER 26

Telerehabilitation in Disasters

Colleen O'Connell

Introduction

A disaster is an event or situation that causes great damage, destruction, and human suffering; overwhelms local capacity; and can necessitate requests for national or international assistance.[1] In its 2019 Global Assessment Report, the Head of the United Nations (UN) Office for Disaster Risk Reduction states that "the human race has never before faced such large and complex threats."[2] With the launch of the Global Humanitarian Overview 2021, the UN Secretary-General has quoted:

> Conflict, climate change and COVID-19 have created the greatest humanitarian challenge since the Second World War… together, we must mobilize resources and stand in solidarity with people in their darkest hour of need.[3]

Climate change directly impacts health through the injuries, displacements, and deaths associated with floods, storms, wildfires, and heat-related illnesses.[4] Occurrences of extreme weather events have doubled since the year 2000, with disasters associated with natural hazards having affected 60 million people in 2018 alone.[5] Between 1998 and 2017, 2 billion people were affected by floods and 125 million by earthquakes.[5] Not limited to natural and environmental events, disasters in the context of human activity, war, terrorism, industrial catastrophe, and pandemics, for instance, demand large-scale coordinated response efforts and attention. In the 21st century, conflicts are increasingly affecting civilian populations; since 2010 the world has reached the highest number of internally displaced persons (IDPs) ever with 51 million IDPs and doubling to 20 million refugees.[6] The global COVID-19 pandemic is reported to have set back decades of development progress, with extreme poverty increasing for the first time since 1990.[3]

Reducing the risks and minimizing negative impacts of disasters is approached through comprehensive emergency management.[7] Generally, comprehensive emergency management involves a cycle of four phases: preparedness, response, recovery, and mitigation (Fig. 26.1). During the preparedness phase, planning, training exercises, and resource management activities are conducted. Response in a disaster focuses on saving lives and reducing damage and covers warnings, evacuations, emergency response, medical care, and relief efforts. Evolving to the recovery phase, service restoration, reconstruction, and longer-term care and support are implemented. Mitigation strategies can include evaluation of previous response outcomes, vulnerability identification and awareness, and public education.

DISASTER COORDINATION

Large-scale disasters such as sudden-onset emergencies necessitating international response are typically managed under the auspices of the UN Office for Disaster Risk Reduction, which covers preparedness, response, and recovery measures. Coordination of responses is operationalized

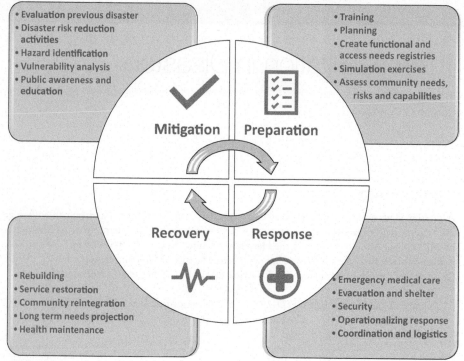

- Evaluation previous disaster
- Disaster risk reduction activities
- Hazard identification
- Vulnerability analysis
- Public awareness and education

Mitigation

- Training
- Planning
- Create functional and access needs registries
- Simulation exercises
- Assess community needs, risks and capabilities

Preparation

Recovery

- Rebuilding
- Service restoration
- Community reintegration
- Long term needs projection
- Health maintenance

Response

- Emergency medical care
- Evacuation and shelter
- Security
- Operationalizing response
- Coordination and logistics

Fig. 26.1 Comprehensive Emergency Management: four phases of the disaster cycle.

through a cluster approach, which groups disaster response into clusters covering each of the main areas of action, including health, shelter, sanitation and water, logistics, and emergency telecommunications. Various humanitarian organizations including UN agencies (such as UNICEF, the United Nations Children's Fund) and nonprofit organizations (International Federation of Red Cross and Red Crescent Societies) are designated by the Inter-Agency Standing Committee (IASC) as lead(s) responsible for each cluster's activities. The IASC was created by the UN in 1991 and is the highest-level humanitarian coordination forum of the UN. The Health Cluster is led by the World Health Organization (WHO), and the Emergency Telecommunications by the World Food Program. The UN response is coordinated with the national authorities, and humanitarian actors should actively engage with and support the national and local authorities to lead or progressively take over the response.[8]

DISASTERS AND DISABILITY

The field of disaster medicine has made important advances in the past 25 years, with formalization of training, education, and clinical competencies.[7] While surgical and acute care are traditionally the focus of emergency medical responses, there is increasing recognition of the critical role of rehabilitation in disaster management.[9–12] Articles 11, 25, and 26 of the UN *Convention on the Rights of Persons With Disabilities* clearly support as a human right the access to rehabilitation for persons with disabilities, including during emergencies and natural disasters.[13] Unfortunately, in many areas affected by disasters, rehabilitation resources and infrastructure are often poorly developed, particularly in low and low-middle income countries.[9, 14] Relative to general populations, persons with disabilities endure higher risks in disaster and emergency situations, including conflicts.[15] Physical and societal barriers include inaccessible transport and shelters, loss of specialized equipment such as wheelchairs and communication aids, deprioritization for emergency services, and absence of disability-specific planning. Hurricane Katrina in the United States exposed such vulnerabilities, with disproportionate death rates for persons with disability.[16]

Notwithstanding the higher risk and vulnerability of persons with disability in disasters, improvement in disaster responses, in general, has resulted in increased numbers of persons surviving severe trauma events, with high numbers of injured survivors relative to mortality.[11] Injuries more commonly occurring in disasters include complex fractures and peripheral nerve injuries, spinal cord and brain injuries, and amputations. Earthquakes result in lower-extremity trauma with amputations, compound fractures, soft tissue, nerve, and spinal cord injuries. Cyclones cause more upper body trauma, with head injuries most common.[17] Wars, conflicts, and terrorist attacks result in blast injuries and gunshot wounds; a report from a hospital in Turkey treating refugees from the Syrian war described firearm injuries as the major cause of injuries needing emergency surgery, with a survival rate of 24% for neurosurgical cases.[18] Between 150 and 750 new spinal cord injuries were estimated to have occurred in each of the earthquakes in Iran (2003), Pakistan (2005), and Haiti (2010).[19]

New disabling or potentially disabling injuries require dedicated, targeted, and timely rehabilitation interventions to reduce impairment and optimize outcomes for the injured, the family, and community.[9] Evidence supports that rehabilitation in disasters improves patient and community outcomes in both the short and long term, reduced disability and complications, improved participation, and quality of life.[9, 11, 12] In Pakistan, rehabilitation professionals and trainees in the military program were able to provide more specialized care for one cohort of spinal cord survivors, which demonstrated improved outcomes relative to those who did not receive specialized rehabilitation care.[20] Following the 2010 earthquake in Haiti, persons with new spinal cord injuries were denied admission to some field hospitals, and one center reported "…we believed it would be incorrect to use our limited resources to treat patients with such a minimal chance of ultimate rehabilitation."[21] While many persons with spinal cord injury did ultimately get treated in Haiti[22] — in fact Haiti was represented at the 2012 Paralympics in London, UK by one such individual — the oft-overlooked yet vital role of rehabilitation in disasters was evident. The aftermaths of the Haitian earthquake, coupled with other relatively recent disasters including the Pakistan earthquake, Sichuan, China earthquake 2008, and Hurricane Katrina 2005, have mobilized efforts of international aid organizations, the WHO, and disability advocates and professions to promote, strengthen, and regulate disaster management in the context of persons with disabilities (Table 26.1). Guidance notes, training resources, and rehabilitation recommendations have been developed, further supporting a more structured approach across the disaster life cycle. Core rehabilitation-specific activities during a disaster response have been proposed, with refinement informed by experience and research (Fig. 26.2).[7,9] In the United States, a "functional-needs approach" has been adopted by the Federal Emergency Management Agency since 2010 in identifying disability-related needs in a disaster. Five areas are considered: communication, medical health, functional independence, supervision, and transportation (C-MIST), recognizing that persons with disabilities as well as other vulnerable groups (children, elderly) may need additional assistance.[23]

Telerehabilitation in Disasters

The goals of rehabilitation in a disaster are not unlike any rehabilitation setting; manage the injury/trauma, prevent secondary complications, apply a holistic approach to functional restoration and recovery, and facilitate community reintegration.

Telehealth strategies have been used effectively in disaster situations for several decades, including human-caused disasters and natural disasters. In 1988 the National Aeronautics and Space

TABLE 26.1 ■ International Organizations Active in Rehabilitation in Disasters.

Organization	Activities/Mission	Resource Examples[a]	Website
World Health Organization (WHO)	WHO works worldwide to promote health, keep the world safe, and serve the vulnerable; including goal to protect a billion more people from health emergencies	World report on disability Guidance note on disability and emergency risk management for health Disability considerations during the COVID-19 outbreak Minimum technical standards and recommendations for rehabilitation (HI, ICRC, WHO, Christian Blind Mission)	http://who.int/health-topics/disability
Humanity and Inclusion (HI)	International aid organization working in situations of poverty and exclusion, conflict, and disaster. Works alongside people with disabilities and vulnerable populations	Early rehabilitation in conflicts and disasters; guide for therapists Responding internationally to disasters: a do's and don'ts guide for rehabilitation professionals	http://hi.org http://disasterready.org
International Committee of the Red Cross (ICRC)	Independent neutral organization ensuring humanitarian protection and assistance for victims of armed conflict and other situations of violence	Exercises for lower-limb amputees Management of limb injuries during conflicts and disasters	http://icrc.org
United Nations Office for the Coordination of Humanitarian Affairs (OCHA)	OCHA contributes to principled and effective humanitarian response through coordination, advocacy, policy, information management, and humanitarian financing tools and services	Relief Web—global online site for timely and accessible resources	https://reliefweb.int/
Médecins Sans Frontières	Nonprofit, member-based organization, provides medical assistance to people affected by conflict, epidemics, disasters, or exclusion from health care	Medical Guidelines: Essential drugs	http://msf.org
International Society of Physical and Rehabilitation Medicine	Professional organization of physicians and researchers in physical and rehabilitation; Disaster Rehabilitation Committee advocates for physical and rehabilitation medicine perspective in minimizing disability, optimizing functioning, and health-related quality of life in persons who sustain traumatic injury, and those with preexisting disability during natural or man-made disasters	Multiple publications on rehabilitation in disasters	http://isprm.org

Continued

TABLE 26.1 ■ International Organizations Active in Rehabilitation in Disasters.—Cont'd

Organization	Activities/Mission	Resource Examples[a]	Website
International Spinal Cord Society	Professional organization of spinal cord injury clinicians and scientists; endeavors to foster education, research, and clinical excellence	International perspectives on spinal cord injury Online education and training modules for health professionals	http://iscos. org.uk http://elearnsci. org
International Society for Prosthetics and Orthotics	Professional organization aiming to improve the quality of life for persons who may benefit from prosthetic, orthotic, mobility, and assistive devices	Implementing prosthetic and orthotic services in low-income settings	http://ispoint. org

[a]Many of these publications are collaborative efforts of multiple organizations.

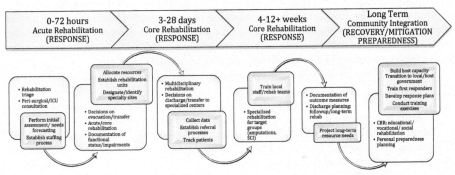

Fig. 26.2 Disaster Rehabilitation Continuum. Key clinical activities are in *unshaded* boxes and nonclinical activities in *shaded* boxes. *CBR*, Community based rehabilitation; *ICU*, intensive care unit; *SCI*, spinal cord injury. (Adapted from Fig. 1. A suggested plan of rehabilitation interventions after a natural disaster, in Rathore FA, Gosney JE, Reinhardt JD, et al. Medical rehabilitation after natural disasters: why, when and how? *Arch Phys Med Rehab.* 2012;93(10):1875–1881 and used with permission from Chapter 24, Gosney J and O'Connell C. Rehabilitation of disaster casualties. In: *Koenig and Schultz's Disaster Medicine: Comprehensive Principles and Practices, Cambridge University Press, 2016.*)

Administration agency deployed a spacebridge to facilitate telerehabilitation support for the earthquake victims in Armenia, and the US armed forces has a long history of employing telerehabilitation support in military humanitarian action.[24] In a review of telerehabilitation and disasters published in 2014, the authors concluded that telerehabilitation systems should be established in disaster-risk areas as a preparedness strategy.[25]

The merits of telerehabilitation approaches have been reported for conditions such as stroke, musculoskeletal and neuromuscular disorders, and are well described in this textbook. However, there is a paucity of literature specific to telerehabilitation in the context of disasters. Drawing on disaster rehabilitation evidence and extrapolating telerehabilitation principles from the general non-disaster field can inform current telerehabilitation approaches across the disaster cycle and identify further research needs. In a special report published in the *Journal of Rehabilitation Medicine,* authors call on the need to develop innovative models of rehabilitation during disasters, including telerehabilitation in order to optimize delivery of timely, cost-efficient, and patient-centered services as needed.[11]

One of the key benefits of telerehabilitation initiatives is the increased ability for persons with disability to access essential health services when physical attendance at a hospital or clinic is not possible or represents a significant burden. A disaster situation presents extreme obstacles to health care access, which telerehabilitation can potentially rectify. Benefits of telerehabilitation during disasters can include:

1. Remote consultations with rehabilitation specialists not available in the field, facilitating earlier assessment and initiation of appropriate interventions, and thus earlier discharge to community,
2. Earlier and informed triage to allow for appropriate transfers, referrals, or evacuations as needed,
3. Peer-to-peer support for patient assessment and management,
4. Avoiding the need patients to be transported through dangerous or unstable territory,
5. Assessment and management direct to consumer reducing burden to overwhelmed health facilities,
6. Training and mentoring of local health providers in more specialized care needs, and providing longer-term capacity and skills development, and
7. Technical evaluations facilitating specialized rehabilitation interventions, for example, three-dimensional scanning of residual limbs to generate a custom prosthesis offsite.[26]

Another consideration is that telerehabilitation services could reduce strain on a medical system burdened due to ongoing disaster, where a patient could receive ongoing rehabilitation services from home, freeing up hospital beds potentially in need for emergency circumstances. In pandemics, as the world has recently experienced, telerehabilitation can:

1. Allow for patients and families to maintain "lockdown" practices while still accessing health services,
2. Reduce burdens and risks to health facilities and personnel by reducing in-person contacts,
3. Be used for triage assessment to determine if in-person visit is required.[27]

Through the disaster continuum (Fig. 26.1), rehabilitation-specific roles have been described.[7,9] Considering such activities in the context of telerehabilitation allows for identification of strategies across all four phases of disaster management.

PREPAREDNESS

Effective planning is based on awareness of how a disaster will affect health and anticipating the tasks and resources that will be required. Telehealth information technology and mobile communication technology should be adapted for disaster preparedness and training purposes; it should be tested in advance with appropriate training of users. Rehabilitation professionals should look to their professional organizations for vetted and/or accredited training resources specific to disaster management and response.

Preparedness activities that are intended to address needs of persons with existing disability, and those with new injuries and rehabilitation needs include:

- Identify population needs; evaluate telerehabilitation capacities among persons with disability in disaster-risk areas.
- At health systems levels, establish mechanisms to secure electronic health records that can be accessible in an emergency or disaster.
- Train rehabilitation providers and persons with disability on use of telecommunication technologies and applications; identify and test options for use in disaster situations.
- Establish procedures for protection of patient information and confidentiality in a telerehabilitation encounter.
- Train and credential rehabilitation providers in disaster medicine and rehabilitation.
- Incorporate telerehabilitation strategies into disaster response planning and simulation exercises.

- Identify local, regional, national, and international resources for telerehabilitation provision that can take a lead coordinating role in disaster response.
- At local and regional levels, establish mechanisms to register and contact persons with disability in the event of a disaster.
- Develop and disseminate accessible modules for injury-specific telerehabilitation interventions, in keeping with diagnoses likely to be encountered.

RESPONSE

Foremost in a disaster situation, the responding health care provider must be approved and working collaboratively with the local or national health services or designated Health Cluster agencies; credentials should be appropriately vetted and approved by the disaster coordinating body. While telehealth improves access to much-needed rehabilitation services that are often in very short supply, if available at all in disaster situations, it is of paramount importance that such access does not circumvent the coordination and delivery efforts of the national response services and official coordinating centers. The WHO, with guidance and leadership from international aid organizations, has created recommendations for rehabilitation in disaster, as well as minimum technical standards for rehabilitation teams in disasters.[28, 29]

A disaster situation does not allow for reduced considerations of and adherence to proper informed consent and confidentiality, and as such the security and protection of all beneficiaries must be upheld in all response efforts.[30] Further, telerehabilitation providers should be aware of the realities "on the ground" such that recommendations and interventions are feasible, safe, and culturally and socially appropriate.

Recognizing that communications services may be damaged, interrupted, or unreliable, providers must be prepared for contingencies, including options for asynchronous store and forward platforms, simple mobile application–based interfaces, or basic mobile telecommunication. Sharing and storing of electronic health information, including biometric data or imaging, must strive to meet security standards.

Telerehabilitation response activities can include:

- Peer-to-peer support for triage of potentially disabling injuries
- Peer-to-peer support for guidance in specialized rehabilitation assessment and management, including therapy, equipment, referrals, care transitions, for example, in diagnoses such as burns, amputation, spinal cord injuries, and brain injuries (Fig. 26.3)
- Direct-to-consumer support and care for health maintenance including ongoing rehabilitation
- Direct-to-consumer education and self-care training
- Direct-to-consumer guidance and support for navigation during crisis; wellness checks, equipment/supplies logistics, accessible evacuation, and shelters
- Education, training, and capacity building of local providers
- Data collection to inform on telerehabilitation outcomes
- Liaison and cooperation with the Health Cluster and/or designated leads and coordination centers; assist in informing on projected longer-term needs and issues

Following the 2015 earthquake in Nepal, under the leadership of the local experts and directors of the Spinal Injury Rehabilitation Centre, regional humanitarian response was supported by invited telerehabilitation participation of spinal cord injury experts from distant countries including Canada and the United States. Combining synchronous peer-to-peer support through a daily schedule of videoconferencing for complex case management complimented by asynchronous sharing of resources such as pediatric spinal cord injury guidelines was part of a very successful local-managed response to the 100+ numbers of new spinal cord injured persons admitted to the

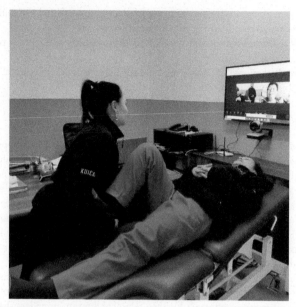

Fig. 26.3 Telerehabilitation services provided to community and outpatient populations during the COVID-19 pandemic by rehabilitation team members of the Spinal Injury Rehabilitation Centre (SIRC) for Nepal. Activities included observation, consultation, and training therapy to caregivers and to patients. (Photo courtesy and with permission, Dr. R. Dhakal, Medical Director, SIRC.)

center.[31] The center has continued to incorporate telerehabilitation into patient care and recently reported on the near seamless transition to telerehabilitation therapy and assessments during a COVID-19 outbreak in their center.[32]

RECOVERY

Perhaps rehabilitation medicine is ideally suited to assume leadership in recovery efforts, as long after acute medical and surgical needs are met, the outcomes of surviving a disabling injury depend on the longer-term efforts of dedicated rehabilitation. Telerehabilitation during the recovery phase facilitates a return to community living at the patient and family level, while at a community level contributes to capacity building and long-term needs projections and planning. Specific tasks can include:

- Counselling and support for discharge to community
- Vocational assessment and counseling
- Patient and caregiver education, training
- Rehabilitation capacity building activities with local providers
- Establish home/community health maintenance including exercise program
- Direct-to-peer ongoing home-rehabilitation therapy and support
- Evaluation of response and outcomes through data analysis
- Supporting community-based rehabilitation

A telerehabilitation effort inclusive of persons with disability is illustrated by an initiative in Pakistan; persons who sustained spinal cord injuries resulting in paraplegia in the 2005 earthquake were offered computer training in order to support their longer-term rehabilitation through telerehabilitation (in-home rehabilitation, counseling, health maintenance), as well as provide skills for employment reintegration. The training was facilitated by the hospitals' own telerehabilitation training centers, thus increasing the utilization of the facilities. Skills included how to use email and capture images as well as to use the telerehabilitation website.[33]

MITIGATION

The experiences from one disaster should be analyzed and inform the next phase of prevention and preparedness activities. Recognizing the risks that persons with disability face in a disaster scenario will guide the education and awareness targets and priorities. Specifically, telerehabilitation actions should address:

- Public awareness and education
- Integration of telerehabilitation into disaster planning and training exercises
- Strengthening of telerehabilitation skills, equipment, training
- Contributions to research efforts to further inform on best practices in telerehabilitation in disasters

The utility of incorporation of telerehabilitation strategies as part of disaster preparedness was illustrated in a case report published following the California Valley Fires in 2015. A spinal cord injury telerehabilitation program provided SCI-specific care to discharged patients through teleSCI visits. Participants were provided with a video-enabled tablet with encryption for security of information. A participant of the program displaced during the Valley Fires was able to receive guidance and support through teleSCI visits when home and equipment was lost. The program was thus able to pivot to provide care during and in the aftermath of this disaster, demonstrating the value of having had services established and integrated into disaster planning.[34]

PRACTICE

While the literature may be scant on specific applications of telerehabilitation in disasters, the experiences of those working in the field can provide a rich appreciation for the creativity and ingenuity that allows dedicated professionals to care for their fellow citizens during periods of disasters and emergencies.

CASE STUDY

Here presented is the experience of humanitarian aid organization **Médecins Sans Frontières (MSF)** in pivoting to **telerehabilitation patient support in the Gaza Strip** in response to restrictions imposed by the COVID-19 pandemic.

INTRODUCTION

In the Gaza Strip MSF is taking care of post-violence trauma, burn injuries, and hand injuries. The rehabilitation department is based on physiotherapy and occupational therapy care, and the rehabilitation team works as a multidisciplinary team. MSF has four outpatient clinics, one plastic surgery and dressing unit, and one inpatient unit.

With COVID-19 spread in the community, on August 20, 2020, all the Gaza strip went into a lockdown. The clinic remained open with 30% of activity for the critical patients, with highly protective measures in place. In physiotherapy approximately 250 patients were remotely followed.

THE SYSTEM, TOOLS, AND RESOURCES

The remote telerehabilitation systems were based on phone calling and social media. The physiotherapy supervisor distributed case lists to the physiotherapist, each list consisting of 15 to 20 patients with case details and phone numbers for communications. A OneDrive video library of 550 short videos for burn rehabilitation, trauma rehabilitation, assessment techniques, hand rehabilitation, and occupational therapy is shared among the team's therapists. To track the patient progression, an online SOAP (Subjective, Objective, Assessment, Plan) note system was created using a DropBox shared folder, containing physiotherapy records and progress note for each patient file. The physiotherapyexercise.com website was used to share with the patient a handout of the home exercises recommended.

CASE STUDY —cont'd

One therapist served as the focal point for data entry, tracking patient status, recording daily sessions, and referring patients from and to the clinics.

REMOTE TREATMENT SESSIONS

The physiotherapist and the occupational therapist call the patient on twice-weekly basis, consisting of the following components:

- **Introduction of service and provider:** to ensure the time is suitable for the patient to receive the sessions, and to introduce themselves.
- **Assessment:** for patients with WhatsApp the session is provided via a WhatsApp call; the patient sends a photo to the therapist of their current condition. The therapist may at times assess the patient by video calls.
- **Session:** the therapist tracks what the patient did at home since the previous session and instructs the patient on the current recommended exercise; the therapist either demonstrates the treatment on video for the patient or shares with the patient the videos needed for treatment. If the patient only has a phone, the therapist tries to conduct the session over the phone.
- **Finalization of the call:** the therapist ends the call by telling the patient what exercise tasks should be performed at home until the next call. The therapist also determines if the patient needs rehabilitation materials (bandages, pressure tools, exercise tools) and, if so, provides a clinic appointment to receive the kits. The patient is then provided with the next call appointment.
- **Record:** the therapist documents a progress note for the patient in the remote progress file and calls the data focal point to record the session details.
- **Referral if needed:** the physiotherapist refers the patient according to need to other multidisciplinary team members such as health promoter for health education, social worker and counselor for psychological support, medical doctor and pain doctor for medications, or nursing department to support wound care.

DIFFICULTIES AND CHALLENGES FACED WITH REMOTE REHABILITATION

The telerehabilitation team encountered some difficulties during the remote rehabilitation sessions, such as:

- Some patients had no internet connections or smartphones. It was thus difficult to provide the exercise hand-outs and videos, with sessions limited to phone calls.
- There was some difficulty to ensure the patient commitment to follow the exercises prescribed, which was gauged by patient reevaluations documenting progression.
- Demand from patients for medications and analgesics was sometimes greater than interest in doing therapeutic exercises or physical training programs, especially among patients with chronic pain.
- Some patients faced a shortage of their rehabilitation materials (cohesive bandage, pressure garment) during the first period of full closure; however, the remote contact aided identifying such patients and arranging for rehabilitation kits to be sent to their homes.

RESULTS AND OUTCOMES FOR THE REMOTE REHABILITATION SYSTEM

The MSF team conducted a satisfaction survey of patients and the therapists regarding the remote physical therapy treatments:

- 88% of patients reported that they are committed to the sessions and the instructions.
- 60% were satisfied with the remote rehabilitation sessions.
- 26% of physiotherapists faced difficulty related to patient commitments, while 30% of the therapists faced difficulty related to communication and resources.
- 78% of the physiotherapists felt satisfied about the resources they received.

To study the patient outcomes of the remote rehabilitation sessions, patients attended in-person clinics for a full reevaluation after 2 months of treatment. Patients were sent to the clinics in groups (maximum 10 per day). During the in-person session, the patient's overall condition was reviewed, including assessment of changes in range of motion, muscle power, and functional abilities. Findings included:

- 65.5% of the patients had improved.
- 29.2% of the patients remained unchanged.
- 5.2% of the patients had deteriorated.

Overall, the MSF team concluded that their remote telerehabilitation system helped their patients to improve their conditions, or at least avoid deterioration, and although it could not replace hands-on physical therapy, telerehabilitation was a good temporary system for use in crises situations when the patient is out of reach.

Special Considerations

Privacy concerns are paramount in any interaction between consumer and health provider, and national standards and regulations, such as Personal Information Protection and Electronic Documents Act in Canada, or Europe's General Data Protection Regulation law must be adhered to.[28] In a disaster, maintaining such standards may pose particularly challenging due to reduced privacy in field hospitals, loss of secure or encrypted telecommunications and health records, rapid turnover of responding to health and logistics workers, and the presence of transient populations in mass migrations. In certain emergency situations, such as wars or refugee crises, identification of beneficiaries could predispose one to security risks; hence, there may be fear, reluctance, or even refusal to participate in telerehabilitation. Recognition and contingencies for such situations are important and should be considered in preparedness and response activities.

Relatively unique to disaster situations, there is a tendency for individuals and groups to "want to help." Perhaps this is amplified in instances where an event is both well publicized and accessible. Hundreds of organizations, many uninvited and without a local partner or designated role under the UN response, arrived in Haiti in the weeks following the 2010 earthquake. Such efforts, while usually well-meaning, diverted resources and complicated an already logistically challenging operation, particularly when responders were unprepared or not trained in the skills needed. Telerehabilitation is intended to broaden the accessibility of rehabilitation services, both to consumer and to peer. However, this could have negative consequences if such access is unregulated or unchecked, resulting in service offerings by untrained or noncredentialed providers. Further, it is imperative that telerehabilitation providers have skills training and education that is specific to disaster context; recommendations for therapy and treatment must be informed by the local realities, including what resources are available, the safety and accessibility of the environment, and cultural and linguistic practices.

Recommendations

Historically, rehabilitation medicine evolved as a specialty from responding to the needs of war-wounded survivors with amputations, spinal cord injuries, and brain injuries. Although essential, the role of rehabilitation has been underrepresented both in the literature and in action, in disaster management across all phases. Intentional efforts to study and optimize specific strategies for incorporating telerehabilitation throughout the disaster cycle are needed. Such information can then inform on policy, for both disaster rehabilitation and telerehabilitation procedures. Such research efforts and eventual policy frameworks must be inclusive of persons with disability.

Guidance materials for the provision of telerehabilitation in disasters, based on available evidence and vetted through experienced and credentialed disaster response and professional organizations, would be welcomed by the international community. Such materials would be complimented by training programs specific to rehabilitation disaster response inclusive of telerehabilitation service provision. Alexander et al. reported on the results of a survey of rehabilitation professionals on providing disaster-related services for persons with spinal cord injury; of the 125 respondents from six continents, 28% reported using telemedicine for either or both emergencies and routine practice; however, 76.8% indicated they were interested to learn more about telemedicine, and just over half were interested in information on disaster preparation.[35] Another international survey of rehabilitation health professionals evaluated effects of the COVID-19 pandemic on rehabilitation services. Of the 60% who reported use of telemedicine, only 39% reported having been educated on the appropriate use of the technology.[36]

Finally, every effort must be made for ensuring far greater participation of persons with disabilities in all phases of the disaster planning and response process: *Nothing about us, without us.*

Telerehabilitation has tremendous potential to improve care for persons with disability and at risk of disability in disaster situations. With improved technologies that are increasingly affordable, secure, and globally accessible, no person with a disability should be left out of reach. Telerehabilitation can facilitate expert and specialized assessment, mentoring and support in regions where such services are not available. Remote scanning technologies for off-site prostheses fabrication are being explored to improve access to quality prosthetic devices in humanitarian settings.[26] Persons in need of rehabilitation in conflict zones can access care without increased risk of exposure during travel. The COVID-19 pandemic has propelled telerehabilitation to the forefront of health delivery options, accelerating translation of telerehabilitation into practice. Rehabilitation is essential in any disaster, and the integration of telerehabilitation in all phases of disaster management will lead to improved outcomes, including survival, reduced disability, and greater quality of life for persons affected by disasters throughout the world.

References

1. Centre for Research on the Epidemiology of Disasters. EM-DAT: The International Disaster Database. https://www.emdat.be/glossary; Accessed 04.10.21.
2. United Nations Office for Disaster Risk Reduction. Global assessment report on disaster risk reduction, Geneva, Switzerland. 2019. https://gar.undrr.org/report-2019; Accessed 13.11.20.
3. United Nations Office for the Coordination of Humanitarian Affairs. Global humanitarian overview. 2021. https://www.unocha.org/global-humanitarian-overview-2021; Accessed 01.12.20.
4. Perrotta K, ed. *Climate Change Toolkit for Health Professionals*. : Canadian Association of Physicians for the Environment; 2019.
5. Centre for Research on the Epidemiology of Disasters. United Nations Office for Disaster Risk Reduction. 2018: Extreme weather events affected 60 million people. 2019.
6. United Nations Refugee Agency. Refugees. https://www.un.org/en/sections/issues-depth/refugees/; Accessed 25.01.21.
7. Koenig KL, Schultz CH, eds. *Disaster Medicine: Comprehensive Principles and Practices*. 2nd ed. New York, NY: Cambridge University Press; 2016.
8. UNHCR The United Nations Refugee Agency. Emergency handbook. 4th ed. The Cluster Approach (IASC). https://emergency.unhcr.org; Accessed 29.12.20.
9. Khan F, Bhasker A, Lee SY, et al. Rehabilitation in disaster relief. *Phys Med Rehabil Clin N Am*. 2019;30:723–747.
10. Mills J, Durham J, Packirisamy V. Rehabilitation services in disaster response. *Bull World Health Organ*. 2017;95:162–164.
11. Amatya B, Galea M, Li J, et al. Medical rehabilitation in disaster relief: towards a new perspective. *J Rehabil Med*. 2017;49(8):620–628. https://doi.org/10.2340/16501977-2250.
12. Reinhardt JD, Li J, Gosney J, et al., On behalf of the International Society of Physical and Rehabilitation Medicine's Sub-Committee on Rehabilitation Disaster Relief. Disability and health-related rehabilitation in international disaster relief. *Glob Health Action*. 2011;4(1):1–9.
13. United Nations General Assembly. Convention on the rights of persons with disabilities: resolution/adopted by the General Assembly. 2007. A/RES/61/106. https://www.refworld.org/docid/45f973632.html; Accessed 25.01.21.
14. Lathia C, Skelton P, Clift Z, eds. *Early Rehabilitation in Conflicts and Disasters*. 1st ed. : Humanity and Inclusion; 2020.
15. Humanity and Inclusion. Factsheet – accessing rehabilitation services: a challenge to overcome. 2019. www.hi.org; Accessed 29.12.20.
16. Fox MH, White GW, Rooney C, et al. Disaster preparedness and response for persons with mobility impairments: results from the University of Kansas Nobody Left Behind study. *J Disabil Policy Stud*. 2007;17(4):196–205. https://doi.org/10.1177/10442073070170040201.
17. Rotheray KR, Aitken P, Goggins WB, et al. Epidemiology of injuries due to tropical cyclones in Hong Kong: a retrospective observational study. *Injury*. 2012;43(12):2055–2059. https://doi.org/10.1016/j.injury.2011.10.033.

18. Kocamer Şimşek B, Dokur M, Uysal E, et al. Characteristics of the injuries of Syrian refugees sustained during the civil war. *Ulus Travma Acil Cerrahi Derg*. 2017;23(3):199–206. https://doi.org/10.5505/tjtes.2016.95525.

19. Burn AS, O'Connell C, Rathore FA. Meeting the challenges of spinal cord injury following sudden onset disaster – lessons learned. *J Rehabil Med*. 2012;44:414–420.

20. Rathore FA, Farooq F, Muzammil S, et al. Spinal cord injury management and rehabilitation; highlights and shortcomings from the 2005 earthquake in Pakistan. *Arch Phys Med Rehabil*. 2008;89(3):579–585.

21. Merin O, Ash M, Levy G, et al. The Israeli field hospital in Haiti – ethical dilemmas in early disaster response. *NEJM*. 2010;e38:1–3.

22. Landry MD, O'Connell C, Tardif G, et al. Post-earthquake Haiti: the critical role for rehabilitation services following a humanitarian crisis. *Disabil and Rehabil*. 2010;32(19):1616–1618.

23. Kailes JI, Enders A. Moving beyond "special needs": a function-based framework for emergency management and planning. *J Disab Pol Studies*. 2007;17(4):230–237.

24. Nicogossian AE, Doarn CR. Armenia 1988 earthquake and telemedicine: lessons learned and forgotten. *Telemed e-Health*. 2011;17(9):741–745. https://doi.org/10.1089/tmj.2011.0118.

25. Latifi R, Tilley EH. Telemedicine for disaster management: can it transform chaos into an organized, structured care from the distance? *Am J Disaster Med*. 2014;9(1):25–37.

26. Moreau P, et al. 3D technology and telemedicine in humanitarian settings. *Lancet Digit Health*. 2020;2(3):e108–e110.

27. Reebye R, Finlayson H, May C, et al. Practical guidance for outpatient spasticity management during the Coronavirus (COVID-19) pandemic: Canadian spasticity COVID-19 Task Force. *Can J Neurol Sci*. 2020;47(5):589–593. https://doi.org/10.1017/cjn.2020.104.

28. Responding internationally to disasters: a do's and don'ts guide for rehabilitation workers. Handicap International; 2016. https://wfot.org.

29. Emergency medical teams: minimum technical standards and recommendations for rehabilitation. Geneva: World Health Organization; 2016. Licence: CC BY-NC-SA 3.0 IGO.

30. Tedeschi C. Ethical, legal, and social challenges in the development and implementation of disaster telemedicine. *Disaster Med Public Health Prep*. 2020:1–8. https://doi.org/10.1017/dmp.2020.118.

31. Personal correspondence, Dr. R. Dhakal, Medical Director of the Spinal Injury Rehabilitation Centre, Nepal. January 25, 2021.

32. Dhakal R, O'Connell C, Gurung JB, et al. A team effort in Nepal: experiences from managing a large COVID-19 rehabilitation hospital outbreak. *Spinal Cord Ser Cases*. 2021;7(5):1–4. https://doi.org/10.1038/s41394-020-00374-2.

33. Gul S, Ghaffar H, Mirza S, et al. Multitasking a telemedicine training unit in earthquake disaster response: paraplegic rehabilitation assessment. *Telemed J E Health*. 2008;14(3):280–283. https://doi.org/10.1089/tmj.2007.0042.

34. Pasipanodya EC, Shem K. Provision of care through telemedicine during a natural disaster: a case study. *Spinal Cord Ser Cases*. 2020;6(60):1–5.

35. Alexander M, Alexander J, Arora M, et al. A bellwether for climate change and disability: educational needs of rehabilitation professionals regarding disaster management and spinal cord injuries. *Spinal Cord Ser Cases*. 2019;5(94):1–6.

36. Gustafson K, Stillman M, Capron M, et al. COVID-19 and spinal cord injury and disease: results of an international survey as the pandemic progresses. *Spinal Cord Ser Cases*. 2021;7(13):1–5.

CHAPTER 27

Educating Health Care Professionals About Telerehabilitation: Developing a Curriculum Map for High- and Low-Resource Settings

Carl Froilan D. Leochico

Introduction

Mother Teresa once said, "I alone cannot change the world, but I can cast a stone across the waters to create many ripples." Rehabilitation professionals are agents of change, capable of transforming disability into "this ability." In line with the 2030 Agenda for Sustainable Development, the 17 internationally agreed goals led by the United Nations to transform the world include "good health and well-being," with particular emphasis on the inclusion and development of persons with disabilities (PWD).[1] Current and up-and-coming physiatrists and allied health professionals can work together to promote rehabilitation as a vital means of achieving the Sustainable Development Goals, while ensuring that PWD and health care settings with limited resources are not left behind.

The Global Burden of Disease Study 2019 estimates that 2.41 billion people are living with disabilities and require rehabilitation.[2] Despite the absence of specific data on disability in developing countries, the World Health Survey shows that disability prevalence estimates are highest in low- and middle-income countries (LMIC).[3] Unfortunately, as the global need for rehabilitation continues to rise, many challenges to face-to-face delivery of or access to physical medicine and rehabilitation (PM&R) services remain unaddressed, especially in resource-limited countries.

Recognizing the vastly unmet need for rehabilitation, the World Health Organization's Rehabilitation 2030 Call for Action cites the lack of rehabilitation workforce (i.e., PM&R doctors, physiotherapists, occupational therapists, speech and language therapists, prosthetists and orthotists, nurses) as a pressing challenge.[4] In many low- and lower-middle-income countries, the density of skilled rehabilitation professionals is below 10 per 1 million population.[4] Meanwhile, challenges to face-to-face rehabilitation in developed and developing countries alike may include geographical landscape, lack of nearby rehabilitation facilities, traffic, transportation and logistical concerns, disability-related limitations, direct and indirect costs of services, long waiting times, lack of awareness, poor compliance, caregiver fatigue, and loss of productivity, among others.[5-7]

Telerehabilitation—which is the use of information and communication technologies (ICTs) to provide remote rehabilitation services across a continuum of care—has the potential to address the aforementioned challenges.[8,9] Although internet connectivity and costs are commonly reported as challenges to synchronous telerehabilitation, asynchronous techniques—such as short messaging system (SMS) using certain low-cost mobile phone models—are feasible and practical, despite their inherent limitations (e.g., data privacy, patient safety, medicolegal liabilities).[10-13] In any health care setting, especially when catering to patients with limited resources and in geographically isolated and disadvantaged areas, telerehabilitation in the form of internet-independent, low-cost, and locally available technologies should also be accessible.

Telerehabilitation in Low-Resource Settings

In developing countries, there is a general scarcity of publications on telehealth, more so on telerehabilitation.[14] The majority of available reports leverage the technology to link health care providers, usually in geographically isolated and disadvantaged areas with urban-based specialists.[14,15] Despite the worldwide growing evidence for telerehabilitation, adoption of this emerging technology in developing countries has been slow because of various interrelated factors, such as: a lack of acceptance among patients and rehabilitation providers; inadequate digital knowledge, skills, and resources; the noninclusion of telehealth in the educational curriculum of current and future health care professionals; a lack of adequate telehealth training and experience; the long-standing history and culture of in-person clinical encounter; a lack of clear national guidelines; legal and ethical considerations; and a shortage of studies documenting safety and cost-effectiveness.[10,11,14] Nonetheless, the value of telerehabilitation cannot be overemphasized in times like the COVID-19 pandemic or certain disasters, which have moved previous nonadopters to reconsider alternative means to connect with patients or health care providers when physical encounters are not possible.

As of 2020, there are no systematic reviews summarizing the extent of telerehabilitation experiences in different developing countries. This may be due to a lack of interest by senior practitioners, limited acceptance of new technologies, and reservations about allocating budget for procedures that have not been widely studied. In the Philippines, the telerehabilitation literature is limited to feasibility studies and case reports, and telerehabilitation is done mostly in academic institutions or university hospitals that provide free educational and clinical support to rural communities in either doctor-to-doctor or doctor-to-community health worker format as an alternative to community-based rehabilitation.[14,16,17] Community-based rehabilitation, an "ongoing evolutionary process," adapts to the changing times by taking advantage of locally available technology (i.e., telerehabilitation through mobile phones) to cater to the needs of PWD.[7,18] Over 5 billion people worldwide own either a smartphone (>50%) or any mobile phone.[19] As the text capital of the world, the Philippines has more than 110 million mobile subscriptions, possibly implying that low-cost digital tools can be leveraged to provide universal access to health care.[20] Text messaging or SMS generally remains the most common method of remote referral, monitoring, and support service in the Philippines, similar to other LMIC.[21] However, the limited capacity to accurately and comprehensively conduct remote examination using SMS should be carefully considered.

Unlike telemedicine, telerehabilitation does not provide remote consultations only. Winters' four conceptual models of telerehabilitation service delivery, aside from teleconsultation, included telehomecare (i.e., remote support), telemonitoring (i.e., remote assessment), and teletherapy (i.e., remote coaching of exercises).[22] While these services have evolved and expanded over the past 18 years to safely and adequately deliver care—particularly teleconsultations and teletherapy—synchronous videoconferencing requiring a reliable internet bandwidth is advantageous. Nonetheless, as the internet has continued to improve in LMIC compared to earlier years, real-time interactive telerehabilitation has become more feasible.[23]

In 2019, more than half of the world's population was using the internet.[24] In developed or high-resource countries, 87% and 81% of people had internet access in urban and rural areas, respectively. In contrast, 65% and 28% of people in developing or low-resource countries had internet access in urban and rural areas, respectively. Internet access remains unevenly distributed, particularly in geographically isolated and disadvantaged areas in developing countries, where setting up internet infrastructures may not be profitable.[25] Nevertheless, with the sustained efforts of government and private sectors to improve internet availability, the internet-of-things (IOT), including telehealth, continues to diffuse to developing countries at a faster rate than before.[25] As a corollary, incorporation of telerehabilitation in clinical practice, teaching, and research has the potential to become widespread.[26, 27]

Even though internet speed lags in many developing countries, there is a huge potential for telehealth. While it is true that the extent of using digital technology is largely dependent on internet speed, the minimum bandwidth speed of 4 megabits per second (Mbps) recommended for a single physician telerehabilitation practice may be achievable in several LMIC.[28] This recommended speed enables high-quality video consultation between a physician and a patient, noncontinuous remote monitoring, access to electronic health or medical records, email, and web browsing, but does not allow real-time image downloads.[28, 29] Higher bandwidth speeds are required to support larger telerehabilitation practice settings (e.g., rural health clinic and nursing homes: up to 10 Mbps, hospital: 100 Mbps, academic medical center: 1000 Mbps).[28] Even though the Philippines and India are reported to have the lowest average internet speeds among surveyed countries in the Asia-Pacific region, at 5.5 and 6.5 Mbps respectively (which are below the global average of 7.2 Mbps), they continue to develop and improve telehealth programs.[30]

Aside from the internet, however, there are several health issues and needs unique to LMIC that may affect their uptake of telerehabilitation or telehealth in general. Examples of this include poverty, civil unrest, workforce shortage, inability to "build the capacity to build capacity," substandard health care, limited health information systems, expensive telecommunication costs, low average educational and technological literacy, inadequate political support, or poor electrical supply.[31] To help address these, the second global survey on eHealth presented four strategies that could enable telehealth implementation, namely (1) governance, (2) policy, (3) scientific development, and (4) evaluation.[27]

Governing bodies formed through multisectoral collaborations have the paramount role of developing legal, regulatory, and capacity-building requirements that can guide telehealth initiatives. Administrative and monetary support from the government, health care institutions, and professional organizations is crucial in the success of telehealth in any country. Substantial planning is required to facilitate telehealth, particularly telerehabilitation, at the national level.[27, 32]

Clear and comprehensive telerehabilitation policies are required to direct rehabilitation professionals in designing, implementing, and evaluating telerehabilitation solutions appropriate for their respective health care settings.[27] The choice of telerehabilitation method should fit the health care setting's purpose, clientele, technical resources and support, workforce eHealth skills, and financial capacity, among others.[33] Policies founded on a combination of local best practices and lessons learned from other countries should start with the need for telerehabilitation, operational definitions, and scope of services, followed by administrative, clinical, technical, and ethical principles.[8] When the need for telerehabilitation is accurately assessed, documented and communicated with various stakeholders (i.e., patients, families, health care providers, policymakers), relevance and sustainability of related programs can be ensured. Telerehabilitation policies should be "designed and established organically within the context and setting in which they will be applied."[31] Carefully contextualized policies may help improve the adoption and implementation of telerehabilitation.

Colleges of rehabilitation sciences, medical schools, and teaching hospitals are potential drivers of the scientific advancements of telerehabilitation in any country, including LMIC. Through the expertise of clinicians and academicians, along with institutional resources dedicated to research and development, telerehabilitation can be systematically applied and evaluated.[27] Furthermore, telehealth experts can be involved in the education and training of current and future generations of doctors and allied health professionals. For instance, since 2017, Philippine General Hospital (PGH), the country's national university hospital, has incorporated telerehabilitation in its teaching-learning activities for third- to fifth-year medical students prior to and during their rural community immersion.[16,17] In unprecedented times, such as during the COVID-19 pandemic, knowledge and skills on telehealth—or telerehabilitation in particular—of both educators and students prove to be practical and socially relevant.

Conducting systematic and regular program evaluations is an indispensable step in ensuring telerehabilitation success.[27] Results of these evaluations—including satisfaction of various stakeholders, safety, and cost-effectiveness—must be communicated within and among professional organizations, and translated to policy changes whenever possible. Given the scarce empirical evidence of telerehabilitation especially in LMIC, studies of any research design are encouraged to be submitted for peer review and publication to make their data accessible to other local and international rehabilitation professionals and policymakers.

Educating Health Care Professionals About Telerehabilitation

Following the World Health Organization's International Classification of Functioning, Disability, and Health (WHO-ICF) framework, telerehabilitation and its related contextual factors are appropriate to incorporate in the holistic evaluation of patients. Identifying these factors can help a health care professional to plan a telerehabilitation approach suitable to the patient's needs, considering relevant medical, clinical, functional, environmental, and personal backgrounds. Using the WHO-ICF as a guide can facilitate individualized patient care, stimulate multidisciplinary research, and ultimately update health policies.[34] Table 27.1 lists the factors to consider prior to engaging in telerehabilitation with a patient.

Telerehabilitation stays true to the purpose of PM&R, which is essentially "the prevention, medical diagnosis, treatment, and rehabilitation management of persons of all ages with disabling

TABLE 27.1 ■ Patient-Centered Factors to Consider in Individualizing Telerehabilitation Based on the WHO-ICF.

Domains of WHO-ICF	Factors Influencing Telerehabilitation
Health condition	Primary medical and/or surgical condition/s Comorbid condition/s Clinical phase in the continuum of care (e.g., preventive, acute, subacute, chronic, palliative, preoperative, postoperative, wellness)
Body functions and structures	Neurocognitive status Functional strength Cardiopulmonary endurance Visual and auditory capacities Hand-eye coordination Language and communication Integrity of somatosensory system Balance
Activities	Ability to perform basic and instrumental activities of daily living (e.g., functional mobility, communication device use, health management and maintenance, safety procedures, and emergency responses) Capacity for self-monitoring of response to exercise

Continued

TABLE 27.1 ■ **Patient-Centered Factors to Consider in Individualizing Telerehabilitation Based on the WHO-ICF.—cont'd**

Domains of WHO-ICF	Factors Influencing Telerehabilitation
Participation	Position and responsibilities in the family Work or vocation Leisure Role in the community
Environmental factors	Immediate setting (e.g., inpatient care, outpatient department, skilled nursing or rehabilitation facility, community, home, workplace) Distance to the nearest health care facility for emergency cases or face-to-face referral Distance to the nearest rehabilitation facility Privacy (e.g., shared room, number of people in the household) Safety (e.g., outdoor civil unrest, indoor fall hazards) Availability of home-monitoring devices or wearable sensors (e.g., blood pressure monitor, heart rate monitor, pulse oximeter, smartwatch, smartphone application) Availability of home remedies (e.g., warm compress, cold compress) Availability of home rehabilitation equipment (e.g., electrical stimulation device, elastic bandages, exercise gadgets, makeshift weights, adaptive devices like built-up handles, assistive devices like splints and mobility aids) Ambient temperature and lighting Electrical supply Network coverage Internet coverage Local telecommunication costs Availability of social service or support from community health workers
Personal factors	Age Sex Civil status Educational background Language/dialect Awareness of the need for rehabilitation Attitude toward telerehabilitation Compliance Access to telecommunication device (e.g., landline phone, mobile phone, smartphone, tablet, computer) Internet access and speed Internet source (e.g., dial-up, fixed wired or wireless broadband, mobile broadband, hotspot) Choice of telecommunication method (e.g., text message, phone call, instant message, online call with or without video) Choice of telecommunication platform (e.g., web-based application, mobile or desktop application, social media platform) Digital knowledge and skills Technical and physical assistance from a family member/caregiver Family support Financial resources Psychological predisposition (e.g., depression, anxiety)

WHO-ICF, World Health Organization—International Classification of Functioning, Disability, and Health framework.

health conditions and their comorbidities, specifically addressing their impairments and activity limitations in order to facilitate their physical and cognitive functioning (including behavior), participation (including quality of life), and modifying personal and environmental factors," albeit performed virtually within the apparent limitations of telehealth.[35] Similar to in-person setups, telerehabilitation can be provided by a patient-centered multidisciplinary team of rehabilitation professionals, namely, physiatrists or medical doctors who specialized in PM&R, physiotherapists, occupational therapists, speech and language therapists, psychologists, prosthetic and orthotic technicians, rehabilitation nurses, social workers, and dieticians, among others. Ideally, any of these rehabilitation professionals can be called to provide distant support to PWD within the scope of their professional practice and jurisdiction. Currently, however, few active rehabilitation professionals, especially those in LMIC, have been trained to perform remote "assessment, monitoring, prevention, intervention, supervision, education, consultation, and counseling," which are the services of telerehabilitation.[8] Telerehabilitation and even telehealth, in general, are not part of the curriculum in many medical and allied health schools in the Philippines, India, and other developing and developed countries.[14,23,36]

Fast internet speeds, virtual reality, wearable devices, remote physiological sensors, haptics, or other high-cost technologies being researched for telerehabilitation in advanced health care settings are not common in LMIC and other areas in developed countries. Nonetheless, telerehabilitation can still be conducted using locally available technologies.[26,33] Many PM&R interventions, such as therapeutic exercises, functional training, occupational and vocational activities, cognitive and sensorimotor training, speech-language treatments, seating and wheelchair prescriptions, and environmental modifications can benefit PWD through telerehabilitation, despite the lack of highly advanced technologies. However, open-mindedness, creativity, resourcefulness, careful planning, and proper implementation are necessary.[7,9] According to limited published data on telerehabilitation from LMIC, the doctor-to-doctor setup and preference for former over new patients have always been the common practice in teleconsultations to address various concerns, such as patient safety due to the lack of an initial face-to-face physical examination. However, during the COVID-19 pandemic when in-person delivery of nonessential services including rehabilitation was not feasible, many patients, health care practitioners, and institutions had to find ways to adapt and reconsider means to provide optimal care for PWD, while observing adequate risk mitigation. This included seeing patients for both initial and follow-up evaluations through telehealth, and expanding various forms of rehabilitative treatments based on clinical judgment as opposed to research.[11,37]

Within the context of the patient, telerehabilitation goals and treatment planning can be directed toward addressing the functional consequences of the health condition (Table 27.1). Telerehabilitation can be useful for a wide spectrum of medical and/or surgical conditions in different phases of care, from wellness and prevention to acute, subacute, chronic, and perioperative rehabilitation. It is commonly accessed by outpatients from the comfort of their homes, but it may also be available to inpatients, such as those isolated due to COVID-19, in some hospitals even in LMIC, wherein the scarcity of personal protective equipment, medical resources, and health workforce contributes to the temporary suspension of face-to-face rehabilitation services for patients with confirmed or suspected COVID-19.[11]

Several human (e.g., stakeholders' apprehensions, health care providers' unreadiness) and organizational (e.g., lack of national guidelines) challenges hindering the emergence of telerehabilitation in developing countries may be rooted in the widespread lack of education, training, and clinical opportunities on telehealth for health care professionals.[14,38] Especially amid the COVID-19 pandemic, the urgent need to "build the capacity to build capacity" for telerehabilitation becomes evident.[31] One way of building the capacity of LMIC is by collaborating with an international academic institution, as exemplified by the Botswana-University of Pennsylvania Partnership and many others that provide underserved communities with necessary telerehabilitation equipment and expert-level care.[39]

The rehabilitation workforce is the major driver of telerehabilitation and must therefore acquire relevant knowledge, skills, and experience. The curricula for undergraduate (i.e., medical and allied health schools) and graduate medical education (i.e., residency training in PM&R) vary worldwide, and many of these, whether in high- or low-resource countries, have not included telehealth.[40,41] Since telerehabilitation implies a shift from traditional in-person care to virtual evaluation and management, which is used either as an adjunct (i.e., follow-up care) or an alternative health care delivery (i.e., during pandemic or disasters, or if with constraints to face-to-face access), there should be appropriate education and training for current and future practitioners. Current practitioners can engage in continuing professional development (CPD) or continuing medical education (CME) on telehealth or telerehabilitation. For more comprehensive training, current and future practitioners may enroll in classroom-based or online telehealth courses or modules offered by certain academic centers, most of which are located in developed countries like the United States, United Kingdom, Australia, and France.[41] Formal university courses, such as Health or Medical Informatics, are also available. Moreover, the School of Health and Rehabilitation Sciences at the University of Queensland in Australia offers workforce training programs on telerehabilitation.[42] In general, however, a training curriculum specific to telerehabilitation is not currently available in the literature. Therefore telehealth core competencies and syllabi from developed countries can be adapted and contextualized with respect to the unique health care needs and resources in LMIC. Nonetheless, there is little publicly accessible information from undergraduate medical schools in developed countries that explains how to integrate telehealth in preclinical or clerkship curricula.[43] Moreover, it is unknown if, and how, telehealth is officially incorporated in schools and universities in LMIC.

At the PGH the Department of Rehabilitation Medicine has developed a stepwise curriculum on telerehabilitation for medical students. The curriculum is incorporated in the students' learning activities when they rotate into the Department, beginning in the third-year or preclinical level, wherein students are introduced to the "what, who, where, when, why, and how" of telerehabilitation during a 2-hour combined lecture and case-based small group discussion with a consultant practicing telerehabilitation (Table 27.2). This basic orientation is then reinforced during the

TABLE 27.2 ■ Stepwise Telerehabilitation Curriculum Map for Undergraduate Medical Education.

Learning Outcomes *At the end of the PM&R rotation, the student is able to:*	Levels		
	Preclinical Year/s	Clinical Clerkship	Clinical Internship
1. Discuss the definition and value of telerehabilitation for various stakeholders (i.e., patient, family, community, health care provider, health care organization, society)	I	P	D
2. Explain the limitations and risk-mitigation measures of telerehabilitation for each aforementioned stakeholder	I	P	D
3. Differentiate locally available telerehabilitation platforms in terms of advantages and disadvantages	I	P	D
4. Evaluate relevant international and local (if any) laws and bioethical principles related to telerehabilitation	I	P	P

5. Summarize the step-by-step processes involved in telerehabilitation[a]:
  a. Before the session: orienting the patient/family, securing consent, preparing the virtual clinic, procuring exercise equipment, scheduling, test call
  b. During the session: screening first for emergency symptoms or need for immediate face-to-face clinical encounter, introducing attendees, setting ground rules, patient evaluation and management, ensuring understanding
  c. After the session: proper documentation, gathering feedback, billing[a]
	I	P	D

Continued

TABLE 27.2 ■ Stepwise Telerehabilitation Curriculum Map for Undergraduate Medical Education. —cont'd

Learning Outcomes At the end of the PM&R rotation, the student is able to:	Levels		
	Preclinical Year/s	Clinical Clerkship	Clinical Internship
6. Set up a basic telerehabilitation clinic in both sites (health care provider and patient), observing privacy, proper lighting, safety, and so on	I	P	D
7. Perform trouble-shooting strategies for common technical issues (e.g., connectivity, audiovisual quality)	P	D	D
8. Conduct a tele-evaluation (virtual physiatric history-taking and examination)	I	P	D
9. Create a prioritized rehabilitation problem list based on the WHO-ICF framework	I	P	D
10. Formulate the rehabilitation goals for the patient	I	P	D
11. Recommend a teledisposition (plan-of-care based on the rehabilitation goals)	I	P	D
12. Demonstrate remote intervention, supervision, education, counseling, or exercise-coaching, depending on the teledisposition	I	P	D
13. Discuss the biopsychosocial issues experienced by a person with disability	I	P	D
14. Describe the role of each member of the multidisciplinary telerehabilitation team	I	P	D
15. Develop "webside" manners, professionalism, and a caring attitude	I	P	D

[a]The sequence and specific steps may vary depending on the policies of clinicians or institutions. For example, billing may occasionally be a prerequisite to the actual telerehabilitation session.
D, Demonstrated—knowledge and skills are manifested; *I*, introduced—basic concepts are introduced; *P*, practiced—knowledge is reinforced and/or skills are acquired; *PM&R*, Physical Medicine and Rehabilitation; *WHO-ICF*: World Health Organization—International Classification of Functioning, Disability, and Health.
Adapted from (1) Leochico and Mojica (2017);[18] (2) Papanagnou et al. (2015);[44] (3) Govindarajan et al. (2017);[45] (4) Verduzco-Gutierrez et al. (2020);[37] and (5) McIntyre et al. (2020).[46]

fourth year or clinical clerkship level, when students rotate again into the Department and engage in a more in-depth discussion of the socioeconomic, technical, ethical, and legal aspects of telerehabilitation. The students end their usual 2-week rotation in the Department with a telerehabilitation role-playing exercise, wherein the small group is divided into two teams: (1) telecommunity team pretending to be the telepresenters in the remote spoke, and (2) telerehabilitation team pretending to be in the hub. Each team is in a separate, private room and connected only by the internet or alternative form of telecommunication. The telepresenters, acting as health care providers in the community, are tasked to refer a co-located sample patient to the telespecialists. On the other hand, the telerehabilitation team, acting as Rehabilitation Medicine providers in PGH, is tasked to receive, evaluate, and manage the referral over the simulated physical distance. The telerehabilitation team is composed of the following: (1) rehabilitation medicine consultants, who remotely provide clinical support to the community, and (2) allied rehabilitation professionals who demonstrate specific home exercises and provide concrete tasks and environmental modifications appropriate for the case. Meanwhile, an actual rehabilitation medicine consultant is also present in PGH to observe the telerehabilitation simulation and highlight teaching points or clinical pearls to the students on physiatric principles and proper conduct of telerehabilitation. The curriculum culminates in the fifth year or clinical internship level, wherein students can apply their prior knowledge and skills on telerehabilitation when they rotate in the community. The students get the chance to telepresent actual patients in the outpatient clinic of the rural health unit to the telerehabilitation team in PGH. In this way, interns receive e-supervision in their evaluation and management of PWD in the community, while fostering interprofessional training and collaboration with other members of the rehabilitation team.[16,17]

For each telerehabilitation session, whether simulated or actual, students are assigned specific roles, which may overlap depending on the number of the students in the group. Aside from the telepresenters, telephysiatrists, and teletherapists, the following roles and corresponding tasks should also be delegated beforehand:

1. Telemoderator—formally opens, facilitates, and ends each telerehabilitation session;
2. Receptionist—coordinates the schedule of the initial and follow-up telerehabilitation sessions;
3. Clinic manager—obtains and files the informed consent from the patient, ensures the telerehabilitation session goes smoothly in the hub and spoke, ensures proper electronic or physical charting in both sites, organizes and keeps medical records, obtains feedback from both sites after each session to improve the conduct of telerehabilitation, and manages any complaints; and
4. Technical support—offers in-person or remote technical assistance to the hub and spoke, ensures audiovisual clarity for videoconferencing, troubleshoots technical problems, and suggests alternative methods of telecommunication (i.e., other internet sources, other videoconferencing platforms or applications, phone call, etc.), if needed.

During the telerehabilitation role-playing exercise, students in PGH are evaluated based on the following: (1) adequacy and accuracy of the remote physiatric history-taking and examination; (2) appropriateness of the proposed physiatric plan-of-care; (3) observance of the clinical, technical, and ethical principles of telerehabilitation, ensuring data privacy and patient safety; (4) professional execution of assigned roles; and (5) "webside" manners. The actual telerehabilitation consultants give quantitative and qualitative feedback to the students after each telerehabilitation role-playing exercise.

Developing a Telerehabilitation Curriculum Map

Studies in high- and even low-resource countries, such as Ghana, India, Iran, and the Philippines, indicate the growing need to educate health professionals on telehealth or telerehabilitation in rural and urban areas.[11,23,31,36,47] More than awareness campaigns, adequate community-based training for rural-based health workers and inclusion of telerehabilitation in undergraduate, graduate, and continuing education for all rehabilitation providers, who are currently in training or in practice, can improve access to quality telecare for PWD.

In order to address the state of unpreparedness for telerehabilitation among current and future practitioners, training should move beyond general orientation on the basics of telerehabilitation (i.e., purpose, scope, process, advantages, disadvantages), and seek to provide a deeper understanding of the complex governmental, socioeconomic, cultural, medicolegal, and ethical principles applicable to their health care setting.[43] While aligning telerehabilitation solutions with the "glocal" (global and local) health system and the needs and culture of the people they serve, rehabilitation providers should be equipped to conduct telerehabilitation "professionally, safely, and in an evidence-based manner."[31,43]

According to the World Health Organization, there are four elements germane to telemedicine that are also applicable to telerehabilitation: (1) it provides clinical support; (2) it overcomes barriers, such as geography; (3) it uses various types of ICTs; and (4) it improves health outcomes.[27] These elements can serve as the foundation of an outcome-based telerehabilitation curriculum, as currently there is neither a widely recognized standard for telemedicine nor telerehabilitation training for undergraduate and graduate education in the fields of medicine and allied health (e.g., physical therapy, occupational therapy, speech and language pathology, psychology, prosthetics and orthotics, nursing).[48, 49]

Incorporating telerehabilitation into an already exhaustive medical or allied health curriculum may be challenging for both teachers and students. The key is to weave telerehabilitation competencies through existing teaching-learning topics and activities. For instance, when teaching history-taking and physical examination, a case-based small group discussion may highlight the role of telerehabilitation and technique of virtual physiatric evaluation of a sample or real patient residing in a remote area without access to in-person rehabilitation services. Depending on the level of telerehabilitation competency (i.e., introduced, practiced, demonstrated) expected per year, various possible learning outcomes may be achieved from the case. A sample telerehabilitation curriculum map is presented in Table 27.2.

The Accreditation Council for Graduate Medical Education (ACGME) endorses the following core competencies for residency programs: (1) patient care, (2) medical knowledge, (3) practice-based learning and improvement, (4) interpersonal and communication skills, (5) professionalism, and (6) systems-based practice.[50] The American Medical Association (AMA) and the Association of American Medical Colleges (AAMC) recently recommended the inclusion of telemedicine as a core competency across undergraduate and graduate programs.[49] Telerehabilitation, in particular, can be integrated in various existing curricula, while achieving the six core competencies of ACGME. Including telerehabilitation either as a required or elective course, and either as a separate or integrated topic, depends on the national priorities, regulations, and capacities of local professional boards and academic institutions.

Teaching-learning activities appropriate for each learning outcome and competency per year level should be carefully planned by the faculty. For example, a reflection paper after watching a video of an actual telerehabilitation session may be adequate to *introduce* the uniqueness of conducting a virtual physiatric examination to junior-level medical or allied health students. For higher-level students, however, the skill of performing a virtual physiatric examination can be *practiced* through role-playing and *demonstrated* through a tele-encounter with an actual remote patient (Table 27.2).

Lastly, evaluating whether or not a specific learning outcome and year-level competency are adequately achieved can be performed through one or more of the following assessment tools: "direct observations; global evaluation; audits and review of clinical performance data; multisource feedback from team members, including peers, nurses, patients, and family members; simulation; in-service training examinations (ITE); self-assessment; and others."[50]

Conclusion and Recommendations

While the face-to-face clinical encounter will remain as gold standard for evaluating and managing patients in the field of PM&R, the compelling need for telerehabilitation cannot be underestimated. Among the urgent challenges that must be overcome in high- and low-resource settings is the lack of telerehabilitation training for current and future health care providers. Integration of telerehabilitation into existing educational curricula and clinical workflows can be facilitated by a coordinated, interprofessional, multilevel, and multisectoral approach, prioritizing the health care needs of PWD. Inclusivity through telerehabilitation may be achieved after comprehensive assessment of the needs, resources and capacity-building in various geographically isolated and disadvantaged areas. Nonetheless, leveraging locally available low-cost technologies should be accompanied by context-specific guidelines that ensure quality rehabilitation care, patient safety, and data privacy.

Previous studies and experiences on telerehabilitation worldwide contain a plethora of knowledge that various academic and clinical institutions can learn from. However, there is a lot more to discover, share, and translate into practice. For instance, future research may be geared toward finding evidence-based answers to the following questions:

- "What are the components and characteristics of effective telerehabilitation education and training?"
- "Which specific components of a standard physiatric examination are most appropriate for telerehabilitation?"
- "What function-based rehabilitation goals can be effectively and safely achieved through telerehabilitation?"
- "Which specific PM&R outcome measurements can be performed accurately and safely through telerehabilitation?"

Rehabilitation professionals should aim to become enablers who find ways to facilitate effective treatment for persons with "this ability." Addressing the challenges to the emergence of telerehabilitation across the globe can improve access to a multitude of rehabilitation services throughout the continuum of care, and strengthen linkages with underserved communities.

Acknowledgment

The author expresses his sincerest gratitude to Dr. Jose Alvin P. Mojica, MHPEd and Dr. Sharon D. Ignacio of the Department of Rehabilitation Medicine, College of Medicine and Philippine General Hospital, University of the Philippines Manila for their inspiring vision for and works on telerehabilitation.

References

1. Wiman, Ronald; Helander, Einar; Westland, J. *Meeting the needs of people with disabilities - new approaches in the health sector (English)*. 2002. http://documents.worldbank.org/curated/en/514921468763472468/Meeting-the-needs-of-people-with-disabilities-new-approaches-in-the-health-sector.
2. Cieza A, Causey K, Kamenov K, et al. Global estimates of the need for rehabilitation based on the Global Burden of Disease study 2019: a systematic analysis for the Global Burden of Disease Study 2019. *Lancet*. 2020;396(10267):2006–2017. https://doi.org/10.1016/S0140-6736(20)32340-0.
3. World Health Organization. The global burden of disease 2004 update. World Health Organization. 2004. https://doi.org/10.1038/npp.2011.85.
4. World Health Organization. Rehabilitation 2030 a call for action: the need to scale up rehabilitation. 2017. Retrieved March 29, 2020. https://www.who.int/disabilities/care/NeedToScaleUpRehab.pdf.
5. Bundoc JR. The challenges of "walking free" from disability. *Acta Med Philipp*. 2010;44(2):13–16.
6. Eldar R, Kullmann L, Marincek C, et al. Rehabilitation medicine in countries of Central/Eastern Europe. *Disabil Rehabil*. 2008;30(2):134–141. https://doi.org/10.1080/09638280701191776.
7. Leochico CFD, Valera MJS. Follow-up consultations through telerehabilitation for wheelchair recipients with paraplegia in a developing country: a case report. *Spinal Cord Ser Cases*. 2020;6(1):58. https://doi.org/10.1038/s41394-020-0310-9.
8. Brennan D, Tindall L, Theodoros D, et al. A blueprint for telerehabilitation guidelines. *Int J Telerehabilitation*. 2010;2(2):31–34. https://doi.org/10.5195/IJT.2010.6063.
9. Schmeler MR, et al. Telerehabilitation and clinical applications: research, opportunities, and challenges. *Int J Telerehabilitation*. 2015:12–24. Retrieved from https://telerehab.pithttps//telerehab.pitt.edu/ojs/index.php/Telerehab/article/view/701/951t.edu/ojs/index.php/Telerehab/article/view/701/951.
10. Kay M, Santos J, Takane M. Telemedicine: opportunities and developments in Member States. *WHO Global Observatory for EHealth Series*. 2010. https://doi.org/10.4258/hir.2012.18.2.153.
11. Leochico CFD. Adoption of telerehabilitation in a developing country before and during the COVID-19 pandemic. *Ann Phys Rehabil Med*. 2020;63(6):563–564. https://doi.org/10.1016/j.rehab.2020.06.001.

12. Patdu ID, Tenorio AS. Establishing the legal framework of telehealth in the Philippines. *Acta Medica Philippina*. 2016;50(4):237–246. Retrieved from https://actamedicaphilippina.upm.edu.ph/index.php/acta/article/view/763.

13. Pramuka, M., Van Roosmalen, L. Telerehabilitation technologies: accessibility and usability. *Int J Telerehabilitation*. 1(1), 85–98. https://doi.org/10.5195/IJT.2009.6016.

14. Leochico C, Espiritu A, Ignacio S, et al. Challenges to the emergence of telerehabilitation in a developing country: a systematic review. *Front Neurol*. 2020;11:1007. https://doi.org/10.3389/fneur.2020.01007.

15. Macabasag RL, Magtubo KM, Marcelo PG. Implementation of telemedicine services in lower-middle income countries: lessons for the Philippines. *J Int Soc Telemed EHealth*. 2016;4(e24):1–11. Retrieved from https://journals.ukzn.ac.za/index.php/JISfTeH/article/view/168.

16. Supnet IE, Mojica JAP, Ignacio SD, Leochico CFD. Development of an evaluation tool for the assessment of telemedicine courses. *Asia Pac Scholar*. 2021. (In Press).

17. Leochico CF, Mojica JA. Telerehabilitation as a teaching-learning tool for medical interns. *PARM Proceedings*. 2017;9(1):39–43.

18. World Health Organization. CBR, a strategy for rehabilitation, equalization of opportunities, poverty reduction and social inclusion of people with disabilities: joint position paper. 2004. Geneva.

19. Pew Research Center. Smartphone ownership is growing rapidly around the world, but not always equally.

20. Wavecell, an 8x8 C. Customer engagement in the Philippines: texting capital of the world. 2019. https://medium.com/@wavecell/customer-engagement-in-the-philippines-texting-capital-of-the-world-ceab-271d775a.

21. Gavino AI, Tolentino PAP, Bernal ABS, et al. Telemedicine via short messaging system (SMS) in rural Philippines. *AMIA Annu Symp Proc*. 2008:952. http://www.ncbi.nlm.nih.gov/pubmed/18998858.

22. Winters JM. Telerehabilitation research: emerging opportunities. *Annu Rev Biomed Eng*. 2002;4(1):287–320. https://doi.org/10.1146/annurev.bioeng.4.112801.121923.

23. Ayanikalath S. *Telerehabilitation in resource constrained countries*. 2019. Retrieved from https://insights.omnia-health.com/hospital-management/telerehabilitation-resource-constrained-countries

24. International Telecommunication Union. Measuring digital development: facts and figures. 2020. https://www.itu.int/en/ITU-D/Statistics/Documents/facts/FactsFigures2020.pdf.

25. Dahlman, C., Mealy, S., Wermelinger, M. Harnessing the digital economy for developing countries. https://doi.org/10.1787/4adffb24-en.

26. World Health Organization. World Report on Disability - Summary. 2011. https://gsdrc.org/document-library/world-report-on-disability-summary/.

27. World Health Organization. Telemedicine: opportunities and developments in member states: report on the second global survey on e-health. Global Observatory for E-health Series – Volume 2. NLM classification. 2010. W 26.5. ISBN 9789241564144. ISSN 2220–5462. Geneva.

28. Office of the National Coordinator for Health Information Technology. What is the recommended bandwidth for different types of health care providers? 2019. https://www.healthit.gov/faq/what-recommended-bandwidth-different-types-health-care-providers.

29. Isip-Tan, I.T., Sarmiento, F.I., Fong, M., et al. Telemedicine: guidance for physicians in the Philippines. 2020. https://www.philippinemedicalassociation.org/wp-content/uploads/2020/05/1-Telemedicine-for-Health-Professionals.pdf.

30. Akamai. Akamai's state of the internet Q1 2017 report (Vol. 10). 2017. https://www.akamai.com/fr/fr/multimedia/documents/state-of-the-internet/q1-2017-state-of-the-internet-connectivity-report.pdf.

31. Scott R, Mars M. Telehealth in the developing world: current status and future prospects. *Smart Homecare Technol Telehealth*. 2015:25. https://doi.org/10.2147/SHTT.S75184.

32. Khan F, Amatya B, Groote W, et al. Capacity-building in clinical skills of rehabilitation workforce in low- and middle-income countries. *J Rehabil Med*. 2018;50(5):472–479. https://doi.org/10.2340/16501977-2313.

33. Shenoy MP, Shenoy PD. Identifying the challenges and cost-effectiveness of telerehabilitation: a narrative review. *J Clin Diagnostic Res*. 2018. https://doi.org/10.7860/JCDR/2018/36811.12311.

34. Jette AM. Toward a common language for function, disability, and health. *Phys Ther*. 2006;86(5):726–734.

35. European Physical and Rehabilitation Medicine Bodies Alliance White book on Physical and Rehabilitation Medicine (PRM) in Europe. Chapter 1. Definitions and concepts of PRM. *Eur J Phys Rehabil Med*. 2018;54(2):156–165. https://doi.org/10.23736/S1973-9087.18.05144-4.

36. Bali S. *Barriers to Development of Telemedicine in Developing Countries.* In: *Telehealth,* Thomas F. Heston, IntechOpen. 2018. http://dx.doi.org/10.5772/intechopen.81723. Available from: https://www.intechopen.com/chapters/64650.

37. Verduzco-Gutierrez M, Bean AC, Tenforde AS, et al. How to conduct an outpatient telemedicine rehabilitation or prehabilitation visit. *PM&R.* 2020;12(7):714–720. https://doi.org/10.1002/pmrj.12380.

38. Scott Kruse C, Karem P, Shifflett K, et al. Evaluating barriers to adopting telemedicine worldwide: a systematic review. *J Telemed Telecare.* 2018;24(1):4–12. https://doi.org/10.1177/1357633X16674087.

39. O'Shea J, Berger R, Samra C, et al. Telemedicine in education: bridging the gap. *Educ Health.* 2015;28(1):64. https://doi.org/10.4103/1357-6283.161897.

40. DeLisa J, Berbrayer D, Guzman J, et al. The education of the specialist of physical and rehabilitation medicine: graduate medical education in residency training. *J Int Soc Phys Rehabil Med.* 2019;2(5):58. https://doi.org/10.4103/jisprm.jisprm_15_19.

41. Edirippulige S, Armfield N. Education and training to support the use of clinical telehealth: a review of the literature. *J Telemed.* 2017;23(2):273–282. https://doi.org/10.1177/1357633X16632968.

42. School of Health and Rehabilitation Sciences - The University of Queensland. Telerehabilitation. 2020. Retrieved August 22, 2020. https://shrs.uq.edu.au/research/telerehabilitation.

43. Waseh S, Dicker AP. Telemedicine training in undergraduate medical education: mixed-methods review. *JMIR Med Educ.* 2019;5(1):e12515. https://doi.org/10.2196/12515.

44. Papanagnou D, Sicks S, Hollander JE. Training the next generation of care providers: focus on telehealth. *Healthcare Transformation.* 2015;1(1):52–63. https://doi.org/10.1089/heat.2015.29001-psh.

45. Govindarajan R, Anderson ER, Hesselbrock RR, et al. Developing an outline for teleneurology curriculum. *Neurology.* 2017;89(9):951–959. https://doi.org/10.1212/WNL.0000000000004285.

46. McIntyre M, Robinson LR, Mayo A. Practical considerations for implementing virtual care in Physical Medicine and Rehabilitation: for the pandemic and beyond. *Am J Phys Med Rehabil.* 2020;99(6):464–467. https://doi.org/10.1097/PHM.0000000000001453.

47. Movahedazarhouligh S, Vameghi R, Hatamizadeh N, et al. Feasibility of telerehabilitation implementation as a novel experience in rehabilitation academic centers and affiliated clinics in Tehran: assessment of rehabilitation professionals' attitudes. *Int J Telemed Appl.* 2015;2015:1–8. https://doi.org/10.1155/2015/468560.

48. Pathipati AS, Azad TD, Jethwani K. Telemedical education: training digital natives in telemedicine. *J Med Internet Res.* 2016;18(7):e193. https://doi.org/10.2196/jmir.5534.

49. Theobald M, Brazelton T. STFM forms task force to develop a national telemedicine curriculum, from STFM. *Ann Fam Med.* 2020;18(3):285–286. https://doi.org/10.1370/afm.2549.

50. Accreditation Council for Graduate Medical Education (ACGME). The milestones guidebook. 2020. https://www.acgme.org/Portals/0/MilestonesGuidebook.pdf.

CHAPTER 28

Telehealth Practice Standards With Emphasis on the United States: What Telerehabilitation Providers Need to Know

Kyle Y. Faget

Telehealth has taken the spotlight with the onset of the global COVID-19 pandemic, which rendered traditional, in-person health care visits potentially unsafe in the face of a highly communicable virus. Because many conditions can be adequately diagnosed and treated via telehealth, the use of this mechanism of health care delivery became palatable for telehealth providers, including those providing telerehabilitation, and patients alike. Concurrently, a myriad of laws and regulations governing health care practice were relaxed in an attempt to make use of telehealth easier for telehealth providers and patients. Nonetheless, there is a patchwork of varying standards governing the practice of telehealth, including telerehabilitation, across the globe and in the United States, which makes practicing telehealth potentially confusing for the newly initiated. This chapter will focus on discussing laws pertaining to the practice of telehealth in the United States; readers from other countries are reminded to ensure that including telerehabilitation they have followed the rulings of their particular country and region of practice.

Licensure

Before a telehealth provider can treat a patient, they must be appropriately licensed. All telehealth providers, including telerehabilitation providers, must comply with the applicable licensure requirements in the jurisdiction in which they are licensed. In the United States, this means that a telehealth provider must comply with the licensure requirements of the state in which he or she is licensed. Telehealth adds a layer of complexity to licensure in the United States. Telehealth providers, including telerehabilitation providers, generally must be licensed in the state in which the patient is located. Licensure requirements vary from state to state and can be more or less onerous. In many cases, it can take upward of 1 year for a physician to obtain a license to practice in a given state. To the extent a telehealth statute does not address licensure requirements specifically, it is safe to assume that the telehealth provider needs to be licensed in the state in which the patient is located. Barring a telemedicine special purpose license or an exception, if a telehealth provider intends to provide services in multiple states, he or she must be licensed in those multiple states.

A number of states have implemented a telemedicine special purpose license, permit, or registration. For example, Florida recently enacted a telehealth law establishing a telehealth registration for out-of-state telehealth providers, including telerehabilitation providers; Florida-licensed

---

[1] *See* Fla. Stat. § 456.47(4).

health care providers are not required to register. The law prohibits an out-of-state telehealth provider from opening an office in Florida and providing in-person health care services to patients located in Florida.[1] The Florida Department of Health publishes on its website a list of all out-of-state telehealth registrants.[2] As another example, Georgia's Medical Practices Act requires a medical license of persons physically located in another state who, through the use of telecommunication, perform acts that are part of patient care services in Georgia, but the out-of-state physician may obtain a license if he or she has a full and unrestricted medical license in another state and with no disciplinary actions being taken against him or her by any other state jurisdiction.[3]

In addition to telemedicine special purpose license, permit, or registration, there are exceptions to the general rule that a telehealth provider must be licensed in the state in which a patient is located. For example, Virginia provides license reciprocity for physicians providing telemedicine services to patients in Virginia if the physician is licensed in a bordering state, which includes Maryland, Washington DC, North Carolina, Tennessee, Kentucky, and West Virginia.[4] This exception is familiarly known as the bordering state exception.

Another exception, the peer-to-peer consultation exemption, allows for an out-of-state physician to consult with a physician in a given state without needing to be licensed in that state. Here, the out-of-state physician typically must be licensed in the state where he or she is located, and the in-state physician must be licensed in the state where he or she and the patient are located. The in-state physician is held responsible for maintaining the physician-patient relationship, whereas the out-of-state physician's services are only for secondary consultation purposes. Although the in-state physician has primary responsibility for patient care, some states with peer-to-peer consultation exceptions enable the out-of-state physician to have direct contact with the patient provided that the contact is not frequent and/or is at the direction of the in-state physician.

The contours of the peer-to-peer consultation exception vary among the states that recognize this exception. In Minnesota, for example, an out-of-state physician providing telemedicine services is exempt from licensure in Minnesota if she is licensed in another state and (1) provides services less than once a month or to less than 10 patients per year or (2) provides services in consultation with a Minnesota-licensed physician who "retains ultimate authority over the diagnosis and care of the patient."[5] Contrast this with Iowa, where the state law specifically requires that a physician "practices in Iowa for a period not greater than 10 consecutive days and not more than 20 total days in any calendar year" to be exempt from licensure requirements.[6]

Over 20 states across the United States have joined the Interstate Medical Licensure Compact (the "IMLC"), which offers a voluntary expedited pathway for licensure for physicians seeking to practice in multiple states.[7] In order to be eligible for the IMLC route, a physician must (1) hold a full, unrestricted medical license in a member state, and either live, work, or conduct at least 25% of their practice of medicine there; (2) have graduated from an accredited medical school or an eligible international medical school; (3) have successfully completed Accreditation Council for Graduate Medical Education- or American Osteopathic Association-accredited graduate medical education; (4) have passed each component of the United States Medical Licensing Examination, Comprehensive Osteopathic Medical Licensing Examination of the United States, or equivalent in no more than three attempts; (5) hold a current specialty certification or time-unlimited

---

[2] *See* Fla. Stat. § 456.47(4)(h) (as enacted by HB 23, eff. July 1, 2019).

[3] *See* Ga. Code Ann § 43-34-31(a).

[4] Va. Code § 54.1–2901(A)(7).

[5] Minn. Stat. §147.032.

[6] Iowa Admin. Code § 653-9.1.

[7] *See* Interstate Medical Licensure Compact, available at https://www.imlcc.org/.

certification by an American Board of Medical Specialties or American Osteopathic Association/ Bureau of Osteopathic Specialists board; (6) have no history of disciplinary action toward his medical license; (7) have no criminal history; (8) have no history of controlled substance actions toward his medical license; and (9) not currently be under investigation. Physicians who are not eligible for the expedited process can still seek additional licenses in member states using the traditional state-by-state process. In addition to the IMLC, a majority of states belong to Nurse Licensure Compact ("NLC"), which allows registered nurses and licensed practical nurses to practice in other NLC states without having to obtain additional licenses.[8]

It is worth noting that many states have, in response to the COVID-19 public health emergency, waived licensure requirements for a portion of or for the duration of the public health emergency. Many states accomplished this by governors issuing executive orders. For example, Minnesota authorized out-of-state health care professionals who hold an active, relevant license, certificate, or other permit in good standing issued by a state of the United States or the District of Columbia to render aid in Minnesota during the peacetime emergency declared in Executive Order 20-01, but only to the extent those health care professionals are engaged with a health care system or provider, such as a hospital, clinic, or other health care entity located in Minnesota.[9] The Minnesota state of emergency was extended through February 12, 2020, unless rescinded, terminated, or extended.[10] Similarly, on December 16, 2020, Hawaii's governor issued the Seventeenth Proclamation related to the COVID-19 emergency:

> *Section 453-1.3, HRS, practice of telehealth, to the extent necessary to allow individuals currently and actively licensed pursuant to Chapter 453, HRS, to engage in telehealth without an in-person consultation or a prior existing physician-patient relationship; and to the extent necessary to enable out-of-state physicians, osteopathic physicians, and physician assistants with a current and active license, or those who were previously licensed pursuant to Chapter 453, HRS, but who are no longer current and active, to engage in telehealth in Hawaii without a license, in-person consultation, or prior existing physician-patient relationship, provided that they have never had their license revoked or suspended and are subject to the same conditions, limitations, or restrictions as in their home jurisdiction.[11]*

The Proclamation further declared "that the disaster emergency relief period shall continue through February 14, 2021, unless terminated or superseded by a separate proclamation, whichever shall occur first."[12]

Not all states have licensure waivers in effect, however. For example, in Michigan, the governor authorized all "health care professionals" who are "licensed in good standing" in any US state or territory to practice in Michigan. This applied to health care professionals licensed under Articles 7 and 15 of Michigan's Public Health Code, which specifically includes the categories of

---

[8] *See* National Council of State Boards of Nursing ("NCSBN"), https://www.ncsbn.org/compacts.htm.

[9] *See* Emergency Executive Order 20-46 (Apr. 25, 2020), https://www.leg.mn.gov/archive/execorders/20-46. pdf. The Minnesota Medical Board issued a press release on April 27, 2020 announcing Executive Order 20-46, which currently remains posted on Minnesota's Board of Medical Practice website. Minnesota Board of Medical Practice, Governor Tim Walz' Emergency Executive Order 20-46 (Apr. 27, 2020), https://mn.gov/boards/assets/EO%2020-46%20Out%20of%20State%20Heatlhcare%20Workers%20-%20 FINAL%20-%2004272020_tcm21-429904.pdf.

[10] *See* Executive Order 20-100 (Dec. 14, 2020), https://www.leg.mn.gov/archive/execorders/20-100.pdf.

[11] *See* Seventeenth Proclamation Related to the COVID-19 Emergency (Dec. 16, 2020), https://governor. hawaii.gov/wp-content/uploads/2020/12/2012088-ATG_Seventeenth-Proclamation-Related-to-the-COVID-19-Emergency-distribution-signed.pdf.

[12] *Id.*

medicine, nursing, social work, psychology, counseling, and physical therapy and does not require individuals to apply for or be granted an exception. The Executive Order provided:

> *The restrictions of MCL 500.3476 requiring telehealth services to be provided by a health care professional who is licensed, registered, or otherwise authorized to engage in his or her health care profession in the state where the patient is located is hereby suspended to the extent necessary to allow a medical professional licensed and in good standing to practice in a state other than Michigan to use telehealth when treating patients in Michigan without a license to practice medicine in Michigan. A license that has been suspended or revoked is not considered a license in good standing, and a licensee with pending disciplinary action is not considered to have a license in good standing. A license that is subject to a limitation or restriction in another state is subject to the same limitation or restriction in this state.*[13]

However, on October 2, 2020, the Michigan Supreme Court held the governor did not have the authority to extend the state of emergency.[14] The result is that the Michigan state of emergency is no longer in effect and Executive Order 2020-138 has been rescinded.

On a national level, before COVID-19, Medicare required that health care providers be licensed in the state in which the patient is located. In response to the COVID-19 pandemic, Centers for Medicare & Medicaid Services (CMS) waived Medicare's requirement that physicians and nonphysician health care providers be licensed in the state where they are providing services when the following four conditions are met:

- The health care provider is enrolled in the Medicare program.
- The health care provider possesses a valid license to practice in the state that relates to his or her Medicare enrollment.
- The provider furnishes services—whether in person or via telehealth—in a state in which the emergency is occurring in order to contribute to relief efforts in his or her professional capacity.
- The health care provider is not affirmatively excluded from practice in the state or in any other state that is part of the 1135 emergency area.[15]

It is important for telehealth providers, including telerehabilitation providers, to continue to comply with state-specific licensure requirements regardless of the exceptions provided by CMS applicable to Medicare.

Practice Standards

PROVIDER-PATIENT RELATIONSHIP FORMATION

A threshold issue for any telehealth provider, including telerehabilitation providers, is how something as basic as forming a valid provider-patient relationship may be done compliantly, which is a requirement before a provider may prescribe any drugs or render any medical treatment.

---

[13] *See* Executive Order 2020-138 (June 29, 2020), https://www.michigan.gov/whitmer/0, 9309, 7-387-90499_90705-533221--, 00.html.

[14] *See* Statement from Governor Whitmer on Michigan Supreme Court Ruling on Emergency Powers (Oct. 2, 2020), https://www.michigan.gov/whitmer/0, 9309, 7-387-90499-541283--, 00.html.

[15] *See* Department of Health and Human Services, Interim Final Rule, Medicare and Medicaid Programs; Policy and Regulatory Revisions in Response to the COVID-19 Public Health Emergency (Mar. 26, 2020), https://www.cms.gov/files/document/covid-final-ifc.pdf; Waiver or Modification of Requirements Under Section 1135 of the Social Security Act (Mar. 13, 2020), https://www.phe.gov/emergency/news/healthactions/section1135/Pages/covid19-13March20.aspx.

Establishing a valid physician-patient relationship, for example, requires the physician to take a history and perform a physical examination adequate to establish the diagnoses and identify underlying conditions and/or contraindications to the treatment recommended or provided. Treating patients via telemedicine necessarily includes use of various communication technologies to facilitate patient consultation, diagnosis, education, treatment, and general patient management. The modality through which a physician may establish a valid physician-patient relationship depends on the language of the applicable jurisdiction, which in the United States is state law, and the specific clinical situation. These treatment modalities include, but are not limited to, live video with audio capabilities, store and forward, and mobile health, such as apps.

The treatment modality that may be used to create the physician-patient relationship varies by state. For example, Arkansas regulations provide, "For purposes of this regulation, a proper physician/patient relationship, at a minimum requires that: (a) The physician performs a history and an 'in person' physical examination of the patient adequate to establish a diagnosis and identify underlying conditions and/or contraindications to the treatment recommended/provided; or (b) The physician performs a face to face examination using real time audio and visual telemedicine technology that provides information at least equal to such information as would have been obtained by an in-person examination; or (c) The physician personally knows the patient and the patient's general health status through an 'ongoing' personal or professional relationship".[16]

Importantly, "'Professional relationship' does not include a relationship between a health care professional and a patient established only by the following: (1) An internet questionnaire; (2) An email message; (3) Patient-generated medical history; (4) Audio-only communication, including without limitation interactive audio; (5) Text messaging; (6) A facsimile machine; or (7) Any combination thereof."[17] Moreover, "A pharmacist practicing within or outside Arkansas may not fill a prescription order to dispense a prescription-only drug to a patient if the pharmacist knows or reasonably should have known under the circumstances that the prescription order was issued on the basis of: (A) An Internet questionnaire; (B) An Internet consultation; or (C) A telephonic consultation."[18] These restrictions are aimed at prohibiting what is commonly referred to as internet prescribing.

The modality required to form a physician-patient relationship may or may not be the standard applied to other health care professionals. For example, real-time audio and visual telemedicine technology that provides information at least equal to the information that would be obtained in person, and appropriate follow-up provided or arranged, when necessary, at medically necessary intervals is the standard applied to advance practice registered nurses (APRNs). *See* Code Ark. R. 067.00.4-XIII(A), providing:

A. The APRN shall establish a proper APRN/patient relationship prior to providing any patient care.

B. A proper APRN/patient relationship, at a minimum requires that:

1. The APRN perform a history and an "in person" physical examination of the patient adequate to establish a diagnosis and identify underlying conditions and/or contraindications to the treatment recommended/provided; OR

2. The APRN perform a face-to-face examination using real-time audio and visual telemedicine technology that provides information at least equal to such information as would have been obtained by an in-person examination; AND

3. Appropriate follow-up be provided or arranged, when necessary, at medically necessary intervals.

---

[16] *See* Ark. R. 060.00.1-2(8).

[17] Ark. Code Ann. § 17-80-403(c).

[18] Ark. Code Ann. § 17-92-1004(c).

The Board of Nursing's Telemedicine regulations provide, "An APRN/patient relationship shall be established in accordance with Chapter 4, Section XIII before the delivery of services via telemedicine. A patient completing a medical history online and forwarding it to an APRN is not sufficient to establish the relationship, nor does it qualify as store-and-forward technology."[19] Further, the Arkansas Telemedicine Act, which applies to "health care professionals," including NPs, states that in order to provide care to a patient located in Arkansas via telemedicine, either (1) a "professional relationship" must exist between a health care professional and the patient or (2) the health care professional otherwise meets the requirements of a professional relationship.[20] For purposes of the Act, "health care professional" means a person who is licensed, certified, or otherwise authorized by the laws of this state to administer health care in the ordinary course of the practice of their profession, and would include NPs.[21] As noted earlier, the Board of Nursing regulations allow a NP-patient relationship to be formed via telemedicine.[22]

Telehealth providers, including telerehabilitation providers, must always bear in mind that not all clinical situations are appropriate for telemedicine, regardless of what a given state law says, and it is incumbent on the physician to use his or her informed medical judgment to not only comply with the language of the applicable law, but to also meet the expected standard of care in the community in which care is being rendered.

After creating a valid physician-patient relationship, the telemedicine physician must also conduct an appropriate examination and assessment prior to issuing a medically necessary prescription. Some states, for example, require the use of interactive audio-video technology to establish a valid physician-patient relationship, but after the relationship has been created, the state's law allows the use of interactive audio (e.g., a telephone) or store and forward (e.g., email) telerehabilitation for subsequent prescribing. For example, in Arkansas, "Once a professional relationship is established, a healthcare professional may provide healthcare services through telemedicine, including interactive audio, if the healthcare services are within the scope of practice for which the healthcare professional is licensed or certified."[23] Here, "telemedicine" means the use of electronic information and communication technology to deliver health care services, including without limitation the assessment, diagnosis, consultation, treatment, education, care management, and self-management of a patient."[24] Additionally, "telemedicine" includes store and forward technology and remote patient monitoring.[25]

Finally, all medical practice via telemedicine (whether treatment, diagnosis, prescribing) must comply with the applicable standard of care similar to in-person services. The Arkansas Telemedicine Act provides, for example, "Healthcare services provided by telemedicine, including without limitation a prescription through telemedicine, shall be held to the same standard of care as healthcare services provided in person."[26] If a physician does not have sufficient information available to render a diagnosis, treatment recommendation, or prescription, the physician should not continue with the telemedicine examination. Instead, the physician should instruct the patient to provide more information, laboratory test results, images, or schedule an in-person examination as appropriate.

---

[19] *See* Code Ark. R. 067.00.4-XIV(A).

[20] *See* Ark. Code Ann. § 17-80-403(a).

[21] *See* Ark. Code Ann. § 17-80-402(2).

[22] *See* Code Ark. R. 067.00.4-XIII(A)(2), (3).

[23] Ark. Code Ann. § 17-80-404(a)(2).

[24] Ark. Code Ann. § 17-80-402(7)(A).

[25] Ark. Code Ann. § 17-80-402(7)(B).

[26] Ark. Code Ann. § 17-80-404(c).

INFORMED CONSENT

Many US states, via licensing and practice statutes, administrative codes, medical board guidance, and/or Medicaid laws and policies, require health care providers to obtain an informed consent that is specific to telehealth. These states typically require the telehealth provider, including the telerehabilitation provider, to inform the patient concerning the treatment methods and limitations of treatment using a telehealth platform and, after providing the patient with such information, obtain the patient's consent to provide telehealth services. Most consent procedures must also provide the patient with alternatives to receiving care via telehealth. Some states have explicit requirements that the telehealth provider instruct the patient concerning appropriate follow-up care in the event of needed care related to the treatment. Often, informed consent must be documented in the medical record. The content and format of such required consent can vary and must meet the prevailing standard of care.

In Delaware, for example, physicians who utilize telemedicine are statutorily required to obtain appropriate consent from requesting patients after disclosures regarding the delivery models and treatment methods or limitations, including informed consent regarding the use of telemedicine technologies, which includes discussing with the patient the diagnosis and the evidence for it, and the risks and benefits of various treatment options.[27] In contrast, Iowa's regulations provide, "A licensee who uses telemedicine shall ensure that the patient provides appropriate informed consent for the medical services provided, including consent for the use of telemedicine to diagnose and treat the patient, and that such informed consent is timely documented in the patient's medical record."[28] In Kentucky, the applicable statute provides that a treating physician who provides or facilitates the use of telehealth shall ensure that the informed consent of the patient, or another appropriate person with authority to make the health care treatment decision for the patient, is obtained before services are provided through telehealth.[29] The Kentucky Board of Medicine, however, has much more robust requirements. Here, an appropriate informed consent should, as a baseline, include the following terms:

- Identification of the patient, the physician, and the physician's credentials
- Types of transmissions permitted using telemedicine technologies (e.g., prescription refills, appointment scheduling, patient education, etc.)
- The patient agrees that the physician determines whether or not the condition being diagnosed and/or treated is appropriate for a telemedicine encounter
- Details on security measures taken with the use of telemedicine technologies, such as encrypting data, password protected screen savers and data files, or utilizing other reliable authentication techniques, as well as potential risks to privacy notwithstanding such measures
- Hold harmless clause for information lost due to technical failures
- Requirement for express patient consent to forward patient-identifiable information to a third party[30]

State informed-consent requirements evolve as telemedicine becomes integral to mainstream medical practice. It may happen that over time telehealth-specific informed consent will be done away with as telehealth becomes more mainstream. If this occurs, then the informed-consent requirements applicable to telehealth would be the same as those observed in in-person health

---

[27] See Del. Code Ann. tit. 24, § 1769D.

[28] Iowa Admin. Code r. 653-13.11(10).

[29] *See* Ky. Rev. Stat. Ann. § 311.5975.

[30] Kentucky Board of Medicine Opinion Regarding the Use of Telemedicine Technologies in the Practice of Medicine (June 19, 2014).

care visits. In meantime, it is important for telehealth providers to understand and comply with applicable state informed-consent requirements.

RECORD REQUIREMENTS

Telehealth providers, including telerehabilitation providers, must comply with state laws relating to medical record documentation and retention requirements. Generally, telemedicine documentation retained in a patient's medical record must be as detailed as an in-person office visit. In Texas, for example:

1. Patient records must be maintained for all telehealth services. Both the distant site provider and the provider or physician at the established medical site must maintain the records created at each site unless the distant site provider maintains the records in an electronic health record format.
2. Distant site providers must obtain an adequate and complete medical history for the patient prior to providing treatment and must document this in the patient record.
3. Patient records must include copies of all relevant patient-related electronic communications, including relevant provider-patient email, prescriptions, laboratory and test results, evaluations and consultations, records of past care, and instructions. If possible, telehealth encounters that are recorded electronically should also be included in the patient record.[31]

Compare Texas' standard with Iowa's, which provides, "A licensee who uses telemedicine shall ensure that complete, accurate and timely medical records are maintained for the patient when appropriate, including all patient-related electronic communications, records of past care, physician-patient communications, laboratory and test results, evaluations and consultations, prescriptions, and instructions obtained or produced in connection with the use of telemedicine technologies. The licensee shall note in the patient's record when telemedicine is used to provide diagnosis and treatment. The licensee shall ensure that the patient or another licensee designated by the patient has timely access to all information obtained during the telemedicine encounter. The licensee shall ensure that the patient receives, upon request, a summary of each telemedicine encounter in a timely manner."[32] Each state has its own way of managing record-keeping requirements with respect to telehealth. Knowing the nuances of these requirements in an applicable state is important for compliant telehealth practice.

SPECIAL NOTICE/DISCLOSURES AND PATIENT IDENTITY VERIFICATION REQUIREMENTS

There are a number of states that have requirements that go above and beyond the requirements typically observed in an informed consent and have patient identity verification requirements. For example, in Arkansas, "The following requirements apply to all services provided by physicians or physician assistants using telemedicine... Services must be delivered in a transparent manner, including providing access to information identifying the physician or physician assistant in advance of the encounter, with licensure and board certifications, as well as patient financial responsibilities."[33] In Kansas, when a patient consents to receiving care via telehealth and has a primary care or other treating physician, the person providing telemedicine services is required to send within 3 business days a report to such primary care or other treating physician of the treatment and services rendered to the patient in the telemedicine encounter.[34]

---

[31] Tex. Admin. Code § 279.16(g)(3).

[32] Iowa Admin. Code r. 653-13.11(14).

[33] Ark. Admin. Code 060.00.1-38.

[34] *See* Kan. Stat. Ann. § 40-2, 212(2).

In addition to several nuanced state consent requirements, many states require some form of patient identity verification in advance of providing telehealth services. Maryland, for example, requires telehealth practitioners to develop and follow a procedure to verify the identification of the patient receiving telehealth services; confirm whether the patient is in Maryland and identify the practice setting in which the patient is located; and identify all individuals present at each location and confirm they are allowed to hear personal health information.[35] The Oregon Medical Board states, "A licensee is expected to maintain an appropriate provider-patient relationship. At each telemedicine encounter, the licensee should: verify the location and identity of the patient, provide the identity and credentials of the provider to the patient, and obtain appropriate informed consents from the patient after disclosures regarding the limitations of telemedicine."[36]

Privacy

HEALTH INSURANCE PORTABILITY AND ACCOUNTABILITY ACT OF 1996

The Health Insurance Portability and Accountability Act of 1996 (HIPAA)[37] and its implementing regulations (the "Privacy Rule," the "Breach Notification Rule," and the "Security Rule")[38] establish security and privacy standards to ensure the confidentiality and integrity of Protected Health Information (PHI).[39] The HIPAA standards apply to "Covered Entities," such as health plans, health care clearinghouses, and health care providers that "engage in electronic standard transactions," and their "Business Associates." "Electronic standard transactions," generally speaking, means that the health care provider communicates electronically with health plans, such as to seek reimbursement from the health plan. Health care providers that do not seek reimbursement from health plans are generally not HIPAA Covered Entities.

A subsection of telehealth provider entities is not currently regulated by HIPAA as a Covered Entity. Moreover, if no PHI is being exchanged, then HIPAA does not apply. Many patients and telehealth providers use mobile technologies, such as smartphones or tablets, to communicate and share data. Developers of these applications frequently are not Covered Entities subject to HIPAA rules, that is, they are not health insurers or health care clearinghouses, and they also do not qualify as Business Associates of Covered Entities such that HIPAA would apply. However, even if HIPAA does not apply, telemedicine providers must ensure that they comply with applicable state law, as an increasing number of states have their own privacy and security statutes that can be broader than HIPAA. Additionally, it is best practice for every telehealth provider to respect the privacy of patient health information and to voluntarily comply with HIPAA as completely as is feasible.

Telehealth providers that do engage in electronic standard transactions must fully comply with HIPAA. An important HIPAA requirement is compliance with the administrative, technical, and physical security standards established by the Security Rule, which typically requires a provider

---

[35] *See* Md. Code Regs. 10.32.05.04.

[36] Board's Statement of Philosophy on Telemedicine (last rev. Oct. 2020), available at https://www.oregon.gov/omb/board/Philosophy/Pages/Telemedicine.aspx.

[37] The Health Insurance Portability and Accountability Act of 1996 (HIPAA), P.L. No. 104-191, 110 Stat. 1938 (1996), Public Law 104-91.

[38] 45 C.F.R. 164, Subparts A and C, D, and E.

[39] The Privacy Rule protects all "individually identifiable health information" held or transmitted by a Covered Entity or its Business Associate in any form or media, whether electronic, paper, or oral, with exclusions for employment and educational records. The Privacy Rule calls this information "Protected Health Information." 45 C.F.R. § 160.103.

organization to conduct a security risk analysis of the risks and vulnerabilities to the Electronic Protected Health Information (ePHI) that the organization creates, receives, maintains, or transmits. Moreover, the general rule is that a Covered Entity cannot use or disclose PHI without written patient authorization. There are, however, numerous exceptions, including for treatment, payment, and health care operations' purposes. HIPAA also requires a Covered Entity to comply with various "patient's rights" provisions (e.g., the right to provide access to PHI). Additionally, a Covered Entity may not disclose PHI to a Business Associate unless it enters into a Business Associate Agreement (BAA) that includes each requirement of 45 C.F.R. § 164.504(e).

The granular details of HIPAA compliance are beyond the scope of this chapter. It is important to appreciate that compliance with HIPAA and its implementing regulations generally includes conducting a HIPAA security risk analysis and developing written HIPAA Security Policies and Procedures, implementation of the HIPAA Privacy Policies and Procedures, appointing a HIPAA Privacy Officer and HIPAA Security Officer, workforce training on HIPAA, and negotiation and execution of BAAs with Business Associates.

COMPLYING WITH THE TELEPHONE CONSUMER PROTECTION ACT CONSENT REQUIREMENTS

The Federal Communications Commission (FCC) is responsible for overseeing both interstate and international communications and thus regulates communication devices transmitting medical data. The FCC also administers the Telephone Consumer Protection Act (TCPA), which was enacted to protect consumer privacy by restricting unsolicited contacts from automated telephone calls, fax machines, and automatic dialers. The TCPA generally restricts telephone calls to residential lines and cell phones under certain circumstances without first obtaining prior written consent. Telehealth providers, however, can place artificial/prerecorded voice and text messages to cellphones, without the patient's prior express consent, written or otherwise, in order to convey important informational "health care messages" as defined and covered by HIPAA. These exemptions include the following health care–related messages:

- appointments and examinations;
- confirmations and reminders;
- wellness checkups;
- hospital preregistration instructions;
- preoperative instructions;
- laboratory results;
- postdischarge follow-up intended to prevent readmission;
- prescription notifications; and
- home health care instructions.

These exceptions do have restrictions, however. For example, voice calls and text messages can only be sent to the telephone number provided by the patient and must not include any telemarketing, solicitation, advertising, accounting, billing, or financial content. Additionally, a telehealth provider, including a telerehabilitation provider, may only initiate one message per day (up to three per week) and each message must be concise in length. These messages must also include an easy way for patients to opt out of messages. Providers must honor these opt-out requests immediately.

Given the myriad of laws and regulations applicable to data privacy and security that affect the telemedicine industry, it is important that telehealth providers address privacy and security proactively by taking such steps as developing privacy policies to ensure that patient data are adequately protected. Telehealth providers, including telerehabilitation providers, are well advised to inform patients about what specific data are collected and the purposes for which the data are being used. Privacy policies also ideally inform patients about whether any patient-provided data are shared with third parties and the circumstances in which information may be disclosed. It is also wise to inform patients of the risks in using telemedicine services and provide patients with a mechanism for reporting suspected or actual breaches of security to the telemedicine provider.

Because of the number of state and federal laws and regulations applicable to data privacy and security in commerce, including in the health care context, it is important for those in the telehealth industry including telerehabilitation to stay up to date on the relevant laws affecting the areas in which they provide services.

Worldwide View

Telehealth, including telerehabilitation, is expanding across the globe, especially in response to the worldwide COVID-19 pandemic. The US system is difficult for telehealth providers to navigate because the United States has a unique system of state and federal laws governing various aspects of practice. In other countries, barriers to entry can be as simple as lack of sufficient communication devices or broadband infrastructure to conduct telehealth on the one hand, or more onerous regulations, especially where privacy is concerned, on the other. Regardless of jurisdiction, it is critical that telehealth providers take time to understand the rules and regulations governing telehealth practice before practicing telehealth.

Page numbers followed by *f* indicate figures, *t* indicate tables, and *b* indicate boxes.